Third Edition

Essentials of
Nephrology

Third Edition

Essentials of
Nephrology

R Kasi Visweswaran

Former Professor
Department of Nephrology
Medical College
Thiruvananthapuram

Consultant in Nephrology
Ananthapuri Hospitals and Research Institute
Thiruvananthapuram
Kerala

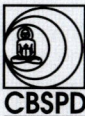

CBSPD

CBS Publishers & Distributors Pvt Ltd

New Delhi • Bengaluru • Chennai • Kochi • Kolkata • Lucknow • Mumbai
Hyderabad • Jharkhand • Nagpur • Patna • Pune • Uttarakhand

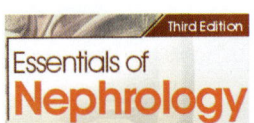

ISBN: 978-93-88527-73-6

Third Edition   **2019**
   Reprint 2023
First Edition   1994
Second Edition   2009

Published by Satish Kumar Jain and produced by Varun Jain for

CBS Publishers & Distributors Pvt Ltd

4819/XI Prahlad Street, 24 Ansari Road, Daryaganj, New Delhi 110 002, India.
Ph: 011-23289259, 23266861, 23266867   Website: www.cbspd.com
Fax: 011-23243014   e-mail: delhi@cbspd.com; cbspubs@airtelmail.in

Corporate Office: 204 FIE, Industrial Area, Patparganj, Delhi 110 092
Ph: 011-4934 4934   Fax: 011-4934 4935   e-mail: publishing@cbspd.com; publicity@cbspd.com

Branches

- **Bengaluru:** Seema House 2975, 17th Cross, KR Road, Banasankari 2nd Stage, Bengaluru 560 070, Karnataka, India
  Ph: +91-80-26771678/79   Fax: +91-80-26771680   e-mail: bangalore@cbspd.com
- **Chennai:** 7, Subbaraya Street, Shenoy Nagar, Chennai 600 030, Tamil Nadu, India
  Ph: +91-44-26680620/26681266   Fax: +91-44-42032115   e-mail: chennai@cbspd.com
- **Kochi:** 42/1325, 26, Power House Road, Opp KSEB, Ernakulam 682 018, Kerala, India
  Ph: +91-484-4059061-65   Fax: +91-484-4059065   e-mail: kochi@cbspd.com
- **Kolkata:** 147, Hind Ceramics Compound, 1st Floor, Nilgunj road, Belghoria, Kolkata 700 056, West Bengal, India
  Ph: +91-33-25633055/56   e-mail: kolkata@cbspd.com
- **Lucknow:** Basement, Khushnuma Complex, 7-Meerabai Marg (behind Jawahar Bhawan), Lucknow 226 001, Uttar Pradesh, India
  Ph: +91-552-4000032   e-mail:tiwari.lucknowi@cbspd.com
- **Mumbai:** PWD shed, Gala No. 25/26, Ramchandra Bhatt Marg, Next to JJ Hospital Gate No. 2, Opp. Union Bank of India, Noorbaug, Mumbai 400 009, Maharashtra, India
  Ph: +91-22-66661880/89   e-mail: mumbai@cbspd.com

Representatives

• **Hyderabad**	0-9885175004	• **Jharkhand**	0-9811541605	• **Nagpur**	0-9421945513
• **Patna**	0-9334159340	• **Pune**	0-9623451994	• **Uttarakhand**	0-9716462459

Printed at: HT Media Ltd, Greater Noida, UP, India

Contributors

Almeida Alan
Former Professor
Department of Nephrology
KEM Hospital, Mumbai
Hinduja Hospital, Mumbai

Abraham Sebastian
Additional Professor
Department of Nephrology
Medical College, Kottayam

Agarwal Sanjay
Professor
Department of Nephrology
AIIMS, New Delhi

Alexander Suceena
Professor
Department of Nephrology
Christian Medical College, Vellore

Almeida Richard Savio Fernandes
Resident in Internal Medicine
MacNeal Hospital, Bengaluru

Augustine Rohan
Consultant Nephrologist
Manipal Hospital, Bengaluru

Bagai Sahil
Additional Professor
Department of Nephrology
PGI, Chandigarh

Bagchi Soumita
Associate Professor
Department of Nephrology
AIIMS, New Delhi

Ballal Sudarshan
Head
Department of Nephrology
Manipal Hospital, Bengaluru

Balasubramaniam J
Consultant in Nephrology
Medical Center, Tirunelveli, Tamil Nadu

Behera Vineet
Senior Resident
Department of Nephrology
AIIMS, New Delhi

Bhat Suresh
Professor and Head
Department of Urology
Medical College, Kottayam

Bhowmik Dipankar
Professor
Department of Nephrology
AIIMS, New Delhi

Bonu Ravi Shankar
Senior Consultant
Department of Nephrology
Manipal Hospital, Bengaluru

D'Cruz Sanjay
Professor
Government Medical College and Hospital
Sector 32, Chandigarh

Durai C Rakesh
Senior Resident
Department of Nephrology
Madras Medical College, Chennai

Fernando Edwin M
Professor
Department of Nephrology
Government Stanley Medical College
Chennai

George Jacob
Professor
Department of Nephrology
Medical College, Thiruvananthapuram

Gomathy S
Professor
Department of Nephrology
TD Medical College, Alleppey

Gopalakrishnan N
Professor and Head
Department of Nephrology
Madras Medical College, Chennai

Gulati Sanjeev
Pediatric Nephrologist
Fortis Escorts Hospital, New Delhi

Gupta KL
Professor and Head
Department of Nephrology
PGI, Chandigarh

Gurudev KC
Professor
Department of Nephrology
MS Ramiah Medical College, Bengaluru

Hema R
Hon Consultant
Govindan's Hospital, Thiruvananthapuram

Former Professor
Department of Pediatric Surgery
SAT Hospital, Medical College
Thiruvananthapuram

Jain Deepak
Professor
Department of Medicine
Pt. BD Sharma University of Health Sciences
Rohtak, Haryana

Jayakumar KP
Professor
Department of Nephrology
Medical College, Kottayam

Jayaraman Muthu
Former Professor
Department of Nephrology
Government Stanley Medical College
Chennai

Jha Vivekanand
Former Professor
Department of Nephrology
PGI, Chandigarh

Visiting Professor
Oxford University

Kalra OP
Vice-Chancellor
Pt BD Sharma University of Health Sciences
Rohtak (Haryana)

Kher Viay
Chairman
Kidney and Urology Institute, Medanta—The
Medicity, Gurugram

Kohli Harbir Singh
Professor
Department of Nephrology
PGI, Chandigarh

Kumar Sampath
Head
Department of Nephrology
Meenakshi Medical Mission Hospital, Madurai

Lekha H
Pediatric Nephrologist
Ananthapuri Hospitals and Research Institute
Thiruvananthapuram

Madken Mohit
Consultant in Nephrology
Fortis Escorts Kidney and Urology Institute
Fortis Escorts Hospital, New Delhi

Mathew Thomas M
Chief Consulatant
Department of Nephrology
Baby Memorial Hospital, Kozhikkode

Former Professor
Department of Nephrology
Medical College, Kozhikkode

Mehrothra Sonia
Department of Nephrology
SGPGI, Lucknow

Mohandas MK
Additional Professor
Department of Nephrology
Medical College, Thiruvananthapuram

Mukhopadhyay Pinaki
Professor
Departmet of Nephrology
NRS Medical College, Kolkata

Muthusethupathy MA
Aswanee Soundra Nursing Home
Chennai

Former Professor
Department of Nephrology
Madras Medical College, Chennai

Nainan Georgy K
Consultant in Nephrology
Lakeshore and PVS Hospitals, Kochi

Narayen Girish
Former Professor
Department of Nephrology
Osmania Medical College, Hyderabad

Pahari Dilip
Professor and Head
Department of Nephrology and Director
Medica Institute of Kidney Diseases, Kolkata

Parameswaran Sreejith
Professor and Head
Department of Nephrology
JIPMER, Puducherry

Phadke Kishore
Former Professor
Department of Pediatric Nephrology
St. Johns Medical College, Bengaluru

Pinnmaneni Venkat Siva Tez
Consultant Nephrology
Department of Nephrology
Venkateshwar Hospital, Dwarka, New Delhi

Prasad Narayan
Professor
Department of Nephrology
SGPGI, Lucknow

Rajeev R
Consultant Nephrologist
Sunshine Hospitals, Secunderabad

Rajesh R
Professor
Department of Nephrology
Amrita Institute of Medical Sciences, Kochi

Rajendran Suguna
Nephrologist
Aswanee Soundra Nursing Home, Chennai

Ram R
Professor and Head
Department of Nephrology
SVIMS, Tirupathi, AP

Ramachandran Raja
Additional Professor
Department of Nephrology
PGI, Chandigarh

Raman Anuradha
Former Professor
Department of Nephrology
Osmania Medical College, Hyderabad

Ramasubramanian V
Professor
Department of Nephrology
Tirunelveli Medical College
Tirunelveli, Tamil Nadu

Rao Namrata
Assistant Professor
Department of Nephrology
Dr Ram Manohar Lohia Institute of Medical
Sciences, Lucknow

Rathi Manish
Additional Professor
Department of Nephrology
PGI, Chandigarh

Roychoudhury N
Consultant in Nephrology
Medica Institute of Kidney Diseases, Kolkata

Sahay Manisha
Professor and Head
Department of Nephrology
Osmania Medical College, Hyderabad

Sai Sameera N
Senior Resident
Department of Nephrology
SVIMS, Tirupathi

Sakhuja Vinay
Chief Consultant and Head
Department of Nephrology and
Transplant Services
Max Hospital, Panchkula

Former Professor
Department of Nephrology
PGI, Chandigarh

Sathyapriya Aruna
Chief Dietician
Department of Nephrology
Government General Hospital, Chennai

Sathyasagar K
Senior Resident
Department of Nephrology
Madras Medical College, Chennai

Satish Balan
Consultant in Nephrology
KIMS Hospital, Thiruvananthapuram

Sethi Jasmine
Senior Resident
Department of Nephrology
PGIMER, Chandigarh

Sharma RK
Director and HOD
Medanta Awadh, Lucknow

Former Director
SGPGI, Lucknow

Sharma Umesh (Surgeon Vice Admiral)
Chief Consultant (Medicine and Nephrology)
Director General AFMS
(Organization and Personnel)
Office of DG AFMS
Ministry of Defence, 'M' Block
Defence HQ, New Delhi

Sivakumar V
Professor and Head
Department of Nephrology
SVIMS, Tirupathi, AP

Sreelatha M
Professor
Department of Nephrology
Medical College, Kozhikkode

Sunnesh A
Senior Resident
SVIMS, Tirupathi

Thomas Mathew Jayanth
Professor
Amala Institute of Medical Sciences, Trichur

Unni V Narayanan
Chief
Department of Nephrology
ASTER Medicity, Kochi

Former Professor
Department of Nephrology
AIMS, Kochi

Uthup Susan
Professor
Department of Pediatric Nephrology
SAT Hospital, Medical College, Thiruvananthapuram

Varughese Santhosh
Professor of Nephrology
Christian Medical College, Vellore

Varma PP Lt Gen (Retd)
Head
Department of Nephrology
Venkateshwar Hospital, Dwarka, New Delhi

Vimala A
Senior Consultant
Cosmopolitan Hospital, Thiruvananthapuram

Former Professor
Department of Nephrology
Medical College, Kottayam

Vishvanath S
Head
Consultant in Nephrologist
Manipal Hospital, Bengaluru

Visweswaran R Kasi
Consultant in Nehprologist
Ananthapuri Hospitals and Research Institute
Thiruvananthapuram

Former Professor
Department of Nephrology
Medical College, Thiruvananthapuram

Preface

The developments in nephrology have been rapid over the last half century. However, the exposure of the medical student to kidney diseases during the undergraduate medical curriculum is limited mostly because of lack of dramatic clinical findings. Renal diseases are very common and the health administration and the community are more aware of the need for prevention, early diagnosis and timely management of chronic kidney disease. Understanding the disease at the molecular level has paved the way for strategies for targeted treatment at the subcellular level. Population studies and hospital statistics show an alarmingly high incidence of renal diseases. As per the available data, patients with renal diseases often seek specialist consultation only when more than 80% of the renal function is deranged. The progressive loss of renal function can be arrested or the progression delayed by early diagnosis and timely management. Although most of the information is available through the medium of 'internet' or medical journals, it is impossible to get a concise review in such medical sites. It is in this context that textbooks become important. Diabetes and hypertension are common particularly in old age and the population of the elderly is increasing throughout the world. The prevalence of CKD may be even up to 10% in the general population and much more among the elderly.

The third edition has been thoroughly revised to include chapters starting from understanding molecular biology, applied anatomy, physiology, common illnesses in clinical nephrology and the pathological changes as relevant. Separate sections and chapters have been allotted for 'approach to common kidney problems' and the management of fluid, electrolyte and acid–base disorders which should help the practicing clinician to manage the cases in a rational fashion. As the longevity of life increases, the problems associated with aging also increase. Separate chapter on aging and kidney has been included in this volume. Diseases like diabetes and obesity have assumed epidemic proportions and renal involvement is common in both. Obesity-related renal disease is also included as a separate chapter.

The contributors are highly experienced nephrologists who are actively involved in teaching, research and clinical services and have been chosen from all major teaching institutions and the armed forces in the country.

Let me quote the concluding paragraph from the Foreword to the second edition by late Prof KS Chugh, who has been considered the 'Father of nephrology in India'.

"Out of myriad and mushrooming hefty books in nephrology, Dr R Kasi Visweswaran has come up with a book which would be enjoyed by students, fellows, and residents preparing for their undergraduate and postgraduate examinations in medicine and nephrology and by practising physicians and nephrology consultants who are keen to improve the care of their patients. I trust that the second edition of *Essentials of Nephrology* will remain their guide and friend for many years to come."

As predicted by him, 'after many years', the third edition is ready but Prof Chugh, unfortunately, is no longer with us. This book is dedicated to late Prof KS Chugh, Emeritus Professor of Nephrology, Postgraduate Institute of Medical Education and Research, Chandigarh, the mentor and guiding light to most of the contributors in this edition, including myself.

R Kasi Visweswaran

Contents

Section VI: TUBULAR DISEASES

Section VII: INFECTIONS OF THE URINARY TRACT

Section VIII: HYPERTENSION

Section IX: PREGNANCY AND KIDNEYS

General

General

Structure of Kidneys and Urinary System

• Susan Uthup

STRUCTURE OF KIDNEYS AND URINARY TRACT

i. Location and relationship
ii. Surface marking and gross anatomy
iii. Nephron structure
iv. Zones in the kidney and relationship to nephron segments
v. Renal circulation, lymphatics and nerve supply
vi. Microscopy and ultrastructure
vii. Structure of ureter, urinary bladder and urethra

i. Location and Relationship

Kidneys are a pair of bean-shaped organs situated obliquely in the retroperitoneum on either side of the vertebral column extending from the 12th thoracic vertebra to the 3rd lumbar vertebra. The upper poles are normally oriented more medially and posteriorly than the lower poles. The adult kidney measures approximately 11.5 × 6.5 × 3.5 cm and weighs about 150 g each. The right kidney is at a lower level than the left due to interposition of the liver between the kidney and the diaphragm. Left kidney is slightly longer and narrower than the right kidney (Fig. 1.1). In some cases,

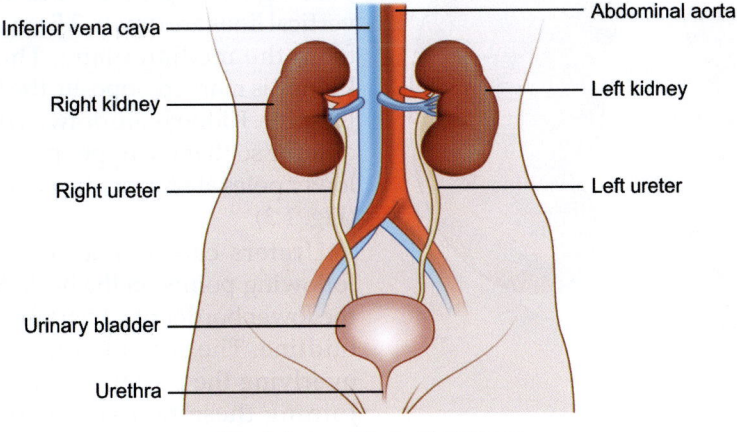

Fig. 1.1: Location of kidneys

3

the left kidney may have a hump-like projection on the lateral border, called "dromedary hump". Kidneys are highly vascular and receive one-fifth of the total cardiac output under normal conditions.

The upper one-third of the posterior surface of both kidneys is in contact with the diaphragm. The lower two-thirds are related to psoas major, quadratus lumborum and transversus abdominis muscles on both sides (Fig. 1.2). The 11th and 12th ribs lie behind the diaphragm posterior to the adrenal glands and upper poles of the kidneys bilaterally. Any injury that produces fracture of lower ribs, especially posteriorly, must be evaluated for potential renal injury as well. The kidneys move during inspiration due to the descent of the diaphragm. Since the pleura and the lower ribs lie more superficial to the diaphragm, removal of the lower ribs during renal surgery may injure the pleura.

Medially, the kidney is in relation to the inferior vena cava. The left kidney is related anteriorly to spleen, stomach, tail of the pancreas, splenic flexure of the large intestine and jejunum. The left suprarenal gland is situated superomedially at the upper pole of the kidney. The right kidney is related anteriorly to the liver. Suprarenal gland is closely related to its upper pole. During operations on the kidney, unless proper care is taken any of the above structures can be injured. Because of its close relation to the gastrointestinal system, kidney diseases may present with misleading gastrointestinal symptoms.

Kidneys are supported by the perirenal fat, the renal vascular pedicle, abdominal muscle tone and the general bulk of the abdominal viscera. The average vertical mobility of the kidney on inspiration or on assuming upright position is 4–5 cm (one vertebral body height). This mobility may be restricted or absent when the kidneys are fixed as in perinephric infections and malignancies. Occasionally the kidneys may be excessively mobile (floating kidney, mobile kidney).

At birth, the kidneys measure approximately 4.5 cm in length and are irregular in contour with multiple lobulations called 'fetal lobulations' which usually disappear in the first year of life. The kidneys and adrenals are larger relative to the body size in children. Because of relative larger size, mobility and lesser amount of perinephric fat, kidneys are more susceptible to injury in children.

ii. Surface Marking and Gross Anatomy

The kidneys can be mapped out by the *Morris parallelogram*. Draw two horizontal lines passing through D11 and L3 spine. Two vertical lines are drawn 2.5 cm and 9.5 cm each from the median plane. The hilum of the kidney is marked opposite the lower border of L1 spine. Kidneys are drawn with the long axis oblique so that the upper poles are nearer and lower poles are farther from the median plane. (Fig. 1.3).

Ureters can be marked by joining the following points on the back. Mark a point at the lower border of L1 vertebra, 4 cm from the midline. The second point is at the dimple overlying the posterior superior iliac spine. Joining these two points give the surface marking of ureter.

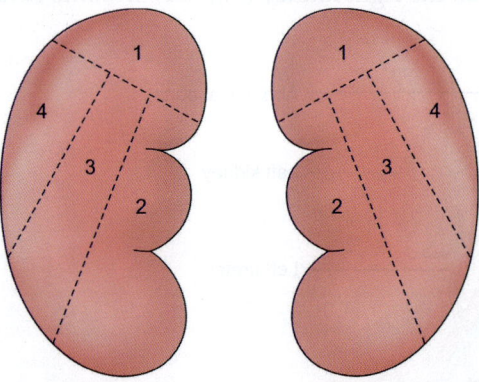

1. Diaphragm
2. Psoas major
3. Quadratus lumborum
4. Transverse abdominis

Fig. 1.2: Posterior relationship of kidneys

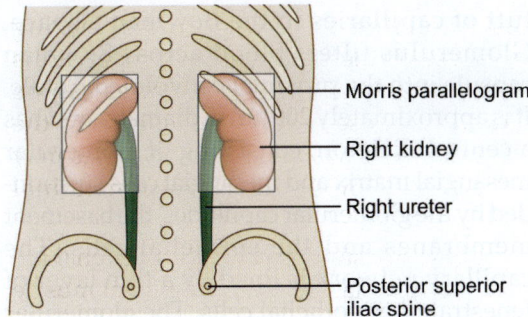

Fig. 1.3: Surface marking of kidneys

Each kidney has an upper pole, a lower pole, an anterior surface, a posterior surface, a convex lateral border and a concave medial border. The upper poles are closer to the midline than the lower poles aligning with the lateral border of the psoas muscle. The kidney is covered by a tough fibrous capsule which can be easily peeled off the surface of the kidney. In renal infections, it becomes adherent to the kidney. Outside this capsule and the perinephric fat, is the fascia of Gerota. It has an anterior layer and a posterior layer. Since the layers fuse on all the sides except at the inferior pole, any perirenal fluid collection tracks only downwards. The concave medial border has a slit-like aperture through which the renal vessels, nerves and pelvis traverse and is called the "renal hilum". The hilum communicates with a flattened space inside the kidney called the "renal sinus". It is filled with fat, through which the pelvicalyceal system, blood vessels, nerves, lymphatics enter or leave the kidney. These structures produce the 'central echogenic complex' on ultrasound. The renal pelvis branches into major and minor calyces in the renal sinus.

On longitudinal cut section, the kidney has 3 distinct parts, the cortex, the medulla and the pelvicalyceal system. The cortex is the outermost part which is homogenous and dark red in color. It is about 2–3 cm wide and contains the glomeruli, tubules, blood vessels and the interstitium. The medulla contains the loop of Henle, the vasa recta, and the collecting ducts

in addition to interstitial space called the "renal medullary interstitial space". The renal medulla can be further subdivided into outer zone adjacent to cortex and inner zone that includes papilla. The outer zone of medulla is subdivided into inner and outer stripe representing the location of various segments of renal tubules. The inner medulla is slightly paler and consists of 8–18 conical masses called renal pyramids and intervening cortical tissue called renal columns of Bertin. The base of the pyramid is at the corticomedullary junction. The tip of the pyramid called the "papilla" extends into the renal sinus and is capped by the funnel-shaped minor calyx. There are two types of papillae: Simple papillae and compound papillae. The upper and lower poles usually contain compound papillae. Compound papillae are prone for intrarenal reflux and scars due to vesico-ureteral reflux. Such scars are commonly seen at the poles. The minor calyx collects the urine drained from the kidney into the extrarenal collecting system.

The innermost region in the pelvicalyceal system is a hollow space lined by transitional epithelium. The spaces between the pyramids are called minor and major calyces. The minor calyces are cup-like structures collecting urine from the papillae. They join to form three or four major calyces which in turn unite to form the renal pelvis. Renal pelvis is the funnel-shaped expanded upper portion of the ureter that drains urine into the urinary bladder (Fig. 1.4).

iii. Nephron Structure

The nephron is the basic functional unit of the kidney. There are approximately 1 million nephron in each kidney. The nephron consists of an ovoid renal or malpighian corpuscle (comprised of the glomerulus and Bowman's capsule) and a hollow tubule of approximately 50 mm length that drains into the collecting duct system. The different segments of the nephron are as follows (Fig. 1.5).

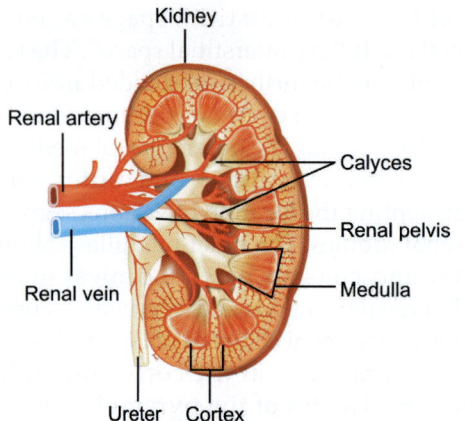

Fig. 1.4: Longitudinal cut section through kidney at hilum

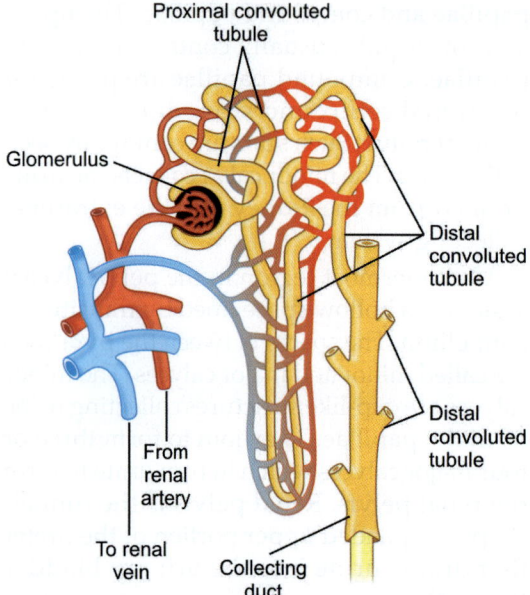

Fig. 1.5: Nephron—the functional unit of kidney

- Glomerulus and Bowman's capsule
- Proximal convoluted tubule
- loop of Henle (LOH)
- Distal convoluted tubule
- Collecting duct (which opens into the renal papilla)

The glomerulus is formed by the invagination of the bulbous, blind proximal end of the nephron by the afferent arteriole forming the tuft of capillaries in the Bowman's space. Glomerulus filters blood across Bowman capsule into the proximal convoluted tubule. It is approximately 200 μm in diameter and has a central skeleton, consisting of glomerular mesangial matrix and mesangial cells surrounded by the glomerular capillaries, the basement membranes and the epithelial cells. The capillary network is lined by a thin layer of fenestrated endothelial cells. The glomerular basement membrane is composed of a central dense layer, the lamina densa, an outer lamina rara externa and an inner lamina rara interna. The Bowman's capsule is lined on the inside by visceral epithelial layer and on the outside by the parietal cell layer. The urinary space is in-between two epithelial cell layers. The visceral epithelium is continuous with the parietal epithelium at the vascular pole, where the afferent arteriole enters and the efferent arteriole exits the glomerulus. At the urinary pole, the parietal cell layer is modified and continues as the proximal tubular cell.

The visceral epithelial cell or podocyte is the largest cell within the glomerulus. Podocyte has a main cell body containing the nucleus and cytoplasmic extensions, which divide, forming small finger-like processes that interdigitate with similar structures from adjacent cells and cover the capillaries. These interdigitations have numerous projections called 'foot processes' which rest on the basement membrane of the glomerular capillaries. The space between adjacent foot processes is known as the filtration slit. The adjacent foot processes are joined together by a thin membrane known as the slit-pore diaphragm. As the blood flows through the glomerulus, an ultrafiltrate of plasma is produced. The filtration barrier is composed of the fenestrated endothelium, glomerular basement membrane (GBM), and the slit pores between the foot processes of the visceral epithelial cells (Fig. 1.6).

The proximal tubule (PCT) consists of an initial convoluted portion, the pars

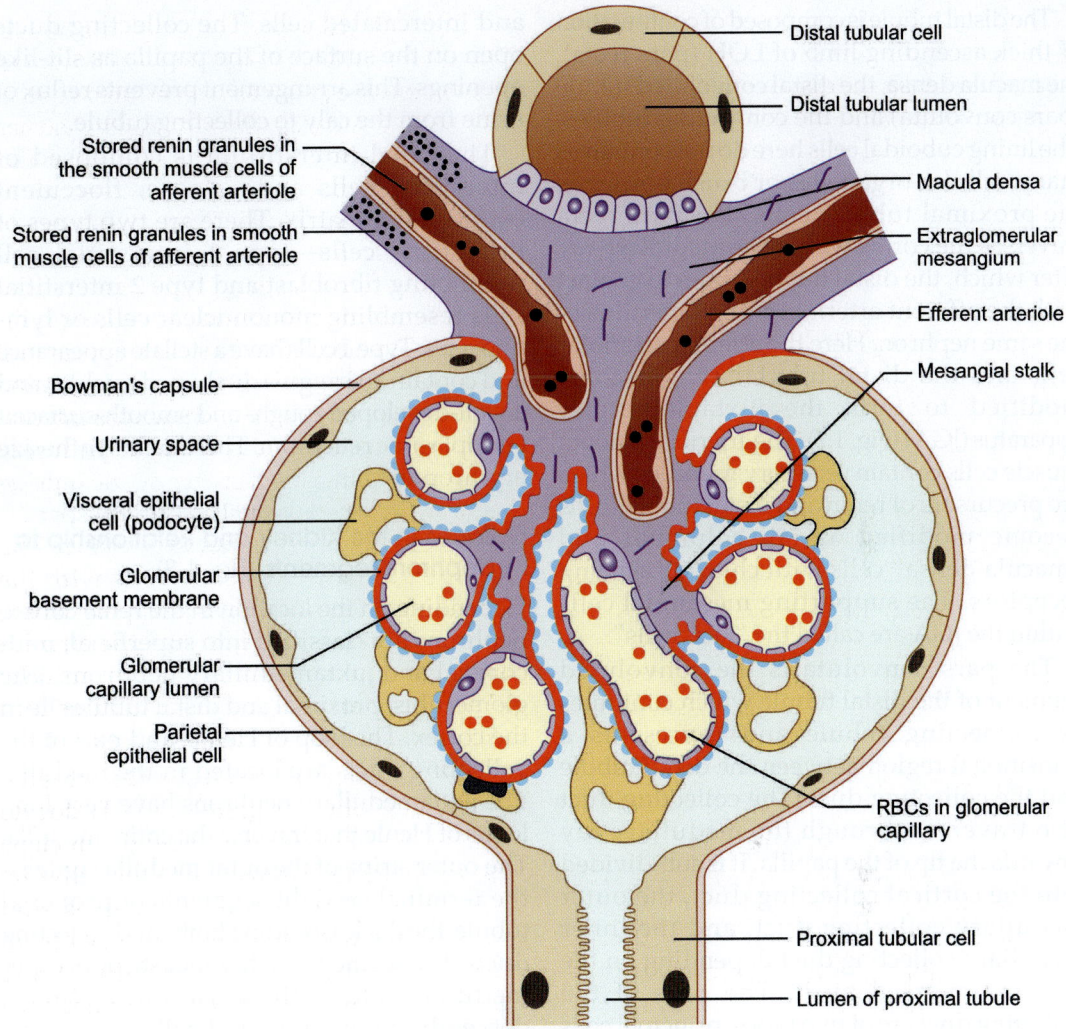

Fig. 1.6: The glomerulus

convoluta, located in renal cortex and a straight portion, the pars recta, located in the outer stripe of outer medulla. The portion of the cortex which contains the straight portions of proximal and distal tubules and collecting duct is called 'medullary ray'. The PCT is lined by metabolically active cuboidal cells that contain a number of cellular organelles like mitochondria. The luminal aspect of the proximal tubular cell has minute finger-like projections giving the appearance of a brush border.

The loop of Henle (LOH) is a U-shaped bend in the nephron. The straight segment of the proximal tubule ends as a narrow tube lined by flattened cells. This is the thin descending limb of LOH and it travels from the corticomedullary junction towards inner medulla where it forms the loop. The thin limb continues in the reverse direction towards the corticomedullary junction for a variable distance as thin ascending limb. In the outer medulla, the cells become cuboidal and form the thick ascending limb and proceed to the cortex.

The distal tubule is composed of continuation of thick ascending limb of LOH (pars recta), the macula densa, the distal convoluted tubule (pars convoluta) and the connecting tubules. The lining cuboidal cells here do not contain as many cellular organelles or brush border as the proximal tubular cells. The pars recta traverses the cortex within the medullary ray after which, the distal tubule comes in contact with the afferent arteriole and glomerulus of the same nephron. Here the afferent arteriolar cells and the distal tubular cells become modified to form the juxtaglomerular apparatus (JGA) (Fig. 1.7). The arteriolar smooth muscle cells contain secretory granules which are precursors of renin and distal tubular cells become modified as tall columnar and "macula densa" cells with chloride sensing receptors. The supporting mesangial cells within the JGA are called the "lacis cells".

The pars convoluta is the convoluted segment of the distal tubule which continues as connecting tubule and represents a transitional region between the distal tubule and the collecting duct. The collecting duct also traverses through the medullary ray towards the tip of the papilla. It is sub-divided into the cortical collecting duct, the outer medullary collecting duct, and the inner medullary collecting duct depending on the region traversed by it. The cells of the collecting duct are of two types, principal cells and intercalated cells. The collecting ducts open on the surface of the papilla as slit-like openings. This arrangement prevents reflux of urine from the caly to collecting tubule.

The renal interstitium is composed of interstitial cells and a loose, flocculent extracellular matrix. There are two types of interstitial cells—type 1 interstitial cell resembling fibroblast and type 2 interstitial cells resembling mononuclear cells or lymphocytes. Type 1 cells have a stellate appearance and contain an irregularly shaped nucleus and a well-developed rough- and smooth-surfaced endoplasmic reticulum. These cells synthesize erythropoietin.

iv. Zones in the Kidney and Relationship to Nephron Segments (Fig. 1.8)

Depending on the location in the renal cortex, nephrons are classified into superficial, mid-cortical and juxtamedullary nephrons. The glomerulus, proximal and distal tubules lie in the cortex. The loop of Henle, and part of the collecting ducts are located in the medulla. The juxtamedullary nephrons have very long loops of Henle that traverse the entire medulla. The outer stripe of the outer medulla contains the terminal straight segments of proximal tubule, the thick ascending limbs and collecting ducts. The segments in the inner stripe of outer medulla include thick ascending limbs, descending thin limbs and collecting ducts.

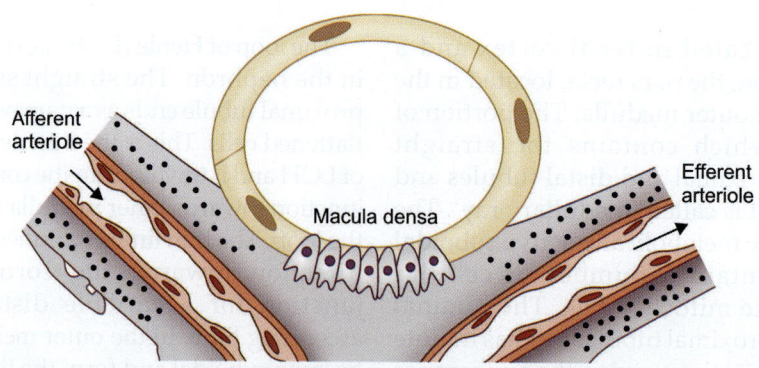

Afferent arteriole

Efferent arteriole

Macula densa

Fig. 1.7: Juxtaglomerular apparatus

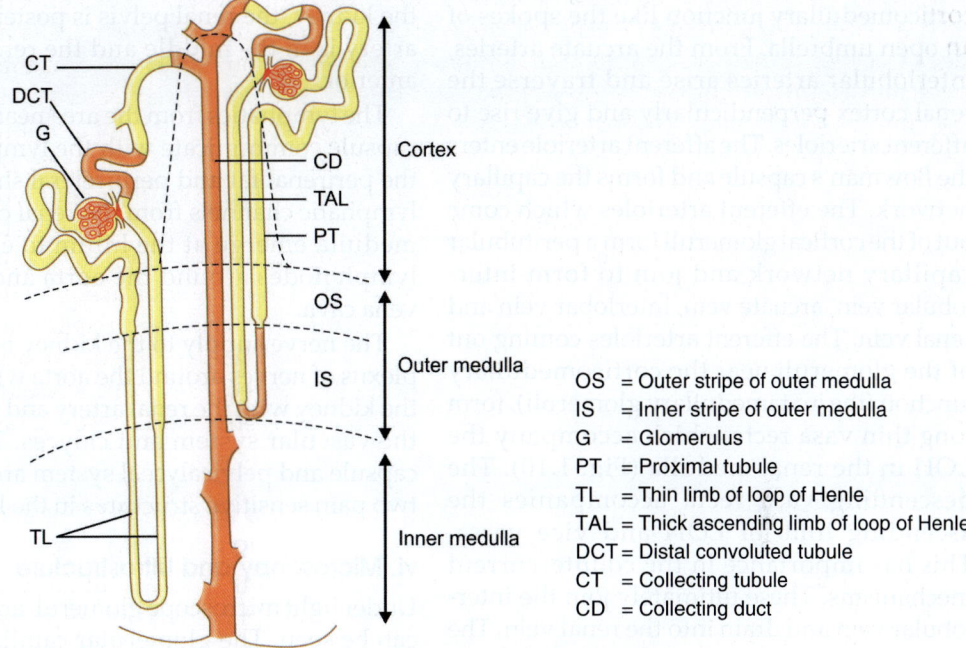

Fig. 1.8: The nephron in relation to zones in renal cortex and medulla

OS = Outer stripe of outer medulla
IS = Inner stripe of outer medulla
G = Glomerulus
PT = Proximal tubule
TL = Thin limb of loop of Henle
TAL = Thick ascending limb of loop of Henle
DCT = Distal convoluted tubule
CT = Collecting tubule
CD = Collecting duct

The inner medulla contains both descending and ascending thin limbs and the collecting ducts. The osmolality of the inner medulla is maintained very high (about 1200 mOsm/kg) by the countercurrent mechanism (Fig. 1.9). The location of various segments of tubules in their respective cortical and medullary zones is of utmost importance in maintaining the concentration gradient and maximally concentrating the urine by the countercurrent system.

v. Renal Circulation, Lymphatics and Nerve Supply

Kidneys are highly vascular and receive one-fifth of the total cardiac output under normal conditions. Renal artery arises from the abdominal aorta and enters the kidneys through the real hilum. It divides into about 6–8 interlobar arteries which pierce the renal medulla to reach the corticomedullary junction. Here, they divide into a number of

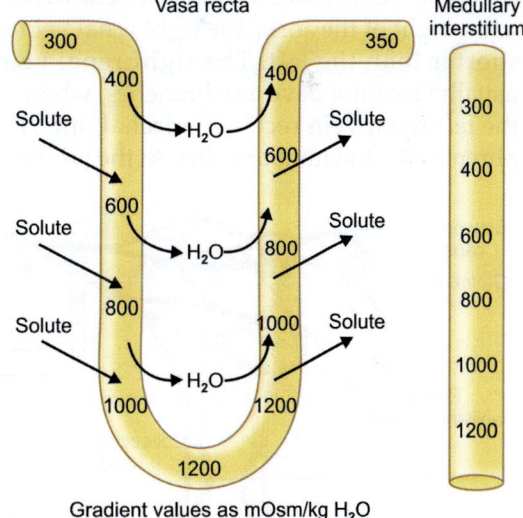

Gradient values as mOsm/kg H_2O

Fig. 1.9: Changes in osmolality along the nephron and various parts of renal interstitium

arcuate arteries which travel in all the directions from the point of origin at the corticomedullary junction like the spokes of an open umbrella. From the arcuate arteries, interlobular arteries arise and traverse the renal cortex perpendicularly and give rise to afferent arterioles. The afferent arteriole enters the Bowman's capsule and forms the capillary network. The efferent arterioles which come out of the cortical glomeruli form a peritubular capillary network and join to form inter-lobular vein, arcuate vein, interlobar vein and renal vein. The efferent arterioles coming out of the glomeruli near the corticomedullary junction (the juxtamedullary glomeruli), form long thin vasa recta which accompany the LOH in the renal medulla (Fig. 1.10). The descending vasa recta accompanies the ascending limb of LOH and vice versa. This has importance in the countercurrent mechanisms. These ultimately join the inter-lobular vein and drain into the renal vein. The renal arteries are end arteries and obstruction can lead to infarction of the corresponding area of the kidney. In contrast to this, there are plenty of communications between the intrarenal veins. Since the inferior vena cava is to the right of the aorta, the right renal vein is shorter than the left. The right renal vein usually does not have any branches, whereas the left renal vein receives adrenal, inferior phrenic and 2nd lumbar veins. At the hilum of

the kidney, the renal pelvis is posterior, renal artery is in the middle and the renal vein is anterior.

The lymphatics from the area near the renal capsule communicate with the lymphatics of the perirenal fat and periureteral sheath. The lymphatic channels from the renal cortex and medulla emerge at the hilum to end in the lymph nodes around the aorta and inferior vena cava.

The nerve supply to the kidney is from the plexus of nerves around the aorta which enter the kidney with the renal artery and innervate the vascular system and calyces. The renal capsule and pelvicalyceal system are the only two pain sensitive structures in the kidney.

vi. Microscopy and Ultrastructure

Under light microscope glomeruli and tubules can be seen. The glomerular capillary loops will be thin and delicate. Endothelial and mesangial cells and epithelial cell number together will be 2–3 per capillary loop. The surrounding tubules will be arranged in a back to back fashion with a little interstitium seen in between the tubules. Under electron microscopy, it will be possible to identify the cells, the fenestrations in the endothelium, the layers of basement membrane, the foot processes of the visceral epithelial cells and help to study the changes in various disease conditions.

vii. Structure of Ureter, Urinary Bladder and Urethra

The ureters are long muscular conduits, transporting urine from the renal pelvis to the urinary bladder. They are composed of helically arranged smooth muscle fibers. The transport of urine down the ureter is by the peristaltic waves that have been generated in the pacemaker cells of the minor calyces. The ureters traverse through the bladder muscula-ture and submucosa obliquely. The oblique course and the firm underlying detrusor support prevent the reflux of urine into the

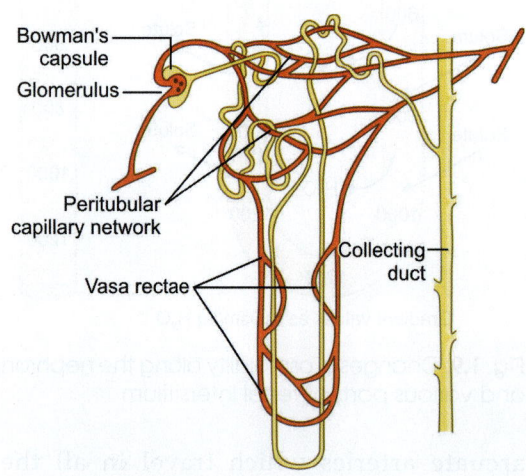

Bowman's capsule
Glomerulus
Peritubular capillary network
Vasa rectae
Collecting duct

Fig. 1.10: Renal circulation

ureters. The ureters are lined by transitional epithelium.

The urinary bladder is hollow muscular organ, storing urine at a low pressure of 5–10 cm of water. This low pressure allows for continuously receiving urine from the ureters and storing the same. When about 400–600 ml of urine accumulates in the bladder, the individual gets an urge to void. If the circumstances are appropriate, voiding occurs with a flow rate of about 20–25 ml/second. If the circumstances are inappropriate, the urge to void can be suppressed. Normal voiding is complete with no residue at the end of micturition. Urinary bladder is composed of smooth muscles called detrusor. They are arranged in a haphazard fashion except at the bladder neck where the detrusor is arranged to form the proximal smooth muscle sphincter (internal sphincter). At rest, the proximal sphincter plays the major role in retaining the urine. This sphincter is ablated during prostatectomy and the continence is maintained by the distal skeletal muscle sphincter at the membranous urethra (the external sphincter). The voluntary initiation of micturition is by relaxation of the levator ani muscle. The urinary bladder is lined by transitional epithelium which has 3–7 layers. More than 7 layers are seen in urothelial malignancies.

The male urethra is about 20 cm long. It is divided into posterior urethra and anterior urethra by the urogenital diaphragm. The posterior urethra consists of prostatic and membranous urethra, whereas the anterior urethra consists of bulbous urethra and penile urethra. In the membranous urethra and distal prostatic urethra, special skeletal muscle fibers are present. These constitute the distal sphincter (rhabdosphincter). Though composed of skeletal fibers this sphincter is also involuntary. The posterior urethra, distal anterior urethra and the intermediate urethra are lined by transitional, squamous and pseudostratified columnar epithelium respectively.

The female urethra is about 4 cm long. The distal sphincter in females is weak. The proximal urethra is lined by transitional and distal urethra by squamous epithelium.

Functions of Kidneys

• V Narayanan Unni

Kidneys are the principal excretory organs of the human body. In addition to this important and vital excretory function (urine formation), these organs have certain regulatory, metabolic and secretory functions as well.

A. EXCRETORY FUNCTIONS AND FORMATION OF URINE

Waste products of cell metabolism, toxins and drugs are excreted through urine. Three processes, namely glomerular filtration, tubular reabsorption and tubular secretion are involved in urine formation.

1. Glomerular Filtration

As blood passes through the glomerulus, the plasma is filtered and the filtrate contains water along with electrolytes, other small molecular weight substances, nitrogenous waste products, toxins and drugs. Thus, the glomerular filtrate is an ultrafiltrate of plasma, without major proteins. The factors which influence the glomerular filtration are renal blood flow, glomerular capillary hydrostatic pressure (60 mm Hg), glomerular capillary oncotic pressure (30 mm Hg), hydrostatic pressure in the Bowman's space (20 mm Hg) and glomerular capillary permeability. Permeability of the glomerular capillary filtering mechanism is controlled by:

i. Size selective barrier in which substances more than 6–8 nm size are not allowed to pass through.

ii. Charge selective barrier due to the presence of negatively charged particles like sialic acid residue which lines the filtration surface. The negative charge repels the negatively charged particles like albumin.

iii. Capillary surface area also affects the filtration rate.

The normal glomerular filtration rate is about 120 ml per minute per 1.73 sq.m body surface area. This amounts to around 180 liters of glomerular filtrate in 24 hours. Out of this, over 178 liters are reabsorbed by renal tubules, so that the final urine volume is about 1.5 to 2 liters in a day. The filtration increases when the glomerular capillary hydrostatic pressure increases. To a great extent, this is controlled by renal blood flow, blood pressure and the tone of the afferent and efferent arterioles of the glomerulus. It is easy to imagine that when the efferent arteriolar tone is increased, the blood flow decreases and the glomerular capillary hydrostatic pressure increases.

2. Tubular Reabsorption

The renal tubule is responsible for maintenance of the milieu intérieur by adjusting the amount of water, electrolytes and other substances that need to be excreted from the plasma. Based on the intake, body stores and the need, the tubules regulate the amount to be excreted. The process of reabsorption of solutes is achieved by different processes which include active transport (ATP is consumed), facilitated diffusion and passive diffusion. Each segment of the nephron functions in a different fashion and the orchestrated function of all the segments put together effectively maintains the normal fluid, electrolyte and acid–base balance.

The proximal tubule reabsorbs nearly 95% of glucose, bicarbonate and amino acids and 65% of water, electrolytes like sodium, chloride, and potassium. Hence, the fluid leaving the proximal tubule is iso-osmotic with glomerular filtrate (plasma).

The remaining ultrafiltrate enters the loop of Henle. The descending limb is freely permeable only to water and impermeable to solutes. Since this segment of the nephron passes through the renal medulla where the osmolality progressively increases towards the deeper parts of the medulla, water is reabsorbed in this segment and the osmolality of the ultrafiltrate equals the osmolality of deeper medulla nearly 1200 mOsm/kg. The ascending limb of loop particularly the thick portion is impermeable to water but an active transport of sodium and chloride occurs in this segment. This segment of the nephron is also called the diluting segment since about 25% of electrolytes like sodium and chloride are reabsorbed actively and no water is reabsorbed. Thus, the fluid leaving the loop of Henle is hypo-osmolar (50–100 mOsm/kg) or dilute.

In the distal tubule reabsorption of electrolytes including sodium and chloride continues. The hormone aldosterone controls sodium absorption. Finally the fluid enters the collecting duct which traverses the renal cortex and medulla to open into the calyx. The permeability of the collecting duct to water is regulated by the antidiuretic hormone (ADH) secreted by the posterior pituitary gland. Under normal conditions, numerous water channels called aquaporin 2 channels remain dormant in the cytoplasmic vacuoles within the cells of the collecting duct. When the body has to conserve the water, the ADH is released from the pituitary which causes the dormant water channels to move and attach themselves to the cell wall. When more water channels are inserted to the luminal wall, more water is reabsorbed and the fluid leaving the collecting duct (urine) is concentrated and lesser in volume. In situations of the need to eliminate from the body, the channels move back into the cell and significant water reabsorption will not take place in the collecting duct. Such urine will be higher in volume and dilute. The urine osmolality can vary from 50 to 1200 mOsm/kg water. Normal functiong of the loop of Henle, medullary interstitium and the hormones aldosterone and ADH are essential for a proper concentration and dilution of the urine to occur. A counter current exchange system and counter current multiplier system help to attain and maintain the osmolality of the interstitium of renal medulla high all the time.

3. Tubular Secretion

The tubule has the capacity to secrete electrolytes like potassium, hydrogen ions, creatinine, uric acid, many drugs and other excretory products. The ability to secrete hydrogen ions is essential to maintain the acid–base balance. The alpha intercalated cells in the distal tubule are capable of secreting H^+ ions into the lumen where they are taken up by ammonia or phosphate buffer and eliminated in the urine.

B. REGULATORY FUNCTIONS

The kidneys are reponsible for regulation of:
  i. Water content in the body
 ii. Concentration of electrolytes
iii. Maintenance of acid–base status.

i. Maintaining Water Balance

Water content in the body is maintained within a specific range in order to keep the tonicity of the body fluids within a narrow range (normal osmolality of plasma is 285 to 295 mOsm/kg). This is achieved due to fine balance between water intake and water excretion. Water intake is determined by availability of water, thirst mechanism and environmental temperature. A very small rise in plasma osmolality by 2% would stimulate thirst, thus increasing the fluid intake and returning the plasma osmolality to normal range. As explained earlier, water excretion is regulated by the kidneys under the influence of the hormone, ADH. An increase in plasma osmolality stimulates secretion of ADH resulting in lesser water excretion and a fall in osmolality suppresses ADH secretion and promotes water loss. In the presence of normal renal functions, ADH action is through 'exocytic insertion' of aquaporin channels in the luminal membrane of the collecting tubular cells making them more permeable to water.

ii. Regulation of Electrolytes

Depending on the intake, body stores and serum levels, the kidneys can regulate the excretion of all electrolytes. Sodium, potassium, calcium and magnesium are the main cations (positively charged ions) and chloride and bicarbonate are the main anions (negatively charged ions).

Sodium is reabsorbed predominantly in the proximal tubules (65%), ascending limb of loop of Henle (25%) and in the distal tubule. In the proximal tubule, sodium reabsorption occurs with water, glucose and bicarbonate. In the ascending limb of the loop, an active transport mechanism (NKCC) reabsorbs sodium, potassium and two chloride ions together. In the distal nephron, the reabsorption of sodium and simultaneous secretion of potassium are regulated by the adrenal hormone, aldosterone. Hypovolemia, fall in blood pressure or hyperkalemia stimulates secretion of aldosterone which increases reabsorption of sodium and excretion of potassium. Calcium and Magnesium are mostly reabsorbed along the paracellular pathways in the loop of Henle and the amount excreted in urine depends on their plasma levels. The filtered bicarbonate is completely reabsorbed by the renal tubule, the bulk of the reabsorption occurring in the proximal tubule.

iii. Maintenance of Acid–Base Balance

Acids enter the body mainly through diet. The non-vegetarian diet contains more acid load in the form of sulphates and phosphates from meat and meat products. In the case of vegetarians, the diet may have lesser acid load. On an average, the cell metabolism in body produces around 15,000 moles of volatile acids and 1 mEq per kg body weight of non-volatile acids in 24 hours. The acid–base balance maintained by successfully eliminating the accumulated acid by the combined action of

a. *Bicarbonate—carbonic acid buffer system*

This is the most important buffer system and mops up the (H^+) ions by combining with HCO_3 forming carbonic acid. This is called a volatile acid since it splits into CO_2 and water under the influence of the enzyme carbonic anhydrase which is present in the body.

b. *Lungs:* The lungs can eliminate up to 15000 mmols of carbon dioxide every day and help in eliminating the volatile acids.

c. *Kidneys:* The kidneys help to eliminate the water load derived from carbonic acid. More importantly, they have to reabsorb all the filtered bicarbonate and regenerate more bicarbonate that is lost due to excretion of non-volatile acids. Normal kidneys reclaim 100% of the bicarbonate filtered by the glomeruli, so that no bicarbonate is lost in the urine. In addition, kidney secretes H^+ ions into the tubular lumen. These H^+ ions are taken up by phosphate buffer, converted into 'titratable acids' and excreted in urine. Ammonia which is synthesized in the renal cell takes one H^+ ion and forms nonabsorbable 'ammonium' and is excreted. Loss of each H^+ ion in the urine results in regeneration of one molecule of HCO_3. Depending on the need and the acid–base status of the body, the pH of urine can vary from 4.5 to 8.0. The excretion of non-volatile acids by the kidneys helps to maintain the blood pH within the normal range of 7.36 to 7.44.

C. REABSORPTION OF VITAL SUBSTANCES FILTERED BY GLOMERULI

The renal tubules are involved in complete reabsorption and retention of essential and vital substances like glucose, amino acids and vitamins that are filtered by the glomeruli.

D. REGULATION OF BLOOD PRESSURE

Kidneys play an important role in regulation of blood pressure. Salt and water retention is the main mechanism of hypertension in many renal diseases and the normal kidney controls the excretion of salt and water from the body.

Renin is secreted from the juxtaglomerular apparatus (JGA) of the kidney in response to ischemia to the kidney, hypovolemia and hypotension. Renin converts angiotensinogen to angiotensin I, which gets converted to angiotensin II (AT II). AT II is a powerful vasoconstrictor and stimulates secretion of aldosterone from adrenal gland.

Secretion of vasodilatory prostaglandins, kinins and certain other substances also help to maintain the blood pressure.

E. SECRETORY AND HORMONAL FUNCTIONS OF THE KIDNEY

1. *Erythropoietin (EPO):* This is a hormone produced by cells in the renal tubulo-interstitial compartment and stimulates bone marrow to produce red blood cells. It is a glycoprotein. Decreased oxygen availability due to anemia, hypoxia or renal ischemia stimulates EPO secretion. Deficiency of EPO is responsible for the anemia of chronic renal diseases. Rarely some renal diseases also produce excessive EPO which results in polycythemia.

2. Active form of vitamin D_3 otherwise called 1,25-dihydroxycholecalciferol [1,25-$(OH)_2$ D_3) is produced by proximal tubules cells from the precursor 25-hydroxychole-calciferol which comes from the liver. Parathyroid hormone, hypocalcemia and hypophosphatemia stimulate the enzyme which catalyses the synthesis of active form of vitamin D_3.

3. *Renin:* Renin is a renal hormone stored as granules in the muscle layer of the afferent arteriole and is released in response to hypo-volemia, hypotension or renal ischemia. The renin acts on angiotensinogen (renin substrate), converts it into angiotensin (AT) I and later to AT II. This is not only a potent vasoconstrictor but also stimulates secretion of aldosterone form the adrenal cortex. Stimulation of renin-angiotensin-aldosterone system leads to retention of sodium and water and increases in blood pressure.

4. *Prostaglandins (PGs):* PGs are known as local hormones as they act locally and have a short half life. PGs produced by the kidney play a role in excretion of electrolytes like sodium, potassium, as well as water; in addition they have a regulatory role in renal and glomerular blood flow, GFR, renin release and response to anti-diuretic hormone. PGs are released in conditions like volume depletion, hemorrhage and cardiac failure.

F. METABOLIC FUNCTIONS

Kidneys play a significant role in metabolism of peptide hormones like insulin, PTH, calcitonin and others. Many drugs are either metabolized in the kidney or are excreted unchanged in the urine.

Symptomatology and Clinical Approach

• Vinay Sakhuja • Vivekanand Jha

INTRODUCTION

Before nephrology developed as a speciality, renal diseases were described only in terms of life history and the therapeutic interventions were limited. Advances in physiology, pathology, immunology, imaging techniques, dialysis and renal transplantation over the last 7 decades have led to a clearer understanding of the pathogenesis and treatment of the diseases of the kidney and urinary tract. In order to establish an early and accurate diagnosis, the clinician must be aware of the various ways in which a disease of the kidneys or urinary tract can present. This requires careful history taking and physical examination. Examination for proteins and sugar and microscopy of a centrifuged specimen of urine is crucial and should be considered an extension of clinical examination. The information obtained is used for planning a structured investigative approach, commencing with simple screening tests and proceeding to specific diagnostic investigations. Estimation of blood urea, serum creatinine, electrolytes and complete blood count constitute basic investigations and are required in almost all patients. Ultrasound is noninvasive, quick, safe even in pregnant women and relatively inexpensive. This makes it the preferred technique for imaging the kidneys and urinary tract. An accurate classification of renal parenchymal diseases requires study of renal histology. Light microscopy can be done at most centers, but electron microscopy and immunofluorescence studies require specialized setups and available only in selected major centers.

MODES OF PRESENTATION

A patient with disease of the kidneys or urinary tract may seek medical attention for:
a. Symptom(s) or sign(s) pointing towards a renal disease.
b. A systemic disease known to involve the kidneys or urinary tract.
c. No symptoms, but an abnormality indicating underlying renal disease detected by a laboratory investigation.

CARDINAL FEATURES OF RENAL DISEASE

The following features point to the disease of the kidneys or urinary tract.
1. Disorders of urinary composition
2. Disorders of urinary volume
3. Edema and hypertension
4. Pain originating from the urinary tract
5. Disorders of micturition
6. Detection of a renal mass
7. Symptoms related to alteration of renal functions.

Disorder of Urinary Composition

Proteinuria

The normal daily protein excretion in urine is less than 150 mg in adults and 300 mg in children and adolescents. Transient rise in protein excretion may be seen during normal pregnancy, fever and following heavy exertion. Proteinuria is the commonest urinary abnormality associated with renal disease. Abnormal proteinuria is classified according to the underlying pathophysiologic disturbance (glomerular, tubular or overflow), quantity (nephrotic or non-nephrotic), time and posture (constant or orthostatic), associated urinary abnormality (isolated proteinuria or proteinuria with hematuria) and type of protein (selective or non-selective). Pathological proteinuria may be a result of diseases primarily affecting the glomeruli or the tubulointerstitial compartment. Usually, proteinuria of interstitial disease consists of a variety of low molecular weight proteins and the daily urinary loss is less than 2 g/24 hours. On the other hand, glomerular proteinuria is usually >1.5 g/24 hours with albumin as the main constituent. Overflow proteinuria occurs when a protein produced in excessive amounts is filtered at the glomeruli, overwhelms the tubular reabsorptive capacity and thus appears in urine. The kidneys themselves are structurally normal in such cases. The amount excreted may vary from trace to massive quantities. Examples include Bence-Jones proteinuria in multiple myeloma, hemoglobinuria and myoglobinuria. Minor degree of posture-related (orthostatic) proteinuria (urinary protein <1 g/24 hours) may not be clinically significant. This is confirmed by documenting absence of protein in the urine sample passed immediately on rising in the morning but proteinuria appears when the patient has been up and about for some hours. Dye impregnated paper strips that depend on color change of a pH sensitive dye used in dipstix are very good for detection of albumin, but are insensitive to globulins like Bence-Jones proteins. Proteinuria that is dipstick negative but detected on sulfosalicylic acid test indicates light chain excretion. When heavy proteinuria is detected by these strips, it is useful to quantitate protein excretion by timed samples or by comparing the concentration with that of creatinine.

Hematuria

Hematuria is defined as the excretion of abnormal quantities of erythrocytes in the urine. It may arise from any part of the urinary tract from the glomerulus to the urethra. Bleeding disorders may also be responsible for hematuria. Hematuria is conventionally described according to the following parameters:

a. *Gross or microscopic:* The term gross hematuria is used when the urine is obviously discolored. Less than 5 ml of blood can discolor 1 L of urine. At acidic pH, the urine appears brownish red, smoky or cola colored, whereas a bright red colour indicates brisk bleeding or highly alkaline urine. Microscopic hematuria refers to urine that looks normal to the naked eye but has abnormal quantities of RBCs on microscopic examination. Hematuria is defined as excretion of >5 RBCs/HPF in a centrifuged sample. The RBC excretion can go up after vigorous exercise. The count may be spuriously elevated in menstruating females or in urine samples obtained by urethral catheterization. Dilute urine can cause hemolysis and significant reduction in numbers of intact erythrocytes.

b. *Persistent or intermittent:* Hematuria may be described as persistent when all the samples examined show presence of erythrocytes. Intermittent hematuria is diagnosed when the abnormality is seen only on some occasions, the urine being normal in-between.

c. *Symptomatic and asymptomatic:* Hematuria may be symptomatic (associated with pain originating in the urinary system) or asymptomatic (painless).

d. *Initial, terminal or uniform:* Blood seen only at the beginning of micturition suggests bleeding from the bladder neck, prostate or urethra. Terminal hematuria indicates bleeding from the bladder. Uniform bleeding throught the act of micturition suggests renal or systemic causes for bleeding.

True gross hematuria must be differentiated from other causes of brownish or red urine (Table 3.1). Some of the common pitfalls are failure to elicit a history of intake of drugs that discolor the urine and mistaking hemoglobinuria or myoglobinuria for hematuria.

The next step is localization of the origin of hematuria. Presence of a typical unilateral renal colic permits localization to that kidney or ureter. Similarly, suprapubic pain is indicative of disease in urinary bladder. Passage of clots suggests bleeding either from renal tumors or lesions in the renal pelvis, ureter or bladder. Long thread like clots indicate renal origin, whereas small bits of clots point to a bladder origin. The following points suggest the origin of bleeding to be the renal parenchyma rather than elsewhere in the urinary tract.

a. Erythrocyte casts indicate glomerulonephritis or rarely, interstitial nephritis.

b. Concomitant presence of heavy proteinuria (3 to 4+ qualitatively, or >2 g/day) nearly always signifies a glomerular origin for the hematuria.

c. RBCs due to glomerular disease commonly appear fragmented and distorted (dysmorphic) due to the damage sustained as they traverse the nephron. This phenomenon is best seen by phase contrast microscopy. In contrast, red cells due to lesions in renal pelvis, ureter or bladder retain their uniform biconcave circular shape.

d. Concomitant demonstration of eosinophiluria suggests the possibility of drug-induced interstitial nephritis.

After initial localization, additional points in the history or physical examination may provide a clue to the diagnosis. These include history of weight loss (tumor or tuberculosis), edema (nephritic or nephrotic syndrome), loin pain and colic (stones), fever and dysuria (urinary tract infection), joint pain (collagen vascular disease), skin rashes (SLE, Henoch-Schönlein purpura, drug hypersensitivity), renal mass (tumors, polycystic kidney disease), deafness (Alport's syndrome), hemoptysis (Goodpasture's syndrome, microscopic polyarteritis, Wegener's granulomatosis), recent throat or skin infection (postinfectious glomerulonephritis), and heart murmur (infective endocarditis). A family history of renal disease, deafness or bleeding tendency is important. A history of drug ingestion should be elicited carefully, especially prolonged use of analgesics (papillary necrosis), antimicrobials (interstitial nephritis) and cyclophosphamide (hemorrhagic cystitis). Foreign travel in an area with endemic *Schistosoma haematobium* infection should also be excluded.

Patients with evidence of bleeding not arising from the renal parenchyma should

		Table 3.1: Differential diagnosis of red or brown urine			
Disorder	*Orthotoluidine test*	*Heat test (proteins)*	*Color of spun serum*	*Color of spun urine*	*Urine microscopy*
Hematuria	4+	0–4+	Clear	Clear	RBCs
Hemoglobinuria	4+	0	Pink	Red, brown	–
Myoglobinuria	4+	0	Clear	Brown	–
Porphyria	0	0	Clear	Red (chloroform extractable)	–
Exogenous pigment	0	0	Clear	Red	–

have a plain X-ray of abdomen, ultrasound scan of the urinary tract or intravenous urography (IVU). In addition to looking for routine organisms, urine should also be cultured for mycobacteria. Malignant cells due to transitional cell carcinoma of the urinary tract can be picked up on cytologic examination of urine. Cystoscopy is indicated to look for foreign body, vascular anomalies, tumor or ulcers in the bladder and to determine if hematuria is originating in one or both kidneys.

The appearance of urine can also be altered by precipitation of phosphate, urate or uric acid crystals. Phosphates produce a whitish deposit in alkaline urine which increases on warming and dissolves after acidification of urine with acetic acid. Urates and uric acid form faint pink deposits, particularly if the urine is concentrated or acidic. These deposits disappear on warming or adding sodium hydroxide.

Abundant leukocytes and bacteria may give the urine a turbid appearance. Rarely, patients may complain of a gross deposit of yellow-white pus. Chyluria, caused most commonly by filarial infection, is an important cause of milky urine. This can be confirmed by Sudan red stain which colors the fat red. Addition of an equal volume of chloroform, ether or xylol clears the turbidity in chyluria.

Disorders of Urinary Volume

Oliguria and Anuria

Oliguria is a reduction in urine output to less than that required for excretion of the daily metabolic solute load at maximal urinary concentration. Since the average daily solute intake and maximal urinary concentrating ability in adults are 600 and 1200 mOsm/kg respectively, a minimum daily output of 500 ml can achieve this goal. Oliguria is, however, traditionally defined as a urine output of less than 400 ml/24 hours. In situations where the urinary output is monitored with an indwelling catheter, documentation of urine volume less than 20 ml/hour can give an early indication of oliguria in adults. In children, a urine volume of 0.5–0.8 ml/kg/hour is taken as oliguria. Oliguria can be produced by three major groups of disorders: Prerenal, renal and post-renal.

Prerenal oliguria. This is a state where the kidneys and the urinary tract are normal and the reduction in urine volume is due to reduced renal perfusion. Also called functional renal failure, this is produced by a reduction in effective arterial blood flow. This can occur in settings where the total extracellular fluid volume is reduced (blood or fluid losses, sequestration of fluids from the vascular compartment to a third space), normal (sepsis, anaphylaxis, anaesthetic agents) or even increased (congestive cardiac failure, cardiac tamponade, cor pulmonale, severe hypo-albuminemia). It is important to differentiate prerenal azotemia from ischemic acute renal failure quickly; failure to do so may result in development of acute tubular necrosis in those with prerenal azotemia. In absence of obvious fluid overload, a useful method of differentiating prerenal oliguria from other causes of oliguria is to infuse 1–1.5 L of saline followed by 100–200 mg frusemide intravenously. If the kidneys are normal, the urine output should increase to >40 ml/hour. A number of indices helps to differentiate prerenal azotemia from intrinsic acute renal failure and is discussed elsewhere in the book.

Intrinsic renal diseases causing oliguria. A wide spectrum of intrinsic renal diseases produce oliguric acute renal failure, the commonest being acute tubular necrosis (ATN). Some forms of ATN, especially those associated with nephrotoxic injury (aminoglycoside antibiotics, contrast media) and hypercalcemia at times are not associated with oliguria. This is known as nonoliguric acute renal failure. Acute glomerulonephritis and vasculitis may also lead to oliguria. Edema, hypertension, hematuria and RBC casts point to these conditions. Fulminant pyelonephritis or renal papillary necrosis can rarely present with oliguria. Oliguria also occurs in acute rejection, acute tubular necrosis or ureteric obstruction affecting a transplanted kidney.

Postrenal oliguria. Obstruction to urine flow commonly occurs due to calculi or benign prostatic enlargement. Other causes include prostatic carcinoma, retroperitoneal fibrosis, blood clots or sloughed renal papilla. Intermittent obstruction causes oliguria alternating with polyuria. Intrarenal obstruction can be produced by deposition of crystals (e.g. uric acid, cystine or drugs such as sulfonamides or acyclovir) in tubules.

Anuria results from a complete cessation of glomerular filtration and is diagnosed when the daily urinary output is <50–100 ml. Diagnosis requires drainage of previously formed urine from the bladder to document lack of new urine production. The causes of anuria are listed in Table 3.2. Any condition that produces oliguria can present with a transient period of anuria. Occlusion of vascular system or ureters calls for swift management and hence must be ruled out in anuric patients. A distended bladder indicates outlet obstruction. Calculi, accidental ligation of both ureters during pelvic surgery or pelvic malignancies with infiltration of ureters can cause complete obstruction of the urinary tract. Unilateral ureteric obstruction in a solitary functioning kidney also produces anuria. Ultrasonography is the method of choice for evaluation of the urinary tract. Besides evaluation for obstruction, it also gives useful information about kidney size

---

Table 3.2: Etiology of anuria

- Bilateral renal artery occlusion
- Bilateral renal vein occlusion
- Complete obstruction of both ureters
- Bilateral renal cortical necrosis
- Rapidly progressive glomerulonephritis
- Urethral obstruction

---

and renal cortical thickness. Urine microscopy may reveal crystals in patients with calculi or urate nephropathy. Retrograde pyelography may be needed to determine the exact site of upper urinary tract obstruction. A color Doppler or radionuclide scan provides information about patency of renal arteries. Suspicion of rapidly progressive glomerulo-nephritis constitutes an indication for an early biopsy.

Polyuria and Nocturia

Polyuria may be defined as the excretion of excessive amounts of urine. Normally, the daily urine volume varies over a broad range, with an average of 1.6 liters in a healthy adult. Excretion of >3 L urine in a day (2.0 ml/min) suggests polyuria. The 24-hour volume is measured by emptying the bladder at the time of starting collection, collecting, the whole urine including that passed at the same time the following day. Urine can be considered a mixture of water and solute. Measuring urinary osmolality can assess the relative contribution of the two compartments. From a clinical standpoint, the causes of polyuria may be divided into three groups: (a) Water diuresis (osmolality <150 mOsm/kg), (b) solute diuresis (osmolality >300 mOsm/kg) and (c) mixed water-solute diuresis (osmolality 150–300 mOsm/kg). In patients with water diuresis, the water deprivation test determines whether the diuresis is due to decreased antidiuretic hormone (ADH) secretion by the posterior pituitary, central diabetes insipidus or to renal insensitivity to ADH (nephrogenic diabetes insipidus). The causes of solute diuresis are often obvious and determination of the dominant solute in the urine (e.g. glucose in diabetes mellitus) helps in narrowing down the list of possibilities (*see* Chapter 43 on approach to polyuria).

Nocturia increases in ADH secretion limits the volume of urine produced during sleep. The day/night ratio of urine output is 2:1 in healthy adults. This ratio falls with increasing age and is close to unity by the age of 60 years. Nocturia is thus defined as passage of large amounts of urine between 6 PM and 6 AM with the ratio coming close to 1:1 in young adults and below 0.6:1 in the elderly. Nocturia is an early but often overlooked sign of progressive renal disease; history of long-standing nocturia in a patient with recently discovered renal failure indicates chronic renal disease. It can also occur in conditions where the diurnal pattern of urine production is altered (cirrhosis, nephrotic syndrome) or with urological diseases, commonest being benign enlargement of the prostate.

Edema and Hypertension

Edema refers to the accumulation of excess fluid in the interstitial component of the extracellular fluid (ECF). It is produced when the Starling forces controlling the movement of fluid between the capillary and interstitium and back is altered. The lymph also helps to return the fluid from the interstitial to the intravascular space. Edema could be a result of loss of proteins from the intravascular space, avid sodium and water retention by the kidneys or a combination of the two. Edema of renal disease is usually most noticeable in the parts of the body subjected to the highest hydrostatic pressure, such as around the eyes in the morning and ankles in the evening. This variation is lost in the later stages when edema becomes generalized. The edema is pitting in nature and when severe, may be accompanied by ascites and pleural effusion. Edema is common in acute nephritic and nephrotic syndromes, but is less pronounced in the former. The reason for this, and the presence of hypertension, is a lack of peripheral adaptation such as increased compliance of the interstitial space observed in the nephrotic syndrome that protect the intravascular volume from rising. Edema in the late stages of chronic renal failure is due to salt and water retention. Rarely, edema develops as a consequence of intake of drugs such as dihydropyridine

calcium channel blockers (nifedipine, amlodipine) or nonsteroidal anti-inflammatory agents.

Edema of renal disease has to be differentiated from edema due to other systemic causes. History of orthopnea and paroxysmal nocturnal dyspnea and detection of elevated jugular venous pressure, hepatojugular reflux, gallop rhythm and cardiac murmurs suggest the diagnosis of congestive cardiac failure. History of gastrointestinal bleed and signs of chronic liver disease (spider naevi, palmar erythema, gynecomastic testicular atrophy), jaundice and dilated abdominal wall veins suggest cirrhosis of liver.

Patients with advanced chronic renal failure and glomerular diseases often have hypertension, whereas it is less frequent in tubulointerstitial disease. In adult polycystic kidney disease, hypertension precedes renal failure by several years. In diabetic nephropathy, the blood pressure begins to rise before albuminuria occurs.

Pain Originating from the Urinary Tract

The renal capsule and plevicalyceal system are sensitive to pain. Pain produced by acute dilatation of the urinary system as a result of obstruction results in renal colic. Typical renal colic begins as an ache in one flank or loin or along a band about the size of a palm, extending from the side downwards and increases within 20–30 minutes to pain of indescribable severity. At this time, the patient moves about restlessly and may have nausea and vomiting. In contrast to colics originating in other organs that wax and wane, renal colic is continuous and crescendo in character with minor fluctuations. The pain forces the victim to seek medical attention and is usually terminated by medication. The pain may disappear suddenly following spontaneous relief of obstruction.

The site of pain is determined by the site of obstruction. Obstruction at the ureteropelvic junction gives rise to pain in the flank that radiates to the upper abdomen, whereas midureteric pain is felt in the flank, or along a band coursing downward, laterally and inferiorly across the abdomen. Stones that obstruct the lower ureter cause pain in the anterolateral abdomen, groin or ipsilateral testicle or vulva. Obstruction at ureterovesical junction gives rise to symptoms of trigone irritation: Frequency, urethral pain and dysuria.

Renal colic may result from a stone, blood clot, sloughed renal papilla or foreign body (e.g. broken tip of nephrostomy catheter) and needs to be differentiated from pain due to biliary obstruction and appendicitis on the right side; diverticulitis and irritable bowel syndrome on the left and prolapsed inter-vertebral disk, sprain or trauma on either side. The typical characteristics as well as presence of hematuria, leukocyturia or graveluria help to make this distinction. Another type of renal pain occurs due to stretching of the renal capsule. This pain is a nagging and persistent ache or sense of heaviness that worsens on standing. Disease associated with rapid enlargement of the kidneys such as acute glomerulonephritis, acute interstitial nephritis, acute pyelonephritis, renal abscesses, renal vein thrombosis, bleeding into a cyst or a rapidly enlarging renal cell carcinoma cause this type of pain. In diseases giving rise to perinephric inflammation, pain is localized to the flank and is associated with focal muscle spasm and tenderness. Movement of the flank aggravates this pain and the patient prefers to lie quietly. This type of pain may occur with rupture of a renal cyst, perinephric abscess, or hemorrhage or necrosis in a tumor mass.

The initial diagnostic tool in evaluation of pain is renal ultrasound and a straight X-ray of abdomen to detect radiopaque stones. An IVU can help in detection of blood clot, sloughed papilla or uric acid stones that are radiolucent and thus not seen on plain skiagrams. Patients with renal colic should have their urine screened through fine muslin in the hope of capturing stones, clots or necrosed papillae.

Disorders of Micturition

Dysuria and Frequency

Dysuria describes pain or discomfort during micturition. It usually arises as a consequence of bladder, prostatic or urethral inflammation and is described as a burning or tingling sensation felt at the urethral meatus or in the suprapubic region during or immediately following the act of micturition. Frequency is a term used to indicate that the bladder is emptied more often than normal. This may be associated with a decreased or normal urinary volume. Frequency and dysuria often occur together. However, frequency alone may be seen in patients with reduced bladder capacity due to fibrotic contraction or external pressure by a pelvic mass or gravid uterus. The 'frequency-dysuria' complex is seen far more frequently in women than in men. Enquiry regarding the precise site of discomfort has diagnostic usefulness in women. The pain is felt as being 'inside the body (internal dysuria)' with cystitis or urethritis, whereas external dysuria is felt in the labia and indicates vaginitis. In men, perineal or rectal pain suggests inflammation of the prostate. Prostatic localization is also suggested by terminal dysuria and pyuria.

Microscopic evaluation of the urine sediment is the first step in the evaluation for dysuria and frequency. In presence of pyuria, a positive urine culture provides information regarding the infecting organism and its antimicrobial sensitivity. Sterile pyuria is indicative of infection with a fastidious organism (Chlamydia, tuberculosis, viruses) or a chemical irritant. Hematuria is suggestive of stones, hemorrhagic cystitis or tuberculosis of the urinary tract. Cystourethroscopy may be required for complete investigation of patients suspected of having urethral stricture or bladder neoplasms. A voiding cystourethrogram provides information regarding vesico-ureteric reflux or urethral pathology. A combination of frequency, dysuria and urgency in women in whom an infection cannot be documented is termed 'urethral syndrome' and can be due to trauma, use of irritants or systemic diseases (e.g. Reiter's and Behçet's syndromes and Crohn's disease). Prostatic enlargement in elderly males causes the urinary stream to be poor and the voiding time to be prolonged. There may also be difficulty in initiating micturition (hesitancy) or terminal dribbling. When extreme, this may cause complete obstruction leading to urinary retention.

Uremic Symptoms

Kidneys have vast anatomical and functional reserve. They respond to disease or surgical removal by compensatory hypertrophy of remaining tissue. These physiological adaptive mechanisms make it possible for a patient to be asymptomatic despite destruction of as much as 80% of the renal parenchyma. Azotemia indicates accumulation of nitrogenous waste products like urea and creatinine in the blood as a result of reduced renal excretory capacity. Uremia indicates symptomatic renal failure. It may involve virtually any organ system and the presentation is extremely variable. Appearance of uremic symptoms often provides the first indication of the presence of renal disease. Uremic symptoms are discussed in detail in the section on chronic renal failure. Failure of endocrine functions of the kidney produces anemia (reduced erythropoietin production) and bone disease (altered vitamin D hydroxylation). Hypokalemia as a consequence of reduced acidification at proximal and/or distal tubular segment can cause flaccid weakness of skeletal muscles, leading in extreme cases to respiratory paralysis.

Renal Mass

Renal masses may be detected at any age but the incidence is highest in the young (before 10 years) and after the age of 40. The causes may be divided broadly into inflammatory, hereditary and congenital, traumatic and neoplastic disease (Table 3.3). Fever, flank pain and pyuria indicate an acute inflammatory disease. A positive family history and/or associated hepatomegaly suggests polycystic

Table 3.3: Renal masses in children and adults		
Category	*Children*	*Adults*
Inflammatory	Acute focal bacterial nephritis Renal abscess	Xanthogranulomatous pyelonephritis Malakoplakia Renal abscess Tuberculosis
Congenital	Hydronephrosis, ARPKD** Multicystic dysplasia, ADPKD	ADPKD* Hydronephrosis
Trauma	Hematoma	Hematoma
Neoplastic		
Benign	Mesoblastic nephroma Angiomyolipoma Nephroblastomatosis	Simple cyst Fibroma, lipoma Leiomyoma Angiomyolipoma
Malignant	Wilms' tumor Renal cell carcinoma	Renal cell carcinoma Wilms' tumor Sarcomas Secondaries

* ADPKD: Autosomal dominant polycystic kidney disease
** ARPKD: Autosomal recessive polycystic kidney disease

kidney disease (PKD). Features of urinary tract obstruction suggest hydronephrosis. A history of hematuria and rapid weight loss is indicative of a malignant mass. The important steps in evaluation include an ultrasound examination and/or IVU. Presence of multiple cysts on both sides distorting the renal outline confirms the diagnosis of PKD. CT scan or MRI helps to study the nature and extent of renal masses, and whether the draining lymph nodes or blood vessels are involved. In the case of a solitary cyst, these modalities provide a clue as to whether the cyst is benign or malignant. In doubtful cases, cyst puncture and cytologic examination may be necessary to exclude a malignant lesion. Finally, histologic diagnosis of the mass may be obtained by open biopsy or at the time of surgery.

Clinical Examination and Approach to Diseases of the Kidney and Urinary Tract

• Vivekanand Jha • Vinay Sakhuja

Proper history and thorough physical examination are the first steps in the diagnostic approach followed by relevant investigations.

HISTORY

The first step in history is to elicit all the symptoms in clear chronological order. Patients should be encouraged to explain their symptoms in their own words. The precise date of onset and duration of symptoms should be determined wherever possible. Enquiry should be made regarding the cardinal symptoms of renal disease and associated symptoms, e.g. presence and temporal relationship of upper respiratory tract symptoms with an episode of hematuria or sexual activity and dysuria. If the patient has sought medical help previously, the records should be carefully reviewed. Long-standing renal disease often manifests with relatively minor symptoms such as nocturia. Renal involvement can be seen in a number of systemic diseases (e.g. diabetes, hypertension, collagen vascular diseases, multiple myeloma) and their symptoms usually precede those of renal disease by a variable period. Sometimes, however, renal disease is the initial presenting feature and specific enquiries should be made about symptoms of systemic diseases.

Past History

The past history is of particular relevance in patients with unexplained chronic renal failure. Enquiries should be made regarding events in childhood and adolescence with stress on long forgotten symptoms. In very young children, unexplained febrile episodes may be the sole manifestation of urinary infection. A history of protracted nocturnal enuresis may indicate either a structural abnormality of the urinary tract or a disordered concentrating mechanism. A poor urinary stream in a male infant suggests the presence of a posterior urethral valve or neurogenic bladder. History of excessive thirst, salt craving and repeated episodes of dehydration in the first decade of life is highly suggestive of medullary cystic disease. Hypertension detected in the first two decades could be due to renovascular or renal parenchymal disease. Detailed past history of unrelated illness is also important in planning treatment. For example, β-blockers would be deleterious in a patient known to have bronchial asthma.

Drug History

A careful note must be made of recent intake of all drugs including indigenous medicines or drugs of other systems of medicine with details regarding the dose, duration and temporal relation to the clinical manifestations. Drugs can affect the kidneys in several ways. Aminoglycoside antibiotics, contrast media, nonsteroidal anti-inflammatory drugs (NSAIDs), some cephalosporins, cisplatinum and amphotericin B can cause acute renal failure due to acute tubular necrosis. Acute allergic interstitial nephritis can be produced by a single dose of a large variety of drugs. On the other hand, interstitial nephritis due to NSAIDs may develop after several months of administration. Hypotensive drugs, in particular angiotensin converting enzyme inhibitors can precipitate acute renal failure, especially in patients with low cardiac output states or bilateral renal artery stenosis. Drugs that are nephrotoxic on chronic ingestion include analgesics and lithium (chronic tubulo-interstitial nephritis) and gold salts and D-penicillamine (glomerular changes). Elderly patients are particularly susceptible to drug toxicity. Indigenous drugs contain heavy metals and may affect the kidneys. In addition to direct renal damage, drugs can aggravate renal disease by causing elevations in the blood pressure (oral contraceptives) or producing volume loss (diuretics).

Personal History

Occupational factors are important in development of renal disease. Some predisposed groups are: Workers in a hot environment (urinary stone disease), aniline dye workers (urothelial tumors), sewage workers and farm labourers (leptospirosis), those exposed to lead fumes in pain industry or welders (lead nephropathy), exposure to inhalational hydrocarbons (Goodpasture's disease). Intravenous drug addiction exposes the patient to renal complications related to infective endocarditis, hepatitis B, septicemia, human immunodeficiency virus infection and rhabdomyolysis.

Family History

In all patients with renal disease, the family pedigree (including consanguinity) should be established. Some renal diseases that have a genetic predisposition are autosomal dominant and recessive forms of polycystic kidney disease, Alport's syndrome (X-linked), medullary cystic disease (autosomal recessive) and renal tubular acidosis syndromes. Vesicoureteric reflux, congenital nephrotic syndrome, renal tubular acidosis, Fabry's disease and metabolic disorders (primary hyperoxaluria, cystinosis) are also inherited. Familial cases of some primary glomerular diseases (e.g. MPGN, FSGS) have been described. Some forms of hypertension are inherited. Patients with diabetes mellitus or hypertension may also have a familial predilection for renal involvement.

Obstetric History

Renal disease may appear or get aggravated during pregnancy. Pre-existing renal disease can affect the outcome of pregnancy. Enquiries should be made about the duration and outcome of each pregnancy blood pressure throughout pregnancy, and presence of proteinuria. Recurrent fetal losses in a patient with normal renal function could be due to lupus anticoagulant and should raise the possibility of antiphospholipid antibody syndrome. Acute tubular or cortical necrosis may occur in association with complications or pregnancy, such as accidental or post-partum hemorrhage, post-abortal or puerperal sepsis and severe pregnancy induced hypertension. Enquiries should be made regarding antenatal history and findings of obstetric ultrasound examination in neonates with renal disease. Oligohydramnios may suggest renal dysplasia, agenesis or autosomal recessive polycystic kidney disease. Dilated fetal urinary tract suggests obstructive uropathy or vesico-ureteric reflux. Perinatal asphyxia can lead to ischemic medullary necrosis and renal failure.

PHYSICAL EXAMINATION

A thorough general physical examination provides a lot of useful information and must be carried out before going on to specific examination of the kidneys and the urinary tract. The general appearance of the patient may provide a clue to underlying renal disease. Partial lipodystrophy characterized by loss of subcutaneous fat in the upper half of the body may be associated with type II membranoproliferative glomerulonephritis. Similarly, hemihypertrophy and medullary sponge kidney, nail patella syndrome (dystrophic nails, absence of one or both patellae, deformity of elbow joints) and characteristic glomerular changes, are some well-known associations. In children, absent abdominal wall musculature is often associated with cryptorchidism and urological abnormality (prune-belly syndrome).

Both physical and mental growth should be assessed in children. The height should be compared with the expected height for that age and sex from nomograms. Growth retardation often results from chronic renal disease in childhood. Abnormalities in bone metabolism can occur in a large number of renal diseases and give rise to rickets, osteomalacia or secondary hyperparathyroidism. The clinical features vary with age and may even help in timing the onset of the disease. During the first year of life, rapid growth of the skull results in cranial softening, widening of cranial sutures, frontal bossing and flattening of posterior portion of the skull in those with rickets. In young children, rapid growth of the arm and rib cage lead to widening of the forearm at the wrist and costochondral junctions (rickety rosary). Harrison's sulcus, an indentation of the lower ribs at the site of attachment of the diaphragm, may also be seen. In older children, rapid growth of legs leads to development of knock-knees or bow legs. A malunited fracture in the ribs or clavicle may be palpable. In patients with secondary hyperparathyroidism, resorption of the terminal phalanges of fingers and toes leads to loss of pulp (pseudoclubbing).

Ocular examination may reveal perilimbal calcification and conjunctival congestion (red eye) in patients with long-standing uremia. The ocular fundus must be examined in every patient for hypertensive or diabetic retinopathy. Typical fundal abnormalities may also be seen in infective endocarditis, toxemia of pregnancy, retinal artery or vein occlusion and methanol poisoning. In patients with diabetes, absence of retinopathy suggests a non diabetic cause of renal disease. Anterior lenticonus shows up as a drop of oil in a pool of water upon examination with a strong convex lens in patients with Alport's syndrome. Early appearance of cataract is particularly common in patients on long-term corticosteroid therapy. Alport's syndrome may be associated with sensorineural deafness on clinical examination or audiometry. In examination of the mouth, condition of teeth and palate and presence of white patches due to oral candidiasis must be noted. Gum hyperplasia may be present in patients taking cyclosporine A.

The skin in uremic patients is dry and scaly. Scratch marks indicate pruritus. Intradermal deposits of urochrome produce pigmentation in the sun-exposed areas. Precipitation of urea crystals due to high concentration in the sweat gives rise to 'uremic frost' most notably in the bearded areas and skin folds. Uncontrolled nephrotic syndrome may result in protein-calorie malnutrition. Drug side effects may present as facial mooning, central distribution of body fat, purpura, pink striae and acne due to corticosteroids, alopecia due to cyclophosphamide and hirsutism due to cyclosporine. Renal transplant recipients can develop hyperkeratotic skin lesions on sun-exposed areas.

Cutaneous manifestations often provide a window to many systemic disorders. Patients with SLE can have an erythematous rash over the cheeks and bridge of nose (malar rash) or circular raised, depigmented and scaly lesions with follicular plugging (discoid rash). Palpable purpura or infarcts of skin and digits may be present in patients with vasculitis. Systemic sclerosis (firm, thickened and leathery skin bound tightly to underlying skin) Henoch-Schönlein purpura (palpable purpura, usually over buttocks and extensor surface of extremities) are often suspected by typical appearance. In Fabry's disease, small red hyperkeratotic papules (angiokeratomas) are typically seen over the lower half of the abdomen and buttocks. Hamartomatous cutaneous lesions indicate underlying tuberous sclerosis. Secondary sexual characteristics should be looked for as puberty is delayed in uremia.

Transverse parallel white bands flush with the surface (Muehrcke's lines) may be seen in the nails of patients with nephrotic syndrome and indicate periods of protein loss. Their width may give a rough idea about the duration of hypoalbuminemia. Splinter hemorrhages seen as bluish bands along the sides of nails may be visible in patients with vasculitis or infective endocarditis. The so-called 'half-and-half' nail, in which the distal 40–60% of the nail bed is brown or red and sharply demarcated from the dull whitish proximal portion, is typical of uremia.

The jugular venous pressure may be elevated due to fluid overload in an oliguric patient, congestive cardiac failure due to uncontrolled hypertension, infective endocarditis or associated ischemic heart disease. A prominent 'x' descent is noted in patients with cardiac tamponade due to uremic pericardial effusion.

All peripheral pulses should be felt carefully in a hypertensive patient. Absent or asymmetric pulses may indicate aortoarteritis in the young and atherosclerosis in an elderly patient. Auscultation over major vessels (subclavian or carotids) may reveal a bruit at the site of narrowing.

A number of issues should be kept in mind when measuring blood pressure (BP). Attention needs to be paid to (1) correct cuff size, (2) accuracy of the manometer, (3) reliability of the observer, and (4) sufficient number of measurements for a reasonable approximation of average BP. It is good practice to record the BP in supine (or sitting) and standing posture. The arm should rest at the heart level. Generally the systolic BP is same in both positions, but the diastolic blood pressure is lower in supine position, especially in younger individuals. Recent exposure to cold, smoking and eating overestimate the true BP, whereas recent exercise underestimates it. A mercury sphygmomanometer should be used as far as possible. Aneroid apparatuses need to be calibrated once every 6 months. It is important to choose an appropriately sized cuff (width and length of at least 40% and 80% of arm circumference respectively). The standard adult cuff is 23 × 12 cm. The commonest mistake is to use a cuff that is too small, resulting in an overestimation of the BP. In general, using a large, adult sized cuff for all but the thinnest arms can minimize errors. The best site for cuff placement is 2–3 cm above maximum pulsation of brachial artery, with the center of bladder over the vessel. Systolic BP should be measured first by palpation. After infancy, Korotkoff phase V (total cessation of sounds) is used to record the diastolic BP. This phase may be absent in infants, old age or high cardiac output states (anemia, thyrotoxicosis, pregnancy, recent exercise). Phase IV (muffling) is the only reliable index of diastolic BP in these situations. In a hypertensive patient, an increase in diastolic reading on making the patient upright is a feature of essential hypertension, whereas some degree of postural hypotension is often observed in patients with hypertension due to secondary causes, in those on anti-hypertensive therapy and in volume depleted states. The oscillometric technique of measuring BP is based on the observation that the oscillations of pressure in a sphygmomanometer cuff are maximal at the mean intra-arterial pressure. Systolic and diastolic pressures are derived from this value according to complex algorithms. Ambulatory and home BP recorders use this technique.

The BP must be recorded in all the 4 limbs at least once in young or elderly hypertensives and in those with asymmetric pulses so that the diagnosis of aortoarteritis, coarctation of aorta or atherosclerotic vascular disease are not missed. In patients with pericardial effusion, the degree of pulsus paradoxus can be determined by noting the difference between the levels when sounds are heard only during expiration and in both phases of respiration.

The rate and pattern of breathing should be noted. Tachypnea may be an early indication of fluid overload. Deep and rapid breathing is seen in metabolic acidosis. Rales over the lung bases or a third heart sound indicate fluid overload, and a pleural or pericardial friction rub can be present in advanced uremia. In neurological examination, note should be made of the level of consciousness and mental status of the patient. Metabolic flap (asterixis) is an early sign of uremic encephalopathy. It is elicited as irregular, abrupt and brief loss of posture seen in the tongue or outstretched hand with the wrists extended and fingers spread out.

Examination of the Kidneys and Urinary Tract

The clinical examination should follow the standard routine of inspection, palpation, percussion and auscultation.

Inspection. Normally, the kidneys and the urinary tract are not visible. However, massively enlarged kidneys in a patient with polycystic kidney disease may be seen as diffuse ill-defined bulge in the flanks. A full urinary bladder may be seen as an oval swelling in the suprapubic region. The external genitalia must be inspected to rule out congenital anomalies. Vaginal or urethral discharges in women and urethral discharge in men should be inspected with attention to consistency, odor and color.

Palpation. The patient should be lying supine with the arms resting at the sides. For palpating the left kidney, the right hand is placed anteriorly in the left lumbar region whilst the left hand is placed posteriorly in the left loin. The patient is asked to breathe in with the left hand pushing forwards and the right hand backwards, upwards and inwards. The right kidney is palpated in much the same way, with the left hand placed posteriorly in the loin, and the right hand placed horizontally on the anterior abdominal wall to the right of umbilicus. The lower pole of the right kidney may be normally plapated at end inspiration as a firm rounded swelling in very thin individuals. When palpable, the left kidney needs to be differentiated from an enlarged spleen. The presence of a characteristic notch and inability to insinuate a finger between the mass and left costal margin identify it as a spleen. An estimate of size and shape should also be made. The surface may be irregular and knobby in polycystic kidneys. Any tenderness on palpation should be recorded. Costovertebral angle tenderness should be assessed in those with suspicion of acute pyelonephritis.

A full bladder may be palpable as a smooth firm swelling with well-defined upper and lateral borders in the hypogastric region. As it arises out of the pelvis, its lower border cannot be felt. The patient may have an urge to micturate on pressing the swelling.

Percussion. Abdominal percussion is valuable when there is a difficulty in differentiating an enlarged kidney from the liver or spleen. A renal mass has a band of resonance anteriorly over the swelling (due to colon), whereas the other organs are uniformly dull on percussion. The presence of ascites should also be noted.

Auscultation. A bruit arising in the renal arteries should be looked for at initial evaluation in all hypertensives. This is best heard anteriorly about 1" above and lateral to the umbilicus, posteriorly in the loin (opposite

L2 vertebra) and laterally in the flanks. It should be noted whether the bruit is heard only during systole or during both phases of the cardiac cycle. A systole-diastolic bruit and one heard in the loin is most likely to be a renal bruit. A bruit over the renal allograft must be looked for in a post-transplant patient with hypertension, or in a patient who develops hypertension after a renal biopsy (due to an arteriovenous fistula).

Finally, a per rectal examination should be performed in elderly males and all males with symptoms of urinary tract outflow obstruction or UTI to assess the prostate gland. Normally both lateral lobes separated by the median fissure can be palpated as smooth, rubbery and firm bulges on the anterior rectal wall. Though prostatic enlargement may be detected on rectal examination, an accurate estimation of its size may not be possible. In carcinoma of the prostate, its consistency becomes hard, the lateral lobes tend to be irregular and nodular, and there may be distortion or loss of the median sulcus. Prostatic massage provides valuable information in males with chronic UTI. A pelvic examination with palpation of adnexae may be necessary in women with recurrent UTI. Vaginal examination may also reveal carcinoma of the cervix extending laterally to the pelvic wall giving rise to a 'frozen pelvis' in women with unexplained urinary obstruction.

Examination of the external genitalia is indicated in all patients with disorders of the urinary stream. Abnormalities to be looked for include tight phimosis, an ectopic (abnormally placed) or narrowed (pinhole) external meatus. The ectopic location can be anywhere on the dorsum of the penis (epispadias) or on the ventral aspect (hypospadias). Careful palpation along the length of the penile urethra may reveal a firm cord-like segment of urethral stricture.

CLINICAL SYNDROMES IN NEPHROLOGY

Traditionally, presentation of renal diseases has been divided into ten clinical syndromes that serve as useful starting points in patient evaluation. These syndromes are not disease entities by themselves but simply a constellation of symptoms and signs that tend to coexist and identify diseases that present in a similar fashion. This helps in narrowing down the list of differential diagnosis and planning diagnostic and therapeutic strategy. The ten clinical syndromes are as follows:

1. *Acute nephritis.* This syndrome is characterized by a short history of hematuria, hypertension, oliguria, edema and mildly elevated serum creatinine. Glomerular hematuria is the *sine qua non* of this syndrome, and erythrocyte casts or dysmorphic RBCs confirm the nephronal origin of hematuria. The commonest cause of this syndrome is postinfectious glomerulonephritis; the clinical features can be correlated to preceding skin or throat infection. Most cases recover spontaneously. Renal biopsy is necessary only when a cause cannot be found, renal function deteriorates rapidly or if the recovery is delayed beyond 2 weeks.

2. *Nephrotic syndrome.* This syndrome is characterized by massive proteinuria (urinary protein excretion >3.5 g/1.73 m^2/24 hours in adults or >40 mg/m^2/hour in children). There may be associated hypoalbuminemia, edema and hyperlipidemia. This symdrome can be seen in a large number of primary and secondary glomerular diseases. Minimal change disease, the commonest cause of this syndrome in children, responds readily to corticosteroid therapy, and so a therapeutic trial is given first. Nephrotic syndrome may occur in diabetes mellitus, amyloidosis and other systemic disorders. Renal biopsy is necessary for proper classification in most adults and in children not responding to steroid therapy.

3. *Asymptomatic urinary abnormalities.* Asymptomatic patients may be found to have abnormalities during urinalysis done

for routine evaluation for either health insurance, occupational purpose, during pregnancy or medical evaluation for other disorders. These abnormalities can be microscopic hematuria, non-nephrotic proteinuria and pyuria alone or in combination.

4. *Acute kidney injury (AKI).* AKI is a sudden decline in glomerular filtration rate (GFR) leading to accumulation of nitrogenous wastes in the blood, usually following an ischemic or toxic insult to the kidneys. The strongest evidence for AKI is documentation of a rise in blood urea or creatinine over a period of days. Absence of anemia, hypertension and demonstration of normal-sized kidneys on ultrasound constitute strong points in support of acute nature of the disease in a patient presenting with unexplained azotemia. The urine output may be decreases, normal or rarely increased. In most instances, the decline in renal function is completely reversible. An acute deterioration in renal function may occur in a patient with pre-existing renal insufficiency. An aggressive search must be made for factors which can cause such deterioration (ECF volume depletion, hypotension, uncontrolled hypertension, nephrotoxic drugs or urinary tract obstruction).

5. *Chronic renal failure (CRF).* CRF implies that the GFR has been reduced to its present level for a long period so that there is a little hope of significant improvement. The term renal insufficiency is sometimes used to describe patients with milder reduction in GFR before appearance of uremic symptoms. The time course of renal disease before these features appear may extend from months to years. Confirmation requires demonstration of reduced GFR for 3–6 months. In absence of such data, findings suggesting chronicity are: Presence of anemia or hypertension, clinical evidence of neuropathy in absence of any other cause, clinical or laboratory evidence of renal osteodystrophy and small kidneys seen on ultrasound.

6. *Urinary tract infection (UTI).* This syndrome is established by demonstration of significant number of pathogenic microorganisms (usually $>10^5$ colonies/ml) on urine culture. Symptoms of UTI include dysuria, frequency, urgency and suprapubic or loin pain. Most infections are limited to urethra and urinary bladder. Fever with rigors, loin pain, vomiting and nausea suggest involvement of upper tract. Demonstration of WBC casts, impaired urinary concentrating ability and antibody-coated bacteria also favor an upper tract infection. Physical examination and special investigations help to demonstrate any underlying structural abnormality in the urinary tract.

7. *Urinary tract obstruction.* Obstruction in the urinary tract may can occur at many levels: Renal pelvis, ureter, bladder or urethra. Obstruction of lower tract (bladder/urethra) is established by urinary retention or demonstration of residual urine in the bladder after micturition. Associated symptoms may include poor urinary stream, hesitancy, prolonged voiding time, or dribbling with overflow incontinence. Common causes are benign enlargement of prostate in the elderly, urethral stricture or congenital urethral valves in children. Upper tract obstruction is documented by demonstration of a dilated collecting system in the presence of empty bladder on imaging studies.

8. *Hypertension.* Hypertension is defined as persistent rise in diastolic BP to over 90 mm of Hg in an adult. Systolic BP of more than 140 mm Hg with a normal diastolic BP is known as isolated systolic hypertension. Exclusion of all treatable secondary causes is necessary in the young and those over 50 years of age. Appropriate investigations include serum electrolytes

(Conn's syndrome), urinary VMA or catecholamine levels (pheochromocytoma), renal function tests (renal parenchymal disease) and vascular imaging (renovascular disease). Hypertension can adversely affect the heart, kidney, eyes, brain and peripheral vascular system and all hypertensives should be evaluated for target organ damage.

9. *Nephrolithiasis.* This syndrome is defined clinically by a combination of renal colic, hematuria and either stone passage, radiologic visualization of a stone in the urinary tract, or surgical removal of such a stone. The stone should be analyzed to determine its composition. Metabolic studies are needed in recurrent stone formers.

10. *Renal tubular defects.* Although tubule function defects are often seen in association with other renal diseases, isolated disorders of tubule function may be the dominant feature in some inherited or acquired renal diseases. These abnormali-

ties may result from isolated dysfunction of proximal or distal tubules or a combination of the two. The proximal tubule is responsible for reabsorption of glucose, uric acid, phosphate, amino acids and bicarbonate. Dysfunction manifests as increased excretion of these substances in the urine, but is usually clinically silent. Distal tubular defects may present as disorders of urinary concentration, dilution or acidification. Distal renal tubular acidosis may present with muscle weakness (due to hypokalemia), nephrocalcinosis, nephrolithiasis or renal osteodystrophy. Most primary tubular defects present in childhood, and are characterized by failure to thrive, anorexia, polydipsia, polyuria, episodic vomiting, dehydration, unexplained fever, rickets and growth retardation. In adults, symptoms are related to defective bone mineralization (bone pain, fractures), muscle weakness and fatigue.

Investigations in Renal Disease

• R Kasi Visweswaran • KP Jayakumar

1. Collection of urine specimen
2. Physical characteristics of urine
3. Chemical examination of urine
4. Microscopic examination of urine
5. Hematologic tests
6. Renal function tests:
   a. Tests of glomerular function
   b. Tests of tubular function

COLLECTION OF URINE SPECIMEN

A careful examination of a properly collected urine specimen performed by clinician gives a lot of useful information. Hence, urine examination is considered to be an extension of the clinical examination. Accurate urinalysis begins with a proper collection. For this, the bladder should contain at least 200 ml of urine. A midstream urine specimen collected directly into a clean dry container of approximately 50–100 ml capacity is usually sufficient for laboratory purposes. The external genitalia is thoroughly cleaned with a mild antiseptic solution. In males the foreskin is retracted and in females the labia are separated when urine sample collected. The initial portion of urine stream is allowed to escape and the midstream portion is collected into a sterile container for culture. In certain situations, the urine passed as the initial, middle and terminal phases of micturition is collected separately and it helps in differentiating the source of turbidity or bleeding into the urinary tract. Rarely, a catheter drained sample may be needed in woman particularly during the menstrual period. Since catheterization may involve risk of infection, it is not advocated as a routine. In infants and children, suprapubic needle aspiration of the bladder may be used to avoid vaginal and urethral contamination. It can also be used to get a good sample of bladder urine for examination and culture. A simple method for collecting urine in infants and children is as follows. After feeding the child and before it voids, the genitalia is cleaned. The child is then held in the prone position. By stroking the back along the paravertebral muscles, spontaneous voiding usually occurs within five minutes due to stimulation of the spinal reflexes. In women and in pediatric age group, urine collectors attached to the external genitalia may also be used.

As far as possible, urine must be examined in a fresh state preferably within 30 to 60 minutes. The urine samples are also cultured as early as possible. At room temperature the bacteria convert the urea in the urine to ammonia, and change the pH to alkaline levels. The urinary casts may disappear at this pH. If there is a delay in the examination of the urine, it should be preserved so that decomposition does not occur. When urine is to be examined for chemical constituents, addition of 2 ml toluene to 100 ml urine is advised. 1 drop of formalin in 30 ml of urine is a useful preservative for examining the cells in the urinary sediment. Chloroform may be used for inhibiting bacterial growth but it may alter the characteristics of the cellular elements. Addition of one crystal thymol is a good preservative but it may interfere with the acid precipitation test for protein.

Ideally, the morning sample is preferred since the urine will be sufficiently concentrated. Random sample of urine can also be used. Screening for glycosuria is done in a 2-hour postprandial urine sample. Urine urobilinogen is best evaluated in a sample collected early in the afternoon. Timed urine samples are required to quantify substances like creatinine, glucose, proteins, electrolytes and VMA. A 24-hour urine collection is undertaken in most instances. If 24-hour collections are difficult, timed collections of 12 hours, 6 hours or 2 hours may be used. For timed collection, the patient is asked to empty the bladder at the beginning of the collection period. All samples thereafter, including the sample end of the collection period are added to the collection. It is preferable to refrigerate the collected sample during the entire collection period. For some tests, certain regents may be adds to prevent decomposition.

Daily urinary creatinine excretion is 20 to 25 mg/kg in males and 15 to 20 mg/kg in females. Proper and complete collection of urine can be assessed by measuring urinary creatinine.

Collecting urine sample from a long-standing indwelling catheter should be avoided since a 'Biofilm' forms in the catheter and the microorganisms colonizing the catheter may give misleading and false results. In such instances, the existing catheter should be removed and sample for culture sample taken immediately after inserting a new sterile catheter.

PHYSICAL CHARACTERISTICS OF URINE

Color: The color of normal urine is pale yellow, but it is lighter if urine is dilute and darker if it is concentrated. The color depends upon the pigments, viz. urochrome and urobilin. Alterations in the diet, drugs or diseases may lead to changes in the color of urine (Table 5.1). Red urine may be seen after the ingestion of beets and it is due to the betalain pigment.

Appearance. Normal urine is usually clear. It may turn cloudy due to precipitation of amorphous phosphates. This usually disappears when the specimen is warmed. Presence of leukocytes, epithelial cells, and bacteria disappears on acidifying the urine. Amorphous urates also give a cloudy appearance with a slightly, mucous and prostatic secretions may result in turbid urine. A proper microscopic examination helps to identify the leukocytes, epithelial cells, bacteria or prostatic threads in the urine. The urine may be smoky due to the presence of RBCs and this can be identified by a careful microscopic examination of the urine. The presence of fat or lymph leads to milky urine. This condition is called chyluria. Chyle dissolves on adding ether or chloroform to the sample. Staining for fat is confirmatory.

Odor. Freshly passed urine is odorless. It develops the pungent odor due to the splitting of urea to ammonia by the bacteria. The presence of ketones gives rise to a fruity smell. If freshly passed urine has a pungent smell it usually suggests urinary tract infection with urea splitting organisms. In certain congenital metabolic disorders like maple syrup urine disease, phenylketonuria, and hypermethio-ninemia, the characteristic smell of maple syrup, mousy odor and fishy odor respectively may be noted.

Specific gravity. Specific gravity of urine is defined as ratio of weight of urine to that of equal volume of water. It depends on weight of solutes in it and hence it is related to

Table 5.1: Causes of changes in color of urine

Color of urine	Illness or compound responsible
Pink red or orange red	Phenazopyridine, phenindione, phenytoin
	Phenolphthalein, beets, blackberries, Rhubarb, rifampicin, phenothiazines, azathioprine, doxorubicin
Brown black	Nitrofurantoin, metronidazole, sulfonamides, chloroquine, methyldopa, salicylates, levodopa, methocarbamol, phenol, iron, sorbitol
Blue Green	Methylene blue, triamterene, riboflavin, amitriptyline
Red to red brown	Hemoglobin, myoglobin, porphyrins, *Serratia marcescens* infection, amorphous urate
Golden brown	Bilirubin
Green blue	Pseudomonas infection
Brown black	Melanin, homogentisic acid
White	Chyle, pyuria

osmolality. Normally, the specific gravity ranges from 1003 to 1035. The presence of proteins, glucose, contrast media and variations in temperature alter the specific gravity, when it is measured with conventional urinometer. A correction for the alteration in specific gravity can be done by subtracting 0003 for each gram of protein and 0004 for each gram of glucose in the sample. Since the instrument is calibrated for 20°C, 0001 is added or subtracted for every 3°C above or below 20°C. This difficulty is overcome by the use of a temperature compensated refractometer or TS meter where, the specific gravity can be read directly using a drop of urine. Urine is said to be concentrated if specific gravity is 1016 or above. Special chemical impregnated strips are also used for testing the specific gravity.

Osmolality. Osmolality indicates the number of osmotically active particles in a solution. Osmolality does not depend on the molecular weight of the solutes, whereas specific gravity depends not only on the number of particles but also on their molecular weight. Therefore, substances like glucose, protein and dextrans alter the specific gravity more than the osmolality.

Urinary osmolality is a measure of urine concentration and is decided by solutes and the action of ADH. In the absence of ADH,

osmolality varies from 50 to 100 and in presence of ADH osmolality ranges from 900 to 1200. In normal urine, there is a rough correlation between the osmolality and specific gravity. Approximately 40 milliosmols (mOsm) is equal to one unit of specific gravity. Therefore, a specific gravity of 1010, 1020 and 1030 would correspond to osmolality of 400, 800 and 1200 mOsm per kg water, respectively. However, in presence of renal diseases, glycosuria, heavy proteinuria and use of radiographic contrast, this correlation is not reliable. The osmolality of urine varies from 50 to 1200 mOsm/kg water.

Osmolality is measured by noting the freezing point of the solution. A solution which has an osmolality of one osmole or 1000 mOsm/kg water freezes at −1.86°C. Therefore, if a sample of urine freezes at −0.93°C it suggests that the osmolality is 500 mOsm/kg water. When the urine is concentrated, it is generally hyperosmolar and dilute urine is hypo-osmolar.

Measuring osmolality is useful in the following states:
1. *Prerenal vs. acute tubular necrosis:* More than 500 indicate renal, but lower value is not helpful.
2. *Primary polydipsia:* Less than 100 indicate normal suppression of ADH while higher value indicates the presence of ADH.

Urine osmolality is contributed mainly by sodium, chloride, urea and ammonia.

CHEMICAL EXAMINATION OF URINE

pH. Since the kidney is involved in eliminating the acid produced by body as a result of daily metabolism, the urine is usually acidic. The pH of urine can be measured by using pH indicator strips or pH meter. The normal pH varies between 4.6 and 4.8. Immediately after meals, the pH is usually alkaline (alkaline tide). The measurements of pH are also important in the diagnosis and management of urinary tract infections, metabolic acidosis including renal tubular acidosis and renal stones.

1. It is useful in assessing the appropriate response in metabolic acidosis. In metabolic acidosis, expected urine pH is less than 5.3 in adults and 5.6 in children.
2. Efficacy of treatment in metabolic alkalosis.

Protein. The normal daily urinary protein excretion is 150 to 300 mg. This is constituted mainly by the Tamm-Horsfall mucoprotein secreted by the renal tubules, immuno-globulin and β_2-microglobulin. Proteinuria may also occur due to increased protein filtration or in the erect position. A proper evaluation for proteinuria includes 24-hour urinary protein estimation and determination of the type of protein, namely high molecular weight or low molecular weight. Detection of significant proteinuria helps to suspect renal disease, assess its severity, predict the prognosis, monitor the response to therapy or diagnose other systemic disorders with renal involvement.

Examination of the urine for protein can be done by qualitative methods, semiqualitative methods and quantitative methods.

Heat coagulation acetic acid test. This is qualitative test. About 10 ml of the supernatant or centrifuged urine is taken in a test tube up to its two-thirds length. Holding the bottom of the tube, the upper portion of the sample is heated at an angle over the flame with the mouth of the tube facing away from the observer. If cloudiness appears in the heated portion, it indicates the presence of proteins, phosphates or carbonates. 3–5 drops of 5% acetic acid is added and the sample boiled again. If the precipitate disappears, it indicates carbonates or phosphates. If cloudiness persists, it indicates protein. The severity of proteinuria can be roughly graded as 1+ to 4+ as follows:

1+ = Distinct cloudiness, but not granular

2+ = Granular cloudiness, not opaque

3+ = Heavy cloudiness with clumping

4+ = Dense cloud of flocculating curdy precipitates.

Massive doses of penicillin, tolbutamide and radiographic contrast media may result in false positive test. This test does not detect myoglobin and hemoglobin. Small quantities of protein in highly alkaline urine are also missed by the test.

Reagent test strips. This is a semiquantitative method. This dipstick contains tetrabromo-phenol blue in citric acid. When the dipstick with the chemical impregnated in filter paper comes into contact with the urine, the protein binds to the dye and changes the color from yellow to blue. This test is not sensitive if the urine is highly alkaline. It can detect proteins of more than 10 mg/dl but does not detect light chains of immunoglobulin. It is quick, easy and can be used as a screening test for albumin.

Turbidometric test. Substances like sulfo-salicylic acid, trichloroacetic acid and nitric acid cause precipitation of proteins. The extent of turbidity of the sample indicates the severity of proteinuria. These quantitative estimations can also be done by colorimetric. Electrophoresis and immunoelectrophoresis of the urinary protein are the other useful tests.

The 24-hour urine collection may be difficult or inaccurate. Hence, the comparison of the protein–creatinine ratio in a random sample of urine is used to asses the degree of proteinuria. Protein creatinine ratio of 3.5:1 roughly corresponds to 24-hour urine protein excretion of 3.5 g.

Selectivity. Selectivity of proteinuria is the ratio between the excretions of high to low molecular weight protein in urine. Albumin (mol wt 69,000 daltons) or transferrin and IgG (mol wt, 160,000 daltons) are used. An IgG to transferrin ratio of 0.1 or less suggests selective proteinuria which indicates lesser quantity of high molecular weight proteins. This suggests that the glomerular damage is not severe compared to non-selective proteinuria, where the selectivity ratio is more than 0.1.

Bence-Jones protein. Detection of Bence Jones protein in urine helps in the diagnosis of multiple myeloma or paraproteinemias characterized by excretion of light chains of immunoglobulin of urine. When the heat coagulation test is done, the Bence-Jones protein is precipitated with the temperature is >60°C and it redissolves when urine is boiled. As the sample is cooled, precipitation occurs again between 60°C and 40°C and the precipitate redissolves when the urine is cooled to room temperature. This can be tested using a water bath set at different temperatures. Bence Jones protein in urine is suspected if the urine protein is negative by dipstick method and positive by sulfosalicylic acid method. Electrophoresis or immunoelectrophoresis of the urinary protein is perhaps the best method to confirm the presence of Bence-Jones protein. In 1845, McBean the first patient known to have multiple myeloma was referred to Dr Henrey Bence Jones for the opinion of patient's urine and hence the name of Bence Jones protein came to the clinical side. Orthostatic proteinuria is coined when proteinuria in supine posture is less than 50 mg in 8 hours and increased proteinuria in upright position usually less than 1 gm.

Microalbuminuria is defined as daily albumin excretion is in the range of 30 to 300 mg. More than 300 mg albumin is detected by the dipstick method .Microalbuminuria can be tested by 24-hour urine collection or timed collection or random collection. Fever, exercise, heart failure and hyperglycemia may transiently produce microalbuminuria. When urinary albumin creatinine ratio is 0.03 mg/mg, it means that urinary albumin is above 30 mg/day.

Sugar. Urine is tested for reducing substances like glucose. Benedict's test is semiquantitative, where 8 drops of urine are added to 5 ml of the reagent, boiled and cooled. The change in color of the reagent gives an idea about the presence of reducing substances which convert the cuprous oxide to cupric oxide. The reagent changes from its normal blue color to, green, yellow, orange or red depending on the amount of glucose present. Other sugars like galactose, lactose, fructose, mannose, pentose, other reducing substances like dextrans, homogentisic acid, glucuronic acid, and some drugs like aspirin and streptomycin may give positive test for reducing substance. Glucose-oxidase test and clinistix are specific for glucose. Glucose appears in urine when blood level is high or when the tubular reabsorption capacity is limited.

Ketone bodies. Acetoacetic acid, β-hydroxy-butyric acid and acetone are the ketone bodies which may be present in urine in diabetic ketoacidosis or in starvation. They can be detected by Rothera's nitroprusside test, Gerhardt's ferric chloride test or by using reagent test strips.

Bile salts. The presence of bile salts in urine can be tested by Hay's method, where sulphur powder is added to urine. If the sample contains excessive bile salts, the sulphur powder sinks whereas; it remains floating if the urine does not contain bile salts.

Bile pigments. Barium chloride test helps to detect bile pigments. To 10 ml of acidified urine, 5 ml of 10% barium chloride is added and a white precipitate is formed. The sample is filtered and the precipitate dried. To the precipitate, Fouchet's reagent (trichloroacetic acid and ferric chloride) is added. Blue or green color indicates the presence of bile pigments. This test can also be performed by the dipstick method using reagent test strips.

Urobilinogen. To 10 ml of freshly voided urine taken in a test tube, 1 ml of Ehrlich's reagent (containing paradimethylaminobenzaldehyde in concentrated hydrochloric acid) is added. If normal amounts of urobilinogen are present, the solution changes into a pink color which can be observed by looking down through mouth of the tube against a white background. This test can be used as semiquantitative test by diluting the urine to 1:10, 1:20, 1:30 and 1:40. If the pink-colored persists in 1:20 and above, excess urobilinogen is present. If pink color does not appear in spite of warming, it suggests absence of urobilinogen. Porphobilinogen can also be detected in the same test by adding sodium acetate or chloroform. Addition of sodium acetate intensifies the color due to urobilinogen but not porphobilinogen. The addition of chloroform extracts the color of urobilinogen but not of porphobilinogen. Drugs like phenazopyridine and para-aminosalicylic acid may yield a pink color which is indistinguishable from that produced by urobilinogen. Urobilinogen can also be detected by specific reagent test strips.

Hemoglobinuria and myoglobinuria. Hemoglobin and myoglobin in urine can be detected with an orthotoluidine reagent which is oxidized by both the proteins resulting in a blue color. The appearance of a blue color in 30 seconds indicates the presence of hemoglobin or myoglobin. The two can be differentiated by addition of ammonium sulphate which extracts the color due to hemoglobin but not due to myoglobin. Although hematuria also gives a positive test, it can be differentiated easily be demonstrating RBCs under the microscope. Hemoglobin and myoglobin can

also be differentiated by noting color of serum in patients having positive orthotoluidine test. Presence of free hemoglobin in serum gives a pinkish discoloration, whereas the serum will be clear in myoglobinuria. This test can detect a minimum of 15 micrograms/100 ml of hemoglobin.

Test for bacteriuria. The nitrite test is a rapid indirect method for early detection of significant and asymptomatic bacteriuria. The first morning sample urine is tested soon after voiding. If significant bacteriuria is present, the nitrate in the urine is converted into nitrite which can be detected by chemical test.

MICROSCOPIC EXAMINATION OF URINE

Microscopic examination of the centrifuged deposits of a fresh morning specimen of urine is a valuable diagnostic tool. It helps in the detection of cellular elements, casts, bacteria and crystals. About 10 ml of urine is centrifuged in a cleaned tube at 2000–2500 rpm for 5 to 10 minutes. Supernatant 9 ml urine is discarded and the sediment resuspended in the remaining urine. A drop of this is placed on a clean side under a cover slip. The specimen is examined at first with reduced illumination under low power magnification and then switched over to higher magnification. For routine purpose, unstained urinary sediments are viewed under the ordinary light microscope. In some special situations sediments are stained with Wright's, Hansel's Papanicolaou's or Strenheim-Malbin's stain or examined under phase and interference contrast microscope.

Cells which may be present in the urine include erythrocytes, leukocytes and epithelial cells. Erythrocytes or red blood cells (RBCs) are recognized as round, refractile, non-nucleated disc-like structures. Yeast cells are ovoid, frequently contain buds, and do not dissolve in 2% acetic acid. In normal urine, red cells are not detected by microscopy under high power. The presence of more than 2 red cells in a high power field is significant.

Phase contrast microscopy helps to identify dysmorphic RBCs and automated blood cell volume analyzers are useful in differentiating glomerular from nonglomerular hematuria. In patients with glomerular diseases, the RBCs in urine are crenated, irregular or fragmented (dysmorphic) when examined under the phase contrast microscope. Acanthocytes in urine also indicate glomerular origin. In conditions like bleeding into the urinary tract, the RBC morphology is normal (isomorphic). Leukocytes or white cells (WBCs) are larger than red cells, usually rounded and distinguished by the presence of lobed nuclei and Brownian movement of the granules. Addition of 2% acetic acid accentuates the nuclei of the leukocytes. Presence of more than 5 leukocytes in male and 10 in females under a high power field is significant. Usually, urinary leukocytes are neutrophils but eosinophils and lymphocytes may also be seen in certain conditions. Wright's stain and Hansel's stain are useful in identifying eosinophils which are characteristic of allergic interstitial nephritis. Epithelial cells are 2–4 times larger than the red cells and are nucleated. They may be tubular, transitional or squamous epithelial cells. The epithelial cells present in urinary sediment may have originated from renal tubule, pelvis, ureter, bladder or urethra. They look alike in wet preparation under light microscopy (LM). Transmission electron microscopy (TEM) distinguishes renal tubular epithelial cells from transitional and squamous epithelial cells. Presence of squamous epithelial cells is not pathological. Malignant cells are less cohesive are shed in the urine easily. The urine sample for malignant cells is fixed with equal parts of urine and 50% ethanol or a fixative composed of alcohol and formalin. After collection and proper fixation, the sample is centrifuged and the sediment is stained with either 1% toluidine blue or triple strength methylene blue.

Casts. Casts are cylindrical elements formed in the distal and collecting tubules as a result of precipitation of Tamm-Horsfall protein which is the matrix for all types of casts. Presence of numerous casts in the urine indicates renal damage. Casts are recognized easily towards the edge of the coverslip. They are classified on the basis of their appearance and the cellular components in them as hyaline, red cell, white cell, epithelial cell, granular, waxy, fatty, broad or pigmented casts. Hyaline casts are colorless, homogenous, transparent and have rounded ends. A few hyaline casts may be found in normal urine. Red cell casts may be colourless or brown and signify glomerular disease. White cell casts contain white blood cells impregnated in the matrix (Fig. 5.1). The common types of WBCs which appear in casts are usually neutrophils. The cast may contain a few cells or have many cells tightly packed together with their distinct nuclei.

Granular casts indicate renal disease and are often the result of degeneration of cellular casts. It may also occur due to the aggregation of serum proteins into the matrix of Tamm-Horsfall protein. Epithelial cell casts contain epithelial cells. If the epithelial cells are arranged in parallel rows, the cells are from the same segment of the tubule, whereas haphazard arrangement of the cells indicates that they are from different portions of the tubule. Waxy cats are yellow, grey or colorless and have a smooth homogenous appearance with serrated edges. They may be formed by the degeneration of granular casts. Fatty casts are formed by the incorporation of free fat droplets or oval fat bodies and these are also seen in fatty degeneration of the tubular epithelium. Broad casts are two to six times broader than ordinary casts and are formed in pathologically dilated or atrophic tubules and signify chronic renal failure. Bilirubin casts are seen in conditions with hyperbilirubinemia. Hemoglobin casts are derived from degeneration of red cell casts or occur in hemolytic states. Telescoped urine sediment denotes cellular elements derived from glomerular and tubulointerstitial cells.

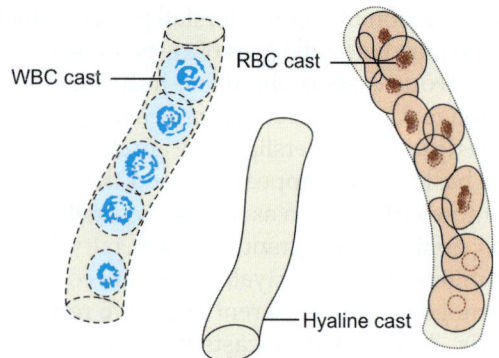

Fig. 5.1: Commonly urinary casts

Bacteria are usually not present in freshly passed urine. However, contamination may occur from the urethra, vagina and other external sources. Presence of bacteria and polymorphonuclear leukocytes denotes urinary tract infection. In suspected bacterial infection, a fresh clean voided midstream specimen of urine is required for culture and sensitivity test. For the detection of tubercle bacilli, the entire urine passed in the early morning is sent to the laboratory. Other non-bacterial organisms like *Trichomonas vaginalis, Enterobius vermicularis* and fungi may also be seen in the urine.

Crystals. Crystals may be visible on microscopic examination and should be interpreted together with pH of urine. Presence of crystals of cystine, leucine, tyrosine and cholesterol are pathological. Presence of crystals may or may not be significant. Calcium oxalate crystals are colorless and appear envelope-shaped oval or as biconcave discs. Uric acid crystals are yellow or red brown with an appearance of rhombic prism, diamond or rosette. Amorphous urates have a yellow red-granular appearance. Triple phosphate crystals are colorless prisms with 3 to 6 sides and oblique ends (coffin lid appearance). Calcium phosphate crystals are long, thin colorless prisms with one pointed end arranged as rosettes or stars or appearing as needles. Cystine crystals are colorless, refractile hexagonal plates with equal or unequal sides and appear singly or in clusters and have layered or laminated appearance. Cholesterol crystals are large, flat transparent plates with notched corners. Figure 5.2 shows the common crystals in urine.

Calcium phosphate is seen I renal tubular acidosis and triple phosphate is seen in infected states.

HEMATOLOGIC TESTS

Hemoglobin, hematocrit and a peripheral smear examination are the usual hematological tests done in renal disease. Normocytic normochromic anemia may be present in many cases of chronic renal failure due to deficiency of erythropoietin and other factors. Microangiopathic hemolytic anemia (MAHA) with thrombocytopenia is typically seen in hemolytic uremic syndrome. Anemia, leukopenia and thrombocytopenia may indicate lupus and thrombocytosis may indicate vasculitis. Serological tests in renal diseases are:

a. Antibodies to exogenous antigens are antibodies to streptococcal exoenzymes, anti-streptolysin O, anti-DNAse, anti-hyaluronidase), hepatitis B/C, HIV virus, anti-CMV, and anti-EBV.

b. Antibodies to endogenous antigens are anti-glomerular basement antibody, antinuclear antibody, anti-neutrophil cytoplasmic antibodies (cANCA, pANCA). Anti-C1q, anti-C3Bb, and anti-phospholipid antibodies.

c. Complement assays

d. Circulating immune complexes

e. Platelet dysfunction may also be demonstrated by appropriate test.

f. A high sedimentation rate may help to suspect collagen disorders or myeloma.

RENAL FUNCTION TESTS

A series of tests are done to assess the various aspect of renal function since no single test gives accurate information about the number of functioning nephrons. The overall renal function can be assessed by combining the

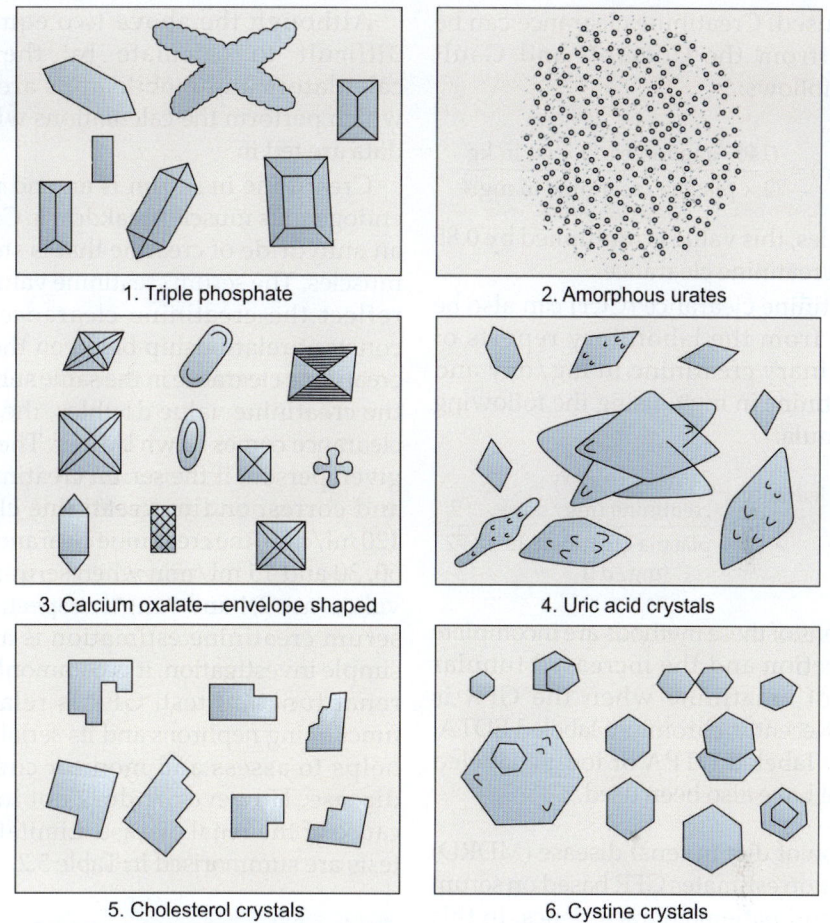

1. Triple phosphate

2. Amorphous urates

3. Calcium oxalate—envelope shaped

4. Uric acid crystals

5. Cholesterol crystals

6. Cystine crystals

Fig. 5.2: Commonly crystals occurring in urine

results obtained by tests of glomerular function, tubular function and maximal capacity of tubules.

Glomerular Function

Since the main function of the glomerulus is the filtration, measurement of glomerular filtration rate (GFR) is the most important test. It can be assessed either by measuring the clearance of or by measuring the blood levels of substances which are excreted by glomerular filtration. Approximately 120 ml of glomerular filtrate is formed every minute and nearly 99% of the filtrate including the substances required by the blood are reabsorbed. For experimental purposes, clearance of inulin, a substance filtered completely by the glomerulus and not reabsorbed or secreted in the tubules is taken as the glomerular filtration rate. Clearance of a substance is the amount of blood which is completely cleared of the substance in unit time and is calculated by the formula, $C \times P = UV$. Hence, $C = UV/P$, where C = clearance in ml/min, U = concentration of the substance in urine in mg/ml, V = urine flow rate in ml/min, and P = concentration of the substance in plasma in mg/ml. For clinical purpose, creatinine, which is completely filtered by the glomerulus and not significantly reabsorbed or secreted into the tubules, is used. Creatinine clearance can be calculated from the Cockroft and Gault formula as follows:

$$\text{Cr Cl (in ml/min)} = \frac{(140 - \text{age in years}) \times \text{wt in kg}}{72 \times \text{plasma creatinine in mg\%}}$$

For females, this value is multiplied by 0.85 to give the creatinine clearance.

The creatinine clearance (CCr) can also be calculated from the laboratory reports of 24-hour urinary creatinine in mg/day and serum creatinine in mg% using the following simple formula:

$$\text{Creatinine clearance (ml/min)} = \frac{\text{24-hour urinary creatinine (mg/day)}}{\text{plasma creatinine in (mg/dl)}} \times \frac{5}{72}$$

Limitations of these methods are incomplete urine collection and the increased tubular secretion of creatinine when the GFR is decreased. Recently, chromium labeled EDTA, technetium labeled DTPA or iodine labeled iothalamate have also been used.

Modification of diet in renal disease (MDRD) study equation estimates GFR based on serum creatinine and patient characteristics. In this equation:

$$\text{GFR (ml/min/1.73 m}^2) = 175 \times (S_{cr})^{-1.154} \times (\text{age})^{-0.203} \times (0.742 \text{ if female}) \times (1.212 \text{ if African American}) \text{ (conventional units)}$$

In adults, chronic kidney disease epidemiology collaboration (CKD-EPI) equation is the most widely used equations for estimating glomerular filtration rate (GFR).

$$\text{GFR} = 141 \times \min (S_{cr}/\kappa, 1)^{\alpha} \times \max (S_{cr}/\kappa, 1)^{-1.209} \times 0.993^{\text{age}} \times 1.018 \text{ [if female]} \times 1.159 \text{ [if black]},$$

where S_{cr} is serum creatinine in mg/dl,

κ is 0.7 for females and 0.9 for males,

α is -0.329 for females and -0.411 for males,

min indicates the minimum of S_{cr}/κ or 1, and max indicates the maximum of S_{cr}/κ or 1.

Although the above two equations are difficult to calculate by the bedside, calculators and mobile apps are available which perform the calculations when simple data are fed in.

Creatinine in serum is an end product of endogenous muscle breakdown. Creatinine is an anhydride of creatine that is stored in the muscles. The serum creatinine values roughly reflect the creatinine clearance. There is constant relationship between the GFR and creatinine clearance in the same subject. When the creatinine value doubles, the creatinine clearance comes down by half. Therefore, in a given person, if the serum creatinine is 1 mg and corresponding creatinine clearance is 120 ml/min, the creatinine clearance would be 60, 30 and 15 ml/min when serum creatinine values are 2,4 and 8 mg% respectively. Since serum creatinine estimation is a relatively simple investigation, it is commonly used as a renal function test. GFR is related to the functioning nephrons and its serial estimation helps to assess and monitor course of the disease. However, it does not indicate the cause of the renal disease. Limitations of the tests are summarised in Table 5.2.

Table 5.2: Limitations of creatinine and creatinine clearance

a. Initial decline in GFR causes only mild elevation of creatinine

b. Progressive glomerular injury may not decrease GFR due to adaptation

c. Tubular secretion may vary with time

d. Rhabdomyolysis increases creatinine disproportionately

e. Trimethoprim, cimetidine, sulphamethoxazole may decrease tubular secretion

f. Acetoacetate, cefoxitin, flucytosine may increase creatinine

g. Extrarenal clearance of creatinine is increased in advanced renal failure

Urea is an end product of protein metabolism. The blood urea also gives a rough idea about the GFR. However, it is not as reliable as creatinine because urea is filtered by the glomerulus and is reabsorbed into some extent in the tubules depending upon the state of hydration and urine flow rate. The rate of production is not constant and high protein intake, gastrointestinal bleeding, increased tissue break down and tetracycline increase the blood urea level. However, blood urea is performed because the uremic symptoms correlate better with the urea than with the creatinine level. When testing for Blood urea nitrogen (BUN). only the nitrogen in the urea molecule is measured. When the blood urea is 60 mg%, the corresponding BUN will be 28 mg or approximately 50% of blood urea. It is not necessary to perform blood urea and BUN test in the same patient since one can be calculated accurately from the other. The urea to creatinine ratio in blood varies from 20–40:1 and BUN/creatinine ratio from 10–20:1.

Uric acid is an end product of purine metabolism and it is excreted by the kidney. The level of uric acid increases as the GFR falls.

Cystatin C is present in all nucleated cells and is produced constantly. It is a cysteine protease inhibitor and having low molecular weight and accumulates in renal failure. Cystatin C (molecular weiht = 13000 daltons) is a protein and has been used as a marker of GFR. The rate of production by nucleated cells is constant. Cystatin C may be a reliable indicator of GFR, it will be clinically useful only after proper standardization, availability and cost reduction.

Renal plasma flow (RPF) can be measured by para-aminohippurate (PAH) clearance. It is however not employed for routine clinical purposes. Radionuclide studies are used to assess the renal perfusion. Radionuclide I-125 iodohippurate and I-131 hippurate may be used for measurement of renal blood flow (RBF), which can be calculated from RPF, by the formula:

$$RBF = \frac{100 \times RPF}{(100 - \text{hematocrit})}$$

Tubular Functions

The functions of the tubules are to reabsorb 100% of the bicarbonate, glucose, amino acids, nearly 99% of water and sodium and prevent the reabsorption and/or secretion of waste products like urea, creatinine and uric acid. The tubules also regulate the reabsorption of calcium, phosphorus, magnesium and potassium. The proximal tubules perform the function of glucose and bicarbonate reabsorption together with reabsorption of nearly 80% of water and sodium. The loop of Henle is concerned with maintaining the hypertonicity of medullary interstitium. The thick ascending limb of loop of Henle called the diluting segment, actively reabsorbs chloride. Since sodium also moves with the chloride, the glomerular filtrate leaving the thick ascending limb of loop of Henle is always hypo-osmotic. In the distal tubule, secretion of hydrogen, ions, reabsorption of sodium in exchange for potassium and variable reabsorption of water depending upon the level of antidiuretic hormone. The adjustments of the pH, osmolality and electrolyte content of urine are completed in the connecting tubules.

Proximal Tubular Function Tests

The amino acids are freely filtered by the glomerulus and 99% of the filtered amino acids are reabsorbed by the proximal tubule. If abnormal function of the proximal tubule is present, generalized aminoaciduria occurs in which all the aminoacids filtered by the glomeruli are present in the urine. Sometimes, the transport mechanisms for some specific amino acids may be defective and may lead to urinary loss of the specific amino acid.

The filtered glucose is completely reabsorbed under normal circumstances. When the blood sugar is very high, the filtered load is also high and its leads to glycosuria because the filtered load has exceeded the maximal reabsorbing capacity for glucose. When there is an abnormal function of the proximal tubule, the capacity of the tubule to maximally reabsorb glucose is diminished and the patient may have glycosuria even though blood sugar is normal.

Since the normal function of the proximal tubules is to reabsorb phosphate, hypophosphatemia and phosphaturia may occur when there is an abnormality in the proximal tubular function. The tests used for determining of the maximum capacity of tubules include estimation T_m PAH, T_m phosphates and T_m bicarbonate (T_m = tubular maximum.).

Distal Tubular Function Tests

Test for the tubule's ability to concentrate the urine is the 'water deprivation test'. When a normal person is deprived of fluids, ADH secretion occurs. In the presence of ADH (antidiuretic hormone), the distal tubules and collecting ducts become freely permeable to water. Since the collecting duct has to pass through the hypertonic renal medulla before opening into the calyces, water reabsorption occurs resulting in production of concentrated urine. If a random sample of urine shows a specific gravity of 1023 or more or an osmolality of more than 900 mOsm/kg H_2O, it signifies normal concentrating ability. If an early morning urine sample after a 'dry' supper on the previous evening show the same values, the concentrating ability can be considered as normal. In other cases the water deprivation test is helpful.

Water deprivation test leads to dehydration, unpleasantness, hypotension and even circulatory collapse in patients with diabetes insipidus (DI). So, it is performed very carefully and helps to confirm and identify the type of DI. The patient is deprived of fluid and weighed hourly. The specific gravity of each urine specimen passed is recorded. The water deprivation under careful monitoring of vital functions is continued for up to 24 hours or until 3–5% of the body weight has been lost or the urine specific gravity rises over 1020 whichever is sooner. In central DI, further improvement of specific gravity occurs after administration of vasopressin.

Ability to dilute the urine is tested in the fasting state if the patient has no cardiac illness or fluid overload. He is made to drink 20 ml/kg body weight water in the course of 10–20 minutes. Urine is collected every hour and the volume is recorded. Specific gravity or osmolality is tested for 4 hours. Normally more than 75% of water excretion takes place in 4 hours and at least one of the samples or urine has a specific gravity of less than 1003 or osmolality <80 mOsm/kg. Smoking, emotional upsets and use of ADH may lead to in accurate results.

The kidneys excrete hydrogen ions as titratable acid or ammonium. By excreting one H^+, the kidney is able to replace one molecule of HCO_3^- to the body. The pH of urine is used to assess the hydrogen ion excretion. In some cases, bicarbonaturia may occur due to renal tubular dysfunction. If the urine pH is less than 5.3 in an early morning or random sample of urine, the acidifying capacity of the kidney may be considered normal. The test for urine pH should be done shortly after collection. If the urine pH is more than 5.5 in the presence of low level of serum bicarbonate, a renal tubular dysfunction is likely.

Ammonium chloride loading test is done to test the ability of the kidneys to maximally acidify urine. Since ammonium chloride is nauseating it is usually given in doses of 0.1 g/kg orally in gelatin capsules with food. The urine is collected at 2, 4 and 6 hours and blood sample is collected for plasma HCO_3^- at 4 hours. If the urine pH is 5.3 or less, it signifies the normal ability of the kidney to acidify urine. If the pH has not come to <5.3 in spite of the plasma HCO_3^- of <18 mmol/L, the test has to be repeated. Measurement of titratable acidity and HCO_3^- in urine may also be used for assessing the ability of the tubules to excrete H^+.

Ability to control sodium excretion can be tested in two ways. The first test, the patient is allowed to have a normal diet containing about 100 mmol of sodium per day for a few days. During the period, the urinary sodium is also measured. This is usually about 15 mmol less than the intake. The dietary intake of sodium is then reduced to about 15 mmol/day and simultaneously the urinary sodium is measured. Within 7 to 10 days, urinary sodium drops down to 10 mmol/day if the tubules are normal. The second test involves 2 mg of 9α-fluorohydrocortisone twice a day for three days when the patient is on normal diet. If the tubules are functioning normally, sodium excretion comes down to <10 mmol/day.

Because of the chances of fatal hyper-kalemia, potassium loading tests are not done. The ability of the tubules to conserve potassium in conditions of potassium depletion can be tested. On a normal diet of 80–100 mmol of potassium per day, the urinary excretion is around 70–90 mmol per day. If the potassium intake is reduced to 20–30 mmol/24 hours, the urinary excretion of potassium also comes down to 20–30 mmol/24 hours, if the tubules are functioning normally. If urinary excretion of potassium is more than 20 mEq/24 hours when serum potassium is less than 3 mEq/L, potassium leak is present.

The calcium content of urine depends on the function of the collecting duct. The daily excretion of calcium on a normal diet is less than three hundred mg in males, 250 mg in females and 4 mg/kg in children. Hyper-calciuria is present when 24 hours urine contains more than 400 mg or in children more than 7 mg/kg/24 hours. Presence of hyper-calciuria is tested by putting the patient on a rice diet (containing 90–130 mg of calcium per day) cooked in distilled water. The 24-hour urine calcium is estimated on the fourth day when it should be less than 200 mg. Normal handling of magnesium by the kidneys parallels that of calcium. Normally, renal conservation of magnesium is extremely efficient. If the serum magnesium is low and the urine contains more than 1–2 mmol per liter of magnesium, urinary magnesium leak is present. The patient with renal failure may be unable to excrete magnesium. Hyperurico-suria is excretion more than 600 mg/day of uric acid. When a person is on purine-free diet and the 24-hour urine excretion is more than 600 mg, it indicates increased endogenous production.

Imaging of Urinary Tract

• J Balasubramaniam

Imaging studies are important tools to evaluate patients with suspected renal or urinary tract disease. These tests are performed in combination to gather anatomical and functional details which help to diagnose and follow-up patients with renal diseases. They help to diagnose renal diseases like urinary tract obstruction, stones, renal cyst/mass, renovascular diseases, vesicoureteral reflux (VUR), abnormalities in size position and echotexture. Imaging studies include:

- Plain X-ray films of the abdomen
- Renal ultrasonography (USG)
- Renal Doppler
- Intravenous urography (IVU) or intravenous pyelography (IVP)
- Voiding cystourethrogram and ascending urethrogram
- Computed tomography (CT)
- Magnetic resonance imaging (MRI)
- Radionuclide scanning
- Renal angiography
- Renal elastography and contrast enhanced sonography (CES)

Common uses and limitations of each of these imaging modalities with particular reference to urinary tract are discussed below.

PLAIN X-RAY

Despite availability of many newer imaging modalities, plain film of the abdomen is still a simple and useful tool used as the basic study in many situations. It assesses the adequacy of bowel preparation and gas distribution pattern before other radiologic/contrast studies are undertaken. Among patients presenting with symptoms suggestive of nephrolithiasis, a plain film of the abdomen can identify calcium-containing, struvite, and cystine stones, but will miss radiolucent uric acid stones, small radiopaque stones and stones overlying bony structures. Phleboliths and fecoliths can be mistaken for renal stones in plain radiography. Hence, reliability of plain abdominal films in detecting a stone in patients with renal colic is limited. The diagnostic tests of choice when stone disease is suspected is an USG and non-contrast CT scan. Nevertheless, X-ray can identify radio-opaque stones anywhere in the urinary tract. Extensive renal parenchymal calcification (Fig. 6.1), stones in the ureter, bladder (Fig. 6.2), prostatic urethra or penile urethra can be identified by Xray. Stones in mid-ureter, bladder neck or urethra may not be easily identified by USG. Plain films not be able to identify soft tissue shadows or tumors of the urinary tract. Yet for a trained eye, this

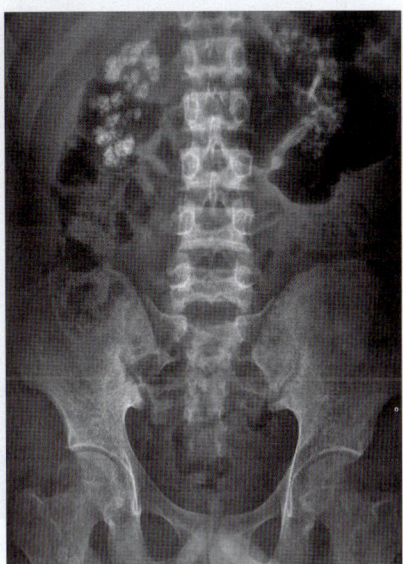

Fig. 6.1: Bilateral nephrocalcinosis. Plain X-ray shows numerous radiopaque shadows in both renal areas suggesting extensive calcification of both kidneys

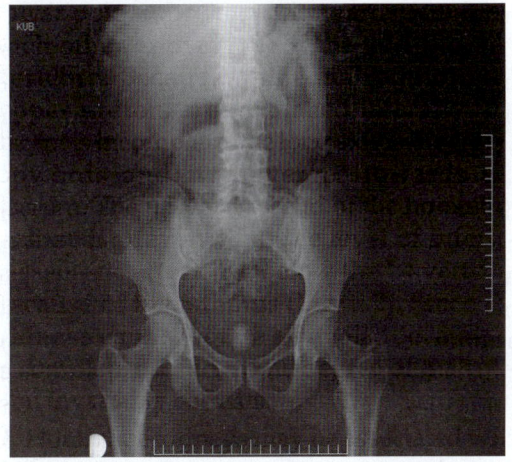

Fig. 6.2: Bladder stone. Plain X-ray KUB showing rounded radiopaque shadow in bladder area—vesical stone

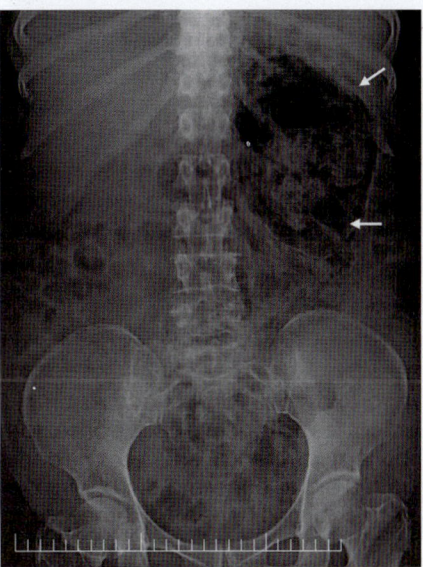

Fig. 6.3: Emphysematous pyelonephritis. Plain X-ray showing gas shadow in and around left kidney (arrows)

imaging technique does provide information regarding kidney size and shape and presence of gas as in emphysematous pyelonephritis (Fig. 6.3) and cystitis.

Chest film can show air under diaphragm, evidence of uremic lung in a case of renal failure presenting with breathlessness or pulmonary edema in a patient with fluid overload. X-ray bones can show features of renal osteodystrophy, secondary hyperparathyroidism, punched out lesions of multiple myeloma.

Limitation: Exposure to radiation precludes use in pregnant women.

RENAL ULTRASONOGRAPHY

Renal ultrasonography has become an invaluable screening test for renal diseases. Variations in renal size, cortical echogenicity and corticomedullary differentiation indicate renal diseases. Cortical echo is compared with that of adjacent liver or spleen and graded. Renal size can be measured and should be corrected for age and body size. It gives information contracted kidney in chronic diseases or enlargement. Cortical thickness can also be measured. Normal adult kidneys (Fig. 6.4) have >1 cm cortical thickness. If the cortex is more echogenic and the corticomedullary distinction is lost, it suggests

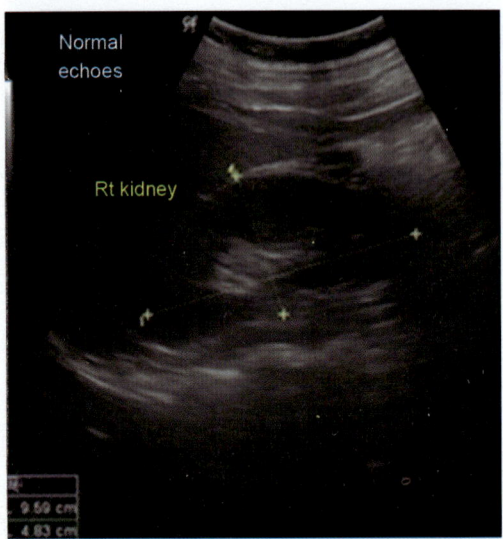

Fig. 6.4: Renal ultrasonography (normal). Renal ultrasonography showing normal cortical echoes and corticomedullary differentiation

significant parenchymal damage (Fig. 6.5). If the size of the kidney is <9 cm in an average built adult, with small kidney, it indicates chronic kidney disease (CKD) (Fig. 6.6). Enlarged kidneys, with normal collecting

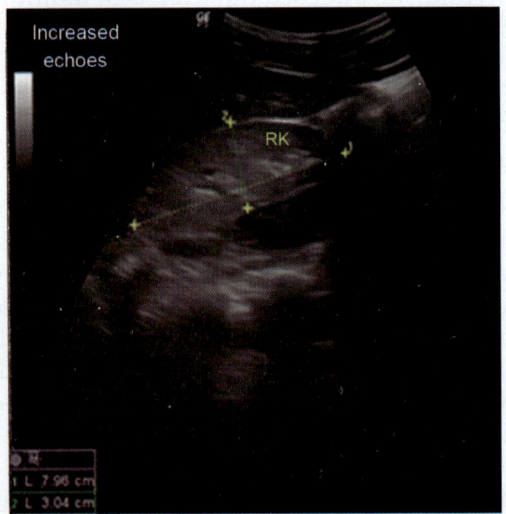

Fig. 6.5: Renal ultrasonography showing increased cortical echoes and loss of corticomedullary differentiation suggesting chronic parenchymal disease

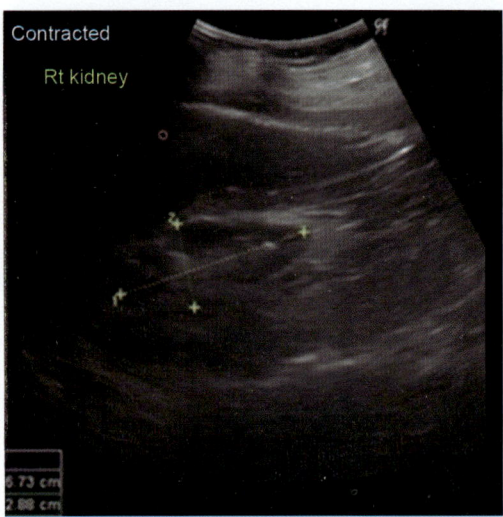

Fig. 6.6: Renal ultrasonography showing contracted kidney (<9 cm)

system, are seen in diabetic kidney disease, infiltrative diseases like malignancy, multiple myeloma and rapidly progressive glomerulo-nephritis.

Urinary tract dilatation is the hallmark of urinary tract obstruction. Dilatation could involve calyces (calyectasis), pelvicalyceal system (hydronephrosis), ureters (hydroure-terosis), or all the three (hydroureteronephrosis) depending on the level of obstruction. Dilatation could be unilateral or bilateral depending upon the site of obstruction. However, one may find dilated collecting system in polyuria and normal pregnancy (gravid uterus can cause partial urinary tract obstruction). Parapelvic cysts may be mistaken for pelvi-caliectasis. Occasionally, no evidence of dilated system may be present in patients with anuria due to acute obstruction.

Renal ultrasonography is the primary investigation to identify kidney stones. Shadowing produced by the stone confirms the presence of stone. USG reliably helps in measuring the size and location of the stone in addition to identifying associated caliectasis/ hydronephrosis. Lately non-contrast computed tomography (CT) is being preferred over USG in the diagnosis of nephrolithiasis because renal stones in certain locations like the mid-ureter and very small stones cannot be identified by USG. Upper UTI/pyelonephritis are diagnosed more easily by noting perinephric inflammatory stranding in USG. Air in the renal tissue/collecting system as shown by bright specks of echoes is diagnostic of emphysematous pyelonephritis and early diagnosis of the serious infection is now possible by USG. This is also the procedure of choice for identifying acquired or hereditary polycystic kidney disease and mass lesions.

Indications

i. Evaluation of renal calculus disease, cystic kidney disease, renal masses

ii. Diagnosis of hydronephrosis

iii. Measurement of kidney size and echogenicity as part of an evaluation of CKD

iv. Detection of renal artery occlusive disease by Doppler study.

v. Evaluation of pregnant women by avoiding exposure to radiation or contrast.

Limitations

i. Interpretation is operator-dependent

ii. Very obese patients with deep seated organs

iii. Restless, breathless patients

COLOR DOPPLER ULTRASONOGRAPHY

Ultrasonography by using color Doppler is used to measure flow or velocity of blood in the main renal artery and its branches (Fig. 6.7). Even if main renal artery is not well imaged, Doppler flow pattern in segmental and interlobar arteries showing parvus tardus pattern indicates renal artery stenosis. Doppler ultrasonography is also used to obtain the renal resistive index.

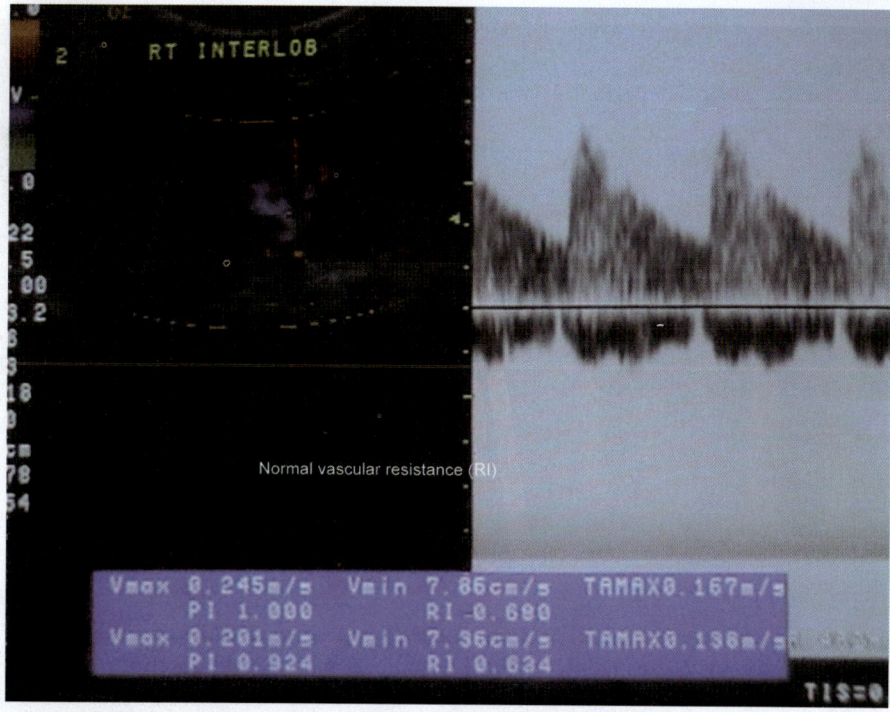

Fig. 6.7: Doppler ultrasonography of segmental renal artery showing normal resisting index (RI) and pulsatile index (PI). Note: (V_{max} or PSV = 24.5) and (V_{min} or EDV = 7.86) see formula below

Formula for calculating RI

$$RI = \frac{[\text{Peak systolic velocity (PSV)} - \text{End diastolic velocity (EDV)}]}{\text{Peak systolic velocity}}$$

Example: Refer to Fig. 6.7

PSV = 24.5, EDV = 7.86.

$$RI = \frac{24.5 - 7.86}{24.5} = 0.68$$

The normal renal resistive index is <0.7. A high renal resistive index is dependent primarily on extrarenal hemodynamics and the resistance caused by the renal edema and fibrosis. As a result, the renal resistive index is less affected in glomerular diseases compared to tubulointerstitial diseases. Resistive index is also commonly measured in transplanted kidneys but is again an insensitive and nonspecific indicator of rejection but is useful as prognostic value. Figure 6.8 shows normal, high resistive index respectively. Combination of prolonged time to peak (>100 ms) and reduced acceleration time (<100 cm/s²) in the Doppler recording of intrarenal artery constitute the 'parvus tardus' pattern which is very typical of renal artery stenosis (Fig. 6.9). Color ultrasonography and Doppler are now used for better identification and assessment of blood vessels for dialysis access creation and periodically assess the functionality of dialysis accesses like AV fistulas and grafts.

INTRAVENOUS UROGRAPHY/PYELOGRAPHY (IVU/IVP)

In the past, IVU was the principal radiologic technique used for evaluation of urinary tract. It provides detailed information concerning calyceal anatomy, the size and shape of the kidney, functional status of the kidney and locate renal stones.

However now, IVP is used less since:
- It requires the administration of contrast, limiting its use in patients with renal failure and persons with iodine sensitivity.

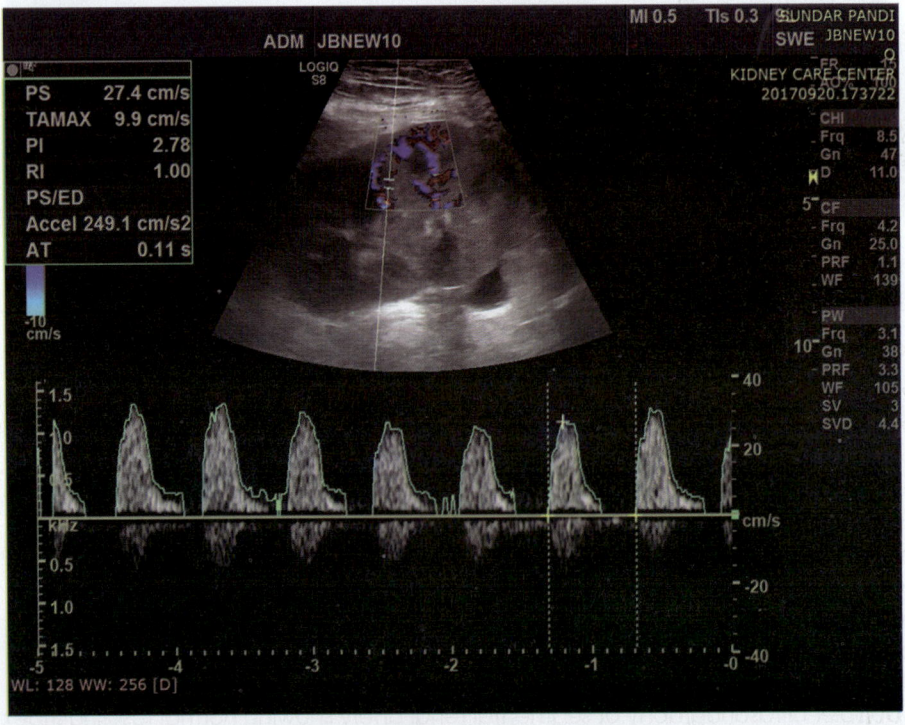

Fig. 6.8: High resistive index (RI). Doppler ultrasonography showing increased resistive index (RI)

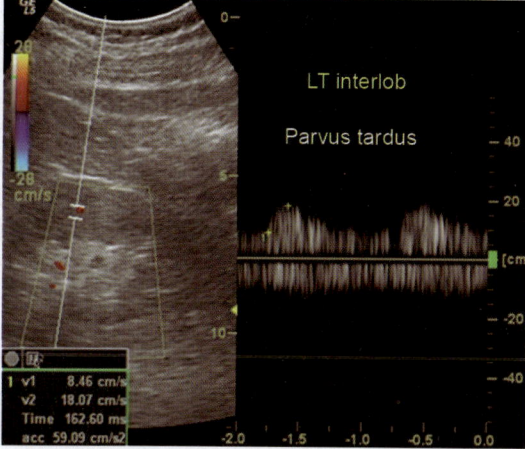

Fig. 6.9: Doppler renal ultrasonography of interlobar renal artery showing prolonged time to peak (162.60 ms) and reduced acceleration time (59.09 cm/s²) pattern called "parvus tardus". This is diagnostic of renal artery stenosis

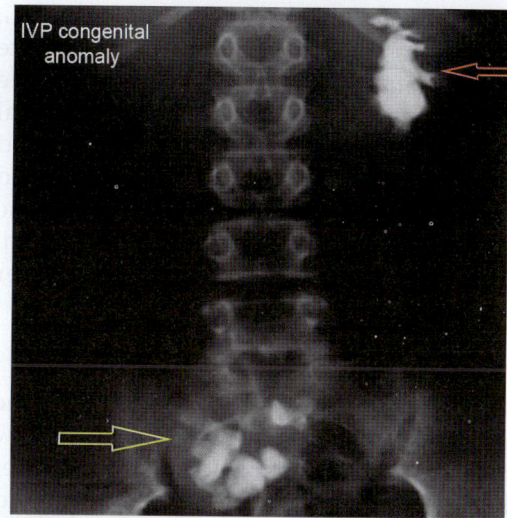

Fig. 6.10: Intravenous urogram showing 2 congenital renal anomalies. 1. Malrotation of left kidney (pink arrow) (*note:* Long axis of kidney almost parallel to spine. 2. Unascended right kidney in the pelvis (yellow arrow)

- Associated with substantial radiation exposure limiting its use in pregnancy.
- Other techniques, such as USG and CT, can provide similar or more detailed information.

IVU is very useful for identifying renal anomalies (Fig. 6.10) and renal stone disease. It also gives information about some functional aspect and data on the degree of obstruction. However, noncontrast-enhanced helical CT scanning is becoming the gold standard for the radiologic diagnosis of renal stone disease.

VOIDING CYSTOURETHROGRAM (VCUG)

Urinary bladder is catheterized and diluted radiocontrast instilled into the bladder by gravity. X-ray of the kidney ureter and bladder (KUB) area taken after removing the catheter. Image of the bladder would give an assessment of the bladder capacity, bladder wall thickness, mucosal irregularity (cystitis, diverticulum) and tumors. It will also be able to identify reflux of urine in the resting state. The patient is asked to void and an X-ray is taken during voiding. The picture during voiding will reveal the lower urinary tract,

and presence of reflux of urine into the ureter if any (Fig. 6.11). The severity of the reflux is

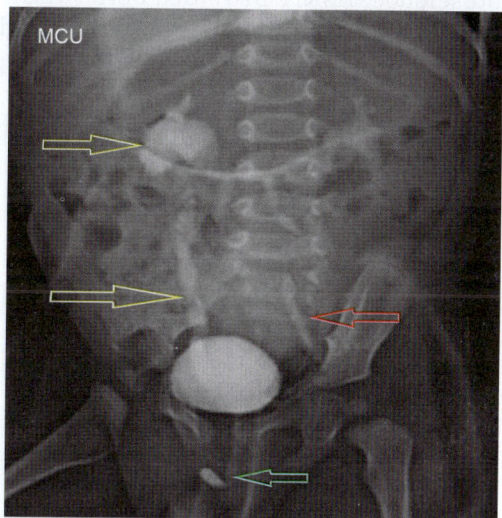

Fig. 6.11: Micturating cystourethrogram showing bilateral vesicoureteric reflux. *Note:* 1. Reflux of dye from bladder into dilated right ureter and renal pelvis (yellow arrows), 2. Reflux into lower part of left ureter (red arrow), 3. Dye in the urethra (green arrow)

graded depending on the findings of VCUG. Dilated posterior urethra and a 'valve'-like tissue distally, blocking the urethra is the characteristic finding in posterior urethral valve. Urethral stricture can also be identified in VCUG. Videocystourethrogram combined with urodynamic studies help to diagnose functional aspects like voiding pattern, voiding pressure and detrusor sphincter dyssynergia.

ASCENDING URETHROGRAM (AUG)

Radiocontrast is injected into the urethra as the radiograph is recorded. This delineates its flow into the urethra and the bladder (Fig. 6.12) better than the voiding urethrogram. Urethritis and strictures are identified well by this method.

COMPUTED TOMOGRAPHY SCANS

Computed tomography (CT) was invented in 1972 by British engineer Godfrey Hounsfield of England and by South Africa-born physicist Allan Cormack, who were later awarded the Nobel prize for their contributions to medicine and science. As CT provides better tissue detail than renal ultrasonography due to high spatial resolution, it is an excellent imaging tool to evaluate renal masses, traumatic injury, stones, and pyelonephritis. CT scanning is useful to differentiate malignant from non-malignant renal masses and helps to evaluate the local spread of renal malignancy. CT angiography is excellent in diagnosis of renal artery stenosis, aneurysms (Figs 6.13 and 6.14) and renal vein thrombosis. CT scanning is superior to ultrasonography in identifying renal cysts, since it can detect small cysts (2–3 mm in diameter). Because of safety and cost, renal ultrasonography is the best imaging option to screen for polycystic kidney disease. With the advent of multislice CT scanning, CT urography is fast replacing intravenous urography. Multislice CT urography is much superior in identifying the etiology of hematuria and identifying urothelial tumors than IVU. It is not only comparable to cystoscopy but provides additional information about extra-urinary extent of the disease.

Indications

- Diagnosing nephrolithiasis
- Evaluating kidney masses and staging renal tumors
- Evaluating polycystic kidney disease

Technique

Plain scan is done to record baseline study of calcifications, stones, and space-occupying lesions in the kidney and urinary tract. Within a minute after injection of contrast, the renal vasculature is delineated. In the nephrographic phase (up to 3 minutes after contrast injection), renal masses can be identified since they are vascular and show 'enhancement'. They can be differentiated from simple cysts which do not enhance with contrast. In the excretory phase (5 minutes after contrast injection), the collecting system—calyx, pelvis, the ureter and bladder are imaged.

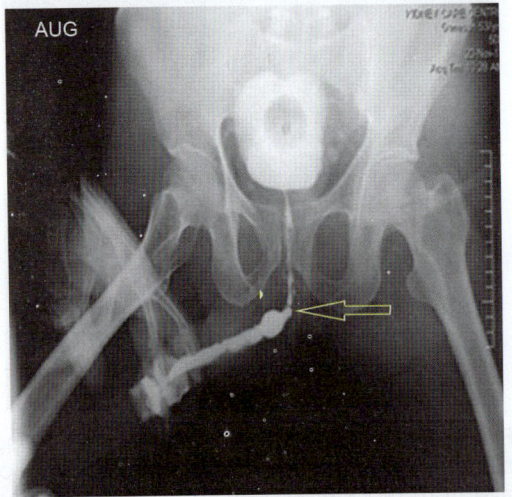

Fig. 6.12: Ascending urethrogram (AUG) showing stricture urethra. *Note:* The narrowing at the beginning of penile urethra (arrow)

Limitations

Risks of radiation and administration of contrast (contrast-induced nephropathy).

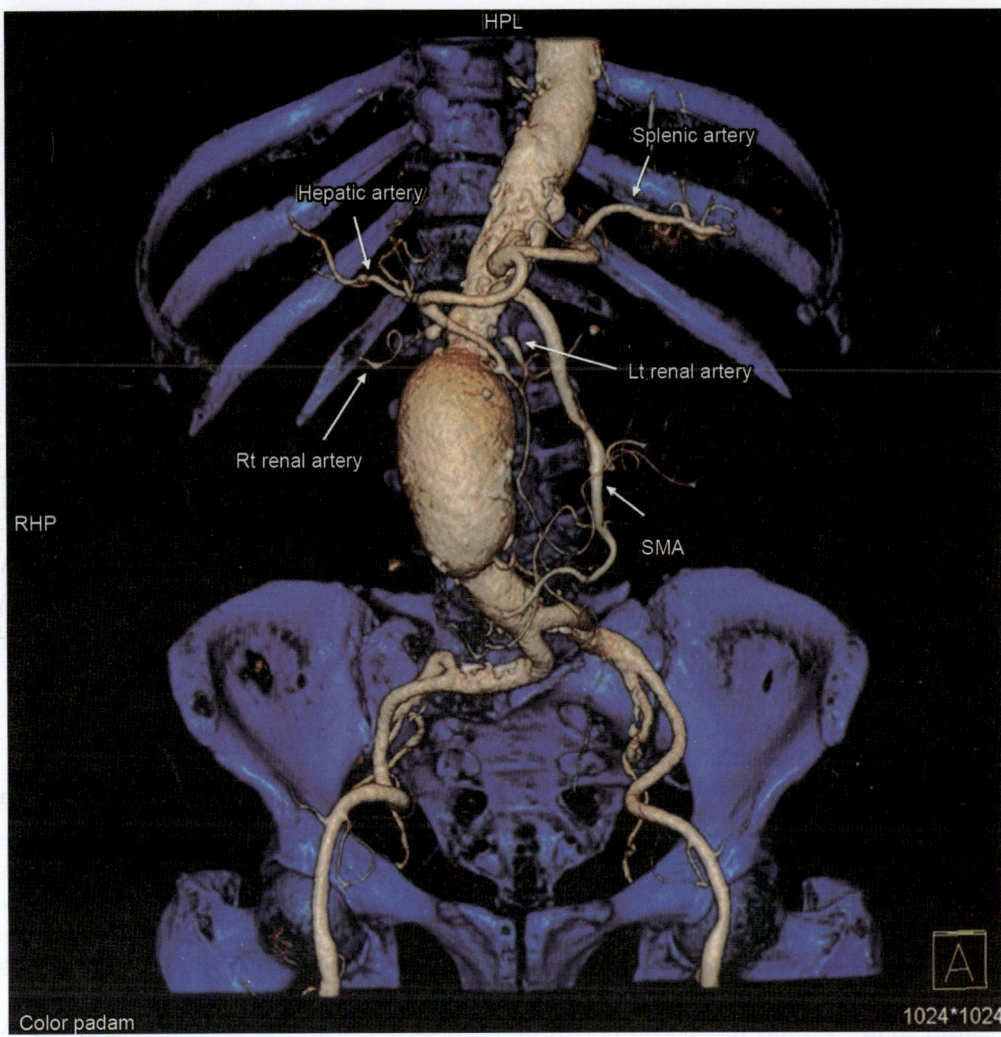

Fig. 6.13: CT angiography after reconstruction showing aneurysm of abdominal aorta and bilateral renal artery stenosis. CT angiogram showing infrarenal aneurysm of abdominal aorta and bilateral renal artery stenosis

Contraindications

Pregnancy, iodine sensitivity, and presence of renal failure.

Contrast-induced nephropathy (CIN) is becoming an important cause of acute kidney injury. With increased use of radiological studies in sick, elderly patients, the incidence of CIN has increased (10–30% in high risk patients). With our understanding of the pathogenesis, it is possible to reduce or prevent morbidity. The types of radiocontrast agents can be high osmolal, low osmolal, iso-osmolal and are either ionic or non-ionic. The dose is 300 mg Iodine/kg body weight. The non-ionic, low or iso-osmolal contrast agent is better and safer and must be preferred particularly in infants/elderly, patients with renal or cardiac failure, diabetics and patients with myeloma/sickle cell disease. It should be avoided if history of allergy to iodine is present.

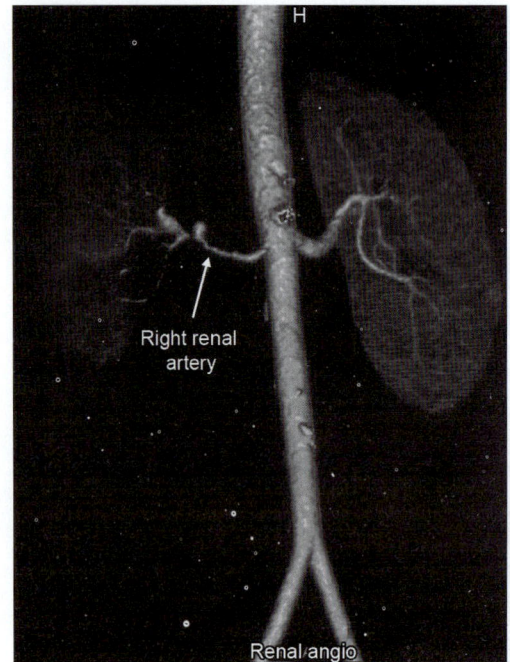

Fig. 6.14: CT abdominal aortic angiogram showing right renal artery stenosis with dilatations due to fibromuscular dysplasia. Note: The 'string of beads appearance of the right renal artery (arrow)'

Methods to prevent contrast-induced nephropathy:

i. Avoid high risk patients
ii. Use lower dose
iii. Use non-ionic low or iso-osmolal agents
iv. Avoid dehydration; use isotonic saline infusion.
v. Other measures like bicarbonate infusion, acetyl cysteine, aminophylline have not proved to be effective.

MAGNETIC RESONANCE IMAGING (MRI)

Magnetic resonance imaging (MRI) (Fig. 6.15) is an imaging modality using non-ionizing radiation from nuclear magnetic resonance to create 2D images. Lauterbur and Mansfield were awarded Nobel prize in 2003 for developing it for clinical use. MRI provides useful alternative to CT scanning in individuals at risk for toxicity from intravenous contrast. MRI is often used as a problem-solving modality when the CT findings are nondiagnostic. It also offers an advantage in the evaluation of small renal masses. Magnetic resonance angiography (MRA) has been found useful in detecting renal artery stenosis especially in the mid and proximal renal arteries.

Gadolinium is usually administered as 'contrast' for MRI scan. Gadolinium is contra-indicated in patients with renal insufficiency. Noncontrast-enhanced magnetic resonance angiography is very useful in detecting lesions in main renal artery but not smaller branches. At best it can be used as a safe non-invasive screening tool. Newer modalities, such as magnetic resonance renography, have shown promising results in assessing morphology and function of the kidneys. Magnetic resonance urography is commonly used in children and pregnant women to avoid the risk of radiation.

Attempts are being made to use MRI for imaging of renal function, including perfusion, glomerular filtration rate and intrarenal oxygen measurement. Blood oxygenation level dependent (BOLD) imaging is an imaging technique used to generate images in functional MRI (fMRI) studies, and relies on regional differences in blood flow to delineate regional activity. Though this was originally conceived to image the brain, now it is being tried in kidneys also.

Indications for MRI

i. Detailed assessment of the kidney anatomy
ii. Non-invasive assessment of kidney function
iii. Estimation of GFR
iv. MR angiography
v. Magnetic resonance renography
vi. Assessment of congenital anomalies of the kidney, bladder, and urinary tract.

Limitations

- MRI takes longer time. Some patients may become claustrophobic. Significant patient cooperation and radiologist supervision is required.

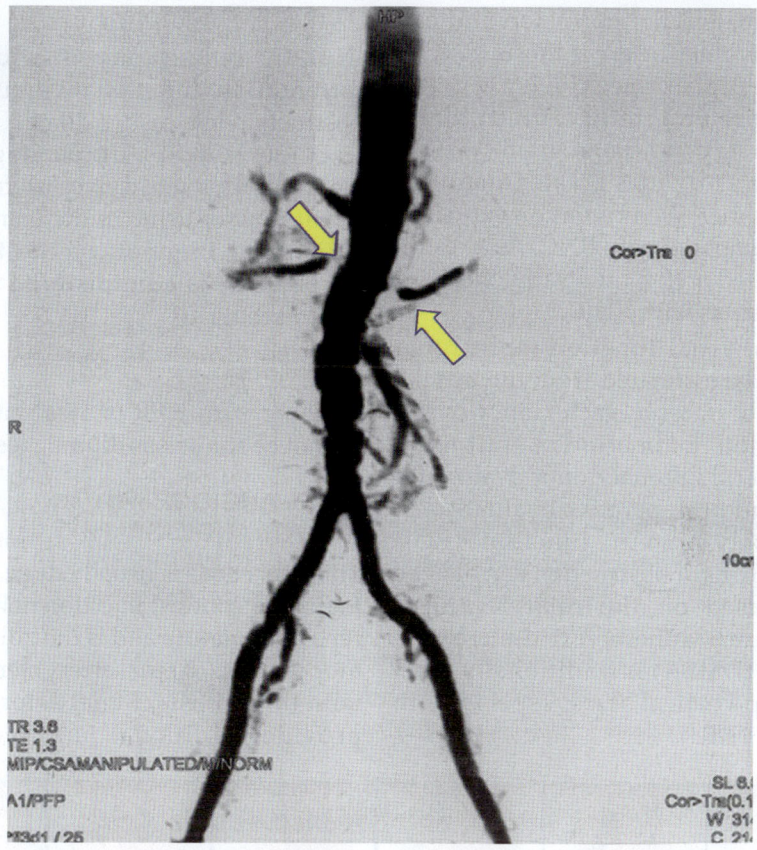

Fig. 6.15: MR angiography—bilateral renal artery stenosis. MR angiogram without contrast showing bilateral severe renal artery stenosis (arrows)

- The image quality is less robust with an undistended urinary system. Use of intravenous fluids, diuretics, compression devices and gadolinium chelate help in improving the resolution of MRI.
- Respiratory and ureteral peristaltic movements may affect image quality. However, forced breath-holding may improve the image.
- MRI is not good at detecting calcifications, although renal calculi can be inferred indirectly from filling defects or ureteral dilatation.
- The sensitivity of MRI in detecting urothelial and renal malignancies is less than that of CT imaging.

Nephrogenic systemic fibrosis (NSF) is a complication of MRI whenever gadolinium was used in patients with renal failure. This disorder was recognized very late since there is a long time gap between the insult and the complication. Although rare, NSF is invariably progressive. Therefore, MRI with gadolinium contrast is to be avoided when serum creatinine level exceeds 2 mg/dl (estimated glomerular filtration rate [eGFR] <30 ml/min). Newer contrast agents at low doses are under investigation to circumvent this problem.

RADIONUCLIDE (RNC) SCANNING

Radionuclide renal scans provide both functional and anatomic information (Fig. 6.16).

RNC can estimate renal perfusion and can reliably identify renal artery stenosis. RNC is widely used in pediatric nephrology to detect early vesicoureteral reflux in children. Although voiding cystourethrogram (VCUG) by radiography provides greater anatomic detail, there is increased radiation exposure with VCUG compared with RNC. As a result, RNC is often used preferentially for follow-up imaging in patients with VUR.

Differential renal function (split renal function) can be estimated from the uptake and clearance of tracer by each kidney over a specified period. Estimation of split renal function is useful in renal donor evaluation and in pre- and postoperative evaluation of congenital pelviureteric junction (PUJ) obstruction. Urinary obstruction can also be identified based on the relative tracer excretion via each kidney. ^{99m}Tc dimercaptosuccinic acid (DMSA) is traditionally used to identify up-cortical scars, especially in children with VUR.

Diuretic Renography

Diuretic renography is widely used to differentiate functional versus anatomical obstruction in a case of dilated upper urinary tract identified by ultrasonography or CT scanning. This study gives useful information about flow of urine in the urinary tract and split renal function of the two kidneys. Furosemide is administered with a radiopharmaceutical.

Limitations

Patients with GFR of less than 15 ml/min cannot be studied as diuretic response is poor.

RENAL ANGIOGRAPHY (DSA/CT ANGIOGRAPHY)

This procedure is usually done in the cathlab. Iodinated contrast injection helps to visualize renal vasculature and is the gold standard for the diagnosis of renal artery stenosis and renal vein thrombosis. Renal arteriography can provide additional information in the

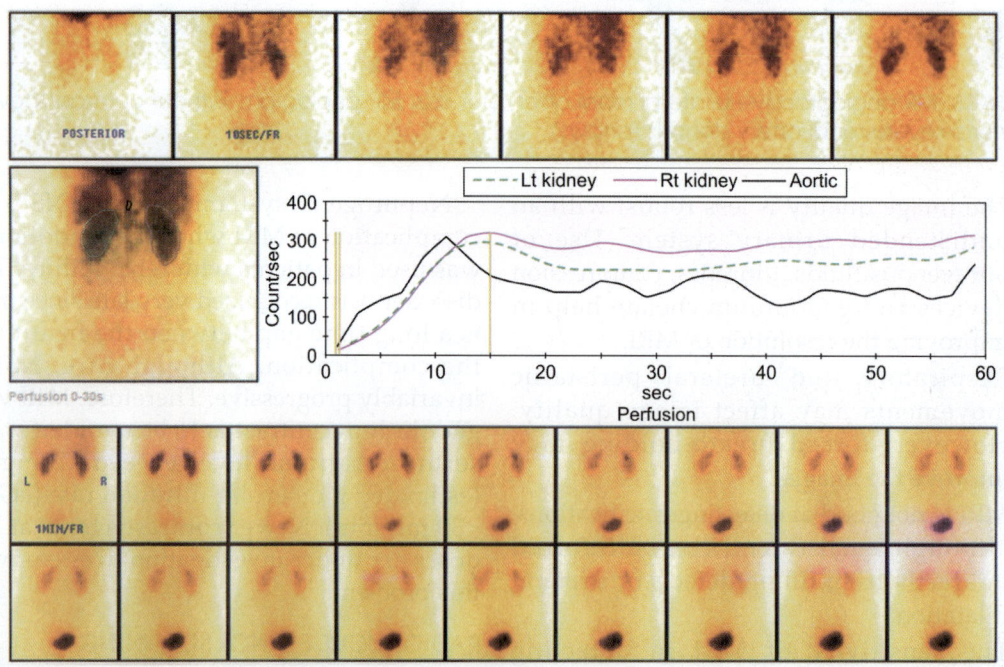

Fig. 6.16: Normal isotope renogram. *Note:* The red and green lines in the graph are identical. The renogram shows identical density of the tracer in both kidneys

preoperative evaluation of a renal mass, its vascularity and operability. The catheter can be introduced into one of the renal arteries to study the artery in detail. Figure 6.17 shows significant stenosis of renal arteries can be identified clearly. With advent of 64 and 128 slice CT scan, CT angiography is fast replacing conventional angiography and has the advantage of avoiding arterial puncture. It also provides provision for reconstructed 3D pictures for evaluation and planning of interventions. Problem of iodine contrast nephropathy remains, precluding these useful tests when there is renal dysfunction (eGFR <60 ml). Still conventional angiography using iodine contrast with standard precautions (using minimum contrast, pre-procedure hydration with IV saline) remains useful in suspected polyarteritis nodosa, fibromuscular dysplasia, demonstrating multiple aneurysms and irregular constrictions in the larger vessels, with occlusion of smaller penetrating arteries.

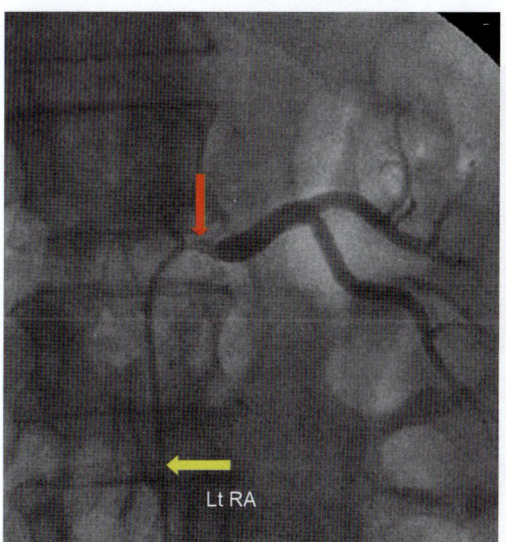

Fig. 6.17: Selective left renal angiogram–left renal artery stenosis. Conventional renal angiogram showing renal artery stenosis. *Note:* Catheter from femoral artery to abdominal aorta and left renal artery (yellow arrow). And stenotic segment in left renal artery (red arrow)

Newer imaging techniques
- Elastography
- Contrast-enhanced sonography (CES)

ELASTOGRAPHY

This is a newer imaging technique where stiffness of a tissue is assessed to study the underlying disease process. Strain (Fig. 6.18) and Shear wave elastography (Fig. 6.19) are two types of elastography using different types of energy (mechanical or ultrasound) to assess the elastic property of the tissue under study. Originally it was used to study thyroid, breast, and liver. Now its usage has been extended to prostate and kidneys. Non-invasive evaluation of renal fibrosis is being attempted. In renal transplantation, elastography appears to be a potential tool in differentiating acute rejection from calcineurin toxicity as the cause of acute renal allograft dysfunction.

CONTRAST-ENHANCED SONOGRAPHY (CES)

This is done by injection of contrast agents which can give more information on micro-vascular renal perfusion than regular USG and color Doppler. This appears to have significant role in study of renal allograft. The ultrasound contrast agent consists of gas-filled microbubbles stabilized by a supporting shell of biocompatible material like protein, lipid or polymer. First-generation agents were filled with room air, which had the disadvantage to diffuse quickly into surrounding plasma. Second-generation contrast agents contain gases of low solubility like sulfohexafluoride or octafluoropropane. These gases do not leak from the protecting shell for several minutes. Due to their small size with a range from 1 to 10 μm, microbubbles reach the capillaries and enable visualization even of the microvascular circulation. Microbubbles act as contrast agent by creating a boundary surface between the fluid phase in blood at the outside and the gaseous phase at the inside. The gas is exhaled through the lungs within 20–30 minutes after

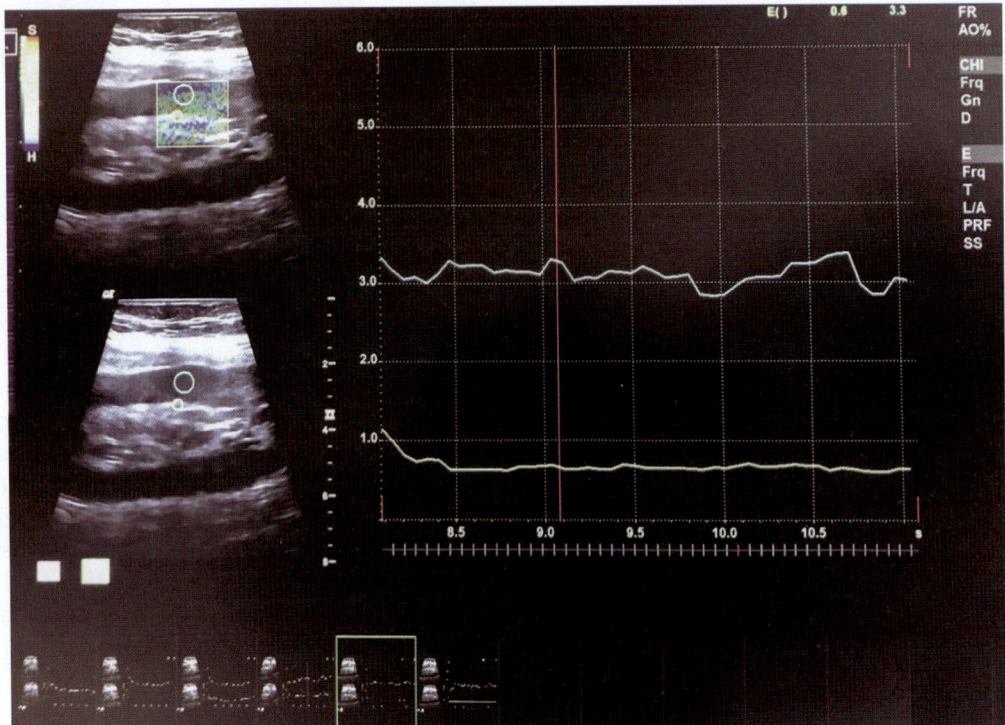

Fig. 6.18: Strain elastography. Strain elastography of renal allograft showing raised stiffness (blue line on top) when compared to sinus area stiffness (yellow line in bottom) suggesting acute rejection

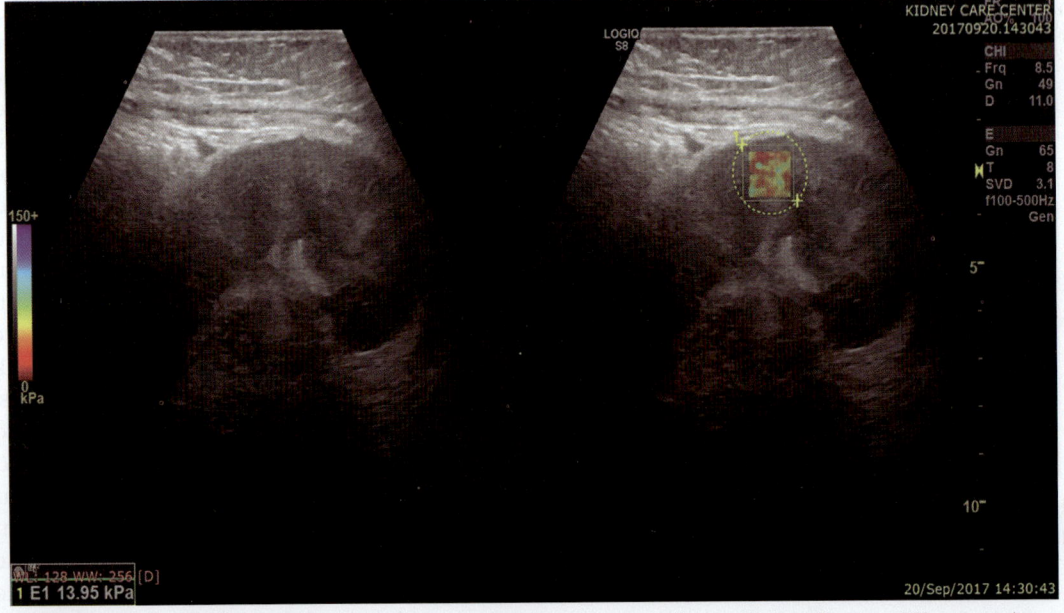

Fig. 6.19: Shear elastography. Shear elastography of renal allograft showing a stiffness value of 13.95 kPa

injection and the shell is metabolized in the liver. Microbubble-based contrast agents are not nephrotoxic and do not interact with thyroid function. In CES, renal infarction can be clearly delineated (Fig. 6.20). CES is also being tried in evaluation of renal allograft dysfunction by studying the time curve of contrast uptake and clearance.

Other imaging studies to help renal evaluation: Hitherto, lung, an air-filled organ was considered for study by USG. Now by ingenious interpretation of the artefacts produced by the lung, diagnosis of interstitial pulmonary edema, alveolar pulmonary edema, pleural effusion and pneumothorax are possible. This is now increasingly used in point of care ultrasonography in critical care nephrology. Imaging the size and collapsibility of inferior vena cava (IVC) in supine position before and after leg raising can throw light on the hydration state of a critically ill renal patient.

Advancements in imaging of the urinary system by the way of newer sensitive equipment and intelligent interpretation of the findings have made diagnosis of renal disease much

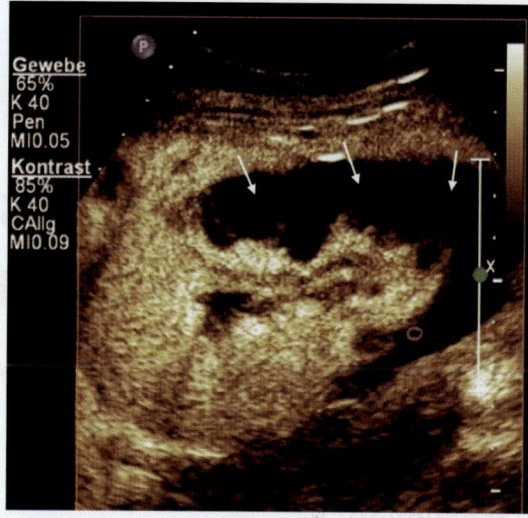

Fig. 6.20: Contrast-enhanced sonography showing absence of perfusion of lower pole due to thrombosis (arrows)

better and easier for the clinician. Still the responsibility of selection of the right investigation at the right time and protection of the patient from potential hazards of exposure to toxic radiations and contrast agents lies on the hands of the physician.

Understanding Molecular Biology

• R Kasi Visweswaran

INTRODUCTION

Understanding of biological processes requires knowledge of the basis of cellular function at the molecular level. Molecular biology is based on the biologic activity between various molecules within the cell, synthesis of proteins and interactions between deoxyribonucleic acid (DNA) and ribonucleic acid (RNA). Whereas biochemistry focuses on proteins and their functions, genetics between genes and functions, molecular biology focuses interactions of genes and proteins (Fig. 7.1). Thus, molecular biology focuses on how is the inherited genetic information is encoded within DNA, how it is regulated and expressed so that highly specialized cells of a multicellular organism develop from a single cell. This understanding of the specialized functions is important for a more in-depth understanding of human diseases.

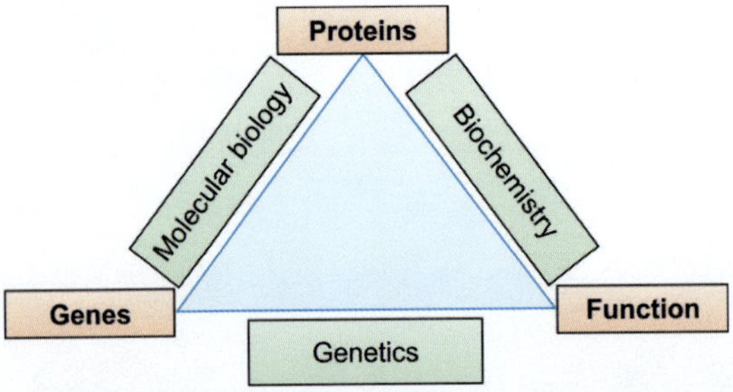

The data from clinical research in molecular biology have helped in the understanding of cellular functions, gene therapy, diagnosis of diseases, targeted drug therapy and nanotechnology. Over the last 2 decades, emerging subfields like bioinformatics, computational biology (interface between molecular biology and computer technology), molecular genetics (study of gene structure and function), cell biology, evolutionary biology, developmental biology, biophysics, population genetics and phylogenetics have evolved and are rapidly advancing.

1. Cell Biology

Knowledge of molecular and cell biology involves understanding of four groups of macromolecules which are essential for structure and function of cell. They are:

a. Carbohydrates made up of carbon (C), hydrogen (H) and oxygen (O) involved in energy storage and form part of receptors and transport molecules.

b. Proteins, which are polypeptide chains containing nitrogen (N), C, O, and H. They provide the basis for structure, act as enzymes, transporters, receptors and co-enzymes.

Fig. 7.1: The inter-relationship between proteins, genes and their functions

c. Nucleic acids, which are polynucleotide or nucleic acid containing N rings, sugar, phosphate and nitrogenous base. They are mainly involved in information storage and transfer.

d. Lipids, which are glycerol and fatty acids containing C, H and O. They are not polymers but involved in maintaining membrane structure, insulation and energy storage.

2. Cell Membrane Structure and Function

The cell is the basic unit of any living organism and the contents are enclosed by the cell membrane, which separates it from the extracellular space. The cell membrane is not just an envelope that encloses the contents of the cell but is a dynamic structure. It is a thin elastic structure 7.5–10 nanometers thick, composed of protein 55%, phospholipids 25%, cholesterol 13%, other lipids 4% and carbohydrates 3%. It consists of a lipid bilayer (2 lipid molecules thick) and continues as a sheet over the surface of all membranes. Movement of the molecules along the surface and matrix of the lipid bilayer is possible.

Each phospholipid molecule is shaped like the 'clothespin' with phosphate forming the 'head' and the lipid forming the 'tail'. Since the hydrophobic tail portion is repelled by water, the lipid ends of 2 molecules mutually attract each other forming a bilayer which form the sheet which envelops the contents of the cell, mitochondria or other cellular organelles

(Fig. 7.2). The lipid bilayer is impermeable to water-soluble substances, ions, glucose, urea etc. but freely permeable to fat-soluble substances like oxygen, carbon dioxide, nitrogen and alcohol.

a. The rounded end is hydrophilic phosphate containing 'head' and tail-like portion is hydrophobic lipid component.

b. The hydrophobic ends of two phospholipids molecule align with each other and become stable in aqueous environment.

c. The lipid bilayer is formed.

Proteins constitute about 50% of the mass of cell membrane. They appear embedded in the membrane as globular units and are large molecules. If the protein chains pass through the whole of the lipid bilayer they are called integral proteins. If they are attached to the surface only, they are called surface proteins (Fig. 7.3).

Integral protein traverses through the lipid bilayer. Surface proteins are attached to outside or inside of the cell membrane. GPI anchor helps to fix the surface protein.

The functions of the protein in cell membrane include:

1. *Act as structural protein*—contributes to structural framework.

2. *Function as pumps*—for active transport of ions.

3. *Function as carriers (carrier proteins)*—transport substances down electrochemical gradient by facilitated diffusion.

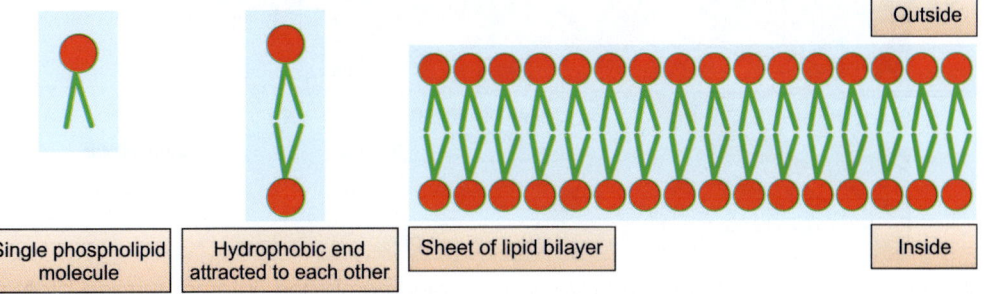

| Single phospholipid molecule | Hydrophobic end attracted to each other | Sheet of lipid bilayer | Outside |
| Inside |

Fig. 7.2: Phospholipid molecule and lipid bilayer

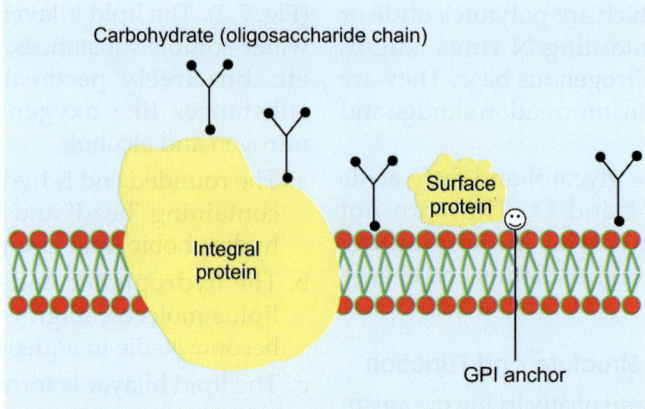

Fig. 7.3: Proteins in the cell wall

The carrier proteins are highly selective:
4. *Act as ion channels (channel proteins)*—
   Permit transport of ions in and out when activated.
5. *Function as receptors*—bind to neuro-transmitters and hormones and activate the intracellular constituents.
6. *Act as enzymes*—catalyse reactions on the surface of the membrane.
7. *Glycoprotein*—function in antibody processing and distinguishing self and non-self.

Carbohydrates invariably occur in combi-nation with proteins or lipids as glycoprotein or glycolipids. Figure 7.4 shows a diagrammatic representation of cell membrane, proteins, glycolipid, and their relationship with cyto-skeleton.

3. Transport of Molecules Across Membrane

Transport of molecules across a cell membrane can be unidirectional or bidirectional. If two or more molecules are moved in the same

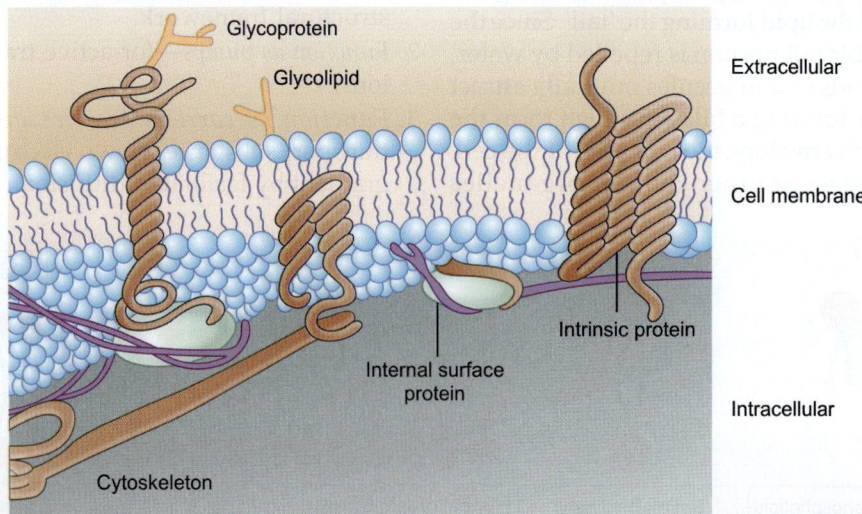

Fig. 7.4: Protein (amino acid chain) traversing the cell membrane, internal surface protein and connection to cytoskeleton of the cell

direction, it is called symport or co-transport (e.g. sodium-glucose co-transport, sodium-potassium, 2 chloride co-transport). If the molecules are transported in opposite directions, it is called antiport or counter-transport (Fig. 7.5). The transport of molecules may occur as a passive process depending on physical forces like pressure, osmotic or concentration gradient. When energy is expended for the transport, it is called active transport.

Figure 7.5 showing (a) antiport (counter-transport) and (b) symport (co-transport).

Transport of two or more different molecules through the same transport protein simultaneously in same direction = symport or co-transport and in opposite directions = antiport or countertransport.

Passive Transport

a. *Simple diffusion:* Simple diffusion occurs due to the random movement of molecules and pass through inter-molecular spaces of permeable membranes.

b. Facilitated diffusion occurs through 'channels' in the integral proteins. Such channels help transport of water and water-soluble substances across the lipid bilayer which has hydrophobic domain in-between.

c. Facilitated diffusion occurs through gated channels. Most protein channels are highly selective for one or more ions or molecules. The selectivity is regulated by the diameter, shape and electrical charge. The 'Gates' are

gate-like extensions of the transport protein molecule which can 'open' or 'close' as a result of re-alignment of the shape of the protein (conformational change). There are two types of gating: (a) Voltage gating and (b) chemical gating.

d. Facilitated diffusion occurs through carrier proteins with the help of a specific carrier protein which facilitates the diffusion, e.g. glucose transport and amino acid transport.

e. *Osmosis:* Osmosis is the process of net movement of water across selectively permeable membrane caused by a concentration difference of solutes (water moves from the side of lower solute concentration to higher solute concentration).

Active Transport

Active transport can be primary or secondary active transport.

a. In primary active transport, the substance is transported across a concentration gradient with the help of energy-often supplied by dephosphorylation of ATP. Sodium-potassium ATPase pump is present in all cell membranes and helps to create and maintain high potassium in the intracellular compartment and high sodium in extracellular compartment. The energy comes from adenosine triphosphate (ATP) which is dephosphorylated to adenosine diphosphate (ADP) (Fig. 7.6).

Figure 7.6 showing active transport.

In the case of calcium, calcium transport pump in cell membrane pushes the Ca out of the cell and another in the mitochondrial membrane pushes calcium into mitochondria. Thus the Calcium content in the intracellular compartment is very low and the mitochondrial calcium concentration is 10,000 times more than the cytosol.

Primary active transport of H^+ ions, occur through pumps are situated mainly in the deep lying parietal cells of gastric mucosa and intercalated cells in distal renal tubule. The gastric glands help to form gastric HCl

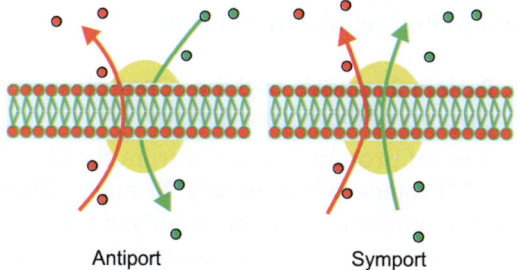

Antiport   Symport

Fig. 7.5: Antiport → transport of molecules in opposite direction. Symport → transport of molecules in the same direction

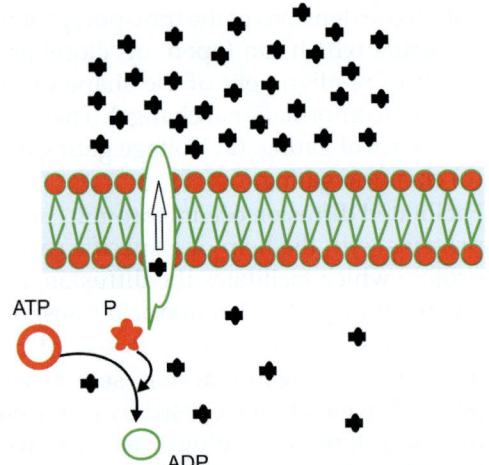

Fig. 7.6: Active transport of molecules with energy obtained from ATP against a concentration gradient

which has a million fold increase of H^+ ions concentration across the parietal cell membrane. The intercalated cells in late distal renal tubule and cortical collecting duct achieve 900 fold increase in H^+ ion concentration in the lumen, thus enabling elimination of the acid load.

b. *In secondary active transport:* In secondary active transport, the energy derived from the primary active transport in the form of ionic concentration difference is used as energy source to transport a different substance against its concentration gradient.

For example, the difference in the concentration of Na across cell membrane attained by sodium potassium ATPase pump is utilized as the "stored energy" for transport of another molecule tagged to it. Since sodium can enter the cell because of the concentration gradient, it can transport a molecule of glucose through the sodium glucose co-transporter facilitating entry of glucose into the cell. Subsequently, sodium is expelled by sodium potassium ATPase pump. The H^+ ion transport in proximal renal tubule (sodium hydrogen symport) is another example of secondary active transport.

Channelopathies are diseases caused due to dysfunction of proteins regulating ion channels.

They may be congenital (due to ion channel mutations) or acquired.

4. Nucleated (Eukaryotic) Cell

All eukaryotic cells contain a nucleus, intracellular organelles and internal membranes. Each section of the cell performs different specialized functions which are vital for the life of the cell. The cell membrane is made of phospholipids, protein and oligosaccharide chains which serve numerous functions outlined in the next section-in addition to forming the envelope like selective boundary of the cell. The nucleus is surrounded by a nuclear membrane with nuclear pores. The nucleus contains chromosomes with DNA and protects the DNA of the cell. The cytoplasm contains endomembrane system consisting of the endoplasmic reticulum, the Golgi apparatus and vesicles in addition to ribosome, lysosome and mitochondria. Ribosomes form the proteins by linking amino acids in the correct sequence. Mitochondria are the sites of metabolism and cellular respiration and transfer energy from food molecules to ATP. The mitochondria are covered by 2 membranes, the outer membrane and the inner membrane. The space between the two is the inter-membrane space. The foldings of the inner membrane form the cristae and it encloses the matrix and DNA. The cytoskeleton is a network of proteins containing actin microfilaments and microtubules. Cytoskeletal proteins support the structure of the cell, help with cell division, and control cellular movements.

5. Protein Synthesis and the 'Central Dogma of Molecular Biology'

The word protein is derived from the Greek word 'Proteos' which means 'Primary'. They are the fundamental components of bacteria, plants and animals. Proteins constitute 75% of the total dry body weight (excluding all water). Hemoglobin, insulin, bone matrix, muscle, collagen, antibodies are all proteins.

Thus, proteins have a leading role to play in maintaining the structure and functions of the body. Proteins are combination of chains of amino acids using peptide bonds. In contrast to the carbohydrates and fats, proteins are compounds containing nitrogen in addition to carbon, hydrogen and oxygen. Permutation and combination of 20 different amino acids give rise to innumerable different proteins in the body.

Chromosomes contain deoxyribonucleic acid (DNA)—a double helical structure containing nucleotides which are tightly coiled (Fig. 7.7). Each nucleotide has a phosphate group, sugar group and a nitrogen base. The four nitrogen bases in the DNA are adenine, thymine, guanine, and cytosine (ATGC). The first step in the protein synthesis is the splitting of the double helix to a single strand of DNA by the DNA polymerase in the nucleus. From this, by the process of transcription, ribonucleic acid (RNA) is formed.

Reverse transcription of RNA to form new DNA occurs in infection with retroviruses such as human immunodeficiency virus. There is reverse transfer of information and is important in viral replication. Antiretroviral drugs act by inhibiting reverse transcriptase enzyme and prevent viral replication.

The nitrogen bases in RNA are adenine, uracil, guanine, and cytosine (AUGC). The relevant portions are 'spliced' and form messenger RNA (mRNA). The mRNA leaves the nucleus and carries the genetic information. The information is transmitted to transfer RNA (tRNA) which conveys the information to ribosome. The ribosome is a globular structure consisting of a large and small sub-unit. The tRNA attaches to the smaller sub-unit and causes synthesis of protein chains in the larger sub-unit. Finally, the ribosomal RNA (rRNA) links the amino acids together to form polypeptide chain which is an unfolded protein chain which is released into the cytoplasm. This process is called translation. These unfolded protein chains are taken up by the molecular chaperones. The molecular chaperones are 'doughnut shaped' structures with a lid on top inside the cytoplasm. They act as 'protein folding machines'. The unfolded protein chains enter the chaperones, the lid closes, the proteins are folded to three-dimensional functional form and released from the cell. These chaperones also 'tag' misfolded proteins which are degraded. The lid reopens to release the folded protein.

Properly folded proteins are soluble, functional, degradable by proteolysis and can be re-utilized in protein turnover. Unfolded/

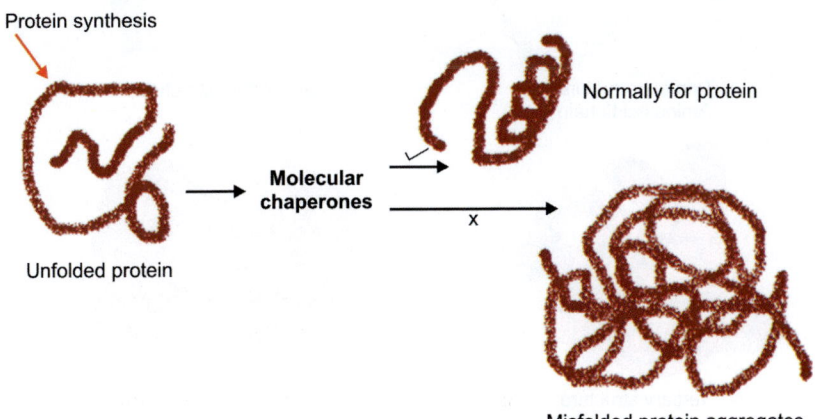

Fig. 7.7: Normal folding of proteins and misfolding

misfolded proteins are non-functional, insoluble, prone to aggregation and deposition and are not degradable. Thus, they may get deposited, compress neighboring tissue and cause death of neighboring cells.

6. Structure of Proteins

The primary structure of protein is a linear chain on a backbone of carbon atoms connected by peptide bonds with other atoms like nitrogen, oxygen, hydrogen and R group attached (Fig. 7.8). The secondary structure is a local substructure on the polypeptide chain. It can be like a coiled ribbon, called alpha helix of pleated sheet-like configuration called β-pleating. The tertiary structure is a three-dimensional configuration with alpha helix and β-pleated sheets folded into a compact globular structure. Quarternary structure is a three-dimensional structure with two or more polypeptide chains functioning as a single unit

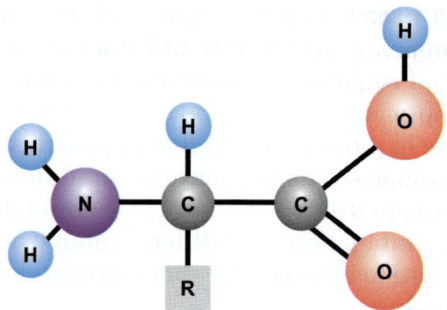

Fig. 7.8: Basic structure of protein containing carbon, nitrogen, oxygen, hydrogen and 'R' group.

(Fig. 7.9). The manner of bonding between the hydrogen ions in the molecule is different between normal and misfolded proteins. External factors like temperature, electric/magnetic field, molecular crowding, limitation of space may influence folding of proteins.

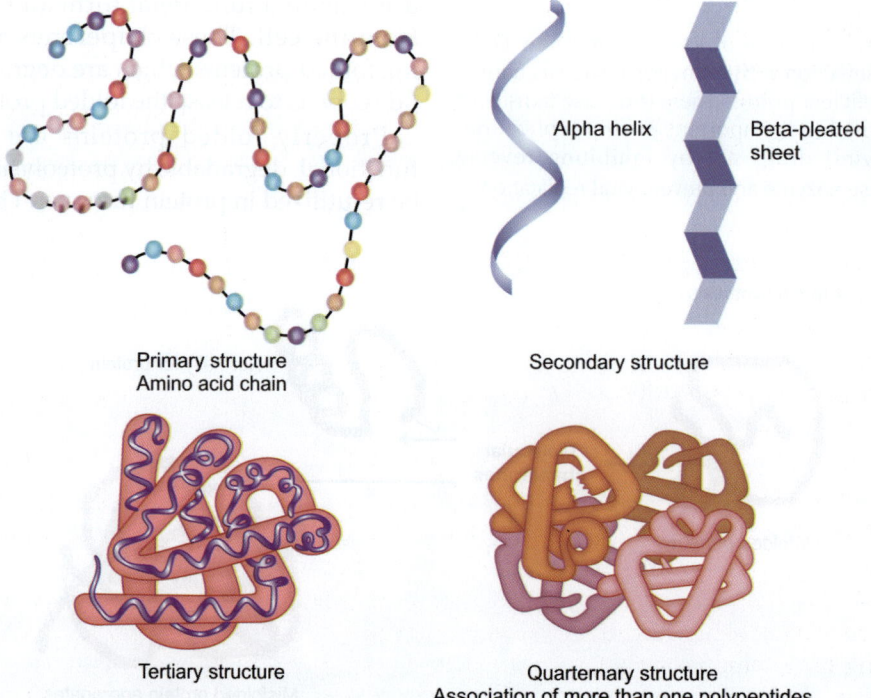

Primary structure
Amino acid chain

Alpha helix   Beta-pleated sheet

Secondary structure

Tertiary structure

Quarternary structure
Association of more than one polypeptides

Fig. 7.9: Structure of proteins—primary, secondary, tertiary and quarternary

7. Proteopathies

A group of disorders have now been identified as due to abnormal protein folding and are called 'proteopathies'. The protein may be misfolded to disease forming configuration, deposited, resist proteolysis and degradation, compress and cause death of surrounding tissue. These abnormal proteins may cause alteration in the normal protein to disease forming configuration by a process called 'permissive templating'. More than 50 disorders due to misfolded proteins have been identified. A few important ones are enumerated here.

a. *All types of amyloidosis (AL/AA/AH (heavy chain)/fibrinogen amyloidosis):* Deposition of abnormal insoluble beta-pleated fibrils, occur in various sites of the body.

b. *Alzheimer's disease:* Deposition of amyloid beta peptide and synuclein in brain.

c. *Taupathies:* Microtubule associated (TAU) proteins are involved in stabilizing the microtubules in the neuronal cells manifesting as dementia.

d. *Parkinson's disease and synucleinopathies:* Variable combination of deposition of amyloid beta peptide, TAU protein and synuclein.

e. *Prion disease:* Prion is a protein that can trigger normal proteins in the brain to fold abnormally and can spread from animals to humans from consumption of infected meat products. Deposition of prion proteins occurs in transmissible spongiform encephalopathies, Jakob-Creutzfeldt disease, etc.

f. *Amyotrophic lateral sclerosis:* Damage to motor neurons caused by probably abnormalities of the enzyme superoxide dismutase.

g. *Type II diabetes:* Due to deposition of islet amyloid polypeptide/amylin which damage the beta cells.

h. *Cystic fibrosis:* Cystic fibrosis is a disease affecting lung, pancreas, skin, kidney and intestine. Caused by mutation of trans-membrane conductance regulator protein (CFTR protein) resulting in abnormal sweat, mucous, intestinal and other body secretions.

i. *Sickle cell disease:* Abnormalities in hemoglobin resulting sickling of RBCs.

8. Molecular Methods

A few molecular methods which are used for research and diagnostics are briefly described below.

a. Gel electrophoresis is the procedure by which DNA, RNA and proteins are separated by means of electrical and size difference. The important ones are agarose gel electrophoresis where electrically charged agarose gel is used to separate DNA and RNA. In SDS-PAGE gel electrophoresis, proteins can be separated based on the size. In 2D gel electrophoresis, the separation based on both electric charge and size is possible.

b. Polymerase chain reaction (PCR) is the technique used in molecular biology to copy a specific DNA sequence, use it as the template and make copies in geometric proportions (2, 4, 8, 16, 32, 64, 128 …) so that millions of copies are made in a short time. Reverse transcription PCR is for amplifying RNA and the recently introduced quantitative PCR is used for quantifying measurement of DNA or RNA molecules.

c. Molecular cloning is the basic technique to study protein function. The DNA coding for a protein of interest is cloned using PCR, carried to the target through a vector and inserted into the genome of the defective cells. These methods may have a role in developing the gene therapy of the future.

d. Hybridization is the method of combining the qualities of two organisms of varieties through sexual reproduction.

e. Southern blotting is a method for probing for a specific DNA sequence in a DNA sample. The name was given after the biologist who invented the test Edwin Southern.

f. Northern blot is used to study patterns of a specific type of RNA molecule. The name is an extension of 'southern' blotting.

g. In Western blotting, proteins are separated (by size) using SDS-PAGE gel electrophoresis and transferred to a membrane. When probed with specific antibody, containing colored solutions, the original protein can be seen by chemiluminescence.

h. Eastern blotting technique is used to detect modifications in proteins after translation (post-translational modification) using specific substrates.

i. DNA microarray or DNA chip is microscopic DNA spots on a solid surface and used to measure the levels of expression of a large number of genes simultaneously.

This chapter is included to sensitize clinicians into this new area of development of medical science which will pave the way for identifying new diseases, investigations and treatment.

Pediatric

Pediatric

Development of Genitourinary System

• H Lekha

Understanding the development of the genitourinary system will help to comprehend the types of congenital anomalies and close associations of the genital and urinary system. Even though functionally the urogenital system is divided into urinary system and genital system, embryologically and anatomically they are intimately interwoven. Both develop from a common tissue, the intermediate mesoderm. The excretory ducts of both systems enter a common cavity, the cloaca initially. In the 3rd week of development, the intraembryonic mesoderm differentiates into 3 distinct parts: Paraxial portion, intermediate mesoderm and lateral plate mesoderm (Fig. 8.1). The urogenital system develops from the intermediate mesoderm derived from the dorsal body wall of the embryo. Nephrogenesis begins around 22 days after fertilization and is complete by 34–36 weeks of pregnancy.

NEPHROGENESIS

During folding of the embryo, the urogenital ridge forms from an elevation of the intermediate mesoderm on either side of the dorsal aorta. The part of the urogenital ridge forming the urinary system is the nephrogenic cord. The kidneys develop from the nephrogenic cord. Three sets of 'nephric' structures develop in a craniocaudal sequence in the urogenital ridge. They are pronephros,

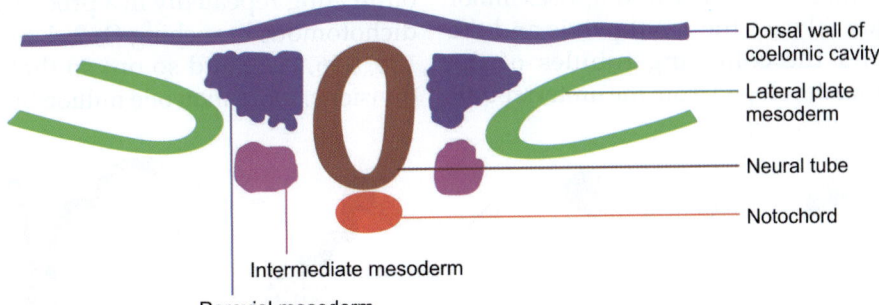

Fig. 8.1: The relationship of intermediate mesoderm in relation to paraxial and lateral plate mesoderm at 3 weeks. The neural tube develops on the dorsal wall of the coelomic cavity. On either side of the neural tube, the paraxial, intermediate and lateral plate mesoderm. Kidneys and gonads develop from intermediate mesoderm

mesonephros and metanephros (Fig. 8.2). Pronephros develops at 22 days in the cervical region and comprises simple nonfunctional tubules and pronephric duct. The pronephros involute by day 25. The cranial part of the pronephric duct also involutes. The remaining portion of the duct elongates and fuses with the cloaca. These units regress as the next set of tubular structures called mesonephric tubules form. Mesonephros is derived from the upper thoracic to upper lumbar segments from around 24th day. The pronephric duct which grows towards the cloaca is now called the mesonephric duct (wolffian duct). The mesonephric tubules are functional between 6 and 10 weeks, produce small amount of urine and involute by 3rd month. In males, some of these tubules are incorporated into epididymis, seminal vesicle and ejaculatory duct and also contribute to formation of efferent duct of epididymis. Metanephros develops by day 32, from the intermediate mesoderm in the sacral region of the embryo. The metanephric blastema is a condensation of the nearby cells. Metanephros develops into the definitive kidney. The development is from two-cell lineages, the ureteric bud which is an outgrowth of the caudal mesonephric duct and metanephric blastema (Fig. 8.3).

Steps in the Development of the Collecting System

The collecting system which comprises minor and major calyces, the renal pelvis and the ureter and the collecting tubules of the nephron are developed from the ureteric buds.

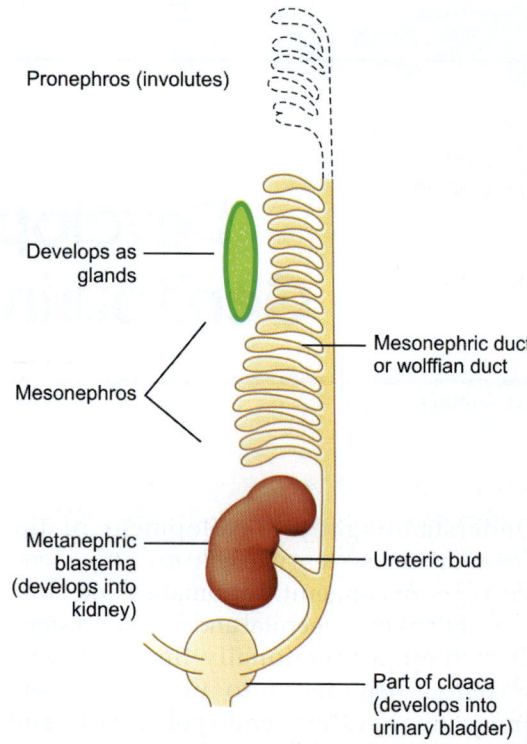

Fig. 8.2: Pronephros, mesonephros and metanephros. These structures develop from intermediate mesoderm. Pronephros involutes. Mesonephric duct persists. Ureteric bud arises from mesonephric duct. Part of the cloaca forms the bladder. Kidneys develop from metanephric blastema

The stalk of the ureteric bud becomes the ureter. By the 6th week, the ureteric bud starts bifurcating repeatedly in a process known as dichotomous branching (1, 2, 4, 8, 16, 32, 64, 128, 256, ... and so on) so that by 16–20 divisions, more than one million branches are

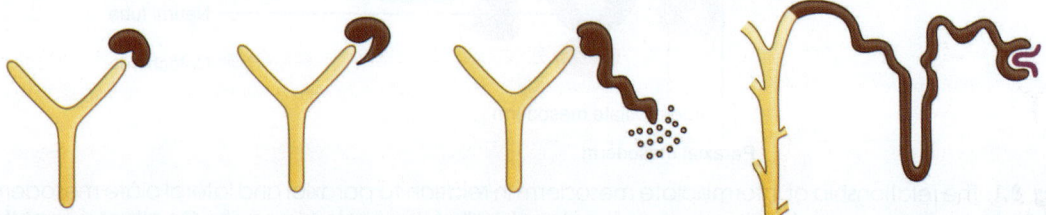

Fig. 8.3: Nephronogenesis. Development of the nephron from ureteric bud (yellow) and metanephric blastema (brown). The red dots represent vascular elements which form the capillary network

Gene	Origin	Action
i. Fibroblast growth factor 2 (FGF2)	Tip of ureteic bud	Mesenchymal proliferation (maintain WT1 expression)
ii. Bone morphogenetic protein 7 (BMP7)	Tip of ureteic bud	Mesenchymal proliferation (maintain WT1 expression)
iii. WNT9B	Branches of the ureteric bud epithelium	Upregulates PAX2 and WNT4 in the mesenchyme (mesenchyme to epithelialize and form tubules)
iv. WNT6	Branches of the ureteric bud epithelium	Upregulates PAX2 and WNT4 in the mesenchyme (mesenchyme to epithelialize and form tubules)
v. –	–	Formation of basement membrane
vi. Laminin, nidogen, agrin		Formation of epithelial cells

formed. By 32nd week, a tree-like branching system consisting of 1 to 3 million collecting tubules are formed (Fig. 8.4). The first four generations of tubules enlarge, become confluent and form the major calyces and the second four generations form the minor calices. Thus, the collecting ducts of the nephron, minor and major calyces and ureter develop from each ureteric bud.

Steps in Renogenesis

Formation of kidneys (renogenesis) is a process of 'reciprocal inductive interactions' between the metanephric blastema and the ureteric bud (UB). The metanephric blastema is of mesenchymal origin. It secretes growth factors that induce growth of the ureteric bud. The ureteric bud (UB) responds by secreting growth factors that stimulates proliferation and differentiation of the metanephric blastema and inducing it to undergo mesenchymal to epithelial transformation (MET).

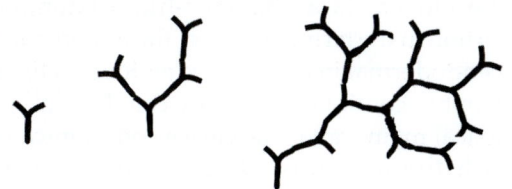

Fig. 8.4: Dichotomous branching of ureteric bud. Branching in geometric pattern—1, 2, 3, 8, 16, 32, 64 ..... for 16–20 times division result in 1–3 million nephrons

This transformation results in the formation of glomeruli and kidney tubules with different types of cells in the nephron with different functions. Cells of the metanephric mesenchyme condense to form a 'tissue cap' around the tip of each branch of ureteric bud (Fig. 8.3). This then undergo a MET to form the renal vesicle. which invaginates to form the comma-shaped and later, an S-shaped body. Capillaries are derived from vascular elements and they grow into the bulbous pocket like proximal end of the 'S' which forms the Bowman's capsule with capillaries, podocyte covering the capillaries, mesangium and ultimately differentiate into glomeruli. Continuous lengthening of the S-shaped excretory tubule results in formation of the proximal convoluted tubule, loop of Henle and distal convoluted tubule. The distal end (near the ureteric bud) forms an open connection with the final branching of the ureteric bud which forms the collecting tubule (Fig. 8.5). A group of cells from the pool of multipotent progenitor cells within the metanephric blastema, do not undergo MET and give rise to interstitial and vascular cells. Urine production begins soon after differentiation of the glomerular capillaries which start to form by 10th week. In humans, the formation of nephrons is completed by 36 weeks. Although maturation of nephrons continue into postnatal life, no new nephrons can be formed after nephrono-

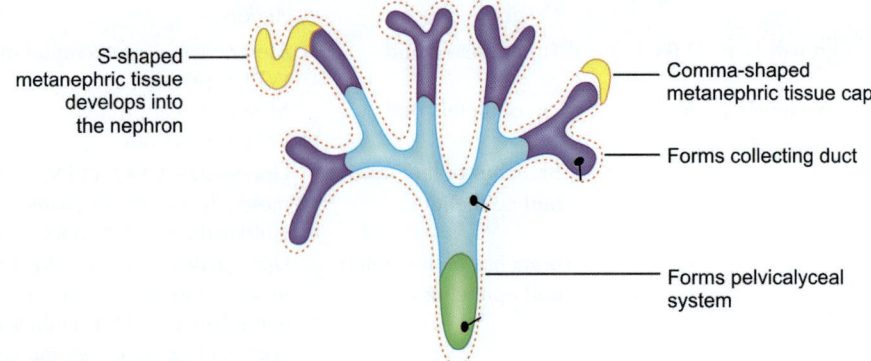

S-shaped metanephric tissue develops into the nephron

Comma-shaped metanephric tissue cap

Forms collecting duct

Forms pelvicalyceal system

Fig. 8.5: Terminal branching of ureteric bud and fusion with collecting duct of nephron. Green and blue part of the terminal divisions of ureteric bud develop into pelvicalyceal system. The purple portions form collecting duct and the yellow metanephric tissue cap develops into the nephron

genesis is complete. Thus, the structures originating from the metanephric blastema are, podocytes covering glomerular capillaries, epithelial cells lining Bowman's capsule, proximal convoluted tubules, the loop of Henle, and distal convoluted tubules.

Molecular Regulation and Genes Involved in Kidney Development

Mesenchymal (metanephric blastema) and epithelial (ureteric bud) elements are involved in the differentiation of cellular elements and formation of the kidney. These interactions are regulated by hundreds of genes involved in renal development. The mesenchyme expresses 'Wilms' tumor 1' gene (WT1) which enables it to respond to induction by the ureteric bud. 'Glial derived neurotropic factor' (GDNF) and 'hepatocyte growth factor' (HGF) genes produced by the mesenchyme interact through their receptors in the ureteric bud epithelium to stimulate growth of the ureteric bud.

Few other genes involved in nephrogenesis are given below.

Ascent of the Kidneys

The kidneys are initially located in the pelvic region. They, ascend to a lumbar site during the sixth to ninth weeks of development.

This ascent is caused by reduction of body curvature and by linear growth in the lumbar and sacral regions caudal to the kidneys. Initially the hilum of the kidneys faces ventrally (anteriorly), but as they ascend they rotate medially by almost 900 and finally the hila are directed almost medially or anteromedially (Fig. 8.6). The position of the kidneys become fixed once they come into contact with the suprarenal glands. Originally the metanephros is vascularized from a pelvic branch of the aorta, the common iliac arteries. However, as the kidneys ascend they are vascularized by a series of arterial sprouts from the dorsal aorta at higher levels. The lower blood vessels usually degenerate.

Development of the Urinary Bladder and Urethra

The cloaca, is a chamber-like distended portion in the terminal part of the hindgut and is endodermal in origin. This endoderm lined chamber continues as surface ectoderm at the cloacal membrane. The cloaca communicates with the allantois. During the fourth to seventh weeks of gestation, a urorectal septum develops dividing the cloaca into urogenital sinus anteriorly and anal canal posteriorly (Fig. 8.7).

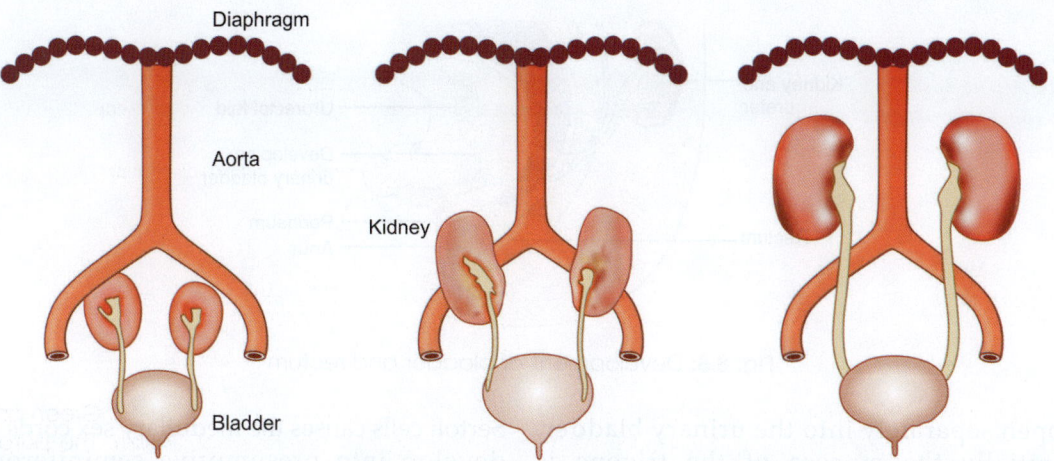

Fig. 8.6: Ascend of kidney from pelvic to lumbar location. The hilum of kidney faces anteriorly in the pelvic location. As it ascends, it rotates medially and the long axis is tilted so that the upper pole is nearer the midline. If the kidney has not ascended completely, the hilum would face anteromedially and the lower pole will be nearer the midline

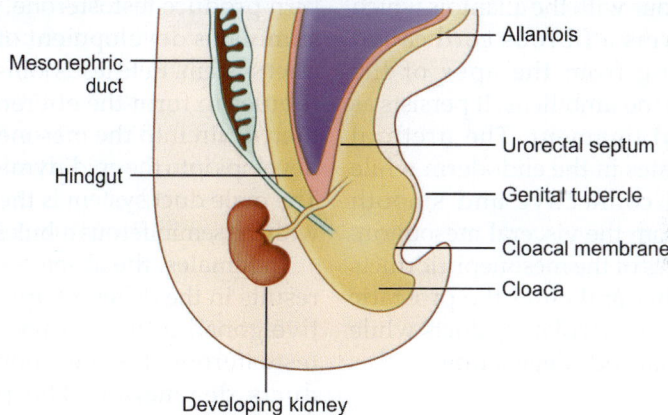

Fig. 8.7: The hindgut, cloaca and urorectal septum. The cloaca is divided into anterior part from which the bladder develops and posterior part which forms the rectum

The urogenital sinus itself is divided into three parts:
1. Vesical part—most of the urinary bladder develops from this part.
2. Pelvic part—the entire urethra in females develop from this part. In males, urethra at the bladder neck, prostatic and membranous urethra develop from the pelvic part of urogenital sinus.

3. Phallic part—grows towards the genital tubercle and develops as clitoris in females and the penis in males.

The urinary bladder develops mainly from the vesical part of the urogenital sinus, but the trigone is derived from the caudal ends of the mesonephric ducts which are absorbed into the wall of the bladder (Fig. 8.8). As the distal mesonephric ducts are absorbed, the ureters

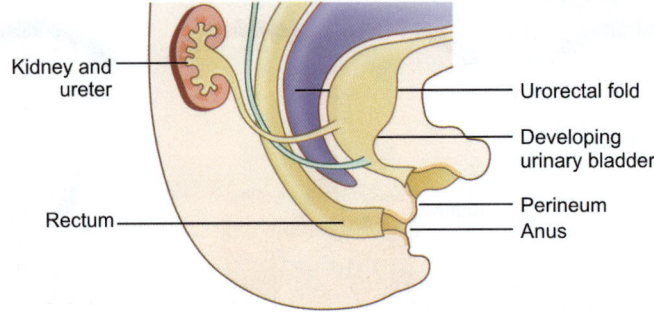

Fig. 8.8: Development of bladder and rectum

open separately into the urinary bladder. Initially the mucosa of the trigone is mesodermal but is replaced by endodermal epithelium similar to the rest of the urinary bladder. The other layers of the bladder wall develop from the adjacent splanchnic mesenchyme. Initially the lumen of the bladder is continuous with the allantois which contracts and forms a fibrous cord called urachus extending from the apex of the urinary bladder to the umbilicus. It persists as median umbilical ligament. The urethral epithelium originates in the endoderm while the surrounding connective and smooth muscle tissue is from the visceral mesoderm. In males, the orifices of the mesonephric ducts move close together and enter the prostatic part of the urethra as ejaculatory ducts while in females, the distal ends degenerate.

Development of Gonads

The male and female reproductive tracts—gonads and internal and external genitalia begin as bi-potential tissues until about sixth week of gestation. The gonads develop from three sources: The mesothelium (coelomic epithelium) lining the posterior abdominal wall, the underlying mesenchyme (intermediate mesoderm), and the primordial germ cells. The mesothelium proliferates to form the genital ridge medial to the mesonephros. From this epithelium primary sex cords penetrate the mesenchyme. In the male, SRY (sex reversal Y) protein produced by the

Sertoli cells causes the medullary sex cords to develop into presumptive seminiferous tubules and rete testis tubules and causes the cortical sex cords to regress. Antimüllerian hormone (AMH) produced by the Sertoli cells then causes the paramesonephric ducts to regress. Leydig cells also develop, which in turn produce testosterone, the hormone that stimulates development of the male genital duct system. Rete testis joins the mesonephros tubules to form the efferent ductules which then drain into the mesonephric duct which develops into the epididymis and vas deferens. The male duct system is therefore continuous with the seminiferous tubules (Figs 8.9 and 8.10).

In females, the absence of SRY expression results in the differentiation of the presumptive gonad into an ovary. In the absence of testosterone, the mesonephric tubules and ducts degenerate. The paramesonephric (müllerian) ducts develop next to the mesonephric ducts. The paramesonephric ducts and sinuvaginal bulb join to form uterus and vagina in females. The paramesonephric ducts (in the absence of AMH) form the fallopian tubes, uterus and upper part of the vagina. The inferior aspect of the uterovaginal canal forms the vagina. This occurs in the presence or absence of ovaries and therefore the internal female reproductive tract is independent of gonadal secretions, and is cell autonomous (Figs 8.9 to 8.11).

Both the testes and the ovaries descend from their original position in the thorax to a much lower level. The testes ultimately descend into the scrotum and the ovaries remain in the pelvis. The descent depends upon a structure called the gubernaculum. In males, testis is attached to gubernaculums, shortening of which brings it down to the inguinal canal and then into the scrotum.

Proliferation of mesoderm and ectoderm around the cloacal membrane produces primordial tissues of the external genitalia in both sexes: The genital tubercle, genital folds, and genital swellings. In males, the urogenital folds fuse, and the genital tubercle elongates to form the shaft and glans of the penis. A small region of the distal urethra is formed by the invagination of ectoderm covering the glans. The labioscrotal folds give rise to the scrotum. In females, the genital tubercle forms the clitoris, and the urogenital folds remain separated to form the labia minora. The labioscrotal folds form the labia majora.

Summary of Male Urogenital Tract Derivatives

- *Ureteric bud:* Ureter
- *Mesonephric ducts:* Rete testis, efferent ducts, epididymis, vas deferens, seminal vesicle, trigone of bladder.
- *Urogenital sinus:* Bladder (except trigone), prostate gland, bulbourethral gland, urethra.

Summary of Female Urogenital Tract Derivatives

- *Ureteric bud:* Ureter
- *Mesonephric ducts:* Trigone of bladder

- *Paramesonephric ducts:* Oviduct, uterus, upper one-third of vagina.
- *Urogenital sinus:* Bladder (except trigone), bulbourethral gland, urethra, lower two-thirds of vagina.

Development of the Suprarenal Glands

The adrenal glands develop from two separate embryological tissues: The medulla is derived from neural crest cells originating in proximity to the dorsal aorta, while the cortex develops from the intermediate mesoderm. The bilateral adrenogonadal primordium (AGP) first appears as a thickening of the coelomic epithelium between the urogenital ridge and the dorsal mesentery. Each AGP contains a mixed population of adrenocortical and somatic gonadal progenitor cells. A subset of AGP cells that express higher levels of steroidogenic factor 1 (SF1) migrate dorso-medially to form the adrenal anlagen ultimately settling ventrolateral to the dorsal aorta.

Development of the adrenal cortex: Arises mostly from intermediate mesoderm in the lumbar region of the embryo.

Development of the adrenal medulla: Trunk neural crest cells migrate into the center of the adrenal glands and develop into the chromaffin cells of the adrenal medulla. These cells are essentially postganglionic sympathetic neurons that release epinephrine or norepinephrine directly into the bloodstream as opposed to innervating a target organ.

Congenital Anomalies of the Kidney and Urinary Tract

• R Hema

Congenital anomalies of the kidney and urinary tract (CAKUT) constitute approximately 20–30% of all anomalies detected in the prenatal period. The broad spectrum of anomalies ranges from mild asymptomatic malformations such as double ureter, unascended kidney, horseshoe kidney or minimal pelviureteric junction obstruction to severe life-threatening pathologies like bilateral renal agenesis or severe renal dysplasia.

The kidney and urinary tract develop from two structures, the metanephros (mesenchymal origin) and ureteric bud (epithelial origin). Three important events are involved in the normal development. They are induction of metanephric tissue, ascend of kidneys from pelvic location to lumbar location and the rotation of kidneys. These three events usually occur in the first 8 weeks of intrauterine life. Abnormality in development can affect the presence, the number and the location of the kidneys. The term "urinary obstruction" is being replaced by the term "urine flow impairment" (UFI) since this term correctly describes the 'functional' obstruction. Congenital disorders causing UFI occur in areas where two or more embryologic structures fuse. For example: Calicotubular junction, pelviureteral junction, ureterovesical junction and vesicourethral junction.

Renal Agenesis, Dysplasia and Abnormal Position

Unilateral or bilateral renal agenesis occurs in approximately 1 in 1000 live births. Bilateral renal agenesis may be sporadic or part of a syndrome like Brachio-oto-renal syndrome. Renal agenesis may be associated with vaginal or rectal atresia. Unilateral or bilateral dysplasia may be associated with cystic changes in the kidneys (Fig. 9.1). Anomalies related to abnormal ascent of kidneys (ectopic kidneys) may result in pelvic, iliac or even thoracic kidney. The orientation, axis and rotation of the kidney are often abnormal and may often be detected as an incidental finding.

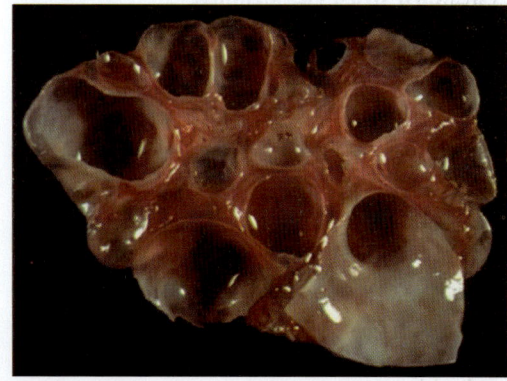

Fig. 9.1: Multicystic dysplastic kidney. Dysplastic kidney in a newborn. *Note:* Small kidneys, cortical cysts and parenchymal thinning

Associated anomalies in other systems or other parts of genitourinary system may also be present. They may remain asymptomatic and be detected incidentally or present with symptoms suggestive of urinary infection, colic, stone formation, obstruction, reflux or hypertension. If these kidneys are associated with impaired drainage or reflux, surgery is indicated.

Horseshoe Kidneys and Fused Kidneys

This anomaly is related to abnormal fusion of the kidneys and the incidence is 1 in 400 to 1800 autopsies. It is more common in males. In 95% of the cases the lower poles of both kidneys are joined by a bridge of tissue (isthmus) consisting of normal or dysplastic renal or fibrous tissue. Most cases have associated anomalies in other systems. IVU is diagnostic and shows malrotation of each kidney. Normally, the axis of the kidney, which represents a line joining the upper and lower pole, if projected upwards will meet each other at the level of the mid-thoracic vertebra. Because of the malrotation, the upper ureters are displaced laterally, the ascent is incomplete, the long axis is divergent upwards and it converges towards the sacrum. The upward ascend of the horseshoe kidney is prevented at the level of inferior mesenteric artery just below the L4 vertebra because of the isthmus (Fig. 9.2). Since the kidneys cannot rotate normally because of incomplete ascend, some degree of malrotation invariably coexists.

Horseshoe kidneys may be associated with pelviureteric junction obstruction or vesicoureteral reflux. The prognosis depends on associated anomalies. Though most cases are asymptomatic, associated PUJ obstruction is common. Nephrolithiasis, abnormal vasculature or dysplastic tissue may produce UTI, pain, hypertension or hematuria necessitating surgical intervention. Horseshoe kidneys are also at increased risk for development of tumors. Associated PUJ obstruction is corrected

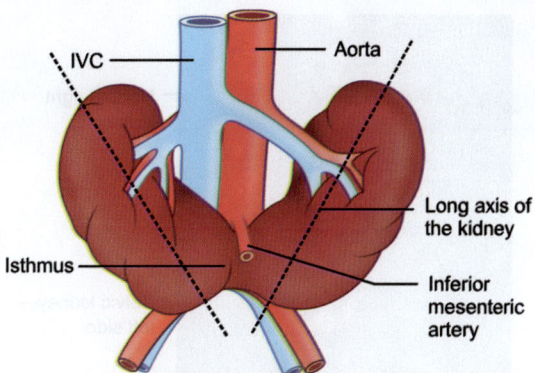

Fig. 9.2: Horseshoe kidney—long axis of normal and horseshoe kidney and arrest of ascend horseshoe kidney. The ascent of the kidney is arrested due to the presence of the isthmus and inferior mesenteric artery. Long axis of normal kidney deviates away from midline inferiorly

by the classical pyeloplasty technique although other alternatives are ureterocalicostomy and endopyelotomy.

Rarely, renal fusion occurs in such a way that both kidneys are on the same side and one of the ureters crosses the midline to join the bladder at the trigone on the opposite side. This is called crossed renal ectopia. The fused kidneys may have different shapes/outlines depending on the site of fusion, e.g. S-shaped kidney or L-shaped kidney.

Ectopic Kidney

Ectopic kidney can be present inside the pelvis, at the pelvic brim, retroperitoneal space below normal location, thorax or even the opposite side. The commonest location is in the pelvis or the pelvic brim (Fig. 9.3).

Ureteral Duplication

Ureteral duplication may be complete or incomplete. Normally, one ureteric bud enters the metanephric blastema resulting in the development of kidney and ureter on each side. Bifid renal pelvis and 'Y' ureter are types of incomplete duplication and result from early or late bifurcation of ureteric bud. Since the lower part of the ureter is single, it opens

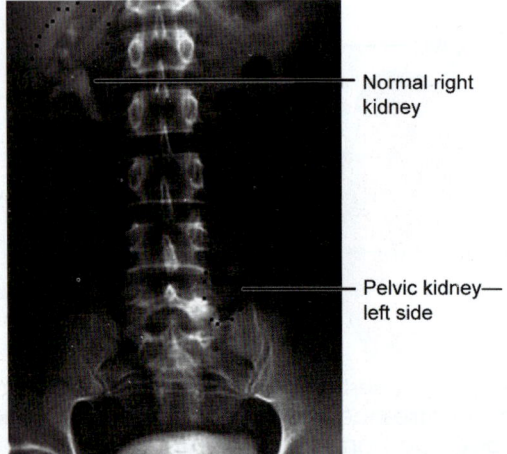

Fig. 9.3: IVU in pelvic kidney. *Note:* Functioning pelvic kidney on left side over the sacrum and side of L5 vertebra (renal outline marked)

into the normal position in the trigone. If the ureteric bud arises in a more cranial or caudal in position, its opening in the bladder is also abnormal (Fig. 9.4).

If two ureteric buds arise on one side and develop completely, complete ureteric duplication occurs. In that case, only one of the ureters

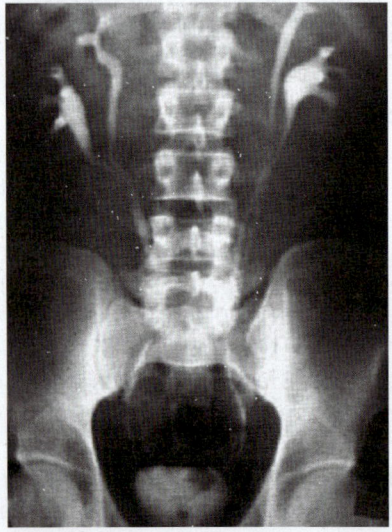

Fig. 9.4: Bilateral ureteric duplication—intravenous urogram. On the right side, both moieties join at midureteric level and on left side, at a lower level

will have the normal opening at the trigone. The other bud opens ectopically. As the mesonephric duct with the ureteric buds is taken up into the urogenital sinus, the distal ureter draining the lower segment is absorbed into the bladder and will then enter the bladder in a higher and lateral position resulting in vesicoureteric reflux. The more cranial bud draining the upper moiety is incorporated into the developing bladder in a more distal location and hence, the ureter draining the upper part of the kidney open in an ectopic position—in the bladder, urethra or vagina in a female or into the bladder, urethra, vas or epididymis in the male. This phenomenon of the ureter draining the upper moiety opening more distally, medially and ectopically and the ureter draining the lower moiety opening cranially, laterally and in the trigone is the 'Weigert-Meyer rule'.

Asymptomatic patients in whom the anomalies are detected incidentally are kept under observation only. In symptomatic patients with recurrent UTI, reimplantation of the ureter may be done. In ureteric duplication, if the affected moiety is nonfunctioning, partial nephrectomy is the treatment of choice. Partial nephrectomy with ureteropyeloanastomosis can also be done laparoscopically.

Ureteroceles

These are dilatations of terminal ureter that project into the bladder (Figs 9.5 and 9.6). It may be unilateral or bilateral and the intravesical projections can be visualized by USG, IVU (Fig. 9.7), MCU or cystoscopy. When there is duplex collecting system, it often involves the ureter draining the upper pole. UTI is the commonest presentation. Uncomplicated ureteroceles are managed by endoscopic deflation whereas; some children may require ureteric reimplantation. If the function of the part of the kidney drained by the affected ureter is sometimes poor and heminephrectomy is indicated.

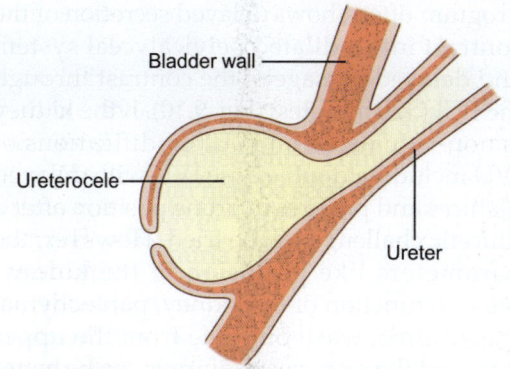

Fig. 9.5: Schematic diagram of ureterocele. Note the dilatation of the terminal ureter before its opening into the bladder

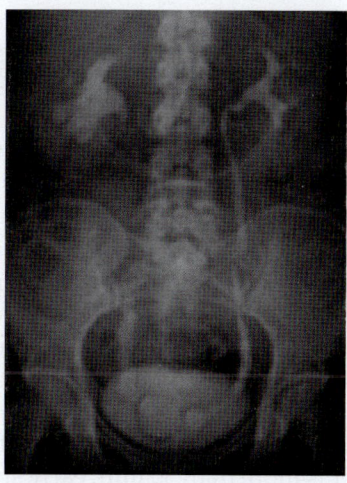

Fig. 9.7: IVU in bilateral ureterocele. Terminal ureteric dilatation inside the bladder due to bilateral ureterocele

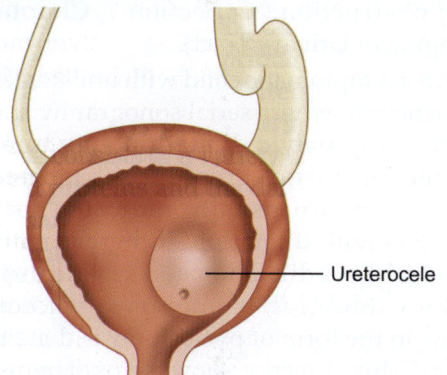

Fig. 9.6: Cystoscopic appearance of ureterocele. Note the bulb-like projection into the bladder lumen due to ureterocele

Ectopic Ureter

Ectopic ureter is more common in females. Urinary dribbling along with normal micturition is the classical symptom. Recurrent UTI may occur. In ectopic single ureters, ureteric reimplantation along with bladder neck reconstruction may be necessary.

Pelviureteric Junction Anomalies

Anomalies of pelviureteric junction are common and occasional familial clustering seen in such cases may be attributed to autosomal dominant inheritance with variable penetrance. Three varieties of PUJ abnormalities

are encountered and are due to intraparietal, parietal and extraparietal causes. Extraparietal causes include extrinsic compression of PUJ by aberrant vessels, kinks, bands and adhesions. The causes in the wall (parietal) are the most common and are caused due to abnormal distribution of muscular and collagen fibers at the junction (Fig. 9.8). Intraparietal causes are

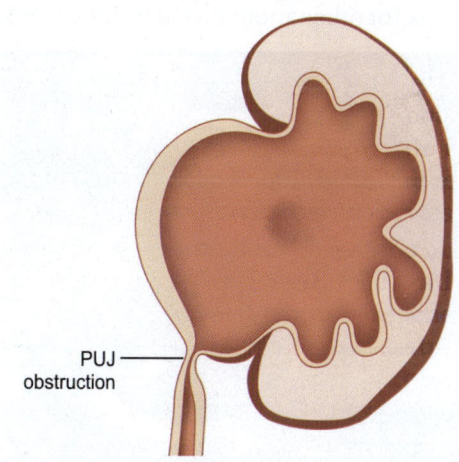

Fig. 9.8: Pelviureteric junction obstruction with dilatation of upper collecting system. Note the narrowing at the junction of renal pelvis and ureter (PUJ) and dilatation of renal pelvis

rare and are due to valves or polyps. Antenatal pelvic dilatation may be physiological or pathological. It is usually considered pathological if it is bilateral, associated with oligohydramnios or persists after 18 weeks of gestation. In such cases, serial ultrasound studies from neonatal period are mandatory.

In children, the common clinical presentations are loin pain, abdominal mass, infection or hematuria following trivial trauma. Serial abdominal ultrasonography and measurement of anteroposterior diameter of the renal pelvis in the transverse axis help to assess the severity and decide the treatment. If the AP diameter is more than 50 mm, early surgery is indicated. If the AP diameter is 20–50 mm, it is suggests moderate dilatation. Early pyeloplasty is undertaken if the relative renal function by renogram is less than 30%. In those with more than 30% renal function, surgery is indicated on follow-up if they become symptomatic, develop urinary infection, have worsening of renal functions on that side or if dilatation increases. The dilated pelvicalyceal system shows the typical "micky mouse appearance" on ultrasound (Fig. 9.9).

The USG also helps to rule out dilation of the ureters, assess the echogenicity of kidneys and look for other anomalies. The intravenous urogram often shows delayed secretion of the contrast into a dilated pelvicalyceal system and delayed passage of the contrast through the PUJ (>20 minutes) (Fig. 9.10). If the kidney is non-visualized on IVU, modifications of IVU including double dose IVU with delayed pictures and pictures in prone position after a diuretic challenge can be tried. However, the parameters like perfusion of the kidney, relative function of the kidney, parenchymal transit time, wash out time from the upper tract and the response to diuretic can be better studied by isotope renography. The renogram curves using Tc 99m DTPA or MAG3 shows decrease perfusion and hold up in the collecting system with an ascending drainage curve in PUJ obstruction (*see* Section 1, Chapter 6: Imaging of Urinary Tract).

An asymptomatic child with unilateral PUJ obstruction, where serial sonography shows decreasing pelvic dilatation may be kept under follow-up. Prophylactic long-term antibiotics are usually indicated for all patients with dilatation. If there is marked pelvicalyceal dilatation and viability of the kidney doubtful, temporary diversion or urine in the form of pyelostomy is done first. If the kidney function shows signs of improvement in 3–4 weeks, pyeloplasty may be

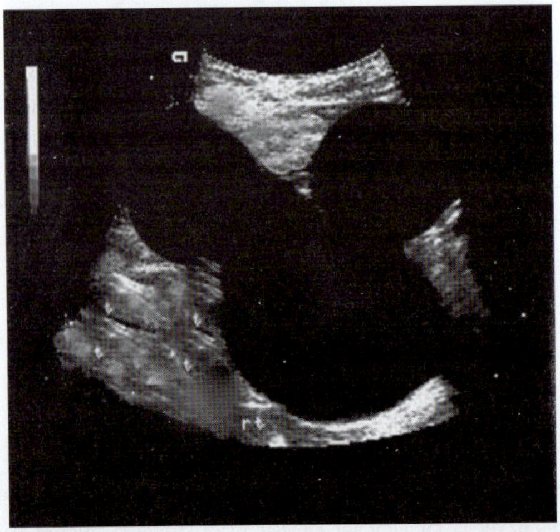

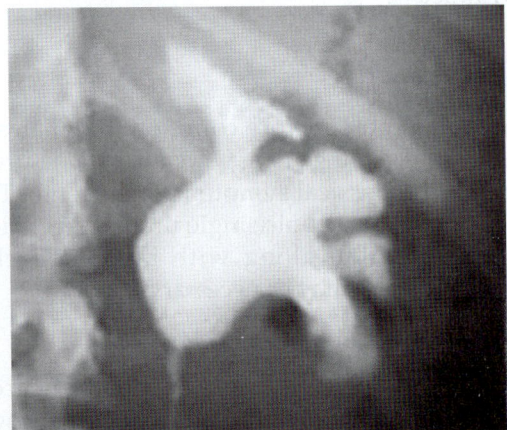

Fig. 9.9: Typical USG in PUJ. "Mickey mouse" appearance in pelviureteric junction obstruction

Fig. 9.10: Typical IVU in PUJ. IVU showing the dilated renal pelvis and clubbed calyces with narrowing at PUJ

undertaken later. In bilateral cases, surgical intervention is done first on the side with lesser function as seen on renogram. Subsequently on serial follow-up, if the dilatation on the opposite side does not subside, pyeloplasty may be considered.

The usual surgical procedures considered for PUJ obstruction are Anderson-Hyne's dismembered pyeloplasty by open technique. The procedure involves excision of reductant renal pelvis along with PUJ and re-approximation of ureter to pelvis in a dependent position. It can be done laparoscopically. Endoscopic procedures are endopyelotomy which involves cutting and enlarging the narrow area with the help of an endoscope and endo-balloon rupture to dilate the narrow segment.

Prune-belly Syndrome

Prune-belly syndrome is characterized by congenital deficiency of the anterior abdominal wall musculature associated with bilateral undescended testes and dilated urinary tract. During intrauterine life, gross dilation of urinary system results in poor development of abdominal wall musculature. Even if the dilated system is corrected the anterior abdominal wall shows a characteristic wrinkled appearance.

Posterior Urethral Valve (PUV)

Posterior urethral valve is the commonest cause of obstruction below the level of the bladder. It is due to the obstruction of lumen of the proximal urethra by mucosal folds arising from the inferior urethral crest. With straining and repeated attempts at voiding, the edges of folds become taut and stretched and the obstruction becomes complete and the posterior urethra dilates (Fig. 9.11). This leads to dysfunction of all the segments of urinary tract. Uncomplicated cases recover completely with early endoscopic ablation of the valves. In complicated cases, the bladder pressure may not return to normal, ureteral drainage may not improve and renal

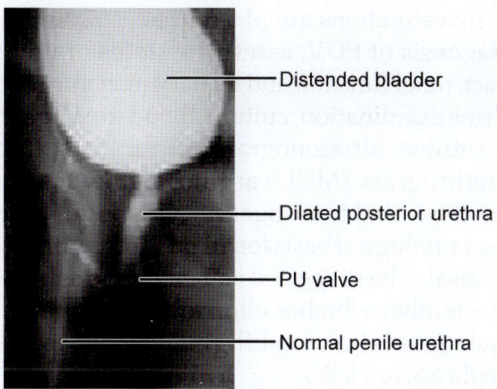

Distended bladder

Dilated posterior urethra

PU valve

Normal penile urethra

Fig. 9.11: Micturating cystourethrogram in posterior urethral valve. Note the dilated posterior urethra, position of posterior urethral valve and near-normal caliber of distal urethra

parenchymal damage may be permanent even if the obstruction is relieved. Antenatal diagnosis of PUV is common these days and early intervention is rewarding. *In utero* procedures are possible in highly developed centers. Those with infections or delayed diagnosis develop end stage renal failure by late teens and others often later. Prognosis improves with early intervention. Antenatally diagnosed cases must be subjected to valve fulguration in the neonatal period itself for best long-term results.

PUV is often suspected in any male child with lower urinary symptoms like weak or interrupted urinary stream, wetting, dribbling and straining, crying at every act of voiding or documented urinary tract infection. Often, other unrelated symptoms may be the presenting manifestation in some cases. Fever, failure to thrive, vomiting, diarrhea, malaise, irritability or convulsions may be the presenting manifestations. Distension of lower abdomen due to enlarged urinary bladder may be noted. Some patients with PUV may present with renal failure, renal rickets, ascites, growth retardation or features of renal tubular acidosis. Others present classically with "three masses" in the abdomen—two hydronephrotic kidneys and an enlarged bladder.

Investigations are planned to establish the diagnosis of PUV, assess the status of upper tract, renal function and urinary tract infection. Urine examination, culture, blood urea, serum creatinine, ultrasonogram, micturating cysto-urethrogram (MCU) and isotope renogram are the initial investigations. MCU provides the radiological basis for the diagnosis of PUV. It can also be suspected in the antenatal period in a mother who has oligohydramnios with a male fetus showing bilateral hydrouretero-nephrosis on USG.

Early infancy is the most important period of development and growth in neonatal kidney and any damage may be permanent. The stasis should be corrected at the earliest so that the renal function may recover. Even antenatal interventions are possible in highly developed centers. After assessment, the newborns with PUV are divided into two groups those with favorable and unfavourable course. Full-term babies with no azotemia, unilateral or no reflux, minimal ureterectasis and good renal function have favorable outcome. They are managed by valve ablation and are put on serial observation. They may be taken up for subsequent reconstructive procedures as needed.

Newborns with azotemia, bilateral VUR, grossly dilated ureters, poor renal function with dysplastic kidneys (loss of cortico-medullary differentiation in USS) constitute the unfavorable group. They are given a trial period of about 5 days with fluid and electrolyte replacement, antibiotics and continuous bladder drainage. Those who respond are managed by diversion of urine from the bladder by vesicostomy. These patients are taken up subsequently for valve ablation and closure of vesicostomy. If the response to bladder catheterization is inadequate, the child is taken up for ureteric diversion followed by valve ablation and reconstructive procedures later.

The short-term prognosis for boys with PUV is very good. Increasing awareness, early diagnosis, timely referral, improvements in diagnostic imaging, anesthetic and neonatal cares have contributed to the improved outlook. The poor prognostic factors for long-term prognosis are:

1. Bilateral VUR at the time of presentation.
2. Daytime urinary incontinence persisting after 5 years of age.
3. Urinary tract infection.

When renal mass is reduced and the number of nephrons cannot increase, there is, hyperfiltration by the surviving nephrons in an attempt to maintain the GFR. Hyperfiltration causes progressive renal damage. So, all patients with PUV are followed up serially throughout childhood, puberty and adult life. Tests for evaluation of proteinuria, renal function, blood pressure, urine culture, ultra-sonogram, isotope renogram and uroflow studies are carried out. The judicious use of antihypertensive drugs, alkali supplements (Shohl's solution or sodium bicarbonate), vitamin D, calcium, antibiotics, diet and other medical lines of treatment supports the patients own renal function and sustain the patients longer. Ultimately many of these patients develop end stage renal failure and may need renal transplantation. Transplantation is performed after the bladder function is thoroughly assessed by urodynamic studies.

Vesicoureteral Reflux (VUR)

This denotes retrograde flow of urine from bladder to the ureter. In mild cases, the reflux may occur only during micturition. In severe cases, urine will enter the ureter whenever the bladder is full. In a patient with UTI, VUR leads to the passage of the infected urine into the ureter and renal pelvis. Thus, the bacteria gain access into the kidney and lead to pyelo-nephritis and renal scars. The irreversible damage to the renal parenchyma leading to focal or generalized renal scaring is called "reflux nephropathy".

The normal vesicoureteric junction prevents the reflux of urine from the bladder to the ureters. The ureter enters the bladder through an oblique submucosal tunnel. The ratio of the submucosal tunnel length to the diameter of ureter is 4:1 or 5:1. Thus, there is a flap-valve mechanism preventing the reflux. In many cases of VUR, the ratio of submucosal tunnel length to the diameter of ureter is less than 3:1 and the flap-valve mechanism is deficient. Anatomically abnormal ureterovesical junction is seen in bladder of children with prune-belly syndrome, paraureteral diverticula, ureterocele and ectopic ureters. In neurogenic bladder, the elevated intravesical storage and voiding pressures often lead to decompensation at ureterovesical junction and VUR.

The residual urine in the bladder predisposes to UTI which further aggravates the VUR resulting in a vicious cycle of events. UTI should be diagnosed at the earliest using a properly collected specimen. This is either a suprapubic aspirated or catheter-collected sample in infants and a clean-catch specimen in older children. Significant bacteriuria is defined as the presence of more than 100,000 colony forming units per ml. Micturating cystourethrography is the radiological investigation of choice and is done 2–3 weeks after control of UTI (Fig. 9.12). Nuclear voiding cystourethrography is better than the conventional MCU because of lesser radiation. The upper tract is evaluated using isotope renograms.

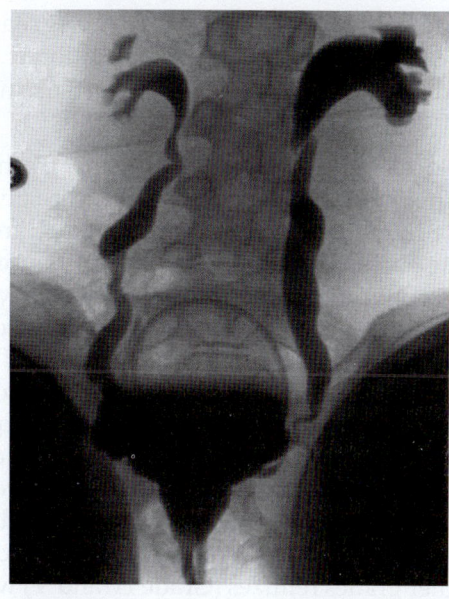

Fig. 9.12: MCU showing bilateral grade 5 reflux. *Note:* Reflux of urine while micturition. Both ureters are visualized full length, are dilated and tortuous with clubbing of calyces

VUR is graded into 5 grades as per the international system based on MCU is shown in Fig. 9.13 .

Grade I	Partial filling of an undilated lower ureter
Grade II	Total filling of an undilated ureter
Grade III	Dilated calyces but fornices sharp

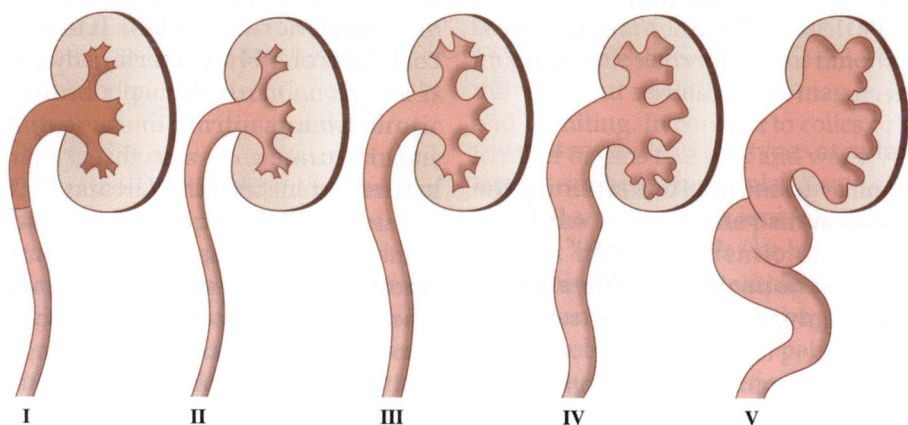

Fig. 9.13: Grading of vesicoureteric reflux

Grade IV   Blunted fornices and greater degree of ureteric dilatation

Grade V   Massive hydronephrosis and dilated tortuous ureter.

Since eradication of UTI prevents fresh or progressive renal injury, antibiotics are given according to sensitivity results obtained from urine culture. In patients with reflux, long-term continuous antibiotic prophylaxis with periodic urinary screening is the cornerstone of treatment. Cases with grade I to III reflux are managed conservatively with antibiotic prophylaxis and multiple micturition technique. In multiple micturition technique the child is trained to perform the micturition act twice or thrice in the same session so that the residual urine if any is expelled out from the bladder. Higher grades refluxes (Grade IV and V) with breakthrough infection, anatomic abnormalities at UV junction and non-compliance with medical management are indications for surgery. Ureteric reimplantation is the surgical method of choice and it relies on the principle of creating a ureteral tunnel with a tunnel length to ureteral diameter ratio of approximately 5:1 (Cohen's transtrigonal technique or Politano-Leadbetter technique). The submucosal injection of Teflon at the vesicoureteric junction through a cystoscope has a success rate of 80% and is gaining popularity. Annual renal imagining with Tc 99m DMSA is performed to monitor renal growth. Patients with documented renal scarring should have a thorough work-up for early detection of renal failure.

Megaureter

Megaureter is abnormally dilated ureter. Ureteroceles and some ectopic ureters also result in megaureters. Megaureters are also seen secondary to posterior urethral valves and neurogenic bladder. There are two main types of megaureters, obstructed and refluxing. Obstructive megaureters result from an intrinsic abnormality in the lower ureter. There is lack of development of muscle in the ureteric wall which results in an adynamic segment and gross dilatation of ureter. UTI is the commonest clinical presentation. Management consists of excision of the adynamic segment, tailoring of the dilated ureter (in severe cases) and ureteroneo-cystostomy. Refluxing megaureter is due to grade 5 vesicoureteric reflux and the management is as for the primary cause.

Antenatally Diagnosed Hydronephrosis

With the advent of antenatal ultrasonography, more and more cases of antenatally detected hydronephrosis are identified. About 1% of all pregnancies may be associated with antenatal hydronephrosis. Howevere, nearly 50% resolves spontaneously and the other cases have to be periodically monitored and surgical treatment undertaken if indicated. The following questions are considered before deciding on the management of these cases.

1. Is an obstruction present?
2. Which kidney will deteriorate and produce symptoms later?
3. How to safety follow-up these children?
4. If surgery is needed, what is the optimum time to carry this out?

There are two groups of patients with antenatal hydronephrosis. One group has unilateral hydronephrosis and the other bilateral hydronephrosis. Hydronephrosis is usually due to posterior urethral valve and vesicoureteric reflux (VUR). It may occur due to bilateral pelviureteric junction (PUJ) obstruction. Once hydronephrosis is confirmed by ultrasonography in the first few weeks of life, micturating cystourethrogram (MCU) is carried out to rule out VUR and PUV. In case of bilateral PUJ obstruction, the side with the greater dilatation or lesser function is operated first. The opposite side may recover spontaneously if compensatory hypertrophy was responsible. Contralateral pyeloplasty is carried out later only if significant hydro-nephrosis persists on that side. In unilateral hydronephrosis, the first postnatal ultrasonogram is performed in the first 72 hours. The anteroposterior (AP) diameter of the kidney in the transverse plane is measured. If it is less than 20 mm, they need regular follow-up with ultrasound study at 1 month, 3 months, 6 months and 1 year to confirm stabilization or to detect a significant increase in hydronephrosis. Isotope study may be combined with USS in those cases with AP diameter between 13 mm and 19 mm to confirm stabilization or deterioration. In case with AP diameter >20 mm, isotope renogram is done at 1 month of age. Further management depends on differential renal function as seen in the renogram. Those with <10% function may end up in nephrectomy and for those with function between 11 and 30% early pyeloplasty is offered. Those with 31–50% renal function are followed up with USS and isotope renogram periodically (at 3 months, 6 months, 1 year and yearly). An increasing hydronephrosis, 10% drop in renal function or drop to <40% or appearance of symptoms warrant surgery in this group.

Renal Cystic Disease

Cystic kidneys in children include:

a. Simple cysts
b. Due to developmental anomalies
   1. Multicystic dysplastic kidneys (MCDK)
   2. Medullary sponge kidney (MSK)
c. Genetic
   1. Autosomal recessive infantile polycystic kidney disease
   2. Autosomal dominant polycystic kidney disease (ADPKD)
   3. Medullary cystic kidney disease.
d. Cysts associated with systemic diseases: Tuberous sclerosis.

Renal trauma accounts for 30–40% of all injuries to the tract. The following anatomical characters of the child's kidneys increase the risk for injury.

1. The kidneys are larger in relation to the size of the child's body and are situated at a lower position in the abdomen.
2. The musculature of the abdominal wall is weaker and the rib cage is incompletely ossified.
3. The renal capsule and Gerota's fascia are less developed creating a greater potential for laceration, bleeding and urinary extravasation.
4. Congenitally abnormal kidneys are more susceptible to trauma and the relative mobility of the kidney causes disruption of PUJ in deceleration injuries.

Injuries in stable patients with hematuria only are managed conservatively. Major injuries like vascular disruption necessitate immediate surgery.

Extrophy Epispadias Complex

Extrophy epispadias complex is more common in males. The basic defect is an abnormal over development of the cloacal membrane. This prevents migration of mesenchymal tissue and proper development of anerior abdominal wall. The separation of pubic symphysis is associated with maldevelopment of the anterior wall of the bladder resulting in visualization of raw red posterior wall of the baldder below the umbilicus. Undescended testis and herniae may occur as associated anomalies. An anteriorly displaced anus, weak pelvic floor and rectal prolapse are also seen. Foreshortened penis in males and bifid clitoris in females are the classical findings. Staged reconstruction is started in the immediate neonatal period followed by the repair of bladder, sphincter and urethral reconstruction.

Tumors

Nephroblastoma (Wilms' tumor) is the commonest renal malignancy in children. Pathologically, the tumor is triphasic and consists of all the 3 elements—blastemal, tubular and stromal elements. Children with various congenital anomalies like sporadic aniridia, Beckwith-Wiedemann syndrome, WAGR syndrome and Denys-Drash syndrome have an increased predisposition to Wilms' tumor. Several tumor-suppressor genes have been associated with Wilms' tumor and inactivation of these genes produce the tumor. Children with Wilms' tumor usually present with a painless, abdominal mass. Contrast-enhanced CT abdomen confirms the diagnosis. X-ray chest or CT chest reveals the presence of the secondaries. Operative removal of the kidney with the tumor (nephroureterectomy) is the treatment of choice during which staging of the tumor is also done. Pathologically, these tumors are grouped into those with favorable and unfavorable histology and subsequent chemotherapy and radiotherapy are planned accordingly.

Common Renal Diseases in Children

• K Phadke • Sanjeev Gulati

- Neonatal nephrology and neonatal AKI
- Infection related glomerulonephritis in children.
- Nephrotic syndrome in children
- Hypertension in children
- Approach to hematuria in children
- Cystic diseases of the kidney
- Renal replacement therapy in children
- Pediatric renal transplantation

In this chapter only some aspects of renal disease specific to children are discussed under the headings as above. For a detailed discussion of these conditions please refer to the specific chapters elsewhere in this book.

NEONATAL NEPHROLOGY AND NEONATAL AKI

Even though nephronogenesis is complete by 36 weeks of gestation, GFR at birth is less than 25 ml/min/1.73 m² body surface area. The GFR increases by 50–100% in the first week of life and reaches the adult value of 125 ml/min/1.73 m² by 2 years. All normal infants void within 48 hours of birth, 90% of them within 24 hours. The average urine output in the first 48 hours is 30–60 ml/day and it increases to about 200 ml/day at the end of first week. The urine concentrating ability of newborns is limited and reaches adult values by 1 year. The GFR at birth is low and the infant cannot excrete large volumes of administered hypotonic fluids like 5% dextrose eventhough the diluting capacity is matured at birth. In preterm babies the GFR at birth is low, about 10–20 ml/min/1.73 m² (Table 10.1). Low birth weight infants usually are oliguric during the first 24 hours and polyuric during the 24–72 hours. Subsequently, an adaptive phase occurs during which the kidney adapts to the volume of fluid intake. The serum creatinine in preterm babies are usually higher than full-term babies.

Serum creatinine in the newborn reflects maternal levels immediately after birth. It takes 3–5 days for serum creatinine to reflect

Table 10.1: Parameters of renal function in neonates and infants

	Preterm baby	Term baby			
	1st 3 days	1st 3 days	2 weeks	8 weeks	1 year
Daily urine excretion ml/kg/day	15–75	20–75	25–120	80–130	40–100
Max. urine osmolality: mOsm/kg	400–500	600–800	800–900	1000–1200	1200–1400
GFR: ml/min/1.73 sq.m	10–15	15–20	35–45	75–80	90–110

Table 10.2: Etiology of neonatal AKI

Prerenal AKI (80%)	Intrinsic AKI (15%)	Post-renal AKI (5%)
Hypovolemia—dehydration, shock	Acute tubular necrosis or cortical necrosis	PU valve
Asphyxia/hypoxia	Renal vein thrombosis	Infravesical obstruction
Low output cardiac failure, coarctation of aorta	Congenital renal anomalies—dysplasia, cystic disease	Bilateral ureteral obstruction
Pharmacologic—ACE inhibitors, NSAIDs, vasodilators (tolazoline)	Toxic nephropathies—radiocontrasts, aminoglycosides, hemoglobinuria/myoglobinuria	Neurogenic bladder, obstruction Acute pyelonephritis

the actual neonatal renal function. In a healthy term baby the serum cretinine at one week is 0.5 mg%. A useful clinical pointer to renal insufficiency in the newborn is the absence of expected postnatal decline in serum creatinine. Blood urea above 40 mg/dl and creatinine above 1 mg/dl in the newborn indicates renal failure.

Because of increased awareness and improved facilities, more cases of neonatal acute renal failure are recongnised now. In the neonatal intensive care units, the incidence of renal failure varies from 8 to 22%. Renal function test have to be monitored serially because the urine output may not indicate the onset or the severity of renal failure. 65 to 75% of ARF in neonates is of the non-oliguric variety. The criteria for oliguria in neonatal period is urine output less than 0.5 ml/kg/hour for at least 24 hours (normal—1.5–3 ml/kg/hour). As in adults, the causes of neonatal ARF are classified as prerenal, renal and post-renal (Table 10.2).

Evaluation

Antenatal history of oligohydramnios or an abnormal antenatal ultrasound is importrant. Potter's facies (Fig. 10.1), ear anomalies, single umbilical artery, imperforate anus, myelo-meningocele and cryptorchidism should be looked for. Urethral obstruction should be ruled out if bladder and kidneys are palpable. Bilateral palpable kidneys in a polycythemic infant of diabetic mother may indicate renal vein thrombosis. Renal hypoperfusion is the

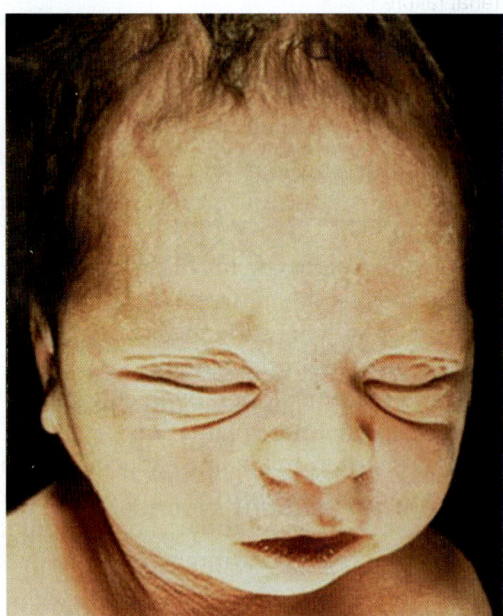

Fig. 10.1: Potter facies. *Note:* Low set ears

commonest cause of neonatal ARF. The baby is assessed for evidence of hypovolemia, hypotension and hypoxia. If the urine output is less than 0.5 ml/kg/hr and there are no signs of volume overload, samples are sent for urinary sodium and osmolality before starting treatment if facilities are available. The baby should be given 20 ml/kg of isotonic saline over 30–60 minutes. If the urine output increases in next 2 hours to (more than 2 ml/kg/hr) the diagnosis of prerenal ARF is likely. When no diuresis ensues, fluid challenge may be repeated if there are no signs of fluid overload. After volume correction a single IV

Table 10.3: Showing the indices in prerenal ARF *vs* established ATN in newborn (corresponding values in older children and adults in bracket)

Parameter	Prerenal	ATN
Urine specific gravity	>1012/(>1020)	<1014/(<1015)
Urine Na (mEq/L)	<20	>50/(>40)
Urine osmolality (mOsm/kg)	>350/(>500)	<300/(<350)
Urine plasma osmolality	>1.2	<0.8–1.2
Blood urea/creatinine	>30	<20
U/P creatinine	>29+16	<10 + 4
FE Na (%)	<3/(<1)	>3 (>1)
Renal failure index	<3/(<1)	>3 (>1)

dose of frusemide (2 mg/kg) is given. If there is no improvement, the diagnosis is intrinsic (established) acute renal failure. The values for Fractional excretion of Na (FE Na) and renal failure index which help to differentiate prerenal failure from acute tubular necrosis are different in preterm and term neonates compared to older children and adults (Table 10.3).

Urinalysis may show RBCs, WBCs, casts and proteinuria in intrinsic ARF. Renal ultrasonography often reveals congenital anomalies, renal size, echogenicity, location, presence of cysts, dilatation of pelvicalyceal system and status of bladder. Mild obstructive lesions can however be missed in the first 3–5 days due to 'non-filled up' urinary tract. The scan may have to be repeated in suspected cases after a week. A DTPA/MAG3 scan can define split kidney function and indicate obstruction. DTPA renogram is unlikely to yield significant information in neonates with renal failure. It will give useful information only after one month of age. Blood urea, serum creatinine, calcium, phosphorus, sodium, potassium and bicarbonate should be serially monitored.

Treatment

The underlying cause of renal failure should be ascertained and treated. The aim is to stabilize the baby and limit complications. It consists of maintaining fluid, electrolyte and acid–base balance, proper nutrition, identification and treatment of complications. Fluids should be restricted to insensible, renal and extrarenal losses. Insensible losses in full-term baby is 20–25 ml/kg per day and in low birth weight infants, >50 ml/kg/day. Strict intake output chart is mandatory. Baby must be weighed 12 hourly. Capillary refill time, core to peripheral temperature gap, BP and CVP monitoring can assess the adequacy of circulation. Improving renal perfusion and urine output by dopamine and/or frusemide (1–2 mg/kg/day) may facilitate maintenance of adequate fluid balance. Hypertonic glucose via central line may be given if fluids need to be limited. Total parenteral nutrition may be started if enteral feeds are contraindicated. Breastfeeds or expressed breast milk should be given whenever possible. Peritoneal dialysis or hemofiltration can be undertaken to allow higher fluid intake if needed. Treatment of hyponatremia, hyperkalemia, hypocalcemia, and acidosis are similar to that in older age groups. Sepsis should be suspected and treated early. Nephrotoxic drugs should be avoided. Dose of nephrotoxic drugs should be adjusted by dose reduction or by interval increasing method.

Timely institution of peritoneal dialysis prevents serious complications in oligoanuric ARF in newborn. The large peritoneal surface area compared to body surface area makes this modality very effective. Vascular access may be a problem in newborns for hemodialysis. The dialysate volume is 30–50 ml/kg/cycle. Adequate attention should be given to ventilation. Dialysate fluid should be pre-warmed to avoid hypothermia. Hypertonic dialysate fluids should be used with caution as sudden fluid shifts can precipitate circulatory collapse. Continuous dialytic therapies especially continuous arteriovenous hemo-filtration (CAVH/CVVH) through the umbilical vessels has been used successfully in neonates. Severe oligoanuria with rising BUN and serum creatinine, encephalopathy, acidosis, severe hypo- or hypernatremia, volume overload with hypertension, hyperkalemia with ECG changes unresponsive to medical therapy, removal of dialyzable toxins and inborn errors of metabolism like hyper-ammonemia are the indications. It is also done to create space for parenteral nutrition or transfusions by removing fluid.

Nonoliguric ARF (33%) carries a good outcome. Poor prognostic factors include intrinsic renal failure with renal malforma-tions, prematurity, multiorgan dysfunction and postsurgical ARF. Overall mortality is 14–73%. Prerenal ARF and ATN has excellent outcome. Obstructive nephropathy carries variable prognosis depending on the extent of renal dysplasia. Long-term sequelae in survivors include impaired concentrating ability, hypertension and impaired renal growth.

Infection-related Glomerulonephritis (Acute Nephritis) in Children

The acute nephritic syndrome consists of hematuria associated with edema, oliguria, or hypertension. The prototype of acute nephritic syndrome in children is post infective glomerulo-nephritis. Post-streptococcal type is the commonest. It follows skin or throat infections with nephritogenic strains of group A β-hemolytic streptococci. Such infections are followed by nephritis in about 15% children. Subclinical nephritis is more common. The usual age group is 5–15 years and male:female ratio 2:1. There is a latent period of 1–3 weeks after the infection. Mini epidemics may occur in crowded areas like dormitories, schools and hostels.

Symptomatology and clinical features may vary from the adults with post-streptococcal acute nephritis. Gross hematuria (24–40%); microscopic hematuria (100%); oliguria (10–50%); hypertension (60–80%); congestive cardiac failure (<5%); oedema (90%); proteinuria (80%; nephrotic range in 4–10%); azotemia (25–40%) are the common features in children. The overall prognosis is better in children compared to adults.

Children with acute nephritis need renal biopsy only if there is family history of renal disease, age is below 2 years, if nephritis occurs within 48 hours of pharyngitis or if manifestations suggestive of systemic diseases are present. Progressive deterioration of GFR or failure of GFR to normalize by 2 weeks, persistent gross hematuria beyond 1 month, persistent hypertension beyond 2 months and persistently low C3 at 6–8 weeks are the other indications for biopsy.

Dietary guidelines for treatment include salt and potassium restriction. Fluid intake is regulated based on the volume of previous day's urine output and insensible loss which is presumed to be 400 ml/m². However, if the atmospheric temperature or child's body temperature is high, appropriate extrafluids are administered. Daily recommended allowance of proteins is 0.6 to 0.8 gm/kg/day mainly as high biologic value proteins. A normal caloric intake is advised. Daily weight record helps to asses the accuracy of intake output chart.

Children with hypertension often have volume mediated hypertension and diuretics remain the mainstay of treatment. Frusemide is given in doses of 1–4 mg/kg/day. Calcium channel blockers are used in the control of blood pressure. Those with hypertensive emergencies need treatment with sublingual nifedipine or parenterally administered hydrallazine, labetalol or sodium nitro-prusside infusions. In those with pulmonary edema, in addition to strict fluid restriction and high dose diuretics, ultrafiltration and oxygen therapy may be required. Hyper-kalemia is managed with appropriate medical measures or dialysis depending on the severity. Antibiotics are indicated only if there is active infection. If there is rapidly increasing blood urea and serum creatinine with development of refractory hypertension, pulmonary edema, severe metabolic acidosis or hyperkalemia, dialysis is done.

Nephrotic Syndrome in Children

Idiopathic nephrotic syndrome in children may be minimal change disease, mesangio-proliferative glomerulonephritis, focal and segmental glomerulosclerosis. The exact etiology is not known. It is considered to be an immune mediated systemic disorder as evidenced by:

a. Response to treatment with steroids/cytotoxic drugs.
b. Association of onset of illness and relapses with any infection
c. Association with atopy
d. Remission following measles (measles supresses cell-mediated immunity)
e. Association with Hodgkin's lymphoma
f. Mediation by lymphokines

In children between 2 and 8 years, minimal change disease is the commonest cause of idiopathic nephrotic syndrome. Above the age of 8 years, FSGS is more common. Treatment of initial episode influences the subsequent relapses in childhood nephrotic syndrome. Steroids are the mainstay of treatment. The infections should be treated before starting steroids. Screening for tuberculosis and assessment of hepatitis B status are important. The management consists of oral prednisolone in doses of 2 mg/kg/day for 6 weeks followed by 1.5 mg/kg every alternate day for the next 6 weeks. This is followed by tapering and

stopping of steroids. In frequent relapsers, along with alternate day prednisolone, levamisole 2 mg/kg is given every other day for 6–18 months and has a weak steroid sparing effect. Cyclophosphamide 2 mg/kg/day for 8 weeks helps to prolong the period of remission. Cyclosporine is recommended for patients who have significant steroid toxicity or fail to benefit from cyclophosphamide. Pefloxacin, an antibiotic with immuno-modulatory effect may be beneficial in doses of 25 mg/kg/day. In steroid dependent NS the dose of steroid is tapered and maintained in the smallest doses for 12–18 months to sustain remission. If the dose needed is more than 0.5 mg/kg alternate day and associated with steroid side effects, alternative drugs are to be considered. This includes 8–12-week course of cyclophosphamide or cycloporine in a dose of 3–5 mg/kg/day. Renal biopsy should be done prior to treatment with cyclosporine. The treatment of steroid resistant nephrotic syndrome is a therapeutic challenge. Various regimens have been tried including oral or IV cyclophosphamide, cyclosporine and pulse methylprednisolone.

Supportive care is important in managing children with nephrotic syndrome. A balanced diet adequate in protein (1.5–2 gm/kg) and calories as recommended for age must be given. Only children prone to malnutrition are given protein in doses of 2–2.5 gm/kg/day. About 30% calories should be derived from polyunsaturated fats. Carbohydrates are best given as complex forms such as starch and maltodextrin. In edematous patients, modest salt restriction of 1–2 gm/day is enforced. Control of edema should be with fluid restriction taking care not to cause intra-vascular volume depletion. Monitoring postural blood pressure is a useful method to detect early volume contraction.

Treatment with steroids often leads to good diuresis in 72 hours. Thus, routine use of diuretics for edema should be avoided. Diuretics should not be used in volume depleted nephrotic children who have vomiting or diarrhea. Administration of frusemide in doses of 1–2 mg/kg/day may be considered in severe and persistent edema. Those who require higher dose of steroids for more than one week should receive spirono-lactone 2–3 mg/kg/day. For refractory edema, infusion of 20% human albumin 100 ml with frusemide 1–2 mg/kg intravenously is beneficial. Refractory ascites may be removed by careful paracentesis if it causes respiratory embarassment. Blood pressure should be monitored and appropriately treated. Children on steroids should be encouraged to have physical activity after attaining remission to prevent excessive weight gain.

Onset of nephrotic syndrome in the first three months of life is congenital and between 3 months to 1 year is infantile. These are heterogenous group of disorders with variable etiology. Congenital nephrotic syndrome may be primary or secondary. Primary congenital nephrotic syndrome may be Finnish type or associated with diffuse mesangial selerosis (DMS). Finnish type is inherited as autosomal recessive and is associated with abnormality in the basement membrane protein called 'nephrin'. The gene is localized to chromosome 19q13.1 (NPHS1). These patients are resistant to steroids and cytotoxic drugs. The cause of death is usually infection or electrolyte imbalance. Bilateral nephrectomy follwed by renal transplantation is the only curative treatement. Appropriate dialytic support and parenteral nutrition allows transplantation to be postponed to 2nd or 3rd year of life. Prenatal diagnosis is possible in subsequent pregnancies. Increased alphafetoprotein in the amniotic fluid and maternal serum is highly suggestive of congenital NS. In infantile nephrotic syndrome minimal change, proliferative glomerulo-nephritis, FSGS and membranous glomerulo-pathy are more common compared to DMS. Secondary congenital NS is usually associated with infections like congenital syphilis,

toxoplasmosis, rubella, CMV, hepatitis, HIV or malaria. Malformation syndromes like Denys-Drash syndrome and cerebral malformation may be seen in some cases of CNS.

Infections are common in children with nephrotic syndrome especially in developing countries. Besides being the commonest cause of mortality, infections result in significant morbidity. They may also be responsible for non-response to steroids or induce a relapse. A knowledge of the spectrum of infections is important not only from the therapeutic point of view, but also for planning preventive strategies like pneumococcal vaccination and prophylactic antibiotics. Peritonitis, urinary tract infection, skin infections and recurrent respiratory infection are common.

Children with nephrotic syndrome are at risk for venous and, rarely, arterial thrombosis. Reduced intravascular volume and coagula-tion abnormalities predispose to thrombus formation. Diuretics should be used judiciously. Puncture of deep vessels should not be done. Renal vein thrombosis is suspected in a patient with oligoanuria, hematuria or flank pain especially following an episode of dehydration. Ultrasound examination of the abdomen may show large kidneys and thrombi in renal veins. Femoral arterial thrombosis may occasionally occur. Deep vein thrombosis of calf veins is less common in children but may lead to pulmonary embolism. Sagittal sinus and cortical venous thrombosis may follow episodes of diarrhea and present with convulsions, vomiting, altered sensorium and neurological deficits. Doppler studies and cranial CT scan are useful in confirming the diagnosis. Patients with thrombotic complica-tions require urgent specialized treatment. The treatment is supportive and consists of correction of dehydration, treatment of sepsis, cautious use of anticoagulants and early mobilization. Hypertension may be noted at the onset of nephrotic syndrome or occur due to steroid toxicity. Therapy may be initiated with ACE inhibitors, calcium channel or β-adrenergic blockers. Hypovolemia may occur due to unsupervised use of diuretics especially if accompanied by septicemia, diarrhea or vomiting. The diagnosis is suggested by the presence of hypotension, tachycardia, cold extremities and poor capillary refill and severe abdominal pain. Blood levels of urea and uric acid are elevated. A rapid infusion of normal saline or plasma in a dose of 15–20 ml/kg, or albumin 1 g/kg is essential. The blood pressure should be monitored carefully. Albumin should be used with caution if the child is hypertensive because of the risk of pulmonary edema. Once adequate hydration is achieved, but the child remains oliguric, a single dose of frusemide (1–2 mg/kg intravenously) may be given. In case no urine is passed despite these measures, the diagnosis of acute renal failure is suspected.

Prolonged high-dose corticosteroid therapy may be associated with significant side effects. Parents and the child should be explained about the side effects of corticosteroids. Steroids result in an increased appetite, cushingoid features, impaired growth, behavioral changes, gastritis, salt and water retention, hypertension and bone demineralization. Children on prolonged treatment with corticosteroids should be monitored for steroid toxicity. Examination for cushingoid features, monthly record of blood pressure, six-monthly record of height and weight, and yearly evaluation for cataract is recommended.

HYPERTENSION IN CHILDREN

Hypertension in a child is defined as blood pressure (BP) above the 95th percentile for age and height. Centile charts showing the 50th, 90th and 95th percentiles for various ages and heights are available in standard textbooks of pediatrics. Convenient approximations for the 95th percentile for various age groups are given below. At birth the BP is 70/40 mm Hg.

- 1–5 years   115/75 mm Hg
- 5–10 years   125/80 mm Hg
- 10–15 years   135/85 mm Hg

The recommended guidelines for measurement of BP in children are as follows. The child should be seated, BP is measured in the right arm after 3–5 minutes rest. The width of the cuff should be at least 40% of the distance between acromion and olecranon and the length should be sufficient to encircle the arm fully. The cuff is inflated to 20 mm above the palpated systolic BP and released slowly 2–3 mm per second. Korotkoff I sound is taken as systolic BP. Korotkoff V is taken as diastolic BP in all age groups. The average of two readings is taken. Automated BP measurement using electronic noninvasive monitors is the most practical method for newborns and young infants.

Most Common Causes of Sustained Hypertension in Children

Age group	Cause
Newborns	Renal artery thrombosis, renal artery stenosis, congenital renal malformations, coarctation of aorta, bronchopulmonary dysplasia
<6 years	Renal parenchymal disease, coarctation, renal artery stenosis, medications like steroids, nasal decongestants like pseudoephedrine, endocrine causes.
6–10 years	Renal parenchymal disease, renal artery stenosis, endocrine causes.
>10 years	Primary hypertension, renal parenchymal disease, renal artery stenosis, white coat hypertension, substance abuse, endocrine causes.

The important points include history of umbilical artery catheterization, trauma, mechanical ventilation, urinary tract infection and voiding problems (reflux nephropathy, obstructive uropathy). Weakness, muscle cramps, or recent weight changes point to endocrine hypertension. History of drugs like amphetamine, antihistaminics, decongestants,

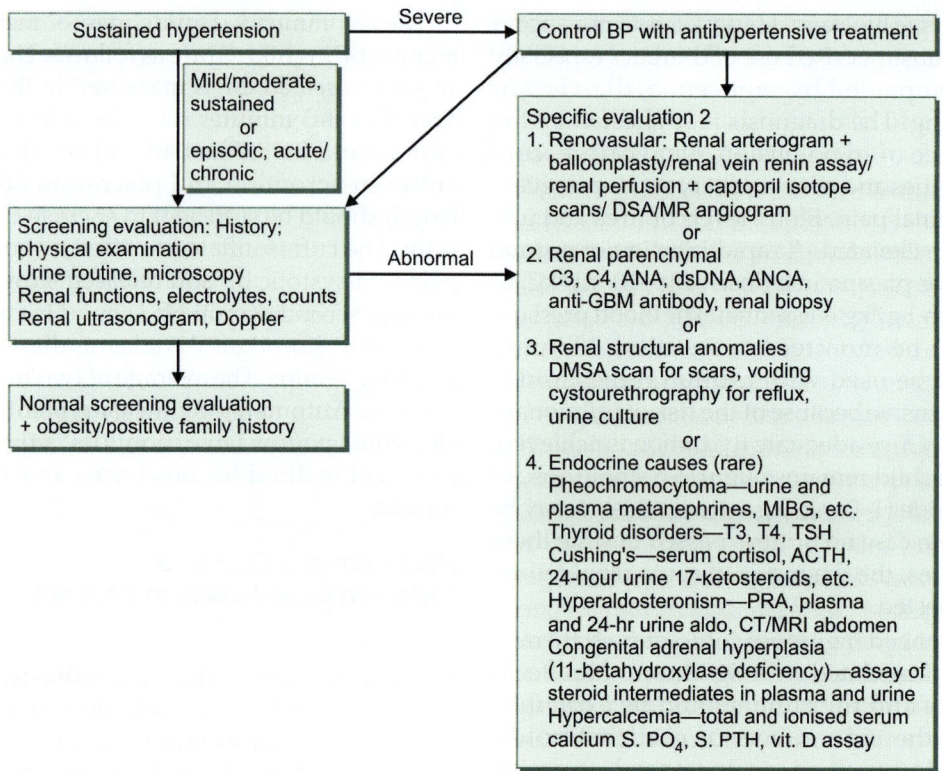

Fig. 10.2: Steps in initial evaluation of hypertension in children

family history of obesity, essential hypertension, hyperlipidemia, early myocardial infarction or stroke, diabetes and renal disease should be obtained. Physical examination should include blood pressures in all four limbs, radiofemoral delay of pulse, café au lait macules, neurofibromas, abdominal bruit, renal and bladder mass. Body mass index, assessment of signs of puberty, external genitalia, cushingoid features and neurocutaneous markers provide important clues to the diagnosis.

The initial evaluation of hypertension in children should ascertain if hypertension is sustained, whether target organ damage or other coexisting diseases are present. Further investigations are done as indicated to identify the cause and curability of hypertension (Fig. 10.2).

APPROACH TO HYPERTENSION

Screening studies include urinalysis, urine culture and sensitivity, serum creatinine, and estimation of creatinine clearance. In children, the Cockroft-Gault formula is not applicable. It can be calculated by Schwartz formula. Creatinine clearance in ml/min = L × K/serum creatinine in mg/dl where L = height in cm, K = the Schwartz constant which is 0.55 in children and 0.45 in infants.

Proteinuria or hematuria indicates possible glomerular disease or reflux nephropathy. Renal ultrasound may demonstrate asymmetric kidneys suggesting renovascular disease, VUR or renal dysplasia. Hyperechoic symmetric kidneys indicate medical renal disease and cysts indicate polysystic kidney or cystic dysplasia. A low serum potassium indicates primary or secondary hyperaldosteronism.

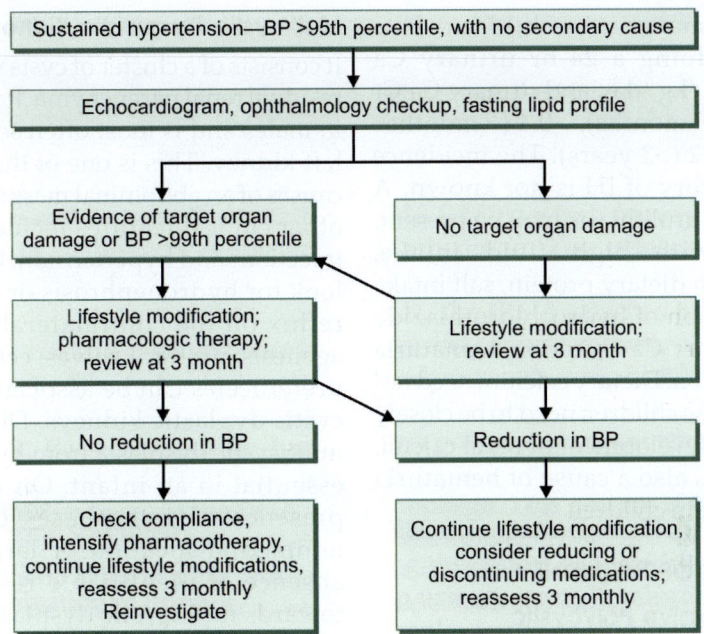

Fig.10.3: Investigations and management strategies for sustained hypertension with no secondary cause

Investigations and management strategies for sustained hypertension with no secondary cause are shown in Fig. 10.3.

Treatment

Curable causes of childhood hypertension.

Renal diseases	Unilateral renal disease (pyelonephritis, hydroureteronephrosis, multicystic dysplasia, segmental renal hypoplasia, tumors)
Cardiovascular	Coarctation of aorta, renal artery lesions (stenosis, aneurysm, fibromuscular dysplasia, thrombosis)
Adrenal	Pheochromocytoma, congenital adrenal hyperplasia, Cushing's syndrome, primary hyperaldosteronism
Miscellaneous	Drug-induced, e.g. glucocorticoids, oral contraceptive pills, decongestants

A scheme for management of sustained hypertension without obvious cause is shown below.

HEMATURIA IN CHILDREN

Hematuria is a common problem in children. The incidence of gross hematuria (macroscopic) is 1.3/1000. Microscopic hematuria is more common and is diagnosed only after a careful microscopic examination of urinary sediment. If microscopic hematuria continues for more than 6 months, it is labeled as persistent hematuria. When urine is colored red due to pigments, drugs, food ingredients or various metabolic disorders, it is called pseudohematuria.

Idiopathic hypercalciuria (IH) is one of the common causes of both recurrent gross or microscopic hematuria in children. It is diagnosed by doing a 24-hr urinary Ca excretion (>4 mg/kg/day and urinary Ca:Cr ratio of >0.8 (0–6 months), >0.4 (6 months– 2 years), and >0.2 (>2 years). The incidence and natural history of IH is not known. A family history of urolithiasis may be present. Management with high fluid intake, avoidance of high dietary protein, salt intake and administration of hydrochlorothiazide will reduce urinary Ca excretion, hematuria and stone formation. Dietary calcium need not be restricted. These children need to be closely followed up for development of renal calculi. Hyperoxaluria is also a cause of hematuria and stone disease in children.

CYSTIC DISEASES OF THE KIDNEY

Autosomal Recessive Polycystic Kidney Disease (ARPKD)

It predominantly manifests in newborns and infants. The prevalence at birth is 1:10,000 and the genetic abnormality is mapped on chromosome 6p21. Congenital hepatic fibrosis and biliary dysgenesis are common associations. Neonates can present with respiratory distress, enlarged kidneys, renal failure and severe hypertension. In due course features of portal hypertension, tubular defects and electrolyte abnormalities are evident. Unilateral or bilateral nephrectomy would be indicated if enlarged kidneys cause respiratory embarrassment. Patients who survive the neonatal period could be stable for many years. Peritoneal dialysis is preferable. Those with hepatic fibrosis may require porto-systemic shunting to prevent complications of portal hypertension.

Autosomal Dominant Polycystic Kidney Disease (ADPKD)

It may be detected incidentally in children during ultrasound evaluation for a non-renal problem. The initial presentation is polyuria and metabolic acidosis and later hypertension followed by renal failure.

Multicystic Dysplastic Kidney

It consists of a cluster of cysts with a little or no residual renal parenchyma. It is more common in males and is most often seen affecting the left kidney. This is one of the most common causes of an abdominal mass in a neonate. The other clinical features include urinary tract infections and hypertension. It is important to look for hydronephrosis or vescicoureteral reflux on the contralateral kidney. Renal agenesis, urethral valves, ectopic ureter and ureteroceles can be associated with multi-cystic dyplastic kidneys. Differentiation of multicystic dysplasia from hydronephrosis is essential in an infant. On ultrasound the presence of interphases between cysts, nonmedial location of largest cysts and absence of identifiable renal sinus point towards multicystic dysplasia. The kidneys tend to decrease in size with age. Uncontrolled hypertension or infection are indications for nephrectomy.

Nephronophthisis-medullary Cystic Disease

It is a heterogeneous disease complex. There are two forms, the juvenile recessive form and adult form. The gene responsible is in chromosome 2q13 (NPH1). The cysts are located at the corticomedullary junction and along the medullary collecting ducts. The histopathology is characterized by irregular thickening of the tubular basement membrane.

Tubular defects associated with salt wasting and polyuria with hypoosmolar urine is common. Small contracted kidneys with anemia and bone disease out of proportion to renal failure by 8–12 years of age suggest the diagnosis of nephronophthisis. Hypertension and significant proteinuria are not common. Associated retinitis pigmentosa and cerebellar ataxia are seen in some children. The treatment involves control of acidosis with bicarbonate, use of calcium and vitamin D supplements and appropriate nutritional support. Renal replacement therapy in the form of dialysis or renal transplantation may be necessary when they develop kidney failure. When renal transplantation is considered from a related donor, the donor should be unaffected and at least 10 years older than the patient.

Glomerulocystic disease can occur in various other cystic diseases like autosomal dominant polycystic kidney disease and certain dysplastic syndromes. It is characterized by glomerular cysts, absence of tubular involvement or urinary obstruction. Recently this has been described in children with an autosomal dominant mode of inheritance.

Medullary Sponge Kidneys

They are characterized by tubular dilatation of the collecting ducts and cyst formation confined to the medullary pyramids. Tubular acidification defect, hypercalciuria, nephrolithiasis, microscopic hematuria and urinary tract infections are the major complications. Rarely renal dysfunction is noted in 3rd or 4th decade as a consequence of recurrent infection and obstruction. Benign simple cysts, acquired cystic disease, multilocular renal cysts and parapelvic cysts are cystic diseases without a genetic basis.

RENAL REPLACEMENT THERAPIES IN CHILDREN

Peritoneal dialysis, hemodialysis and continuous renal replacement therapies like CVVH are employed in children with renal failure based on the patient's needs and facilities available at a particular institution.

Peritoneal dialysis is advantageous in childen in view of near steady state biochemical control, freedom from strict dietary and fluid restrictions, freedom from repeated vene punctures, and better preservation of residual renal function. There will also be better cooperation from the child and the family, rehabilitation, control of anemia and growth. The contraindications for PD are lack of adequate peritoneal surface area as in omphalocele, diaphragmatic hernia or extensive intra-abdominal adhesions or prior episodes of peritonitis.

For continuous ambulatory peritoneal dialysis (CAPD) in children, partial omentectomy is done during the catheter placement. A waiting period of 1–2 weeks is advisable to allow proper healing and prevent leaks. The peritoneal dialysis prescription for children with ESRD depends on the body surface area, peritoneal membrane transport characteristics and residual renal function of the child. The dwell volumes are increased gradually to an optimal level of 1100–1400 ml/sq.m /dwell. The dwell time is 4–6 hours and no of cycles 4–6 per day. Some children need short dwell times and more exchanges and it can be achieved by doing 6–10 exchanges during 8–10 hours at night using a cycler (automated PD/APD/NIPD).

Since optimal growth is to be maintained, 100% of the recommended daily caloric intake for age (RDA) should be provided. The protein requirements for PD based on age are:

- <3 years: 2.5 to 3 gm/kg body wt/day
- 3 years to puberty: 2.0 to 2.5 gm/kg body wt/day
- Pubertal age: 2 gm/kg body wt/day
- Post-pubertal: 1.5 gm/kg body wt/day

At least 60–80% of proteins given should be of high biological value. Periodic growth monitoring and assessment of nutritional status by dry weight, height, weight for height and S. albumin estimation is needed. Normal age-appropriate requirements of fats and vitamins are given.

For hemodialysis, children more than 20 kg can be taken up safely using pediatric kits. Use of machines with precise volumetric control of UF, bicarbonate buffered dialysate, small lines and dialysers, and more biocompatible membranes may help to overcome many of the hurdles. Indwelling catheters for short- or long-term use can be tried in children with ARF or those likely to undergo transplantation within a few weeks. Longer HD planning requires creation of arteriovenous fistulae or grafts by microsurgical techniques.

Catheter sizes are selected according to patient size.

Continuous hemofiltration and its modifications as the renal replacement therapy in infants and children has been limited by technical difficulties. Advances in vascular access and suitable equipment for pediatric use has helped to use these modalities more frequently in children. Pumped circuits of SCUF/CVVH/CVVHD/CVVHDF are preferred to non-pumped circuits of CAVH/CAVHD/CAVHDF.

Renal transplantation is the most optimal way to manage children with end-stage renal disease with good long-term results. Successful transplant permits the child to attend school and to develop normally. Living donors mostly mothers account for most of the pediatric transplants. Transplantation can be done for children weighing >10 kg. All children reaching ESRD are considered candidates for a renal transplant. Pre-emptive kidney transplantation before the child develops dialysis dependent uremia is usually advocated in children so that the need for dialysis does not arise.

Rickets

• Vimala Ammal • Susan Uthup

INTRODUCTION

The bone is a dynamic organ and is constantly formed and reabsorbed by the process of bone turnover. Bone consists of matrix and mineral elements. Matrix consists of collagen and osteoid. Mineral element is mainly calcium hydroxyapatite that gets deposited on the collagen matrix. The epiphyseal cartilage in the growing end of the long bone is transformed into osteoid matrix and mineralization occurs. This mineralization can be seen on X-ray as the mineralization front. The three main cells in the bone are osteoblasts, osteoclasts and osteocytes. Osteoblasts are differentiated mesenchymal cells and they secrete the bone matrix. The activity of osteoblasts is indicated by the level of alkaline phosphatase in the blood. Osteoclasts are differentiated macrophages and are involved in the resorption of bone. They contain enzyme acid phosphatase and its high level in serum indicates increased osteoclastic activity. The bone is remodeled by the coordinated activity of osteoblasts and osteoclasts. Osteoblasts become osteocytes once they are trapped in the bone matrix. Osteocytes are the mature bone cells. They constitute nearly 90% of the cells in the bone. Bone turnover and remodeling involves a complex interplay of calcium, phosphorus, vitamin D, fibroblast growth factor 23 (FGF 23) and parathyroid hormone (PTH).

Osteomalacia is failure of mineralization of osteoid in mature bone. Osteoporosis is reduction of bone mass (both mineral and osteoid). Rickets is a disorder in which there is defective mineralization of the growing skeleton. Since skeletal growth is more during childhood, many disorders involving vitamin D, calcium, phosphorus and renal diseases lead to rickets.

METABOLIC PATHWAY OF VITAMIN D

The precursors of vitamin D are ergocalciferol (vitamin D_2) and cholecalciferol (vitamin D_3). Vitamin D_2 is the active agent in irradiated yeast and irradiated bread. Vitamin D_3 is from animal origin such as in fish liver oil. In human beings vitamins D_2 and D_3 have similar actions qualitatively and quantitatively. Cholecalciferol (D_3) is synthesized from 7-dehydrocholesterol in the epidermis under the influence of ultraviolet light (288–310 nm). This synthesis usually takes about three days. Afterwards it is transported to liver by a binding protein. Vitamins D_2 and D_3 are transported from intestine to the liver. In the liver both vitamins D_2 and D_3 are hydroxylated at the 25th carbon atom to form 25-hydroxy-(25-OH) vitamin D with the help of the enzyme 25-hydroxylase. The 25-OH vitamin D is further converted in the kidney by the enzyme 1α-hydroxylase to the active form, 1, 25-dihydroxy (1, 25 [OH]$_2$) vitamin D. Instead of 1α, if hydroxylation occurs in the 24th carbon atom, an inactive form called 24, 25-dihydroxyvitamin D is produced. Active vitamin D causes an increase in calcium and phosphorus absorption from the intestine and reabsorption in the proximal convoluted tubule. It also increases bone resorption acting synergistically with parathyroid hormone. 1α-hydroxylase is the rate limiting enzyme in active vitamin D synthesis.

FGF23 is a bone-derived hormone that regulates systemic phosphate homeostasis, vitamin D metabolism and α-Klotho expression through a novel bone-kidney axis. Elevated levels of 1, 25[OH]$_2$ vitamin D$_3$ or cholecalciferol (calcitriol) induces FGF23 secretion from osteocytes. Main function of FGF23 is regulation of phosphate concentration in plasma. FGF23 inhibits renal tubular reabsorption of phosphate by decreasing the expression of a sodium-phosphate cotransporter (NPT2) in the proximal tubule. FGF23 also suppress 1α-hydroxylase, reducing its ability to activate vitamin D and subsequently impairing calcium absorption.

PATHOGENESIS OF RICKETS AND OSTEOMALACIA

Defective mineralization of osteoid in a growing bone results in rickets. Normal bone growth and mineralization require adequate calcium and phosphate at the mineralization front. When there is deficiency of vitamin D, there is decreased absorption of calcium from intestine resulting in hypocalcemia. Hypocalcemia stimulates PTH which release calcium from the bone and also acts on kidneys increasing reabsorption of calcium and phosphorus. However in vitamin D deficiency, adequate calcium and phosphorus will not be available for mineralization of osteoid. Accumulation of uncalcified osteoid

occurs due to the failure of mineralization to keep pace with cartilage and osteoid formation. Thus, the growing bone becomes less rigid and bends under the weight of the body or pull of the muscles and the bony deformities of rickets occur. Following treatment, there is deposition of bone mineral in the layer of epiphyseal cartilage adjacent to the distal boundary of rachitic intermediate zone. This is seen on X-ray as a transverse line of increased density called Müller's line or zone of provisional calcification. Over proliferation of osteoblasts in the rachitic intermediate zone leads to the rise in serum alkaline phosphatase. Alkaline phosphatase is invariably elevated in all types of rickets except hypophosphatasia and it returns to normal with healing.

CAUSES AND CLASSIFICATION

Causes of rickets can be classified into two major groups based on the predominant mineral deficiency. Calcium deficiency (calcipenic rickets or and Phosphate deficiency (phosphopenic) rickets. Calcipenic rickets is often associated with low serum calcium levels and is often due to insufficient intake, metabolism or action of vitamin D. End organ resistance to active vitamin D also causes calcipenic rickets and this type does not respond to regular doses of vitamin D. This form of rickets is also called pseudovitamin D deficiency rickets. Phosphopenic rickets is usually caused by renal phosphate wasting. It is characterized by low serum levels of phosphorus. Familial hypophosphatemic rickets, also called vitamin D resistant rickets (VDRR) is a condition associated with phosphaturia and hypophosphatemia. Extremities tend to be predominantly affected in the heritable forms of phosphopenic rickets. VDRR responds only to phosphate supplementation and not vitamin D supplementation.

Nutritional rickets due to vitamin D deficiency was the major cause of rickets in the earlier part of the last century. Non-nutritional rickets is more common now and is associated with disruption of calcium-phosphorus homeostasis, defective metabolic conversion and impaired activation of vitamin D or end organ insensitivity. The classification of rickets is given in Table 11. 1.

CLINICAL MANIFESTATIONS AND EVALUATION

Initial manifestation of rickets is seen at the sites of rapid bone growth. Clinical features depend on the age of onset, severity of rachitic process and the bones involved. In the first 3–6 months of life, softening of parietal and frontal bones cause rachitic craniotabes (soft skull bones) especially at the posterolateral portion of the skull (ping-pong skull). Beyond 6 months there is compensatory thickening of skull. Fontanelle and sutural closure are delayed. Frontal and parietal bones of skull become thickened leading to bossing of classic rickets and 'hot cross bun' appearance. This is due to a deep groove presents over the coronal and sagittal sutures.

Chest deformity develops after 6 months. Earliest changes are thickening of costochondral junction due to overproliferation and lateral spread of un-mineralized chondroosteoid seen as beading along the anterolateral aspects of the chest ("rachitic rosary") (Fig. 11.1). Protrusion of sternum results in 'pigeon chest' deformity. Lower portion of ribcage becomes flared out. Groove like depression at the lower margin of the thorax at the sites of insertion of diaphragm results in 'Harrison's sulcus' (Fig. 11.2). It is caused by the muscular pull of the diaphragm on the weak lower ribs. Greenstick fractures and thoracic kyphosis are also seen.

Deformities of long bones include metaphyseal widening, double malleolus, genu valgum, (knock knee) genu varum or bow legs, cubitus valgus and coxa vara. Deformities of the forearms and posterior bowing of the distal tibia are more common in infants. Genu varum or bow legs is a characteristic finding in the toddler (Figs 11.3 to 11.7). In older children,

Table 11.1: Classification of rickets

I. Calcium deficiency rickets (calcipenic rickets)

a. Lack of vitamin D
- Lack of exposure to sunlight
- Dietary deficiency
- Malabsorption of vitamin D
  - Malabsorption syndromes
  - Cholestatic liver disease
  - Extrahepatic biliary obstruction

b. Transport protein abnormalities
- Absence of transport protein
- Deficiency of transport protein
  - Loss in urine (nephrotic syndrome)

c. Hepatic diseases—defective 25-hydroxylation

d. Increased degradation of 25 (OH) D_3 by enzyme inducers
- Phenytoin
- Phenobarbitone
- Rifampicin

e. Defective 1α hydroxylation
- CKD–MBD (CKD associated mineral bone disorder—previously called renal osteodystrophy)
- Vitamin D-dependent rickets type I—congenital deficiency of 1α hydroxylase enzyme

f. End organ resistance to 1, 25(OH)$_2$ D_3 Vitamin D-dependent rickets type 2

II. Primary phosphate deficiency rickets (phosphopenic rickets)

a. Genetic primary hypophosphatemia (VDRR)

b. Rickets following phosphaturia
- Isolated phosphaturia
- Phosphaturia with glycosuria
- Proximal RTA
- Fanconi syndrome
  - Wilson's disease
  - Cystinosis
  - Tyrosinosis
  - Lowe syndrome

c. Oncogenic hypophosphatemia

d. Phosphate malabsorption—parenteral hyperalimentation

genu valgum or a windswept deformity (valgus deformity of one leg and varus deformity of the other) may be seen. 'Triradiate pelvis' is characterized by protrusion of both acetabula and the sacrum into the

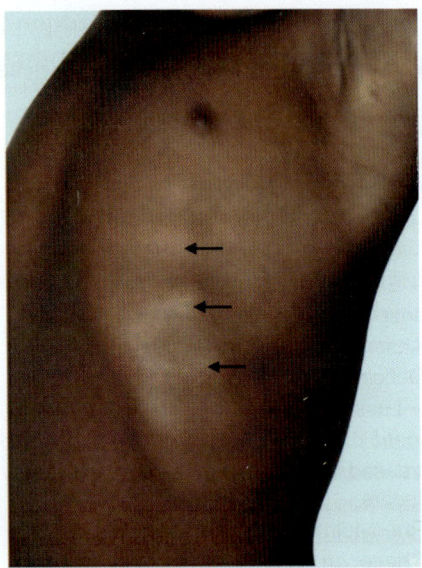

Fig. 11.1: Rachitic rosary. *Note:* The prominence and nodularity of costochondral junction

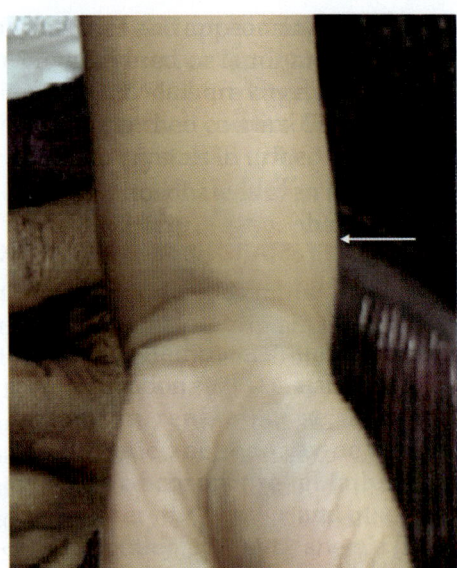

Fig. 11.3: Metaphyseal widening (wrist)

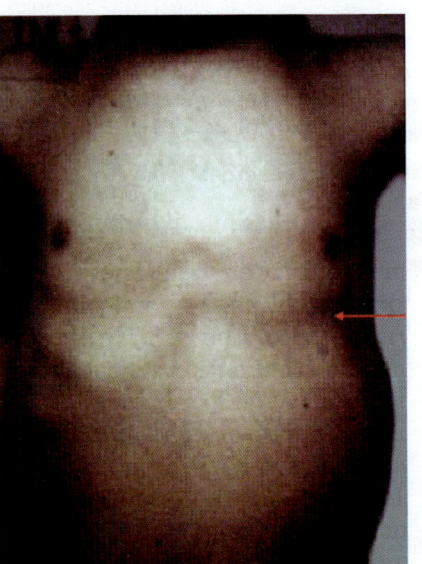

Fig. 11.2: Harrison's sulcus. Note the horizontal groove in lower part of chest (arrow)

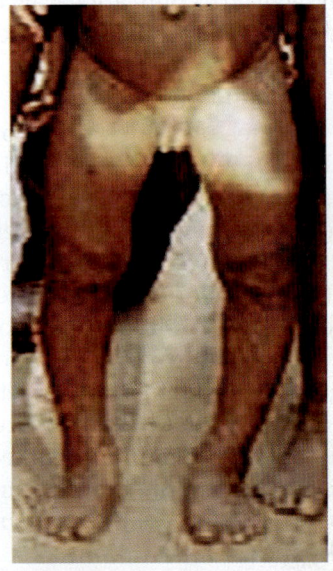

Fig. 11.4: Bilateral genu varum (bow leg deformity)

pelvic cavity causing difficult childbirth. This is only of historical interest now.

In normal dental development, calcium contributes to formation of enamel and phosphorus to dentine. Delayed eruption of deciduous teeth and enamel hypoplasia of permanent dentition are seen in children with severe calcipenic rickets in infancy. Pulp abnormalities, defective dentine and dental abscesses occur more often in hypophosphatemic VDRR. Muscle weakness is also more

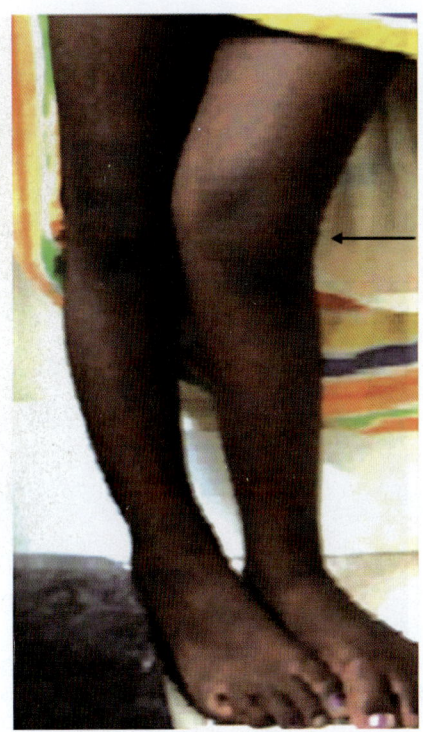

Fig. 11.5: Genu valgum left knee (knock knee)

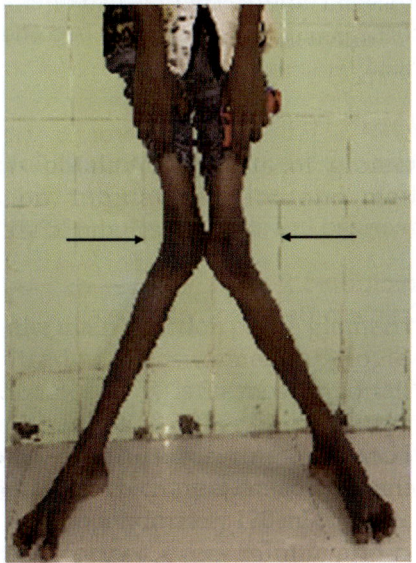

Fig. 11.6: Extreme degree of bilateral genu valgum

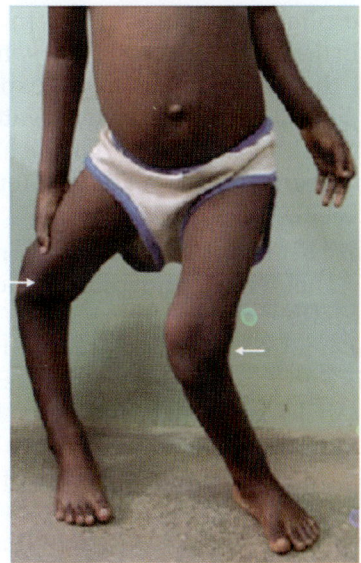

Fig. 11.7: Varus deformity of right leg with valgus deformity of left leg ('wind sweep deformity')

common in VDRR resembling muscular dystrophy. The lower extremities tend to be predominantly affected in the heritable forms of phosphopenic rickets. Nonspecific symptoms include lethargy, irritability, delayed motor milestones, profuse head sweats, muscular hypotonicity, head nodding and laxity of abdominal musculature causing pot belly.

A child with clinical signs of rickets should be evaluated in a systematic manner. A detailed dietary history with particular attention on calcium and vitamin D intake should be taken. Medication history, details on exposure to sunlight and outdoor activities, is important. Biochemical and radiological confirmation is required for the diagnosis if rickets is suspected clinically. Serum calcium, phosphorous and alkaline phosphatase form the basic laboratory investigation to classify the types of rickets. Alkaline phosphatase is required for the mineralization of osteoid and hence is an excellent marker of disease activity. Serum alkaline phosphatase is elevated in all types of rickets except in hypophosphatasia. In hypophosphatasia there is congenital deficiency or absence of alkaline phosphatase resulting in severe rickets. In the heritable forms of phosphopenic rickets, the serum alkaline phosphatase activity tends to be moderately elevated (400 to 800 IU/L). In calcipenic rickets, alkaline phosphatase will often reach greater levels (1000–2000 IU/L).

Serum calcium is usually normal or low in rickets. The serum phosphorus helps to differentiate different types. It is low in Fanconi syndrome, proximal renal tubular acidosis and familial vitamin D resistant rickets (VDRR) and high in chronic kidney disease (CKD) associated mineral bone disease (MBD).Tubular reabsorption of phosphorus is decreased in rickets due to proximal RTA and VDRR. In vitamin D dependent rickets, the level of phosphorus may be low or normal.

Parathyroid hormone (PTH) is elevated in calcipenic rickets while it is normal in phosphopenic rickets. Serum 25-hydroxy-vitamin D [25(OH)D] is low in vitamin D-deficiency. While it is high in vitamin D-dependent rickets (VDDR) type 1. 1,25 dihydroxy D is high in type 2 VDDR. Urinalysis for pH, proteinuria, glycosuria, aminoaciduria and phosphaturia give clues to the diagnosis of renal tubulopathies. High serum creatinine level indicates chronic kidney disease. Ultrasound abdomen shows medullary nephrocalcinosis in distal renal tubular acidosis.

Radiographic evaluation should include plain films of the wrist, hand or knees and long bones to assess the epiphysis and metaphysis. X-rays show characteristic changes at the growing ends of long bones. Distal radius and ulna show fraying, cupping, spur formation, stippling, and spreading at metaphysis end with increased space between epiphyses and metaphyses .This is due to uncalcified osteoid (Fig. 11.8). In severe rickets, pathological fractures and Looser's zones (Milkman pseudofractures) may be noted (Fig. 11.9). There will be delayed appearance of the

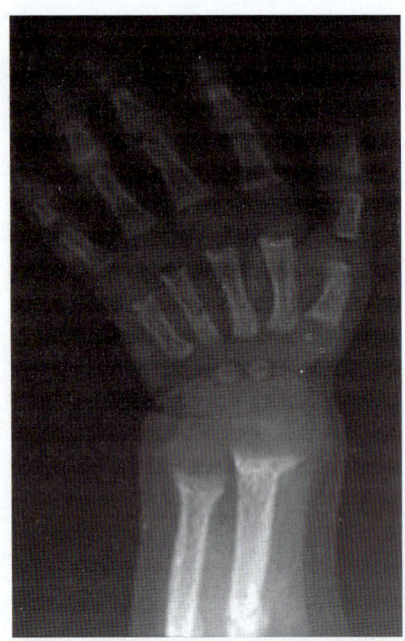

Fig. 11.8: X-ray distal radius and ulna. Radiograph in a 3-year-old boy with rickets. Distal radius and ulna show fraying, cupping, spur formation, stippling, and spreading at metaphysis end with increased space between epiphyses and metaphyses

epiphyseal centers. There is osteopenia and the cortices of long bone shafts become thin. (Fig. 11.10).

COMMON TYPES OF RICKETS

The clinical, biochemical manifestations and treatment in various types of rickets are summarized in Table 11.2.

A. Calcipenic Rickets (Calcium Deficiency Rickets)

1. Nutritional Rickets (Vitamin D Deficiency Rickets)

Vitamin D deficiency rickets is usually associated with malabsorption syndromes and malnutrition. A single large dose of 6 lakh units of vitamin D is given orally or IM (STOSS regimen) and the effect is seen within days. At the end of 1 week, serum phosphorous rises to 5 mg/dl, calcium to 10 mg/dl and alkaline

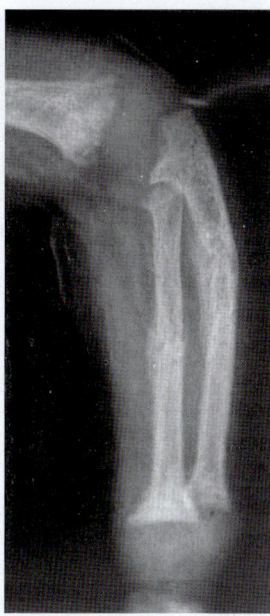

Fig. 11.9: X-ray forearm. Pathological fracture seen at the middle of the shaft of both radius and ulna

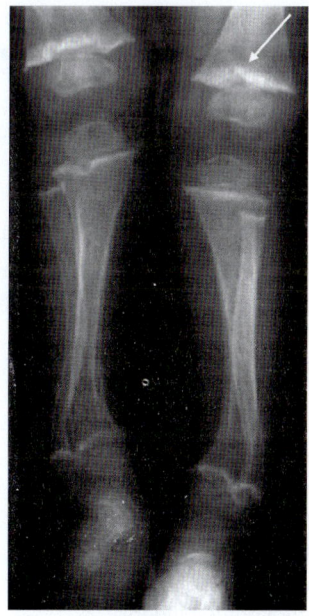

Fig. 11.10: X-ray knees and leg bones. X-ray lower limbs showing thinning and osteopenia of shafts with fraying, cupping, spur formation at metaphysis

phosphatase starts falling. Healing is seen as Müller's line on X-ray within 2 weeks. This rapid response permits differentiation of deficiency rickets from other variants of rickets.

Doses of vitamin D are expressed in 'units' of anti-rachitic activity: 400 units = 10 micrograms. Alfacalcidol and calcitriol (1, 25(OH)$_2$ vitamin D) are not suitable for the management of nutritional rickets and vitamin D deficiency as they can cause hypercalcemia and do not correct the deficiency. These are reserved for patients with severe renal or hepatic impairment. In hepatic disorders there is impaired vitamin D absorption and 25-hydroxylation. Clinical features and biochemistry resemble nutritional rickets. High dose vitamin D along with calcium is the treatment. Vitamin D$_2$ 4000–10000 units or 25(OH)D$_3$ or 1,25(OH)$_2$D3 in doses of 0.25 µg may be given daily along with calcium supplements. In rickets associated with use of anticonvulsants or drugs inducing hepatic cytochrome P450 enzyme, there is increased conversion of 25(OH)D$_3$ to polar inactive metabolites. Use of 500–1000 IU of vitamin D$_2$ daily along with calcium supplements is the treatment.

2. CKD–MBD

CKD associated mineral bone disorder is the result of defective 1α-hydroxylation of 25(OH) vitamin D in the kidney. Secondary hyperparathyroidism, hyperphosphatemia, uremia and attendant acidosis also contribute to the rickets and is discussed in Section 10, chapter 46.

3. Rickets associated with Renal Tubular Acidosis type I (Distal RTA)

In type I or distal RTA, the distal tubule acidification mechanism is defective. There is inability to form acid urine at all levels of serum bicarbonate. There is usually growth failure and rickets towards the end of first year of life. Children are polyuric and dehydrated. Nephrolithiasis is due to bone resorption,

Table 11.2: Clinical and biochemical manifestations of various types of rickets

Type of rickets	Clinical presentation	Salient features	Biochemical features	Treatment	Remarks
Nutritional rickets	Associated with malnutrition or malabsorption	Delayed dentition, craniotabes, 'rachitic rosary'	S. calcium normal or low S. phosphorus normal S. alkaline phosphatase (SAP) increased Generalized aminoaciduria	STOSS regimen (administration of a bolus dose of 6 lakh units of vitamin D orally). After 1 week, SAP starts falling. Müller's line appears on X-ray within 2 weeks	Recent resurgence of nutritional rickets due to lack of sun exposure and consumption of junk food
Vitamin D-dependent rickets I (VDDR I)	Presents in infancy, usually at 3–6 months of age	Hypocalcemic tetany, convulsions, muscle weakness Growth failure, enamel hypoplasia	S. calcium (below 8 mg) S. phosphorous is low or normal Low or undetectable $1,25(OH)_2 D_3$, normal $25(OH)_2$ S. PTH high	Oral calcitriol (0.25–2 µg/day) along with calcium supplements	Defect in 1α-hydroxylase activity. Gene on long arm of chromosome 12 (12q14) Clinical and radiological signs similar to nutritional rickets
Vitamin D-dependent rickets II (VDDR II)	History of consanguinity Presents in infancy	Short stature, alopecia totalis	Hypocalcemia, hypophosphatemia, aminoaciduria very high $1,25(OH)_2 D_3$ (>180 pg/ml)	$1,25(OH)_2 D_3$ (calcitriol) 15–60 µg/day in combination with long-term oral or parenteral calcium supplements	Hereditary end-organ resistance to $1,25(OH)_2 D_3$
CKD-MBD	More common in tubulointerstitial diseases	Anemia, growth failure, metastatic calcification	GFR <30 ml/min low serum calcium, high serum phosphorus and SAP. Low $1,25(OH)_2$ D, high S. PTH high anion gap metabolic acidosis	Oral sodium bicarbonate tablets or Shohl's solution to correct acidosis 1α-hydroxy-vitamin D or 1, 25-dihydroxy-vitamin D 0.25–2 µg/day Calcium acetate and sevelamer as phosphate binders	Dialysis and kidney transplantation in advanced kidney failure

Contd.

Table 11.2: Clinical and biochemical manifestations of various types of rickets (*Contd.*)

Type of rickets	Clinical presentation	Salient features	Biochemical features	Treatment	Remarks
Renal tubular acidosis (RTA)	Presents in infancy	Growth failure dehydration, polyuria	Normal anion gap metabolic acidosis Medullary nephro-calcinosis	Oral sodium bicarbonate tablets or Shohl's solution in doses of 1–3 mEq /kg/ day. 20–50% of alkali can be given as potassium bi-carbonate or citrate	With bicarb supple-ments growth becomes normal and bone starts healing
Vitamin D resistant rickets (VDRR) Familial hypo-phosphatemic rickets Phosphate wasting rickets	Presents between 1 and 2 years	Short stature Dolicocephalic head, rachitic rosary Pronounced lower limb abnormalities. Smooth rather than angular bowing of legs Waddling gait, coxa vara, genu valgum, genu varus Metaphyseal widening at wrist Defective dentine and pulp abnor-malities Periapical and dental abscess	S calcium low or normal, S phosphorus low Serum alkaline phosphatase— increased low 1,25(OH)$_2$ D Urine amino-acidogram normal	Oral phosphate supplement is given 70–100 mg/ kg/day in five divided doses Joule's solution (dibasic sodium phosphate 136 gm and 58.5 gm phosphoric acid in 1 L water (1 ml = 30 mg elemental phosphorus) Dose: 15 ml 5 times daily combined with calcitriol 0.025–0.050 mg/kg/day	Most common type of hereditary rickets Adult height of untreated patients is 130–165 cm

hypercalciuria and decreased level of urinary citrate. Citrate is a chelator of calcium and inhibits stone formation. Renal tubular acidosis (type I) is suspected when there is normal anion gap metabolic acidosis, hyperchloremia, hypokalemia and normal GFR in a child with rickets. In distal renal tubular acidosis, there may be nephro-calcinosis. Acidosis is corrected by giving oral sodium bicarbonate tablets or Shohl's solution in doses of 1–3 mEq/kg/day. About 20–50% of alkali can be given as potassium bicarbonate

or citrate. With treatment growth becomes normal and bone starts healing.

4. Vitamin D-Dependent Rickets (VDDR)

VDDR is an inborn error of vitamin D metabolism. Inheritance is autosomal recessive. There are two types, type I and type 2.

VDDR type 1 (pseudovitamin D deficiency rickets): In type 1 VDDR, the defect is in 1α-hydroxylase activity. Putative gene is on the long arm of chromosome 12 (12q14). Symptoms usually start in 3–6 months of life.

There is growth failure, muscle weakness, hypocalcemia and convulsions. Clinical and radiological signs are similar to vitamin D deficiency rickets. The cardinal feature is hypocalcemia (S. calcium <8 mg). Serum phosphorus is low or normal. Serum alkaline phosphatase is elevated. Oral calcitriol 0.25–2 µg/day) along with calcium supplements is the treatment.

VDDR type 2 (end organ resistance to 1, 25 $(OH)_2 D_3$ hypocalcemic vitamin D resistant rickets): VDDR type 2 is due to hereditary resistance to 1, $25(OH)_2 D_3$ and is seen in children born of consanguineous marriages. There is hypocalcemia, hypophosphatemia, aminoaciduria and rickets in the presence of high circulating levels (>180 pg/ml) of 1,25 $(OH)_2 D_3$. Some patients have short stature and alopecia totalis. Rickets can sometimes be reversed by treatment with $1,25(OH)_2 D_3$ (calcitriol) 15–60 µg/day in combination with long-term oral or parenteral calcium.

B. Phosphopenic Rickets (Phosphate Deficiency Rickets)

Phosphopenic rickets is characterized by low serum phosphorus with normal PTH concentrations. Phosphopenic rickets is almost always caused by renal phosphate wasting, which may be isolated or part of a generalized renal tubular disorder. The common causes include:

1. Genetic primary hypophosphatemia (VDRR or familial hypophosphatemia)
2. Oncogenous rickets
3. Proximal RTA
4. Fanconi syndrome

Genetic Primary Hypophosphatemia (VDRR) (Familial Hypophosphatemia, X-linked Hypophosphatemia)

X-linked hypophosphatemia is the most common type of hereditary rickets, with an incidence of 1 in 20000 births. It is caused by mutations in the phosphate regulating endopeptidase on the X chromosome (PHEX gene) located at Xp22. Mode of inheritance is X-linked dominant. It is characterized by phosphaturia due to reduced activity of renal brush border membrane Na-phosphate cotransporter in the proximal tubule. There is also abnormal regulation of renal 1α-hydroxylase activity resulting in inappropriately low serum level of $1,25(OH)_2 D_3$ relative to the degree of hypophosphatemia.

Most patients present between 1 and 2 years with short stature and bowed legs. Often the head is enlarged and dolicocephalic. Metaphyseal widening at wrist and rachitic rosary are also seen. Abnormalities are more pronounced in the lower extremities. Waddling gait, smooth rather than angular bowing of legs, coxa vara, genu valgum, genu varus, and short stature are common. Adult height of untreated patients is 130–165 cm. Pulp abnormalities, defective dentin, periapical and tooth abscess are common. Urine aminoacidogram and serum PTH are normal. The main biochemical abnormality of X-linked hypophosphatemia is low tubular reabsorption of filtered phosphate in the presence of low serum phosphorus and absence of secondary hyperparathyroidism.

The treatment is by supplementing phosphates to improve hypophosphatemia and active form of vitamin D. Oral phosphate supplement is given 70–100 mg/kg/day in five divided doses. Joule's solution is dibasic sodium phosphate 136 gm and 58.5 gm phosphoric acid in 1 L water (1 ml = 30 mg elemental phosphorus). Dose is 15 ml 5 times daily and is combined with calcitriol 0.025–0.050 mg/kg/day.

Corrective osteotomies are deferred until rickets heals biochemically and roentgenographically. Serum alkaline phosphate should be within the normal range. Patients undergoing osteotomy should stop all vitamin D preparations before surgery and in the postoperative period till full ambulation, to avoid immobilization hypercalcemia. Patient should be monitored regularly with serum calcium, phosphorus and alkaline phosphatase every 3 months, serum PTH every 6–12 months and X-ray knee every year. Ultrasound abdomen should be done to rule out nephrocalcinosis. Complications of treatment include diarrhea, hypercalcemia, hypercalciuria and nephrocalcinosis.

In proximal RTA, oral bicarbonate, phosphate supplements and vitamin D are the treatments. In oncogenous rickets seen in mesenchymal benign tumors, a variety of factors, one of which, FGF23, inhibits the Na-phosphate co-transporters, thus decreasing phosphate reabsorption. Excision of tumor is curative.

Hypophosphatasia is an autosomal recessive disorder resembling rickets. There is deficient activity of alkaline phosphatase and failure of calcium accumulation in mature chondrocytes. No definitive treatment is available for this condition. In primary chondrodystrophy (metaphyseal dysostosis), the patient has short stature, bow legs and waddling gait. In Jansen's type, there is cupped and ragged metaphysis with mottled calcification at distal ends of bone. Spinal deformities may occur. Serum calcium is high (13–15 mg/dl), phosphorous is normal and alkaline phosphatase is increased. Schmidt type is less severe, biochemical parameters are normal and there is no effective treatment.

Normal Micturition and its Disorders

• Suresh Bhat

NORMAL MICTURITION

Normal micturition is an orderly and well coordinated process and is under voluntary control. It requires normal urinary bladder and urethra and with intact nerve supply to the vesicourethral unit. Sphincter like arrangement of the muscle fibers help to hold the urine in the bladder and permit voiding when circumstance permit. The urinary bladder is composed of detrusor smooth muscle fibers which run in all directions. At the bladder neck, they are arranged in 3 definite layers: An outer and inner longitudinal layers and a middle circular layer. These layers constitute the proximal smooth muscle sphincter. The distal sphincter has 2 components, namely an involuntary skeletal muscle component (rhabdo-sphincter) which is more important for continence, and a voluntary skeletal muscle component (deep transverse perineal muscle). The skeletal muscle component controls the voluntary interruption of the urinary stream. The motor supply to the urinary bladder comes from the parasympathetic outflow through sacral S2, 3 and 4 segments. These segments are situated at the level of the vertebral bodies of T12 and L1. They reach the bladder wall through the pelvic nerves and join the vesical plexus at the base of the bladder. The trigone which has a different embryologic origin, gets its innervation from sympathetic outflow from spinal segments, thoracic (T) 11th to lumbar (L) 2nd. They travel down as the hypogastric nerve to the vesical plexus and to the bladder. The voluntary component of the distal sphincter is supplied by somatic nervous system through sacral segments S2, 3 and 4 via pudendal nerve (Fig. 12.1).

The sensation of stretch from the bladder is transmitted along parasympathetic S2, 3, 4 nerves. From the urethra, the sensations travel along somatic S2, 3, 4 through pudendal nerve. The touch, temperature and pain sensations are carried via sympathetic to T9 to L1 segments. Integration of the micturition reflex occurs in the micturition center which is situated in the pons. The cerebral cortex provides the voluntary control over micturition. Functionally, urinary bladder is divided into body and base. The part of the bladder above the openings of the ureters is the body. The part below including the bladder neck and prostatic urethra form the base. The parasympathetic supply is through the cholinergic receptors distributed throughout the body and base. Stimulation of the parasympathetic system acts through the cholinergic receptors and leads to contraction of the detrusor muscle resulting in emptying of the bladder. The α

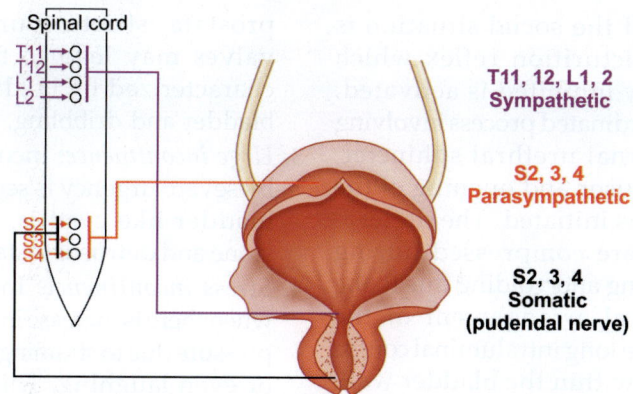

Fig. 12.1: Nerve supply to urinary bladder

receptors of the sympathetic system are present in the base, bladder neck and proximal urethra. Sympathetic stimulation leads to contraction of the proximal sphincter and retention of urine. Blocking of these α receptors produces relaxation of the proximal sphincter and facilitates outflow of urine. Sympathetic β receptors are abundant in the body, base and proximal urethra. Stimulation of β receptors produces relaxation of the smooth muscles and retention of urine (Fig. 12.2).

The two functions of bladder, are storage and expulsion of urine. The normal bladder holds 300–600 ml of urine at a pressure of 5–10 cm of H_2O. This low pressure is maintained during filling because of three factors:

i. Distensibility of the bladder (accommodation)

ii. Action of the sympathetic nerves

iii. Voluntary control of detrusor contractions.

As the capacity of the bladder is reached, an urge to void is transmitted to sensory centers

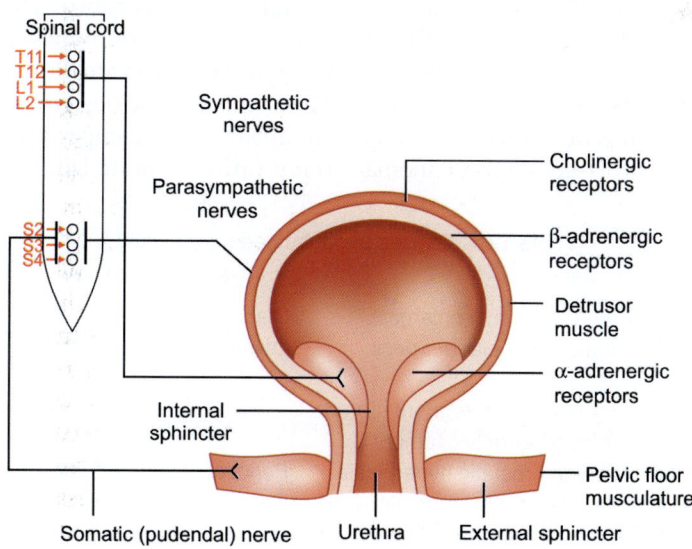

Fig. 12.2: Bladder innervation showing the nerves and the receptors (α, β and cholinergic receptors)

in the cerebrum. If the social situation is acceptable, the micturition reflex which remains constantly inhibited is activated. Thus, voiding, a coordinated process involving relaxation of external urethral sphincter, contraction of detrusor and opening of the internal sphincter is initiated. The uretero-vesical junctions are compressed during normal bladder filling and voiding due to the peculiar anatomical arrangement of the muscle fibers and the long intraluminal course of terminal ureter within the bladder wall. This arrangement prevents vesicoureteric reflux.

CAUSES OF ABNORMAL MICTURITION

Abnormal micturition can either be due to a) obstruction to the flow of urine (Table 12.1) or incontinence of urine.

Causes of Incontinence of Urine

There are 4 types of urinary incontinence.

1. *True incontinence:* In this condition, there is continuous dribbling of urine. Vesico-vaginal fistula, ureterovaginal fistula, ectopic ureteral opening in females and ectopia vesicae are some of the causes of true incontinence. It may also develop as a complication following transurethral resection of the prostate or radical prostatectomy for cancer prostate.

2. *False incontinence* (overflow incontinence): Benign prostatic hyperplasia (BPH), carcinoma prostate, stricture urethra or urethral valves may lead to false incontinence characterized by hold up of urine in the bladder and dribbling.

3. *Urge incontinence:* Incontinence preceded by severe urgency is seen in diseases of the bladder like cystitis, carcinoma *in situ*, stone and detrusor instability or prostatitis.

4. *Stress incontinence:* Incontinence occurs when there is increase in the intra-abdominal pressure due to straining, coughing, sneezing or even laughing. This occurs due to an increase in the intravesical pressure but is not accompanied by detrusor contraction. This is called genuine stress incontinence.

Bladder dysfunction due to neurological causes can be broadly divided into hyper-reflexic bladder and hyporeflexic bladder.

Hyperreflexic bladder (upper motor neuron (UMN) bladder, neurogenic overactive bladder, automatic bladder).

Any lesion in the central nervous system above the S2 segment may lead to UMN bladder. The pons is the co-ordinating center for bladder contraction and sphincter relaxation. The common causes are spinal cord injury due to vertebral fractures, meningomyelocele, spinal tumors, cerebrovascular accidents or parkinsonism. Frequency, urgency, precipitancy and nocturia are the common symptoms. There may also be hesitancy, poor interrupted stream and increasing residual urine and even renal failure due to bilateral hydrouretero-

Table 12.1: Causes of obstructed urinary flow	
Mechanical	*Functional*
a. Causes in the bladder—median lobe of enlarged prostate, bladder stone, tumor near bladder neck, large ureterocele	Diabetes mellitus Lower motor neuron bladder
b. Causes outside the urinary bladder—pregnant uterus, fibroid uterus, ovarian tumor, other pelvic tumors	
c. Causes in the urethra—benign prostatic hyperplasia (BPH), carcinoma prostate, stricture urethra, stone in the urethra, urethral malignancy, urethral valves	Functional bladder neck obstruction Detrusor external sphincter—dyssynergia, spinal trauma, spinal cord tumors, intervertebral disc prolapse (IVDP) and multiple sclerosis

nephrosis and infection. If the lesion is above T6 spinal segment, the patient may also have autonomic dysreflexia characterized by intense sympathetic discharge when the bladder is distended or if procedures like cystoscopy are performed. Prophylaxis with α-blockers or nifedipine before any procedure aborts an episode of autonomic dysreflexia.

Urinalysis, culture, renal function test, ultrasound of the urinary tract, urodynamic studies done periodically are useful in the diagnosis, management and follow-up.

Patients with only detrusor hyperreflexia may be treated with anticholinergics like probanthine 15–30 mg 2 to 4 times daily, dicylomine 20 mg three times a day, oxybutynin 5 mg three times a day or tolterodine 2 mg twice a day. The advantage of tolterodine is that it does not cause dryness of mouth. Mirabegron, a $β_3$-adrenergic receptor agonist is the preferred molecule now. The safety margin and side effects are much less compared to other drugs. The dosage is 25–50 mg. In resistant cases, botulinum toxin is injected into the detrusor muscle. This relaxes the bladder muscle and reduces the pressure. If sphincter dyssynergia is also present, both the bladder and sphincter need attention. Bladder can be treated as above with anti-cholinergics and the back pressure changes can be prevented by clean intermittent self-catheterization (CIC). Instead of CIC, skeletal muscle relaxants like diazepam 5 mg thrice daily, dantrolene sodium or baclofen may be tried. In resistant cases, endoscopic incision of the external sphincter may be performed. Sacral neuromodulation is another procedure to manage this condition.

Hyporeflexic bladder (lower motor neuron bladder, neurogenic underactive bladder, autonomous bladder).

Lesions involving the S2, 3, 4 segments or peripheral nerves supplying the bladder, produce LMN bladder. Common causes are spinal cord injury, diabetes mellitus, inter-vertebral disc prolapse (IVDP), abdomino-perineal resection for carcinoma rectum, myelomeningocele and sacral agenesis. Patients are usually able to void by straining or by applying pressure to the lower abdominal wall (Crede's maneuver). They may also present with incomplete emptying, retention with overflow, recurrent UTI or total incontinence. The investigations as for UMN bladder are done. Patients may be treated by training in performing Crede's maneuver, CIC or by cholinergics like bethanechol 40–150 mg/24 hours in divided doses. In selected patients, sacral neuromodulation gives good results.

APPROACH TO URINARY INCONTINENCE

A detailed clinical history, physical examina-tion and a thorough neurological examination help in the diagnosis. A young female child with normal voiding and incontinence since birth or childhood indicates ectopic ureter. In a male child with distended bladder and dribbling, posterior urethral valve is suspected. All male and female children with incontinence should be examined for spina bifida. Urgency incontinence with dysuria suggests UTI, bladder stone or bladder malignancy. If there is no dysuria, the chance of detrusor instability is high. The diagnosis of vesicovaginal and ureterovaginal fistulae can be confirmed by noting the constant dribbling of urine from the vagina. In a young man, palpable bladder and overflow incontinence is often caused by stricture of the urethra. A previous history of urethritis or trauma to the perineum may be present. In an elderly male similar presentation is likely with, BPH and carcinoma prostate.

1. Vesicovaginal Fistula (VVF)

Vesicovaginal fistula (VVF) is a fistulous communication between the vagina and bladder. This may occur following hyster-ectomy, prolonged obstructed labor, carcinoma cervix and pelvic irradiation. Continuous leaking of urine from the vagina is the symptom and occurs about 1–2 weeks following the event. CT urogram or IVU helps to rule out associated ureteral fistula. Cystoscopy demonstrates the size, site and number of fistulae and associated pathology in the bladder.

Definitive management can be undertaken if the bladder appears healthy cystoscopically. Excision of the fistulous tract and closure of the vagina and bladder separately with absorbable suture material is the treatment. Greater omentum may be interposed between the bladder and vaginal repair especially complicated or large fistulae. This procedure can be done laparoscopically or with robotic assistance.

2. Ureterovaginal Fistula (UVF)

Ureterovaginal fistula may follow injury to the ureter by crushing, clamping, ligature or extensive dissection during hystrectomy. It is usually unilateral. In contrast to VVF, patients with UVF void normally but also have incontenance. Since the injury to the ureter leads to hydronephrosis or pyonephrosis, the patient may have symptoms of loin pain, fever, chills and toxemia. CT urogram, IVU, bulb ureterogram and cystoscopy are the diagnostic investigations. Management depends on the condition of the patient and time of diagnosis. If the fistula is detected within a few days following surgery, ureteric stenting is attempted. If the patient presents late and the general condition is satisfactory, ureteric reimplantation is the treatment of choice. If the patient is toxic, diversion of urine by a nephrostomy is advocated till the condition improves. Later, definitive repair is performed. As in VVF repair, this surgery can also be done using laparoscopy or robot.

3. Stress Urinary Incontinence (SUI)

This occurs often in elderly and multiparous women. Diagnosis is made by demonstrating incontinence during coughing while the patient is in the lithotomy, recumbent or standing position. During the test, careful observation is made to know the time when incontinence occurs and the quantity expelled. In urgency incontinence, there is complete emptying of the bladder and it occurs a little after the act of coughing. Genuine SUI and urgency incontinence may coexist. If the patient gives history of leaking large quantities of urine on minimal straining or has previous history of urethral or anterior vaginal wall surgery, or pelvic irradiation, intrinsic sphincter deficiency (ISD) is suspected. This needs pubovaginal sling surgery or artificial sphincter or endoscopic bulking agent therapy. If neurological cause is suspected, or if incontenance is recurrent, a complete urodynamic study is needed. Mild SUI is treated conservatively with pelvic floor exercises, α stimulants like ephedrine, pseudo-ephedrine or in postmenopausal women with estrogen preparation locally. More severe cases need pubovaginal sling or retropubic suspension procedures.

4. Overactive Bladder (OAB)

OAB is of unknown etiology. Both motor and sensory causes could be responsible. Elderly persons and adult females are usually affected. Patients present with frequency, urgency, urgency incontinence and nocturia. There is no dysuria. Diagnosis is made by excluding other causes. Investigations include urinalysis, urine culture, urine cytology and X-ray for KUB-U. Diagnosis is confirmed by a frequency volume chart (intake and output chart noting the time) and cystometry. Treatment is usually unsatisfactory. Mirabegron gives good improvement. In resistant cases, botulinum injection and sacral neuro-modulation are tried.

5. Enuresis

It is defined as persistence of involuntary voiding beyond the age of anticipated bladder control and includes involuntary voiding during sleep/nap. Daytime wetting is called "diurnal enuresis". Most children achieve normal bladder control by the age of 3 years. Girls gain control earlier than boys. Enuresis is more common in boys. At 6 years of age, 10% of children have enuresis. At 14 years of age, only 5% have enuresis and by 15 years 99% of children are "dry". Enuresis may be broadly classified into primary and secondary. In primary enuresis, the child has never attained bladder control. This type constitutes about 75% of the cases. In secondary enuresis, the child gains bladder control and is dry for at least 6 months and enuresis occurs later.

The etiology is multifactorial and many theories have been proposed. They are: (i) A reduction in the functional bladder capacity, (ii) a developmental delay or a maturational lag in development of CNS, (iii) deep sleep, (iv) genetic factors, (v) psychological factors, (vi) food allergy, (vii) pinworm infestation, and (viii) mild degrees of cerebral dysfunction. A careful history regarding the pattern of wetting and voiding along with a detailed clinical examination including the nervous system, is important. The parents and the child are interviewed separately. In a case of pure nocturnal enuresis, urinalysis and culture may be the only investigations required and are usually normal. Additional investigations in the form of ultrasonogram, intravenous urogram, micturating urethrogram and urodynamic studies are necessary when neurological, structural or spinal abnormalities are suspected or when diurnal enuresis is also present.

Treatment

A variety of treatment modalities is available. Depending on the clinical situation behavior modification, fluid intake regulation, bladder training exercises, conditioning alarms or drug therapy may be chosen. For most children with primary nocturnal enuresis, active therapy is withheld till the age of 5 or 6 years. However, for children with day and night wetting, investigations and appropriate treatment are required at an even younger age.

General Measures

Fluids are restricted after 6 pm. The bladder should be emptied at bed time and the child completely awakened a little before the usual time of bed wetting and taken to the toilet. Drugs like imipramine, in doses of 25 mg in children between 5–8 years and 50 mg in children above 8 years given as a single dose at bed time may be helpful in some cases. Those who wet early in the night may benefit from a later afternoon dose rather than bed time dose. A 2-week trial is generally adequate to assess drug responsiveness. Later, the dose or timing may be adjusted. Imipramine helps by reducing the REM (rapid eye movement) sleep, has antispasmodic properties and stimulates ADH. Anticholinergics like propantheline bromide in doses of 7.5–15 mg at night are useful in some cases. Oxybutynin in doses of 2.5–5 mg/kg at night can also be used. It may cause dryness of mouth and constipation. Desmopressin (DDAVP), an agent affecting the urinary output, in doses of 20–40 μg intranasally cures about 20–40% of children with enuresis. Water intoxication is a major side effect and so the therapy should be supervised.

Behavior modification is very effective in the management of the enuresis. It can be achieved by bladder training aimed at progressively increasing the time interval between voidings, so that the bladder capacity is effectively increased. The child is encouraged to hold urine and void at longer intervals and by conditioning therapy where the urinary alarm awakens the child when the first few milliliters of urine come into contact with the system. Psychotherapy and hypnotherapy may also be beneficial in selected cases.

Glomerular Diseases

Immunopathogenesis of Glomerular Diseases

• Soumita Bagchi • Sanjay Kumar Agarwal

Nephrons are the structural and functional units of a kidney. Each nephron comprises the glomerulus and the renal tubule. The glomerular filtration barrier comprises the fenestrated capillary endothelium, the glomerular basement membrane (GBM) and the visceral epithelial cells (podocytes). Immune mechanisms play a central role in the pathogenesis of majority of glomerular diseases. The glomerular filtration barrier is a chief target of immune mediated injury in these diseases. In the past, the adaptive immunity constituted by the antibodies and T cells alone was considered to be mainly responsible for immune mediated glomerular damage. However, now it is recognized that the innate immune system also plays an important role. The roles played by innate and adaptive immunity in the pathogenesis of glomerular diseases will be discussed in this chapter.

The Innate Immunity

The innate immune response occurs immediately after an inciting event like an infection. It is the first line of defence against pathogens. The constituents of the innate immune system, namely toll-like receptors (TLRs) and the complement system participate in the adaptive immune process as well. In innate immunity, there is no latent period, whereas adaptive immunity, requires time to process and present an antigen to mount a specific immune response.

Toll-like Receptors

Toll-like receptors (TLRs) are present on endosomes in the cytoplasm as well as on cell membranes. Over 10 isoforms of TLRs (serial numbers 1–10) have been identified. They have the capability to recognize molecular patterns. So, they can recognize conserved patterns like peptidoglycans, lipopolysaccharides, bacterial and viral nucleic acids. The TLRs recognize the pathogen-associated molecular patterns (PAMPs) and endogenous molecular patterns known as damage associated molecular patterns (DAMPs) that are derived following autoimmune injury from either dying parenchymal cells or during extracellular matrix remodelling (Fig. 13.1). A large number of cell types in the kidneys including the endothelial, mesangial and tubular epithelial cells express TLRs 1 to 6. Macrophages and neutrophils also express TLRs. Although they are not normally present in the kidneys, they are recruited when there is an inflammatory stimulus. There is a similar type of cytoplasmic receptors called 'nod-like receptors' (NLR) expressed in renal mononuclear phagocytes.

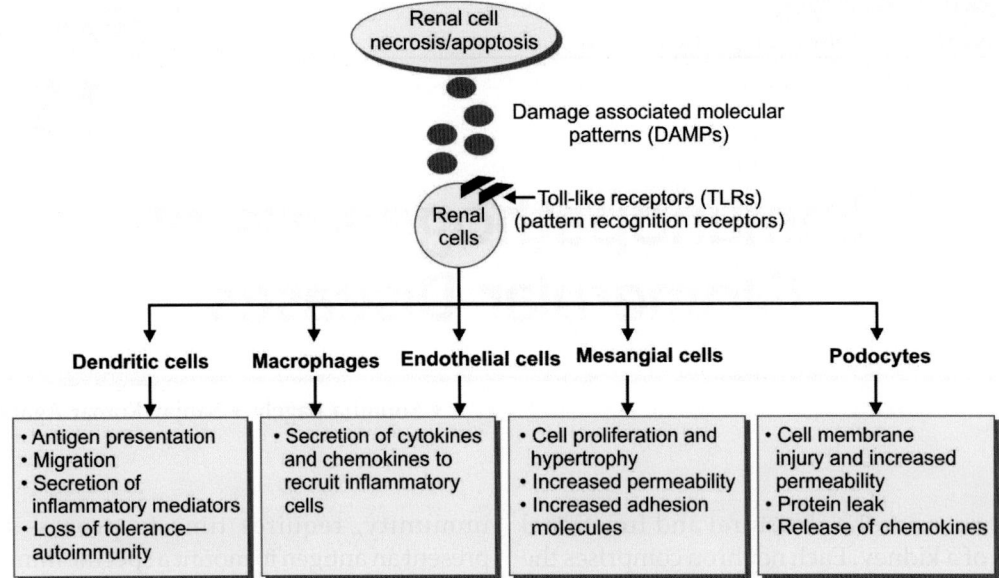

Fig. 13.1: Role of toll-like receptors in glomerular disease

PAMPs and/or DAMPs upregulate TLRs and NLRs and activate multiple intracellular signalling pathways. The signalling pathways control the release of many inflammatory mediators through the nuclear factor κB (NFκB). Mediators like chemokines, cytokines and proteases are released by the inflammatory cells. These mediators activate the resident glomerular cells and other inflammatory cells like neutrophils and macrophages causing glomerular inflammation. Depending on whether the initial stimulus is transient or persistent, the extent of injury and disease pattern varies. Podocyte injury is common and leads to increased glomerular permeability and proteinuria. In the case of adaptive immunity, TLRs promote conversion of dendritic cells to antigen presenting cells.

Complement System

A clear concept about the complement system is essential for understanding the pathogenesis of many renal diseases. The complement system (Fig. 13.2) consisting of its multiple regulatory proteins is an integral part of the innate immune system. It plays a significant role in the pathogenesis of glomerular disease through multiple pathways. There are three pathways by which complement system is activated. They are the 'classical', the 'alternate' and the 'mannose binding lectin (MBL)' pathways.

In the classical pathway, the antigen and antibody (immunoglobulins) combine to form immune complexes (IC) which bind to and activate the complement 'C1 complex' which consists of C1q, r and s. The activated 'C1 complex' splits C4 to C4a and b. The C4b subsequently cleaves C2 to C2a and C2b. The C4b2b complex forms the C3 convertase of the classical pathway and converts C3 to C3a and C3b. The C4b2b3b complex is called the 'C5 convertase'.

The alternate pathway does not rely on IC for its activation. In fact, this pathway remains in a state of continuous activation due to hydrolysis of C3 at a slow and steady rate. However, C3b is rapidly inactivated by factor H and factor I present in the normal serum. When C3 hydrolysis is more than the capacity

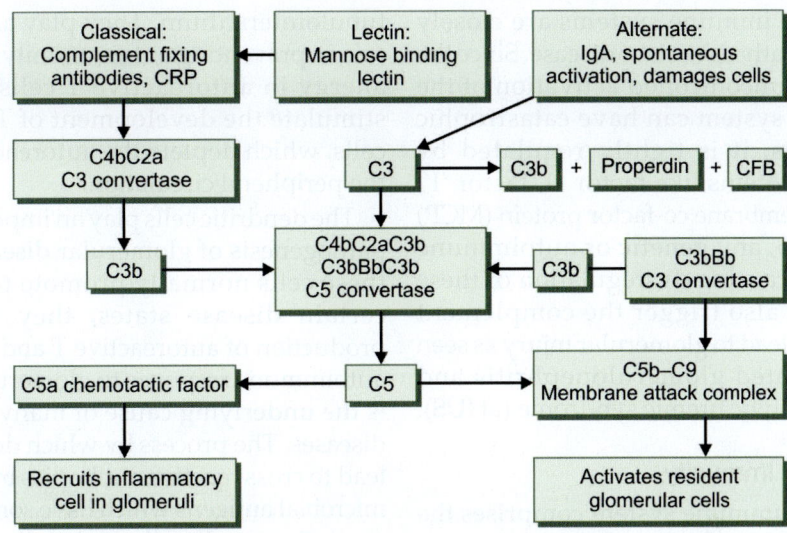

Fig. 13.2: The complement system and glomerular disease

to inactivate, it combines with factor B to form C3bBb which is the 'C3 convertase' of the alternate pathway. Thus, the alternate pathway activation directly acts on C3 and progresses further by activating the downstream events.

The MBL pathway activation is triggered by microbes and binding of galactosyl immuno-globulin G (IgG) to circulating MBL. It acts directly on C4 bypassing the C1 complex and continue the same pattern as the classical pathway.

The rest of the events in the complement cascade are common to all the three pathways. In the next step, C3b cleaves C5 to C5a and C5b and C5a acts as a chemotactic factor to recruits inflammatory cells like neutrophils and macrophages. The C5b combines with other complement components C6, 7, 8 and 9 to form the C5b, 6, 7, 8, 9 or membrane attack complex (MAC). The horizontal line above the numbers suggest 'activated' component of the comple-ment. The MAC drills holes in the cell membrane and cause cell death (Fig. 13.3). It converts resident glomerular cells (endothelial, mesangial and epithelial cells) to local and effector inflammatory cells. Thus, it causes damage to cells with the release of multiple

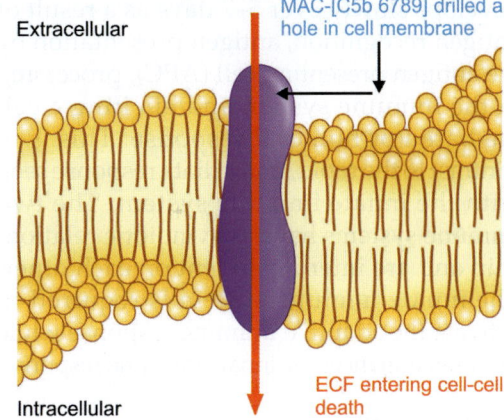

Fig. 13.3: Membrane attack complex. MAC drills a hole in cell membrane and extracellular fluid enters cytoplasm and cell death occurs

inflammatory mediators like cytokines, growth factors, proteases, eicosanoids and oxidants. It also genetically upregulates the production of extracellular matrix components which leads to scarring and sclerosis.

The complement cascade may be activated by specific IC as well as nonspecifically by pathogens and damaged cells. Also the complement component C5a activates the TLRs directly thus suggesting that the innate and adaptive immune systems are closely linked in the pathogenesis of disease. Since the abnormal or uncontrolled activation of the complement system can have catastrophic consequences, it is tightly regulated by number of proteins like factor H, factor 'I', properdin, membrane co-factor protein (MCP) and CD59. So, any genetic or autoimmune abnormality causing dysregulation of these proteins can also trigger the complement pathway and lead to glomerular injury as seen in C3 associated glomerulonephritis and atypical hemolytic uremic syndrome (aHUS).

The Adaptive Immunity

The adaptive immune system comprises the T and B lymphocytes and their soluble mediators. These cells are not present normally, in the glomerulus. Its response develops slowly over 5–7 days as a result of antigen recognition, antigen presentation by the antigen presenting cell (APC), processing in the immune system and eliciting a cell mediated or humoral response. This is in contrast to the rapid, immediate response seen with the innate immune system. The two immune systems have as symbiotic relationship and are interdependent on each other. The innate immune system is required to activate the adaptive immune response while the latter enhances the innate immune response.

Dendritic Cells

Though the dendritic cells are considered to be part of the innate immune system, they play an important role in initiating the adaptive immune response and preventing auto-immunity under normal circumstances. They capture the exogenous antigens like microbes and microbial products and present it through MHC class II molecules to CD4+ T cells. The CD4+ T cells stimulate B cells and plasma cells to produce specific antibodies against these exogenous antigens. Under normal conditions, these dendritic cells are not seen in the normal glomerulus but are widely present in the renal tubulointerstitium. They play an important role in preventing autoimmunity by inducing anergy in autoreactive T cells. They also stimulate the development of T regulatory cells, which deplete the autoreactive cells in the peripheral circulation.

The dendritic cells play an important role in pathogenesis of glomerular disease. Though these cells normally promote tolerance, in certain disease states, they trigger the production of autoreactive T and B cells. This autoimmune response to glomerular antigens is the underlying cause of many glomerular diseases. The process by which dendritic cells lead to cross reactive antibodies by presenting microbial antigens which have some structural similarity to cell antigens is called 'molecular mimicry'. The dendritic cells may sometimes process and present self-antigens derived from dying cells to autoreactive T cells triggering an autoimmune process. The dendritic cells, through a pathway known as 'cross presentation' may present exogenous antigens to CD8 cells which are then activated and differentiate to cytotoxic T cells resulting in glomerular injury.

Immune Mediated Glomerular Injury

Antibody mediated glomerular damage may occur through three pathways:

1. Antibodies react with fixed glomerular antigens like components of the glomerular basement membrane or the podoctye. Anti-GBM antibody reacts with type 4 collagen in the GBM and leads to anti-GBM disease. Antibodies to podocyte protein M-type phospholipase A_2 receptor (PLA2R) lead to primary membranous nephropathy.

2. Antibodies bind to antigens which are trapped in the glomeruli like microbial antigens (components of HBV or HCV, drugs, nucleosomal antigens and meta-bolites).

3. Circulating preformed ICs are deposited in various sites in the glomeruli depending on their size and other characteristics.

The biologic properties of the antibody and/or antigen influence the pathogenesis of diseases. There are 3 main issues relating to interaction between antigen and antibody. The antibody related issues are:

a. The ability to activate the complement pathway varies with the antibody subclass and isotype. IgM is the most potent activator. IgG1 and IgG3 activate classical pathway. IgG2, IgG4 and normally glyco-sylated IgA are poor activators of classical pathway. However, IgA aggregates [non-glycosylated (abnormal) IgA] can activate the alternate complement pathway and the MBL pathway.

b. Antibodies produced within weeks of antigen exposure have lower affinity for the antigen, while 'late' antibodies produced after 4–6 weeks have higher antigen binding capacity.

c. The antigen's affinity for its specific antibody is determined by the number of epitopes (valence) unique for that antibody carried by the antigen.

The properties of the immune complex also have influence on the immune mechanisms. Factors like the electrical charge and molecular size influence the pathogenicity. Cationic (positively charged) nature of IC favours their deposition in the glomeruli since the glomerular basement membrane is negatively charged. In situations of local glomerular injury, the chances of *in situ* immune complex formation are higher. The other mechanism is trapping of circulating immune complexes within the glomerulus. The severity of disease varies with the size and quantum of IC. The relative concentrations of the circulating antigen and antibody determines the size of the IC. Based on their size, immune complexes (IC) are classified as:

a. *Small sized IC:* These are formed when there is significant antigen excess. They have poor affinity for receptors of the innate immune cells and are poor activators of the complement system. They become patho-genic only when they are deposited on the glomerular capillary endothelial cells or endothelial surfaces of small blood vessels. Here, they trigger type III hypersensitivity reaction, complement activation, recruitment of inflammatory cells and damage the endothelium resulting in acute necrotizing vasculitis.

b. *Medium (intermediate) size IC:* These are formed when there is a slight antigenic excess or nearly equivalent amount of antigen and antibody. They are the most pathogenic ICs as they are powerful activators of the complement system. Acute inflammation and severe glomerular injury results due to their trapping in subendo-thelial and subepithelial locations. They are not efficiently cleared by the phagocytes and thus can cause sustained damage.

c. *Large size ICs:* These are formed when there is antibody excess in the circulation. Extensive crosslinking and formation of large insoluble complexes occur because the immunoglobulins forming the anti-bodies are large molecular weight proteins. Although they can activate the complement pathway, their affinity for Fc receptors on phagocytic cells in spleen and liver enable rapid phagocytosis and clearance from the circulation. Thus, the pathogenic response is limited.

Clinicopathologic Correlation in Immune Mediated Glomerular Disease

The histopathologic pattern and clinical profile of glomerular diseases is determined by the pattern of immune mediated glomerular injury. In inflammatory/proliferative glo-merular diseases, if the ICs are deposited in the subendothelial and mesangial region, following events occur sequentially:

i. Since ICs are exposed to the circulation, complement activation is triggered.

ii. Opsonization of the ICs by C3b, occurs

iii. C3a and C5a recruit inflammatory cells into the mesangium and subendothelium.

iv. Resident glomerular cells stimulated.

v. The mesangial cells produce inflammatory cytokines and chemokines directly.

vi. Exaggerated inflammatory response.

vii. Macrophages and neutrophils infiltrate glomeruli and perpetuate the glomerular injury.

viii. Cytokines promote mesangial cell proliferation and hypertrophy.

ix. Resulting in 'inflammatory' or 'proliferative' glomerular disease.

x. Clinically nephritic or nephritic-nephrotic presentation.

In non-inflammatory/non-proliferative glomerular diseases, the ICs have subepithelial distribution or target an antigen of the podocyte (they are on the other side of the basement membrane). The sequence of events is as follows:

i. The resident cells have no proliferative activity.

ii. The small quantities of the membrane attack complex (C5b–9) causes podocyte injury and effacement.

iii. Increased glomerular permeability.

iv. Significant proteinuria.

v. Subepithelial deposits unable to recruit inflammatory cells from the circulation (located on other side of GBM)

vi. Complement components (C3a and C5a) generated in subepithelial space are rapidly filtered and lost in urine.

vii. No inflammatory cells in the glomeruli

viii. Presents with nephrotic syndrome, e.g. membranous nephropathy.

ix. Example of 'non-inflammatory'/'non proliferative' disease pattern.

In conclusion, majority of glomerulonephritis are results of interplay of innate and adpative immunity. Both systemic and resident glomerular cells are involved. Complement cascade is activated, various cytokines released, proliferation of resident cells in the glomerulus occurs, chemotaxis of neutrophils and monocytes occur and a cascade of events follow. These result in the various manifestations of glomerular disease.

Overview of Glomerular Disease and Classification

• Sanjay Kumar Agarwal

Renal diseases can be approached in two ways: Firstly, based on a symptom like hematuria, proteinuria, oliguria, pain or nocturia and secondly, based on the syndromic approach which based on specific groups of symptoms constituting a syndrome. Syndromic approach is better than approach based on one symptom or sign. Common syndromes in patients with renal diseases are (*see* also Chapter 4):

1. Acute kidney injury
2. Chronic kidney disease
3. Proliferative glomerulonephritis (GN)
4. Rapidly progressive GN
5. Nephrotic syndrome
6. Asymptomatic urinary abnormality (AU)
7. Urinary tract infection
8. Urinary tract obstruction
9. Stone disease
10. Hypertension

If we see above syndrome, glomerular disease can cause following syndromes:

1. Chronic kidney disease
2. Proliferative glomerulonephritis
3. Rapidly progressive GN
4. Nephrotic syndrome
5. Asymptomatic urinary abnormality (AU)

Glomerulonephritis (GN) which represents inflammatory response within the glomerulus has two types of manifestations:

I. *Renal manifestations*
   a. Hematuria
   b. Proteinuria
   c. Alteration in glomerular filtration rate (acutely or rapidly)

II. *Systemic manifestations*
   a. Hypertension
   b. Fluid retention
   c. Hypoalbuminemia
   d. Hypercholesterolemia

The glomerulus consists of endothelial cells, mesangial cells, visceral and parietal epithelial cells, glomerular basement membrane (GBM) and mesangium (Fig. 14.1).

It is useful for the clinician to differentiate whether GN is proliferative or non-proliferative. Proliferative is related to proliferation of one of the resident cells of the glomerulus. There is some correlation between clinical presentation and changes in the morphology (histology) in proliferative and non-proliferative GN (Table 14.1).

If the onset of illness is less acute, and associated with no or minimal hypertension, near-normal renal function and absence of abnormal urinary sediments (RBC and RBC cast) it may suggest non-proliferative GN. Nephrotic syndrome (NS), asymptomatic urinary abnormalities (AU) or early stages of

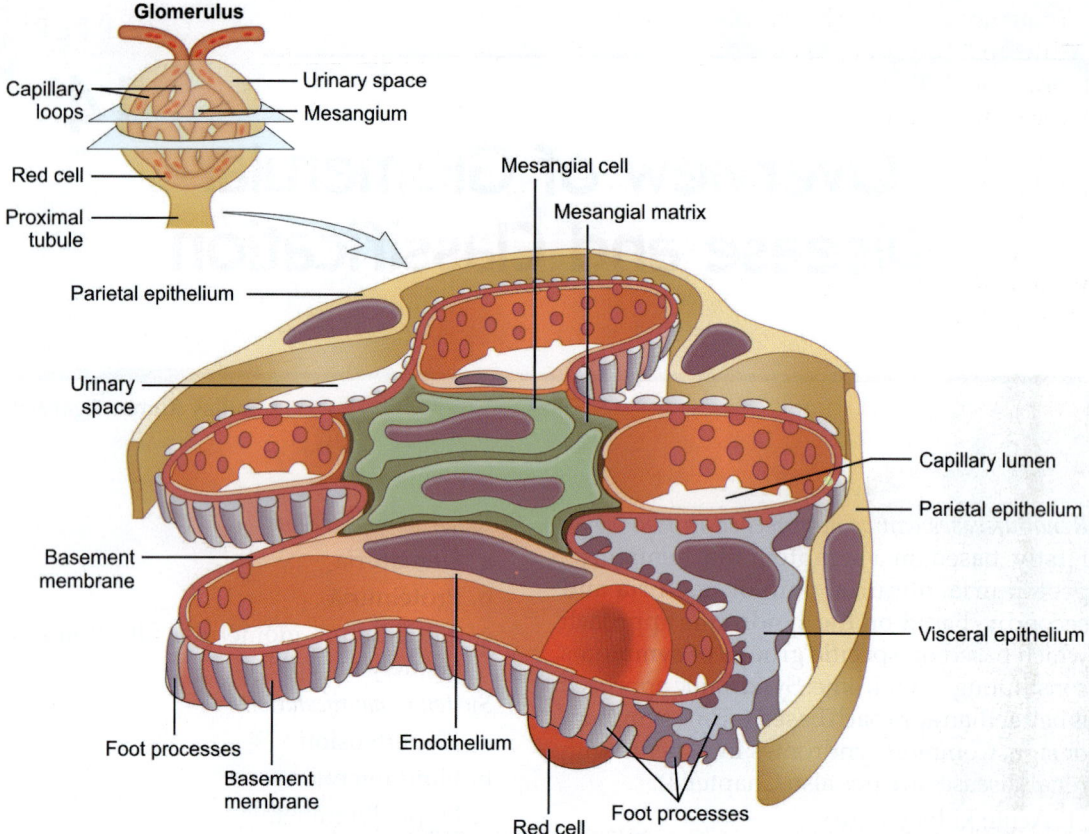

Fig. 14.1: Glomerular structure

Table 14.1: Common causes of proliferative and nonproliferative GN

1. Non-proliferative GN
   a. Minimal change disease (MCD)
   b. Membranous GN (MGN)
   c. Focal and segmental glomerulosclerosis (FSGS)
2. Proliferative GN
   a. Mesangioproliferative GN (MesPGN)
   b. IgA nephropathy (IgAN)
   c. Focal proliferative GN (FPGN)
   d. Crescentic GN (CrGN)
   e. Membranoproliferative GN (MPGN)

chronic kidney diseases (CKD) are the common conditions associated with non-proliferative GN. On the other hand, proliferative GN can present as MesPGN, IgAN, FPGN, MPGN and CrGN. In the case of FSGS,

both the pattern of presentation may be encountered.

In the case of GN, the same etiology can produce different morphological patterns and the same morphological pattern can be caused by different etiologies. Since the approach to diagnosis and treatment may differ, it is necessary to understand both morphology and etiology for deciding proper treatment.

A simple approach to a patient with GN by addressing the following.

Confirm Glomerular Involvement

Any patient with renal disease is said to have glomerular disease if any or more of the following features are found:

1. Significant proteinuria (usually more than 1 g/day) is an evidence of glomerular

proteinuria. (In nonglomerular proteinuria due to tubular diseases or 'overflow' proteinuria due to very high blood levels, the urinary protein excretion is usually less than 1 gm/day.)

2. RBC cast in urine suggests active glomerular disease.

Dysmorphic RBC cast (Fig. 14.2) and dysmorphic RBC (Fig. 14.3) are taken as "active" urinary sediments.

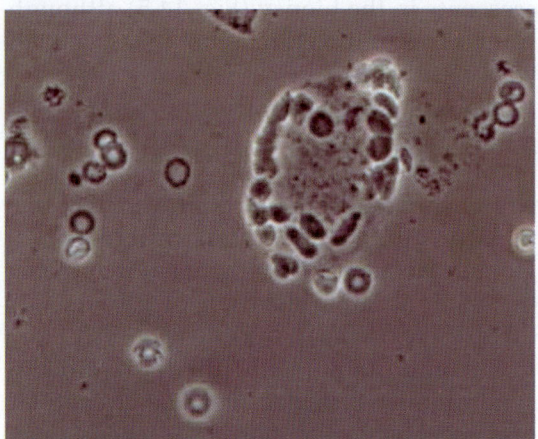

Fig. 14.2: RBC cast. *Note:* RBCs singly and adhering to the cast

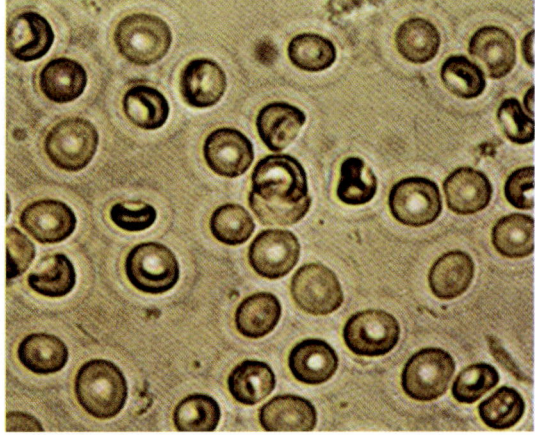

Fig. 14.3: Dysmorphic RBC. *Note:* Shape of RBCs differ and are not uniformly 'biconcave discs' abnormal shapes are seen

Identify the Syndrome

Once presence of glomerular disease is confirmed, it is necessary to identify the clinical syndrome. As discussed earlier, glomerular disease can produce following clinical syndromes:

1. Acute GN or proliferative GN
2. Nephrotic syndrome (NS)
3. Rapidly progressive GN
4. Asymptomatic urinary abnormality (AU)
5. Chronic kidney disease

Acute glomerulonephritis (AGN) is a clinical syndrome characterized by abrupt onset of hematuria (gross leading to smoky urine and or microscopic), hypertension (usually mild), edema, oliguria and fall in GFR. These symptoms occur following an interval of 1–4 weeks after throat or skin infection. The interval between the infection and onset of symptoms may be lesser when following throat infection compared to skin infection. It is common in children with some male preponderance. The body produces antibodies against the streptococcal antigen, the antigen–antibody complexes deposit in the glomeruli and initiate an acute inflammatory response within the glomeruli. This results in the symptoms and signs of acute GN. Histologically, almost all glomeruli are involved, appear swollen, contain numerous cells including polymorphonuclear leukocytes. The capillary lumens may even be occluded partially. This histological picture is described as diffuse endocapillary exudative proliferative GN (Fig. 14.4).

Nephrotic syndrome is a clinicopathological syndrome characterized by glomerular proteinuria of more than 3.5 g/day/1.73 sq.m body surface area, associated with edema, hypoalbuminemia, hypercholesterolemia and hypercoagulability. The degree of proteinuria is usually interpreted while taking GFR and serum protein levels also into consideration. Patients with severe hypoalbuminemia and low GFR may not have more than 3.5 g

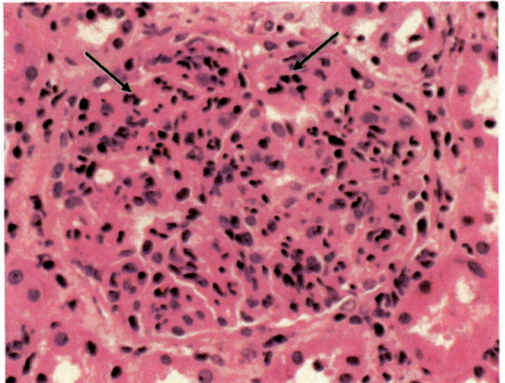

Fig. 14.4: Histology of glomerulus in acute GN. *Note:* Single glomerulus in high power. Most capillary lumens are occluded. The number of cells inside the glomerulus is greatly increased. Many polymorphonuclear cells are also seen

Rapidly progressive GN is a clinical syndrome with evidence of glomerular disease and rapid fall in renal function (GFR) by more than 50% within days to weeks. The onset may not be as dramatic as acute GN but the progression to end stage kidney disease may occur rapidly if not treated in time. In some cases, the progression may occur in spite of treatment. Renal biopsy will help to identify the cause and guide appropriate treatment. The characteristic pathological finding is crescents in the biopsy (Fig. 14.5) although some cases of RPGN may not be associated with crescents.

proteinuria to classify as nephrotic syndrome. We should also differentiate between nephrotic syndrome from nephrotic range proteinuria. There are conditions which have nephrotic range proteinuria but they are not approached like nephrotic syndrome. For example, a patient of amyloidosis may continue to have nephrotic range proteinuria in spite of going into advanced CKD. Similar is diabetes in advance stage may continue to have nephrotic proteinuria but is approached as CKD and not nephrotic syndrome.

Asymptomatic urinary abnormality is a glomerular syndrome in which there is minimal glomerular involvement associated with abnormality in urine in form of proteinuria, usually <1.0 g/day and or (microscopic) glomerular hematuria without any symptoms or systemic manifestation of glomerular disease like edema or hypertension, etc.

Chronic glomerulonephritis is clinical syndrome in which the patient has glomerular disease for a long time and has reached a stage where the disease is unlikely to respond to treatment. This diagnosis is made on the basis of evidence of glomerular disease going on for many months. Depending on the cause, the

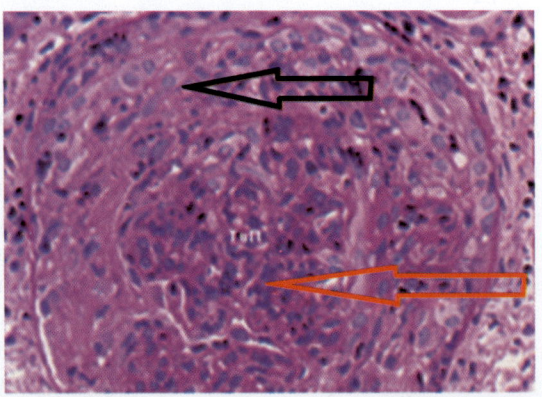

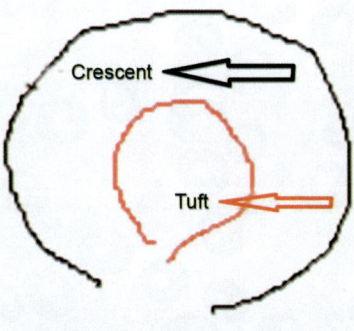

Fig. 14.5: Histology of crescentic GN. *Note:* Single glomerulus under high power. The glomerular capillaries are crowded (red arrow) and compressed by proliferation of parietal epithelial cells in the glomerulus (black arrow) (*see* accompanying line diagram)

patient may or may not have symptoms referable to renal system. This is broad term and includes glomerular disease causing progressive worsening of renal function. The kidneys may be contracted and echogenic on ultrasonography. Renal biopsy if performed, may show sclerosis of glomeruli and tubulointerstitial changes (Fig. 14.6).

Secondary Glomerular Diseases

The next step is to decide is that whether glomerular disease is primary or secondary. Diagnosis of primary GN is made by the exclusion of secondary causes. If extensive appropriate investigations are undertaken, it will be possible to identify the cause in a large number of cases. If no cause found, then GN is labelled as primary or idiopathic. In few situations, the secondary cause can be suspected on the basis of history and clinical examination. Conditions like preceeding throat infection, skin infection, or any other infection, features of rheumatoid arthritis, Henoch-Schönlein purpura, systemic lupus, scleroderma or other collagen vascular disease are easily identified on history and physical examination. In other situations, secondary cause is found only on further investigation. Sometimes secondary cause is suspected only on renal histology as in conditions like amyloidosis, myeloma, monoclonal light chain nephropathy (due to kappa or lambda restriction). In such cases further investigations are planned to confirm the diagnosis and plan treatment (Table 14.2).

Table 14.2: Brief classification of secondary causes of GN

A. Infections
  a Bacterial
    • Streptococcal
    • Staphylococcal
    • Salmonella
    • Other gram-negative infection
  b Viral
    • HBV
    • HCV
    • CMV
    • Enterovirus
    • Parvovirus
  c Parasitic
    • Malaria
    • Filaria
    • Toxoplasma

B. Connective tissue disorders and vasculitis
  a. Systemic lupus
  b. Rheumatoid arthritis
  c. Sjögren syndrome
  d. Progressive systemic sclerosis (PSS)
  e. Cryoglobulinemia
  f. Polyangiitis
  g. Wegner's granulomatosis
  h. Microscopic polyangiitis
  i. Henoch-Schönlein purpura (HSP)

C. Paraproteinemia
  a. Multiple myeloma
  b. Light chain deposition disease
  c. Monoclonal gammopathy of renal significance (MGRS)

D. Malignancy

E. Drugs

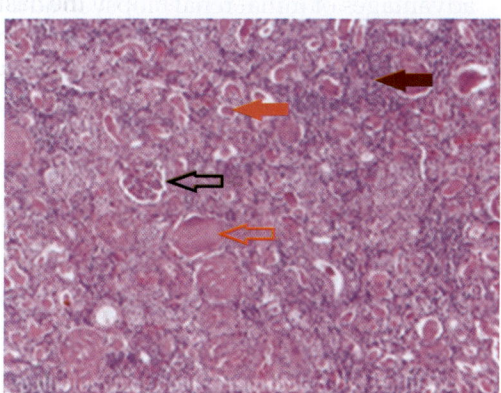

Fig. 14.6: Renal histology in chronic glomerulonephritis. Low power view showing glomeruli, tubules and interstitium
Note: Black open arrow → one viable glomerulus
    Red open arrow → sclerosed glomerulus
    Red bold arrow → atrophic tubule
    Brown bold arrow → interstitium showing lymphomononuclear infiltration

Investigations

As discussed, majority of secondary GN are identified based on investigations. If there is clinical suspicion of a particular disease, then investigations should be restricted to confirming the same. In other situations, a battery of tests is done to diagnose the secondary cause of GN.

Preliminary investigations in all cases of suspected GN:

1. *Urine examination:* Routine urine, urinary sediment and urine protein/creatinine ratio.
2. *Hematology:* Complete hemogram, ESR
3. *Renal function tests:* Blood urea, serum creatinine, Na, K and blood gases (only if indicated or patient is very sick).
4. *Coagulation profile:* Bleeding time, clotting time, activated partial thromboplastin time (aPTT), prothombin time and INR as part of pre-biopsy tests.
5. *Complete serum biochemistry*—Ca, PO_4, alkaline phosphatase, uric acid, total protein, albumin, total cholesterol, triglycerides, LDL, total bilirubin, AST and ALT.
6. *Blood sugar:* Fasting and HBA1c
7. *US abdomen:* Size, echogenicity, CM differentiation, any associated obstruction

Following investigations are done as indicated to identify secondary cause of GN:

1. *For infections:* Antistreptolysin O titre (ASO), complement factor 3 (C3) level, hepatitis B (HB) and hepatitis C (HC) virus, tests for malaria, and cultures of body fluids as needed.
2. *For connective tissue disease:* Tests for antinuclear antibody (ANA), anti-double stranded DNA (dsDNA), rheumatoid factor, cryoglobinemia.
3. *For vasculitis:* Test for antineutrophil cytoplasmic antibody (ANCA) both cytoplasmic 'cANCA' and perinuclear 'pANCA').
4. *For paraproteinemia:* Protein electrophoresis of blood and urine, free light chain assay, bone marrow aspiration/biopsy and immunoelectrophoresis.
5. *For malignancy:* Usually imaging tests and endoscopy are performed depending on symptoms for localising any malignancy.

Indications for Renal Biopsy

Kidney biopsy is a very important investigation in a patient with glomerular disease.

i. If AGN occurs in a child, renal biopsy is not performed initially. However, in an adult, early renal biopsy is a preferred investigation if facilities are available. The usual indications of renal biopsy in all age groups are:
   a. Gross hematuria for >4 weeks
   b. Oliguria persisting for >2–3 weeks
   c. Low complement >8 weeks
   d. Hematuria and proteinuria >12 months
   e. In systemic disease for assessing prognosis and severity
   f. Need for dialysis (biopsy done after stabilizing the patient)

ii. In adults with nephrotic syndrome, renal biopsy on presentation is necessary. The advantages of initial renal biopsy in adults are to enable timely diagnosis of unsuspected secondary causes. Conditions like amyloidosis, monoclonal gammopathy, systemic lupus and IgA nephropathy are diagnosed by renal biopsy. It also helps in planning long-term management and assessing prognosis.

iii. Patients with RPGN always need renal biopsy as an urgent procedure as the biopsy findings help in differentiation of various types of RPGN based on light microscopy and immunofluorescence and line of management is guided by renal histology and other findings.

iv. In AUA, patients are mostly followed up. During follow-up if the condition worsens in term of proteinuria or some systemic feature develop, only then they are subjected to biopsy.

v. Patients with CGN often have advanced disease with contracted kidneys and usually biopsy is avoided. Renal biopsy in CGN is considered if a primary diagnosis can be made so that renal transplantation and post-transplant management can be planned.

Treatment Options

Treatment may be general and specific. General treatment is mostly symptomatic in the form of:

a. Bed rest
b. Diet restriction of fluid and salt
c. Diuretics as needed
d. Antihypertensives as needed
e. Antibiotics or anti-infective agents for infection
f. Specific treatment of systemic disease causing AGN like systemic lupus, which is beyond the scope of this article.
g. Role of immunosuppressive medicine including steroid in post-infective GN is controversial and mostly limited to patients who are progressively deteriorating in terms of renal function or proteinuria.

Management of nephrotic syndrome is divided into symptomatic treatment, specific treatment and immunosuppressive therapy

A. *Supportive treatment*
   a. *Diet:* Salt and fat restriction
   b. Diuretics
   c. Antihypertensive if required
   d. Antilipidemic drugs
   e. Anticoagulant in very specific situation (history of thromboembolism or serum albumin is less than 1.5 g/dl)
   f. IV albumin transiently (during infection, preoperative and massive edema with oliguria)
   g. ACE inhibitor or angiotensin receptor blocker as nonspecific antiproteinuric drugs

B. *Specific treatment*
   • Treatment of specific infections like HBV, HCV, malaria, etc.

• Stopping offending drug in case of drug-induced NS.
• Treatment of malignancy if that is cause.

C. *Immunosuppressive therapy*: In addition to supportive therapy and in the absence of any specific therapy, majority of nephrotic syndrome needs steroid with or without cytotoxic therapy. In most situation steroid is primary line of treatment and cytotoxic drugs are used, if patients do not respond to steroid, or there is frequent relapsing nephrotic syndrome. The common cytotoxic drugs nowadays used in various nephrotic syndromes are:

   a. Cyclophosphamide
   b. Calcineurin inhibitors (cyclosporine and tacrolimus)
   c. Azathioprine
   d. MMF
   e. Rituximab
   f. Plasmapheresis

Management of RPGN mostly require steroid and cytotoxic drugs in addition to supportive treatment as in nephrotic syndrome. In addition to cytotoxic drugs, often these patients do need IVIG and plasmapheresis. Details of RPGN treatment is out of scope of this manuscript.

Management of AUA is mostly observation and follow-up and intervention are required once there is associated systemic symptoms or degree of urinary findings worsen. Then these patients actually fall into another category of glomerular syndrome and managed accordingly.

Management of CGN is primarily management like chronic kidney disease (CKD). These are broadly:

a. Prevent, detect and promptly treat acute factors causing further kidney injury.
b. Avoid nephrotoxic drugs
c. Adjust doses for the degree of renal dysfunction.

d. Conservative treatment of CKD

e. Early and adequate hepatitis B infection

f. Protein restriction to 0.6–0.8 g/kg/day

g. Management of:
- Hypertension
- Anemia
- Acidosis
- Renal bone disease

h. Early elective discussion and preparation of RRT.

Prognosis

Although prognosis of glomerular disease depends on etiology and clinical syndrome, there are certain broad prognostic factors, which are applicable to other glomerular diseases also.

Poor prognostic factors are:

a. Proliferative GN

b. Heavy proteinuria

c. Deteriorating renal function

d. Primary glomerular diseases

e. Chronicity on histology

f. Poor response to treatment

In conclusion, glomerular disease is very common renal disorder, which presents with various clinical syndromes. In addition to different clinical syndrome, there are different etiology of glomerular diseases. Therefore, one must know both the histopathological pattern and etiology of glomerular disease. Overall treatment and prognosis depends on clinical syndrome, etiology and histology of glomerular disease.

Nephrotic Syndrome

• N Gopalakrishnan • K Sathyasagar • C Rakesh Durai

INTRODUCTION

Nephrotic syndrome (NS) is an important manifestation of glomerular diseases and almost always denotes glomerular disease. The term 'nephrotic syndrome' denotes a unique combination of clinical and laboratory phenomena. The 'hallmark' of NS is massive proteinuria (more than 3.5 g/24 hours) and is usually accompanied by edema, hypo-albuminemia, and hyperlipidemia. Nephrotic proteinuria without edema usually implies a secondary cause for glomerular disease. NS, by itself is not a disease. It is the manifestation of a host of pathological conditions. It can be due to primary glomerular diseases (idiopathic NS) or due to various other diseases (secondary NS).

ETIOLOGY

The causes of NS may be primary or secondary (Table 15.1). In addition to the primary causes, NS can occur due to other conditions affecting the glomeruli in other illnesses.

Clinical Features and Pathogenesis

The predominant clinical manifestations of NS are the sequelae following proteinuria, leading to hypoalbuminemia, edema, hyperlipidemia and sometimes lipiduria. Proteinuria occurs when there is damage to the glomerular filtering mechanism consisting of endothelial cell layer, basement membrane and epithelial cell layer (Fig. 15.1). Individual types of NS may have associated features which are discussed in the appropriate sections. The central figure in our understanding of the pathogenesis of many types of NS in the recent times is the role of podocytes. The role of podocytes is briefly discussed here followed by the pathogenesis of various manifestations of NS.

Podocyte (Visceral Epithelial Cell)

The visceral epithelial layer of Bowman's capsule consists of a unique cell type known as podocyte (Fig. 15.2). These are highly differen-tiated and specialized cells attached to the outer surface of the glomerular capillaries. They have a large cell body projecting into the urinary space. From the cell body, long primary processes emerge and project towards the capillaries. Final ramifications of the primary process are known as foot processes and they are attached to the outer surface of the glomerular basement membrane covering the capillaries (Fig. 15.3). The foot processes from different cell bodies interdigitate and the space between adjacent foot processes is bridged by a thin (40 nm width) membranous structure known as 'slit diaphragm'. Podocyte injury seems to play a central role in the pathogenesis

Table 15.1: Causes of nephrotic syndrome

I. Primary glomerular diseases (idiopathic NS)
 a. Minimal change disease (MCD)
 b. Focal and segmental glomerulosclerosis (FSGS)
 c. Membranous nephropathy (MN)
 d. Membranoproliferative glomerulonephritis (MPGN)
 e. IgA nephropathy
II. Secondary NS
 a. *Connective tissue diseases:* Systemic lupus erythematosus, rheumatoid arthritis
 b. *Metabolic diseases:* Diabetes mellitus
 c. *Infections:*
  • Hepatitis B
  • Hepatitis C
  • Human immunodeficiency virus (HIV)
  • Post-infectious glomerulonephritis
  • Infective endocarditis,
  • Quartan malaria and other rare infections
 d. *Drugs:*
  • Gold
  • d-penicillamine
  • Rifampicin
  • NSAIDs
  • Lithium
 e. *Heredofamilial diseases:*
  • Alport's syndrome
  • Fabry's disease
  • Congenital nephrotic syndrome
  • Lecithin–cholesterol acyltransferase deficiency
 f. *Neoplasms:*
  • Lymphoma, carcinoma stomach, colon, breast, lung
  • Leukemia
 g. *Multisystem diseases*
  • Amyloidosis, sarcoidosis
 h. *Miscellaneous:*
  • Morbid obesity
  • Pre-eclampsia
  • Paraproteinemias

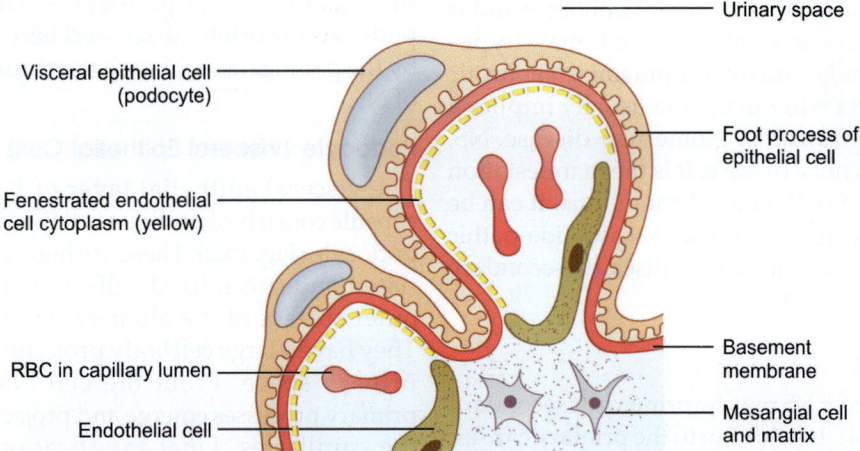

Fig. 15.1: Line diagram of normal glomerular capillary wall showing relationship of mesangium, endothelial cell and visceral epithelial cell

of idiopathic NS. Foot process effacement and disruption of slit diaphragm are common ultrastructural features of glomerular diseases. Podocytopenia is noted in many glomerular diseases. Mutations of podocyte proteins like nephrin and podocin result in congenital NS. Idiopathic membranous nephropathy is due to autoantibody to podocyte antigen 'M-type phospholipase A2 receptor (PLA2R)'. CD80 expression in MCD not in FSGS.

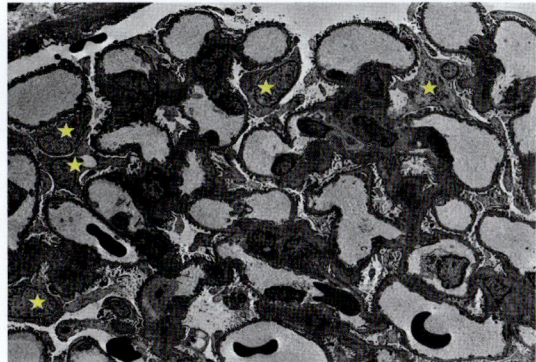

Fig. 15.2: Scanning electron photomicrograph of a normal glomerulus. The yellow asterix indicates podocytes

Proteinuria

The glomerulus acts like a macromolecular sieve, retarding passage of plasma proteins, but allowing free flow of water and small solutes. Proteinuria occurs due to structural and/or functional defect in the glomerular filtration barrier. There are three layers of closely interacting components of glomerular filtration barrier (GFB) (Fig. 15.4).

1. Fenestrated endothelium lining the glomerular capillaries.
2. Trilaminar glomerular basement membrane (GBM)
3. Epithelial cell layer with interdigitating visceral epithelial cells (podocytes) and the 'slit diaphragms' between the foot processes.

The fenestrae in glomerular endothelial cells are permeable to macromolecules in the blood. There is no diaphragm. Because of a negatively charged coating of the luminal surface by glycocalyx, it will repel and prevent negatively charged particles. In the plasma, albumin is negatively charged and filtration of albumin is repelled by the negatively charged glycocalyx. Although the globulins are positively charged, their molecular weight is over 1,50,000 and cannot easily pass through the filtration barrier. GBM is a meshwork of extracellular matrix proteins derived from endothelial cells and podocytes. GBM has no pores but was permeable to small molecular weight solutes. The adjacent space between the foot process of the podocyte and the slit pore is the ultimate filtration barrier.

In health, the total protein excretion in urine is less than 150 mg and urine albumin excretion (in adults) is less than 30 mg/day. So, only <20% of the normally excreted urinary protein is albumin under normal circumstances. Two major factors limit the filtration of albumin and other macromolecules across the GFB.

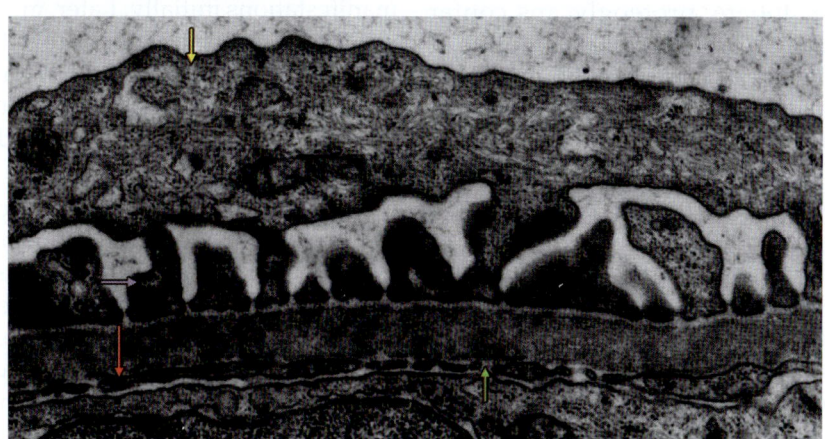

Fig. 15.3: Scanning electron photomicrograph of a single podocyte with its foot processes. Yellow arrow shows cell body of podocyte. Blue arrow shows the foot process. Red arrow shows the basement membrane and green arrow shows the fenestrations in endothelial cell cytoplasm

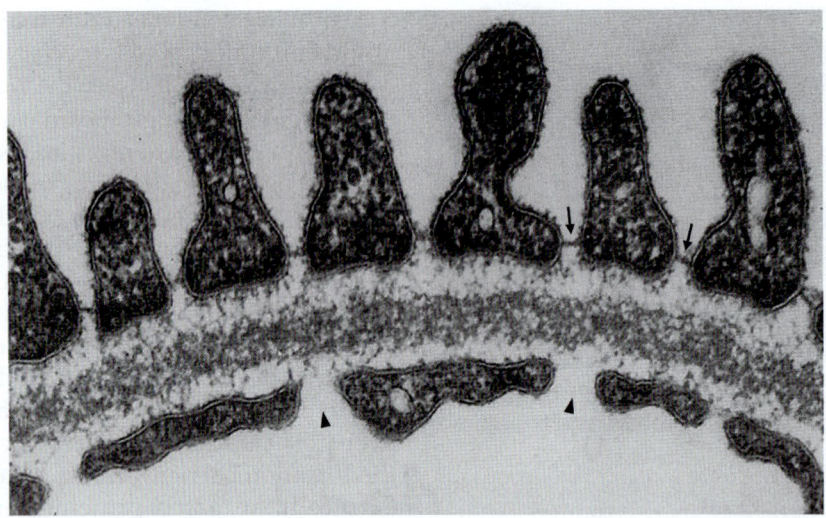

Fig. 15.4: Electron microscopic appearance of normal glomerular capillary filtration barrier. *Note:* The fenestrations in endothelial layer (arrow heads), trilaminar appearance of GBM and foot process between the foot processes of podocyte (bold arrows)

a. *Size selective barrier function:* The pore radius of GFB is about 500 nm. Filtration decreases as molecular size increases. Molecules with >500 nm radius and 1,00,000 daltons molecular weight are not filtered. The location of the size selective barrier is ill-defined.

b. *Charge selective barrier function:* Negatively charged components in the glycocalyx like heparin sulphate, proteoglycans confer anionic charge to GBM. Hence, filtration of anionic molecules is minimized compared to neutral and cationic molecules of same size. Albumin, despite having a radius of only 360 nm and molecular weight of 60,000 Daltons is not filtered due to its negative charge.

If >85% of the protein that is excreted in urine is albumin, it is called 'selective' proteinuria. In milder forms of glomerular diseases like 'minimal change disease', there is mainly disruption of charge selective barrier function. This results in selective proteinuria. In diseases associated with significant structural damage to size selective and charge selective barrier function, larger macromolecules like globulins are lost resulting in 'non-selective' proteinuria. Other proteins lost in urine include immunoglobulin G, complement, antithrombin III, thyroxine-binding globulin and vitamin D-binding globulin.

Edema

Nephrotic edema can be of varying severity. Periorbital and ankle swelling are prominent manifestations initially. Later, gross edema of periorbital region and limbs, genitalia, ascites and pleural effusion may follow. Traditionally, two mechanisms have been proposed to explain nephrotic edema—'underfill' and 'overfill' hypotheses.

a. As per 'underfill' hypothesis, edema is due to movement of fluid from plasma into interstitial space as a consequence of hypoalbuminemia-induced reduction in plasma oncotic pressure. The ensuing fall in intravascular volume would promote compensatory renal sodium retention mediated by activation of renin-angiotensin-aldosterone system, sympathetic activation and release of anti-diuretic hormone.

b. As per the 'overfill' hypothesis, edema is due to enhanced primary sodium retention in the collecting tubules. In nephrotic state, there is a relative resistance to the action of atrial natriuretic peptide (ANP). Natriuretic action of ANP is mediated by the second messenger, cyclic GMP (guanosine mono-phosphate). In nephrotic state, there is elevated levels of phosphodiesterase causing degradation of cyclic GMP with ensuing impedence of ANP activity.

Currently favored hypothesis suggests the role of plasmin that is filtered in the glomerulus. The plasmin in tubular fluid causes activation of epithelial sodium channel (ENaC) on the luminal surface of the tubule (collecting duct), resulting in enhanced sodium absorption.

Hyperlipidemia

Perturbations occur at multiple levels of lipid metabolism and a wide range of lipid abnormalities occur. Elevations in both serum cholesterol and triglyceride are common in NS. Hypoalbuminemia and consequent reduction in the plasma oncotic pressure directly stimulates hepatic cholesterol synthesis. Hypertriglyceridemia is predominantly due to impaired metabolism. Due to reduction in the activity of lipoprotein lipase, conversion of very low-density lipoprotein (VLDL) to intermediate density lipoprotein (IDL) and then to low-density lipoprotein (LDL) is hampered. As per recent observations, plasma level of a protein termed 'angio-poietin-like 4' is increased in NS and it has been shown to inhibit lipoprotein lipase. Also, there is reduction in LDL receptor-mediated clearance of LDL and IDL. Urinary loss of lecithin–cholesterol acyltransferase (LCAT) results in its deficiency. LCAT is essential for reverse cholesterol transport which involves HDL-mediated clearance of cholesterol.

Lipid abnormalities in nephrotic syndrome	
Elevated levels	Total cholesterol
	Triglyceride
	LDL, VLDL
Reduced level	Lipoprotein (A) Apolipoprotein B, C II, and E HDL-2 fraction
Normal (or) reduced level	Total HDL cholesterol

Normalization of even high levels in dyslipidemia occurs when NS enters remission. But, if the glomerular disease persists for longer period, and hyperlipidemia persists in spite of partial remission of NS, intervention is required. The 'atherogenic' lipid profile will have adverse impact on the cardiovascular health. Dyslipidemia may augment underlying glomerular disease. Statins are the preferred lipid lowering agents of choice.

Hypoalbuminemia

Hypoalbuminemia is a prominent feature of NS and it reflects the severity of glomerular disease. The exact mechanism of hypoalbuminemia is not known. Albumin is synthesized in the liver and a normal liver has the capacity to increase albumin synthesis as much as 30 g of albumin per day or more to compensate loss in urine. Cytokines like interleukin-1 and tumor necrosis factor can directly inhibit hepatic albumin synthesis. An unknown amount (presumed to be 6 times more than that lost in urine) of filtered protein is probably taken up by renal tubules and catabolized. Moreover, the amount of protein degraded may be more than the measured urinary protein level.

Complications of NS

Hypercoagulability

Nephrotic syndrome is a hypercoagulable state. Though there is an increased incidence of both arterial and venous thrombosis, risk for deep vein thrombosis (DVT) and renal vein thrombosis (RVT) are particularly increased. The risk of thrombotic complications are greatest in membranous nephropathy. Acute RVT presents with flank pain and hematuria and can result in renal infarction. Bilateral

RVT can cause renal failure. Pulmonary thromboembolism is a potential serious thrombotic manifestation in nephrotic patients. Multiple factors are responsible for the higher risk of thrombosis in NS. The balance between pro- and anticoagulant factors in the blood is altered. Severe hypoalbuminemia correlates with higher risk for thrombosis, particularly in idiopathic membranous nephropathy (MN). Prophylactic oral anticoagulation is recommended in MN if serum albumin is <2 g/dl. The main reasons for hypercoagulable state in NS are:

a. Urinary loss of anticoagulants (antithrombin III, protein C and protein S)
b. Increased levels of procoagulant factors like fibrinogen
c. Decreased level of fibrinolysins (due to urinary loss of plasminogen)
d. Elevated levels of antifibrinolysins (α_2 antiplasmin)
e. Enhanced platelet aggregability contributes for thrombotic tendency.

Infection

There is higher risk for infections in NS due to interference with different components of immune system. Low levels of immunoglobulin G, factors B and I of alternate complement pathway, depressed T cell function, decreased levels of 'opsonins' due to urinary loss, impaired complement activity due to urinary loss of factors B and D, reduced mitogenicity of phagocytes, reduced phagocytic ability of neutrophils and inability to mount specific antibody response have been observed in nephrotic patients. Edema interferes with physical integrity of skin and causes dilution of local humoral defences. Also, edema fluid serves as a culture medium for invading organisms. Corticosteroid and immunosuppressive therapy add to the risk of infection. The risk of infection due to *Streptococcus pneumoniae* is particularly more and is related to defective opsonization. Infections with other organisms such as β-hemolytic streptococci,

haemophilus and gram-negative bacteria are also common in NS. Infections of skin and soft tissue, spontaneous bacterial peritonitis, urinary tract infection and pneumonitis are the common infectious complications. Pneumococcal vaccination is recommended in all nephrotic patients.

Acute Kidney Injury (AKI)

AKI may occur in patients with NS due to multiple factors. Hypovolemia due to shift of fluid from intravascular compartment to ECF as a result of edema and loss of intravascular fluid due to diuretic therapy can result in other causes include use of angiotensin converting enzyme inhibitors (ACEIs) and acute interstitial nephritis due to diuretics and infections. Severe renal interstitial edema causing tubular collapse, referred to as 'nephrosarca' can cause AKI. Ultrastructural changes in the glomerular capillary filtration barrier is being recognized as an important cause of AKI in nephrotic syndrome.

MINIMAL CHANGE DISEASE (MCD)

Minimal change disease is the most common cause of NS in children more than 1 year of age (accounting for 70–90% of patients). In adults, it is the cause of idiopathic NS in about 10–15% of patients. As the name implies, the disease is characterized by absence of histological abnormalities under light microscopy. In clinical practice it is called steroid sensitive NS, especially in children.

Pathogenesis

The basic defect in MCD is linked to dysfunction of podocyte, T lymphocytes and B lymphocytes. The central role of T cells in the pathogenesis of MCD is based on the following observations:

a. Infections like measles which modify cell-mediated immunity induces remission of MCD.
b. Hodgkin's disease, is associated with increased incidence of MCD.

c. Patients with atopy are at a higher risk for MCD.

d. Immunosuppressive drugs which suppress T cell function induce remission of MCD.

Recently, B cell dysfunction also is implicated in the pathogenesis of MCD. This is based on the observation of beneficial role of rituxumab, an anti-CD20 monoclonal antibody in achieving remission in MCD.

A circulating factor of immune origin is believed to cause MCD by acting on podocyte causing neutralization of negative charge. The loss of charge selective barrier function results in proteinuria and MCD. Interleukin-13 (IL-13) is a putative permeability factor causing MCD.

Secondary Causes of MCD

The various secondary causes of MCD are shown in Table 15.2.

Pathology

Kidney biopsy reveals no pathological changes in light microscopy (Fig. 15.5) and no immune deposits in immunofluorescence. However, electron microscopic examination reveals generalized effacement (fusion) of foot processes of the visceral epithelial cells (Fig. 15.6).

Clinical Features

Edema, is the cardinal feature of MCD. Peri-orbital edema and leg edema occur early. Genital edema, edema of scalp and anasarca are common if long-standing and associated with severe hypoalbuminemia. Ascites and pleural effusion may occur causing abdominal protuberance and dyspnea, respectively. Severe edema causes stretching and thinning of skin. Hypertension is observed in 20–30% of adults with MCD. Microhaematuria is rare. Children with MCD are at risk for AKI. Serum complement levels are normal and kidney biopsy is not required in children, whereas it is preferred on diagnosis in all adults with NS. MCD follows a relapsing remitting course. It is

Table 15.2: Secondary causes of MCD

Drugs:
a. NSAID
b. Rifampicin
c. Ampicillin
d. Interferon-α
e. Lithium
f. Sulfasalazine

Allergy:
a. Pollens
b. Bee sting
c. House dust
d. Immunizations

Malignancy
a. Hodgkin disease
b. Thymoma
c. Mycosis fungoides
d. Chronic lymphocytic leukemia

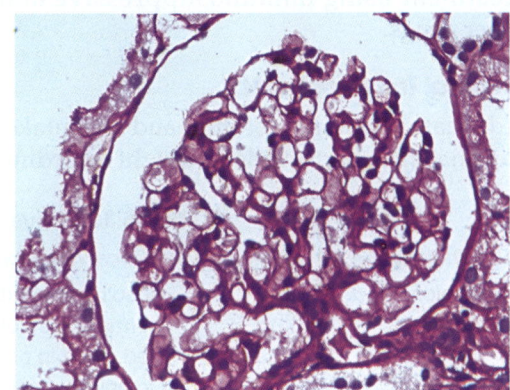

Fig. 15.5: Light microscopy of MCD. High power view showing single glomerulus. (H&E stain). The glomerulus looks essentially normal. Note the open capillary loops, normal mesangium and normal basement membrane. The cellularity is not increased

more common in children. Those presenting at an younger age have more relapses and long disease course. Yet, MCD never progresses to renal failure. The response to corticosteroids is favorable particularly in children. But, relapses are common. Following are the definitions of various terms used in the course and management of MCD (Table 15.3).

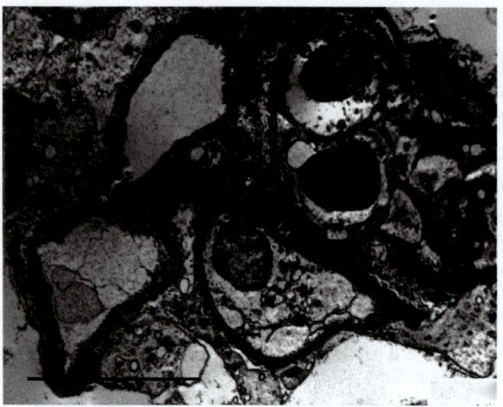

Fig. 15.6: Electron microscopy of MCD. Diffuse effacement of foot process is seen

Treatment

Treatment is broadly divided into general treatment of edematous state and specific treatment using immunosuppressive and other drugs.

General Treatment of NS

Adequate monitoring of fluid and salt intake, fluid balance chart and daily weight recording are important. Fluid intake is restricted so that edema decreases gradually and the weight reduces proportionately. Dietary sodium restriction (about 2 g/day) is recommended. Loop diuretic, frusemide in increasing doses is advocated if fluid restriction fails or edema is gross. Such patients should be observed for evidence of hypovolemia, viz. postural drop in blood pressure, tachycardia and rise in serum creatinine. If these features appear, reduction in the dose or discontinuation of diuretics is required.

In nephrotic state, response to loop diuretics is blunted since frusemide is bound by protein in the tubular lumen reducing availability of free drug at the site of action. In refractory edema, distally acting diuretic like thiazides may be added. Metalozone, a thiazide-like diuretic is widely used in severe edema. Addition of aldosterone antagonist, spironolactone would benefit in some patients.

'Head-out water immersion' (HWI) is an interesting treatment option in resistant nephrotic edema. HWI is done by seating the nephrotic patient for few hours in a water tank

Table 15.3: Various types of responses in NS	
Terminology	*Clinical response*
Remission	Resolution of edema
	Normalization of serum albumin (>3.5 g/dl)
	Reduction in proteinuria
	Complete remission (<0.3 g/day in adults, <4 mg/m²/hr or negative dipstick in children)
	Partial remission (<3.5 g/day and decreased by 50% in adults, <2 g/1.73 m²/day, decreased by 50% and serum albumin >2.5 g/dl in children)
Relapse	Recurrence of proteinuria (>3.5 g/day in adults, >40 mg/m²/hr in children)
Steroid-sensitive nephrotic syndrome (SSNS)	Response to prednisolone 1 mg/kg/day or 2 mg/kg/d every other day, within 16 weeks in adults
	Response to prednisolone 60 mg/m²/day within 4–6 weeks
Steroid-resistant nephrotic syndrome (SRNS)	No response to prednisolone 1 mg/kg/day or 2 mg/kg/d every other day, within 16 weeks in adults
	No response to prednisolone 60 mg/m²/day within 8 weeks in children
Infrequent relapse	<2 relapses per 6 months (or) <4 relapses per 12 months
Frequent relapse	>2 relapses per 6 months (or) >4 relapses per 12 months
Steroid-dependent nephrotic syndrome (SDNS)	Relapse during steroid therapy or within 14 days of discontinuation

Note: In adults with MCD, 40% have frequent relapses, 30% develop steroid dependence and 10% are steroid resistant.

with neck-deep immersion in water. Pressure exerted by water moves interstitial fluid into vascular compartment. Increased intra-vascular volume would enhance ANP release and cause natriuresis. HWI is not widely used due to practical difficulties. Application of non-adhesive elastic crepe bandage to apply graded pressure over the edematous limb helps to redistribute and eliminate the edema fluid from the body.

The specific treatment for MCD in children consists of oral prednisolone 2 mg/kg/day (maximum 60 mg) for 4 to 6 weeks, followed by 1.5 mg/kg every other day continued for 2 to 5 months (minimum duration of 3 months) with tapering of dose. If the child responds, the dose is tapered off and stopped by 6 months. Some children may achieve long-lasting remission. Subsequent treatment depends on the clinical course and whether relapses occur.

In children with infrequent relapse, oral prednisolone 2 mg/kg/day is given till the child achieves remission, followed by 1.5 mg/kg every other day for 4 weeks. In frequently relapsing NS (FRNS)/steroid-dependent NS (SDNS), oral prednisolone at 2 mg/kg/day till remission is achieved followed by alternate day prednisolone at lowest possible dose for 3 months.

Corticosteroid sparing agents are used in FRNS/SDNS patients who develop steroid side effects. Following are the available options—oral cyclophosphamide at 2 mg/kg/day given for 12 weeks after achieving remission with steroids. Cyclosporine at 3–5 mg/kg/day (starting dose) for 12 months or Tacrolimus at 0.1 mg/kg/day for 12 months are also tried. Mycophenolate mofetil at 1200 mg/m^2/day may be tried for 12 months. Patients should be closely followed up if such powerful immunosuppressive drugs are used.

Once steroid resistant NS (SRNS) is confirmed, kidney biopsy should be done even in children. Calcineurin inhibitor (CNI) is the initial choice of therapy for children with SRNS. CNIs should be given for duration of 6 months and should be stopped if no partial or complete remission is achieved. If at least partial remission is achieved, the duration of therapy is extended up to 12 months. All children with SRNS should be given ACEI/ARBs. There is no role for cyclophosphamide in SRNS.

In adults with MCD, the initial episode is treated with prednisolone 1 mg/kg/day for a minimum of 4 weeks and if complete remission is achieved, the steroids are tapered slowly over the next 6 months (from the time of achievement of remission). If no remission is achieved in 4 weeks, the same dose is continued for a total of 16 weeks. This is because the time to attain remission is more in adults compared to children. If no remission is achieved even after 16 weeks of steroid therapy, the patient is classified as SRNS. Other causes must be ruled out. In patients who do not tolerate steroids (uncontrolled diabetes, severe osteoporosis) cyclophosph-amide or CNIs can be used as first line of therapy. The treatment of infrequent relapse in adults is similar to treatment of first episode.

FOCAL SEGMENTAL GLOMERULOSCLEROSIS (FSGS)

FSGS is a histologic pattern of glomerular injury characterized by glomerulosclerosis that is focal (only a few [<50%] glomeruli are involved) and segmental (only a portion of a glomerular tuft [<50%] is involved). It is not an etiological diagnosis. Numerous clinical syndromes present with FSGS pathological pattern. Although it contributes to a minority of cases of idiopathic NS in children, around 35% of NS in adults is due to FSGS and is a major glomerular cause of progressive renal failure.

Etiology

Etiologically FSGS is classified into primary or idiopathic and secondary FSGS. Primary FSGS is postulated to be mediated by circulating permeability factors. The causes for the glomerular changes in secondary FSGS are well defined. The causes of secondary FSGS are broadly classified as familial/genetic, virus associated, drug-related and those mediated by adaptive responses (Table 15.4).

Pathogenesis

The crucial pathogenic event in FSGS is injury to podocyte due to external factors or genetic causes which result in reorganization of actin-cytoskeleton and foot process effacement. Lethal injury result in podocyte depletion and the stress is transferred to the adjacent podocytes results in propagation of damage. Factors like angiotensin II arising out of intrarenal RAAS activation augment injury.

The following observations point to a pathogenic role for circulating permeability factor(s) in idiopathic FSGS.

a. Recurrence of FSGS occurs in 20–50% of patients after renal transplantation. In some patients, proteinuria appears within hours after transplantation.

b. In patients with recurrence of FSGS, proteinuria decreases after plasmapheresis.

c. In experiments, plasma from patients with FSGS has been shown to induces proteinuria in rats.

d. Soluble urokinase-type plasminogen activator receptor (suPAR) level is elevated in plasma of patients with primary FSGS.

Although many putative factors have been considered, a soluble urokinase-type plasminogen activator receptor (suPAR) has received more attention and scrutiny. suPAR is produced by immature myeloid cells in the bone marrow and acts via activation of a crucial adhesion molecule of podocytes which regulate the dynamics of foot processes. Elevated plasma levels are seen in patients with primary FSGS and reduction in the levels occur following plasmapheresis. However, subsequent studies have revealed elevated levels of suPAR in patients with chronic kidney disease due to other causes. Hence,

Table 15.4: Causes of secondary FSGS

1. *Familial FSGS*—(Mutations in genes)
   Nephrin (NPHS1)
   Podocin (NPHS2)
   α-actinin 4 (ACTN4)
   Transient receptor potential cation channel (TRPC6)
   Wilms' tumor suppressor 1 (WT1)
   Inverted formin-2 (INF2)
   Phospholipase C epsilon 1 (PLCE1)
   Risk alleles for apolipoprotein L1 (APOL1)
2. *Virus associated FSGS*
   HIV 1 ("HIV-associated nephropathy")
   Parvovirus B19
   Cytomegalovirus (CMV)
3. *Drug-induced FSGS*
   Heroin ("heroin nephropathy")
   Interferon
   Lithium
   Pamidronate
   Sirolimus
   Anabolic steroids
4. *Adaptive FSGS*–(Reduced renal mass)
   Oligomeganephronia, very low birth weight
   Unilateral renal agenesis
   Renal dysplasia
   Reflux nephropathy
   Sequela to cortical necrosis
   Surgical renal ablation (Partial or unilateral nephrectomy)
   Chronic allograft nephropathy
   Reduction in functioning. Nephrons with renal failure
   Obesity
   Cyanotic congenital heart disease.
   Sickle cell anemia

suPAR cannot be relied upon as a diagnostic biomarker for FSGS.

In the case of secondary FSGS, the pathogenic mechanism is reduction in the number of nephrons. This may be congenital or acquired. The surviving nephrons try to maintain renal function by hypertrophy and hyperfiltration. This adaptive response leads onto sclerosis of glomeruli. Certain toxins may inflict direct injury on podocytes resulting in FSGS.

Clinical Manifestations

FSGS in children results in nephrotic range of proteinuria (70–90%), whereas in adults it is only 50–70%. Secondary forms of FSGS usually have lower levels of proteinuria and normal serum albumin levels and relatively less fluid retention and edema. Nephrotic state, hypertension and microhematuria may occur only in a few patients. Proteinuria is usually non-selective. Complement levels are normal. Some patients have glycosuria, aminoaciduria and phosphaturia indicating tubular damage.

Pathology

As the disease is focal and early disease is confined to juxtamedullary glomeruli there is possibility of missing FSGS lesion in renal biopsy. A biopsy sample with at least 20 glomeruli increases the chance of identifying FSGS lesions. The Columbia classification of FSGS which is based on light microscopy findings has classified FSGS as classic/FSGS, not otherwise specified, perihilar, cellular, collapsing and tip variant.

Classic variant is the most common type and is a diagnosis of exclusion. There is accumulation of extracellular matrix occluding glomerular capillaries segmentally (Fig. 15.7). Adhesions to Bowman capsule (synechiae) are common. Immunofluorescence may show focal and segmental deposition of IgM and C3.

In perihilar variant, hyalinosis and sclerosis, i.e. segmental glomerulosclerosis is seen at the vascular pole. It is frequently seen in secondary forms, especially adaptive type of FSGS.

The cellular variant shows increase in endocapillary hypercellularity in a focal and segmental pattern. It is usually seen in primary FSGS and is thought to represent an early lesion.

Collapsing variant is characterized by at least one glomerulus with segmental or global collapse and overlying hyperplasia of visceral epithelial cells forming 'pseudocrescents'. There is marked tubulointerstitial involve-ment and is frequently observed in FSGS secondary to HIV, parvovirus, interferon therapy or use of pamidronate.

In the tip variant, segmental lesion is in the portion of glomerulus near the origin of proximal tubule (opposite the vascular pole). It is usually seen in primary FSGS. This variant, generally has the best prognosis.

Natural History

Untreated or FSGS not responding to therapy commonly progresses to renal failure. Only 5 to 25% of patients undergo spontaneous remission. 50% of patients reach ESRD by 10 years. The risk factors for progressive renal disease are:

a. Severity of proteinuria
b. Elevated serum creatinine
c. African race
d. Collapsing variant
e. Tubulointerstitial fibrosis
f. Failure to achieve partial or complete remission.

Treatment

Immunosuppressive therapy should be considered only in primary FSGS with clinical features of NS. Corticosteroids are given at

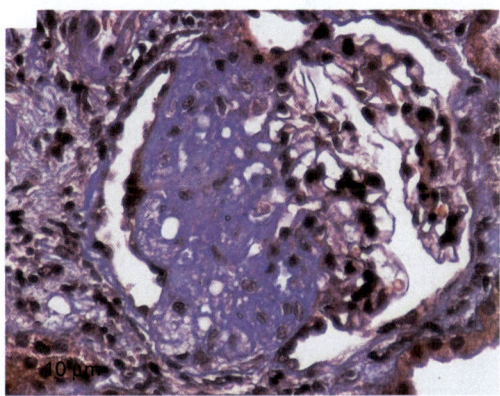

Fig. 15.7: Light microscopy of focal and segmental glomerulosclerosis. Renal biopsy H&E stain showing sclerosed area occupying nearly 50% of the tuft in a single glomerulus under high power. The tuft is adhering (synechiae) to the parietal cell layer in 6–7 o'clock position

dose of 1 mg/kg/day for a minimum of 4 weeks if remission is achieved. It is given for a maximum of 16 weeks if remission is not achieved. After achieving complete remission, steroids are tapered slowly over 6 months. Calcineurin inhibitors can be considered as first line therapy for patients intolerant to steroids. Steroid resistant FSGS is treated with cyclosporine at 3–5 mg/kg/day or tacrolimus 0.05–0.1 mg/kg/ day for a minimum duration of 6 months. If at least a partial remission is achieved therapy is continued for 12 months followed by slow taper.

MEMBRANOUS NEPHROPATHY

Membranous nephropathy (MN) is one of the most common causes of idiopathic NS in adults. Peak incidence occurs during 4th and 5th decades with a male preponderance. MN is characterized by diffuse immune complex deposition in subepithelial location in the GFB. Most of the patients present with NS. This pathological entity is termed 'nephropathy' rather than 'nephritis' since there is no inflammation, cellular proliferation or infiltration. The term membranous refers to prominent, uniform thickening of the glomerular basement membrane.

Etiology

As with other forms of NS, the causes of MN may be either primary or idiopathic or secondary. Table 15.5 shows the secondary causes with some examples.

Pathogenesis

Primary membranous nephropathy is a 'renal-limited' autoimmune disease. In experimental animal models, circulating antibodies against an antigen 'megalin' on podocyte foot processes are formed. The immune complexes deposit in the subepithelial location in the GFB. The complement system is activated and the membrane attack complex C5b–9 gets inserted onto podocyte causing injury. GBM expansion occurs by overproduction of GBM components like type IV collagen and laminin. Podocyte injury results in proteinuria and the characteristic basement membrane thickening. In human kidney, magalin is not present. An endogenous or planted antigen called M-type phospholipase A2 receptor (PLA2R) has been found to cause idiopathic MN in about 70–80% of patients with primary MN. PLA2R is a transmembrane protein located on the podocyte. This antibody is not found in secondary MN and other glomerular diseases. Therefore, antibody to PLA2R is used as a useful biomarker for idiopathic MN. In addition, kidney biopsy staining for PLA2R by immunofluorescence reveals positivity in 60–85% of patients with idiopathic MN.

Thrombospondin type 1 domain-containing 7A (THSD7A) is a transmembrane protein expressed on podocytes and may be the causative antigen in about 10% of patients with idiopathic MN in whom anti-PLA2R antibody is absent. IgG4 antibodies traverse the GBM and form *in situ* immune complexes with PLA2R. The evolution of MN starts with, subepithelial immune complexes, followed by formation of spikes which arise from the outer aspect of GBM, which encircle the immune deposits and incorporate them into the thickened GBM (Fig. 15.8).

Table 15.5: Secondary causes of MN with some examples

Secondary cause	Examples of diseases
Infections	HBV, HCV, HIV, filariasis, malaria
Malignancy (paraneoplastic syndrome)	Ca lung, Ca prostate, CLL, melanoma
Autoimmune diseases	SLE, thyroiditis, rheumatoid arthritis
Drugs	NSAID, d-penicillamine, mercury, gold
Alloimmune diseases	Graft-vs-host disease, transplant glomerulopathy

Pathology

Light microscopy reveals uniformly thickened glomerular capillary wall (Figs 15.9 and 15.10). Immunofluorescence shows diffuse granular deposit of IgG4 along the GBM.

Clinical Features

Most patients present with NS. Hypertension and microhematuria are present in about 30–40% of patients. Male gender, severe proteinuria, persistence of NS for >6 months, low GFR at presentation and hypertension are poor prognostic factors. A detailed evaluation to rule out secondary causes has to be carried out. As mentioned above, MN can occur as a paraneoplastic manifestation and at times, it may precede malignancy. About 30% of patients with idiopathic MN may undergo spontaneous remission.

Treatment

Despite numerous studies, the optimal treatment for primary MN is incompletely defined. Because of the chronic nature and tendency for spontaneous remission (about 30%) the treatment should be tailored for the individual patient. The main therapeutic approaches include:

a. Conservative treatment with RAAS blockade (using ACE inhibitors and ARBs) for their antiproteinuric action. Decision regarding conservative treatment or need for immunosuppression is based on initial response to conservative therapy.

b. Corticosteroids therapy

c. Alkylating agents like cyclophosphamide

Indications for immunosuppression [as per kidney diseases improving global outcomes (KDIGO) guidelines] are:

a. NS with persistent proteinuria >4 g/day despite 6 months of antihypertensive and antiproteinuric therapy.

b. Presence of severe disabling life-threatening symptoms related to NS.

c. Rise in serum creatinine more than 30% within 6 to 12 months from diagnosis but

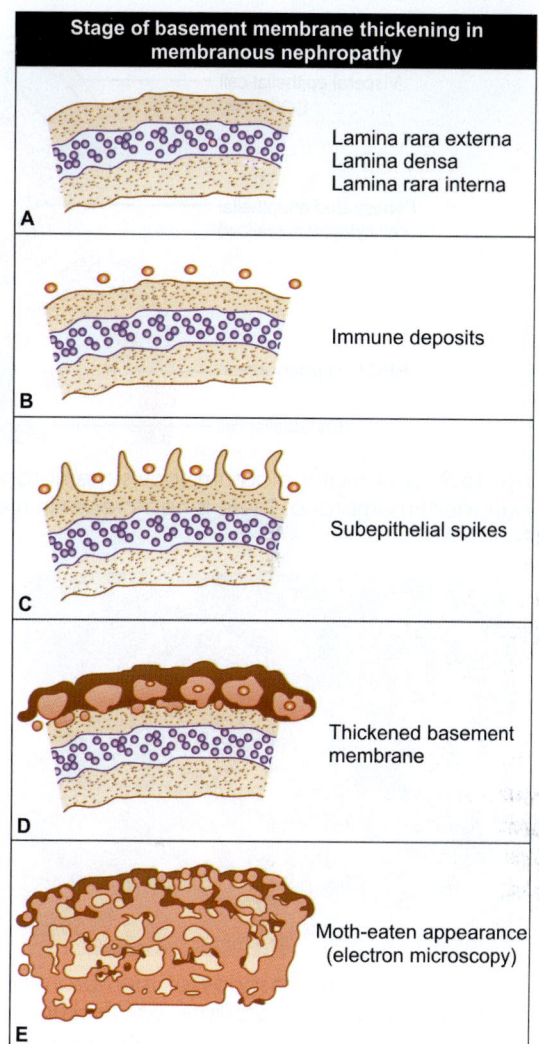

Stage of basement membrane thickening in membranous nephropathy

A — Lamina rara externa / Lamina densa / Lamina rara interna

B — Immune deposits

C — Subepithelial spikes

D — Thickened basement membrane

E — Moth-eaten appearance (electron microscopy)

Fig. 15.8A to E: Stages in pathogenesis of membranous nephropathy. (A) Normal basement membrane; (B) Subepithelial immune deposits; (C) Spikes in the basement membrane between the deposits; (D) Spikes encircling the deposits and thickening of basement membrane; (E) Grossly thickened irregular basement membrane

eGFR not less than 25 to 30 ml min/day/1.73 m^2.

The immunosuppressive regime used is the modified Ponticelli regime. This consists of six month treatment schedule using steroids and cyclophosphamide alternately at monthly

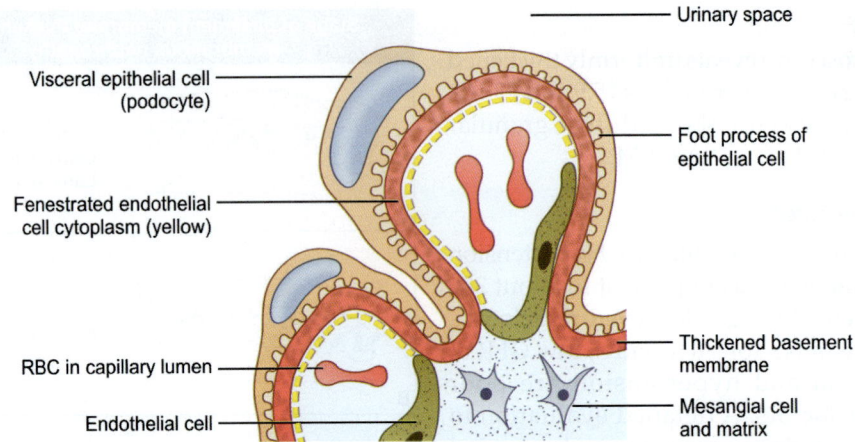

Fig. 15.9: Schematic diagram shows membranous nephropathy. There is uniform thickening of basement membrane. There is no increase in mesangial cellularity

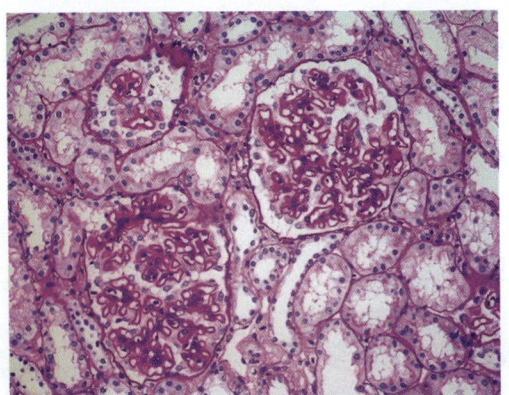

Fig. 15.10: Light microscopy of membranous nephropathy. Uniform capillary wall thickening with open capillary loops and normal cellularity

intervals. During months 1, 3 and 5, intravenous methyl prednisolone 1 g/day is given for the first 3 days followed by oral prednisolone 0.5 mg/kg/day from day 4 to day 30. During months 2, 4 and 6, oral cyclophosphamide (1.5 mg/kg/day) is given for 30 days each. If there is no response in 6 months, it is not advisable to continue immunosuppressive treatment because of infective complications.

In the case of secondary MN, the management is essentially treatment of the underlying disease while continuing general supportive treatment and antiproteinuric measures.

MEMBRANOPROLIFERATIVE GLOMERULONEPHRITIS (MPGN)

Membranoproliferative glomerulonephritis is not a single disease. It represents a pattern of glomerular injury which can be due to a variety of pathogenetically distinct disorders. There are three characteristic pathological changes.

a. Proliferation of endothelial and mesangial cells and expansion of mesangial matrix.
b. Capillary wall thickening due to subendothelial and/or intramembranous immune deposits.
c. 'Double-contour' or 'tram-track' appearance of the capillary wall due to mesangial interposition.

Earlier, MPGN was classified into three subtypes based on the location of immune deposits by electron microscopy as:

a. *Type 1:* Subendothelial deposits and duplication of GBM.
b. *Type 2:* Dense: Intramembranous deposits in the lamina densa of GBM [dense deposit disease (DDD)].
c. *Type 3:* Subepithelial and subendothelial deposits.

The current classification of MPGN is based on pathogenetic mechanism involved as follows:

a. Immune complex-mediated MPGN
b. Complement-mediated MPGN
c. MPGN resulting from mechanisms unrelated to deposition of immune reactants.

Etiology

MPGN may be primary or secondary. The conditions causing secondary MPGN may be following infections, autoimmune diseases, complement-mediated or MPGN without immune deposits (Table 15.6).

Pathogenesis

Immune complex-mediated MPGN is due to deposition of immune complexes in the mesangium and subendothelial space with subsequent complement activation and release of cytokines. Circulating immune complexes have been demonstrated in about 30% of patients.

Table 15.6: Causes of secondary MPGN

a. Immune complex-mediated MPGN
  1. *Infections:*
- Hepatitis B
- Hepatitis C related cryoglobulinemia type II
- Endocarditis
- Hansen's disease
- Visceral abscess
- Shunt nephritis (infected ventriculo-atrial shunt)
- Malaria

b. Autoimmune diseases
- Systemic lupus erythematosus
- Sjögren's syndrome

c. Complement-mediated MPGN
- C3 glomerulonephritis (C3GN)
- Dense deposit disease (DDD)

d. MPGN without immune deposits
  1. Chronic TMA (thrombotic microangiopathy due to radiation nephritis, anti-phospholipid antibody syndrome, nephropathy associated with HSCT (hematopoietic stem cell transplantation)]
  2. Malignancy—lymphoma, leukemia
  3. Paraproteinemias

Complement-mediated MPGN consists of two disease entities collectively known as 'C3 glomerulopathy'. They are C3GN and DDD and occur due to dysregulation of alternate complement pathway resulting in exaggerated complement activation resulting in renal injury. Although the alternate complement pathway is always at a low level of activity, even without a stimulus, this activity is tightly regulated by regulators of complement. Any disease or factor that causes suppression of inhibitors or activation of promoters of complements would result in exaggerated activity of alternate complement pathway. C3 convertase (C3bBb) is the central point in the pathway. The activated complement and complement debris are deposited in the glomerulus causing injury. Pathological activation of alternate pathway can occur due to the following:

a. Inactivating genetic mutations of factor H, factor I, membrane co-factor protein (MCP)
b. Antibody to factor H
c. C3 nephritic factor (C3NeF) (it is an auto-antibody causing stabilization of C3 convertase of alternate pathway). C3NeF is present in about 70% of patients with DDD.

This is in contrast to the classical pathway, which needs a trigger-like immune complexes for activation.

Pathology

Light microscopy reveals glomerular hyper-cellularity due to mesangial and endocapillary proliferation and diffuse, irregular capillary wall thickening. Accentuation of lobularity is a striking feature. The characteristic 'double contour' of the basement membrane is due to interposition of mesangium and formation of new basement membrane (Figs 15.11 and 15.12). Immunofluorescence reveals significant deposits of immunoglobulin and C3 in immune complex-mediated MPGN, but only C3 (in the capillary wall and mesangium) in C3GN. Electron microscopy reveals electron dense, osmophilic deposits in GBM in DDD.

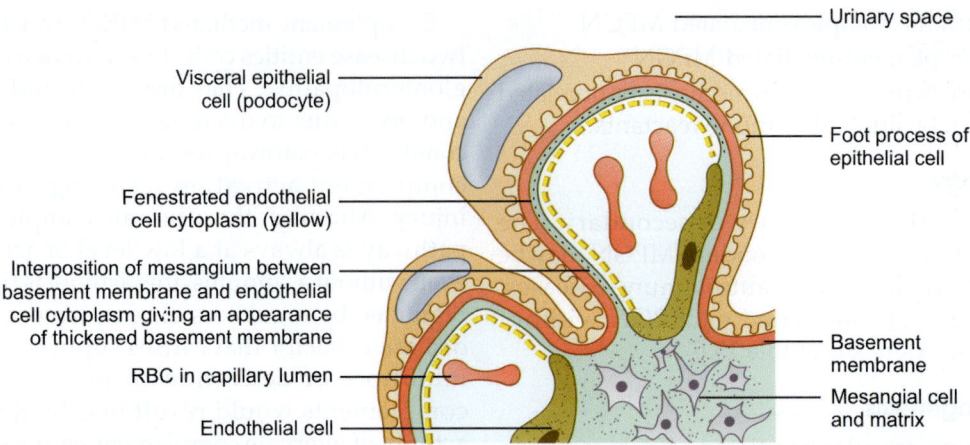

Urinary space

Visceral epithelial cell (podocyte)

Foot process of epithelial cell

Fenestrated endothelial cell cytoplasm (yellow)

Interposition of mesangium between basement membrane and endothelial cell cytoplasm giving an appearance of thickened basement membrane

RBC in capillary lumen

Endothelial cell

Basement membrane

Mesangial cell and matrix

Fig. 15.11: Schematic diagram shows MPGN. Membranoproliferative glomerulonephritis showing increase in mesangial matrix, cellularity and interposition of mesangium between basement membrane and endothelial cell

Electron microscopy is essential to diagnose DDD. In C3GN, electron dense deposits are seen in mesangial and subendothelial areas.

Clinical Features

Idiopathic MPGN and C3 glomerulopathy are more common in children and young adults. The clinical presentation may be variable. Patients may present with acute nephritic

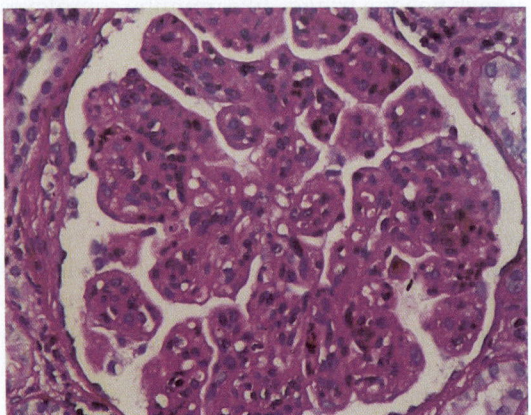

Fig. 15.12: Light microscopy of MPGN. *Note:* Lobular architecture of glomerular capillary tuft, increase in mesangium, apparent thickening of basement membrane and compressed capillary loops

syndrome, NS, recurrent episodes of gross hematuria and rapidly progressive renal failure. Hypertension is present in almost 80% of patients. Patients with DDD may have partial lipodystrophy involving facial muscles. This is due to complement-mediated adipocyte injury. Drusen bodies on fundus examination in a patient with glomerulonephritis should prompt the diagnosis of DDD. Drusen bodies are yellowish deposits in the Bruch membrane of retina and represent complement debris. Low levels of serum complement C3 are common. C4 levels will be normal. Apart from routine investigations, in patients with C3GN, a detailed genetic work-up is essential. Overall prognosis of MPGN is poor.

Treatment

Patients with immune complex MPGN associated with sub-nephrotic proteinuria and preserved renal function require only conservative therapy consisting of control of hypertension, RAAS inhibition and statins. Steroid (prednisolone) therapy is advised for patients with nephrotic proteinuria at a dose of 1 mg/kg/day (maximum of 60–80 mg) for 12 to 16 weeks. If there is response, steroid has to be tapered over 6 to 8 months. If no response, steroid has to be tapered quickly and stopped.

In those with C3 glomerulopathy, milder forms require general measures only. Moderate/severe form of C3GN is treated with steroids and other immunosuppressives like mycophenolate mofetil. In patients with C3NeF or anti-factor H antibody, suggested treatment options include rituximab, plasma exchange and eculizumab (the later in those with elevated plasma levels of soluble membrane attack complex). Intermittent plasma infusion is advocated in patients with genetic mutations resulting in factor H deficiency. There is a high-risk of recurrence of C3 glomerulopathy following renal transplantation.

Nephrotic syndrome is a manifestation of different glomerular diseases of varying etiology. Identification of the cause of nephrotic syndrome is important to assess prognosis and plan therapy.

Acknowledgement: Dr Anila Abraham Kurien, MD, Renal Pathologist, Renopath, Centre for Renal and Urological Pathology, Chennai, for most of the photomicrographs.

Infection-Related Glomerulonephritis

• Krishan Lal Gupta • Sahil Bagai • Raja Ramachandran

INTRODUCTION

Infection-related glomerulonephritis (IRGN) classically included post-streptococcal glomerulonephritis, staphylococcal infection associated glomerulonephritis and glomerulonephritis associated with endocarditis or with viral, fungal, protozoal, or parasitic infections. However, there has been a paradigm shift in the understanding of IRGN. In the past, most cases of bacterial IRGN occurred in children following streptococcal upper respiratory tract or skin infections and were called post-infectious or post-streptococcal GN. Over the past three decades, it has been noted that elderly adults or immunocompromised individuals were more affected. In children, streptococcal infection occurs before the renal disease sets in, which is in contrast to adults in whom infections are often ongoing at the time of diagnosis, so the term IRGN appears more appropriate for adults. The sites of infection in adult IRGN are more heterogeneous than in children and include the upper respiratory tract, skin, lung, heart, urinary tract, teeth/oral mucosa, and bone. In adults, the disease occurs mostly secondary to non-streptococcal bacterial infections, particularly staphylococcal infection seen in 12–24% cases and gram negative bacteria in 22% cases as per one study. In contrast to the favorable course in children, a significant proportion of adults with IRGN, especially the elderly and diabetics, do not recover renal function. Whereas the pathogenesis of post-streptococcal glomerulonephritis has been studied extensively, leading to the identification of two candidate nephritogenic streptococcal antigens, glyceraldehyde-3-phosphate dehydrogenase and pyrogenic exotoxin B, few investigations have focused on IRGN caused by other bacteria. This review will address the current status of sporadic IRGN in the adults.

PATHOGENESIS

IRGN is an immune complex-mediated disease. The infective agent acts as an antigen. It occurs secondary to glomerular deposition of pre-formed circulating immune complexes or formation of immune complex *in situ* due to antigens planted in the glomeruli. In Staphylococcus-associated glomerulonephritis, glomerular deposition of preformed circulating immune complexes is a critical pathogenic mechanism in as the circulating antigens and the antibodies directed against these antigens coexist in the circulation for prolonged periods of time. The prolonged antigenemia, provides more opportunity for immune complexes formation in the circulation, which subsequently activates the complement cascade. The same pathogenesis occurs secondarily to other bacterial, viral or parasitic infections as well. Moreover, specific antigens like staphylococcal antigens may act as 'superantigens', capable of activating T cells which results in polyclonal B cell activation and production of polyclonal IgA, IgG, and IgM.

Epidemiology

In earlier days, post-streptococcal infections occurred as endemic in communities where overcrowding, poor sanitation and lack of personal hygiene predisposed to streptococcal skin or throat infections. Although IRGN is relatively rare, it occurs in middle-aged or elderly patients who are predisposed to infections. Patients with diabetes, alcoholism, cancer or intravenous drug addiction are more prone and the overall incidence is around 1%. Meticulous care while using intravenous lines for fluid or drug administration in hospitals will reduce the chances of sepsis and/or IRGN in hospitalized/ICU patients. In endocarditis, associated GN may occur in up to 20% of cases. Almost, 35–60% of patients with chronic hepatitis C will develop renal manifestations including type I membranoproliferative glomerulonephritis (MPGN), mesangial glomerulonephritis, and focal and segmental glomerulonephritis. The incidence of GN in malaria and is estimated to be around 18%.

Etiology

Infection-related GN may occur in association with bacterial, viral, protozoal, and helminthic or fungal infections. Common causative agents are:

- *Bacterial: Mycobacterium tuberculosis, Mycobacterium leprae*, Staphylococcus, Streptococcus, *Treponema pallidum*, Salmonella, Neisseria.
- *Viral:* Human immunodeficiency, Epstein-Barr virus, cytomegalovirus, varicella, hepatitis B and C.
- *Fungal:* Histoplasma, Candida, Coccidioides.
- *Protozoal:* Leishmania, Plasmodium, Toxoplasma.
- *Helminthic:* Wuchereria, Schistosoma, *Brugia malayi*.

Clinical Presentation

Adults with infection-related glomerulonephritis frequently present with hematuria, proteinuria of varying degrees, rising serum creatinine and edema concurrently with an infective episode. Pedal edema is the presenting feature in up to 50% patients and new-onset hypertension or nephritic range proteinuria in about 33% each. Patients may report fever, night sweats, and rigors. Weight loss is a possible complaint and patients may report arthralgias. Abdominal, chest, or back pain may be caused by a visceral abscess. Unlike post-streptococcal glomerulonephritis, upper respiratory tract infection is not usually seen. IgA nephropathy, also manifests concurrently with an infective episode but here hematuria, rather than edema and hypertension are the prominent feature.

Diagnosis

IRGN should be suspected in patients with clinical manifestations of active glomerulonephritis (e.g. hematuria with or without red cell casts, often accompanied by proteinuria, hypertension and elevation in serum creatinine in conjunction with a known or suspected recent or concurrent infection. Patients can give history of blood transfusion, promiscuity, history of shunt placements for hydrocephalus or presence of vascular graft can hint at IRGN. The investigations done in each case includes complete urinalysis with microscopy for urinary sediments, quantification of urinary protein excretion, complete blood count, serum creatinine, albumin, electrolytes and complement levels (C3 and C4). Even if clinical clues are absent, hypocomplementemia or a positive culture for organism may provide a hint towards the disease. Neutrophilic predominant leukocytosis may point towards acute bacterial etiology, eosinophilia may hint towards bacterial endocarditis or parasitic infection, deranged LFTs might be indicative of hepatitis-associated GN. Renal biopsy helps to confirm the diagnosis in cases of a clinical dilemma. In case of Staphylococcus associated GN the diagnosis can be made if at least two of the following criteria are satisfied in a patient with clinical or laboratory evidence of staphylococcal infection concurrent with the onset of glomerulonephritis.

a. Endocapillary proliferation and exudative glomerulonephritis on light microscopy.

b. Hypocomplementemia (primarily low C3).

c. Immunofluorescence microscopy showing dominant or co-dominant glomerular staining by C3.

However, many patients with Staphylococcus-associated glomerulonephritis have an IgA-dominant or co-dominant disease (together with intense C3 staining). On electron microscopy, hump-shaped subepithelial deposits are seen.

Though the diagnosis of Staphylococcus-associated glomerulonephritis can be made presumptively using the above criteria, these are not specific. Confirmation of the diagnosis of Staphylococcus-associated glomerulonephritis requires that the disease activity (e.g. hematuria, hypocomplementemia if present) to subside after successful eradication of the infection. Elevation of the serum creatinine and proteinuria may persist reflecting irreversible renal injury.

Imaging for localization of visceral infections, echocardiography for bacterial endocarditis are other tests that can help in localization of the infections.

Pathology—Role of Kidney Biopsy

In adults, renal biopsy must be done in all patients suspected of infection-related GN. In cases where there is clear evidence of GN occurring concurrently with culture positive infection, and prompt response to treatment, biopsy may be avoided. However, if there is

clinical suspicion of a systemic etiology or any serological marker that points towards another disease, then a renal biopsy is mandatory. The most common histologic pattern of injury on light microscopy is diffuse endocapillary proliferative and exudative glomerulonephritis. More than 50% of glomeruli may show occlusion of the peripheral capillaries by endocapillary hypercellularity. Numerous neutrophils will be seen in the glomerular capillary tuft (Fig. 16.1). Although few cellular crescents may be seen, they are often not more than 50% to qualify for the diagnosis of crescentic GN (Fig. 16.2). Membranous pattern predominates in patients who have hepatitis B and C related GN.

Immunofluorescence microscopy: In Staphylococcus-associated GN, C3 dominant or co-dominant (with IgA or IgG) glomerular staining is seen. In most cases, there is coarsely granular mesangial and glomerular wall staining, resembling the 'starry sky pattern',

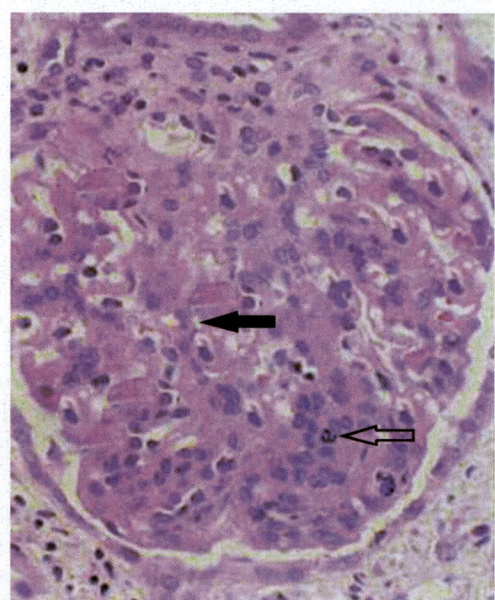

Fig. 16.1: Glomerulus under high power light microscopy H&E stain. *Note:* Increase in the cellularity, occlusion of capillary lumen (bold arrow) and polymorphonuclear leukocytes (open arrow) in the glomerulus

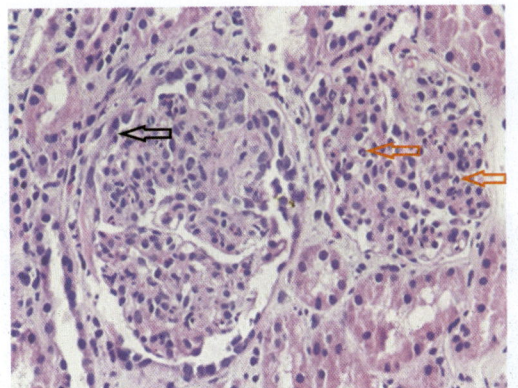

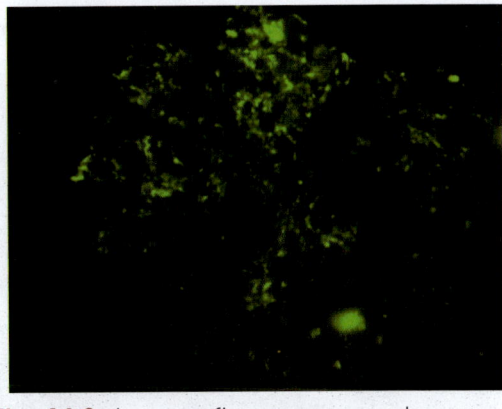

Fig. 16.2: Glomerulus under high power light microscopy H&E stain. *Note:* Partial cellular crescent (4 cell layers thick) in one glomerulus, endocapillary proliferation, mesangial hyper-cellularity and infiltration of neutrophils (red arrows) into the glomeruli. Most of the capillary loops are occluded. Black arrow shows the cellular crescent

Fig. 16.3: Immunofluorescence microscopy (fluorescein isothiocyanate) IgG magnification 40X original. Direct immunofluorescence showing one glomerulus depicting the "starry sky" appearance when stained with fluorescein tagged IgG antiserum

while a minority exhibit predominantly glomerular capillary wall positivity ('garland pattern') or predominantly mesangial staining ('mesangial pattern') (Fig. 16.3). Granular staining of IgG and C3 are seen in viral-associated GN.

IgA dominant staphylococcal IRGN can be differentiated from IgA nephropathy in Table 16.1.

C3GN can closely mimic IRGN and needs to be carefully differentiated from each other.

Following are notable differences between the two.

a. Partial or complete resolution in IRGN but persistence and recurrence in C3GN.
b. Renal histology under light microscopy shows (DPGN) pattern, whereas in C3GN MPGN pattern is seen.
c. Immunofluorescence microscopy showing immunoglobulin with C3 is suggestive of IRGN, whereas in C3GN, only C3 deposits are seen.

Table 16.1: Differences between IgA dominant staphylococcal IRGN and IgA nephropathy

Parameter	IRGN	IgA
a. Age group	Older age	Younger age
b. Associated illness	Present (e.g. diabetes)	Nil
c. AKI on presentation	Yes, often	No, only rarely if associated with gross hematuria
d. Complements	Low	Normal
e. Light microscopy	Diffuse (exudative) proliferative glomerulonephritis (DPGN)	Mesangial proliferative or focal proliferative GN
f. Immunofluorescence	C3 deposits and immunoglobulins in glomeruli	Global mesangial IgA deposits
g. Electron microscopy	Subepithelial deposits (humps) and few subendothelial deposits	Scattered mesangial deposits

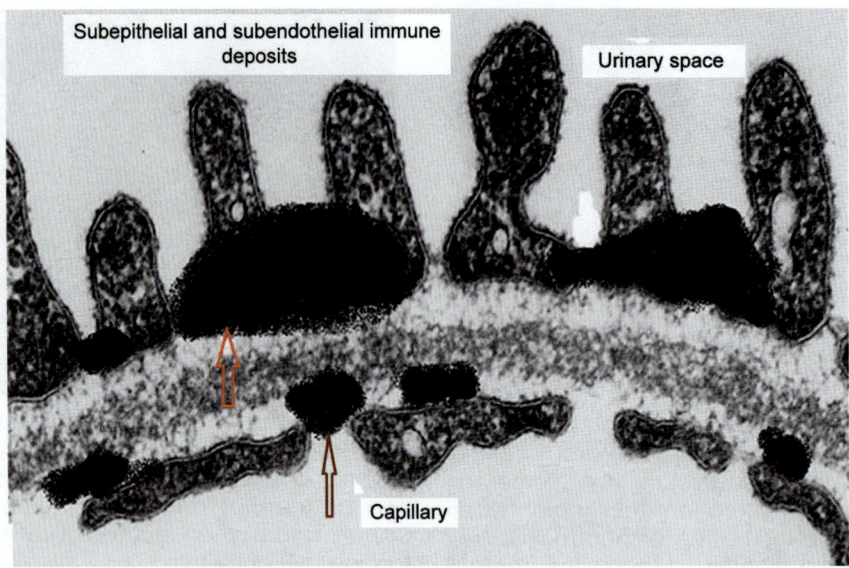

Fig. 16.4: Immune deposits in IRGN electron microscopy. *Note:* Glomerular capillary filtering barrier showing immunoglobulins. As electron dense material of varying sizes in subendothelial (brown arrow) and subepithelial hump-like deposits (red arrow)

Electron microscopy typically shows large, hump-shaped subepithelial electron dense deposits (Fig. 16.4).

Treatment

The first step in the treatment is eradication of infection using appropriate antibiotics. Antivirals are recommended in case of hepatitis B and C related GN. HIV positive patients require highly active antiretroviral therapy in all patients with kidney involvement. Patients with endocarditis or shunt nephritis, who fail medical therapy would require surgical intervention. Antihypertensive drugs and diuretics are used to control hypertension and edema. There is no role of immunosuppressive therapy since it might even cause more harm than help. There was no correlation between glucocorticoid therapy and renal outcomes. If AKI develops, dialysis support may be necessary as indicated.

Prognosis

In adults with infection-associated glomerulonephritis, successful eradication of the infection often results in resolution of the glomerulonephritis.

Depending on the etiology, the outcome of GN associated with infection can be quite variable. Many patients with Staphylococcus-associated glomerulonephritis do not have complete resolution of the serum creatinine to their baseline values and may also have persistent proteinuria. Repeat kidney biopsy is usually not warranted for persistent mild to moderate proteinuria and persistently elevated serum creatinine. Only 'active' urine sediment or persistent hypocomplementemia suggest persistence of the disease process. Findings like persistent proteinuria or elevated serum creatinine represent fibrotic changes or inactive disease.

Rapidly Progressive Glomerulonephritis and Vasculitis

• H Sudarshan Ballal • Vishvanath S • Rohan Augustine

Rapidly progressive glomerulonephritis (RPGN) is a clinical syndrome characterized by a rapid loss of renal function over few days to months along with features of glomerulonephritis (GN), i.e. glomerular hematuria, proteinuria and edema. Patients with RPGN are often oligoanuric. Proteinuria is usually in the subnephrotic range and severe hypertension in not a dominant feature. The clinical picture of RPGN is often synonymous with the histology of crescent formation. RPGN is one of the many causes for rapidly progressive renal failure (RPRF) which is a clinical syndrome characterized by a rapid decrease in the glomerular filtration rate by at least 50% or the doubling of serum creatinine over a short period ranging from few days to <3 months (Table 17.1). Renal diseases other than crescentic GN can cause signs and symptoms consistent with RPRF.

Crescentic GN was first described in 1914 and the term RPGN was introduced in 1942. Subsequently crescentic GN was classified into 3 broad groups depending upon the immunofluorescence findings (Table 17.2).

1. Crescentric GN with linear IgG staining of glomerular basement membrane (GBM)—anti-GBM disease.
2. Crescentic GN with absent or minimal immune deposits—known as pauci-immune crescentic GN.

Table 17.1: Causes of rapidly progressive renal failure

Rapidly progressive glomerulonephritis
- Crescentic GN
- Diffuse proliferative GN
- Mesangiocapillary GN with crescents

Tubulointerstitial disease
- Acute interstitial nephritis
- Acute tubular necrosis (rarely)
- Myeloma cast nephropathy

Vascular diseases
- Thrombotic microangiopathy
- Malignant hypertension
- Hemolytic uremic syndrome
- Progressive systemic sclerosis and renal crisis
- Atheroembolic renal disease
- Thromboembolic disease

3. Crescentric GN with granular pattern of glomerular immune complex deposits—immune complex-mediated crescentric GN which falls into 3 broad sub-groups:
   a. Associated with infection
   b. Associated with systemic illness
   c. Superimposed on primary glomerular disease.

CLINICAL FEATURES

RPGN may have a quite varied presentation. Idiopathic RPGN has an insidious onset with

Table 17.2: Causes of rapidly progressive glomerulonephritis due to crescentic glomerulonephritis

Primary diseases

	Type 1	Antiglomerular basement membrane antibody disease
		1. Anti-GBM Ab mediated without lung involvment
		2. Anti-GBM Ab mediated with pulmonary hemorrhage— Goodpasture's disease
	Type 2	Immune complex-mediated disease
	Type 3	Pauci-immune disease (ANCA positive)
		1. Wegener's granulomatosis
		2. Microscopic polyarteritis
		3. Idiopathic renal limited vasculitis
	Type 4	Mixed anti-GBM and ANCA associated disease
	Type 5	Pauci-immune disease (ANCA negative)
Secondary diseases		**Immune complex-mediated disease**
	Infectious diseases	1. Post-streptococcal glomerulonephritis
		2. Infective endocarditis
		3. Visceral sepsis
		4. Hepatitis B or C infection with vasculitis and/or cryoglobulinemia
	Systemic diseases	1. Systemic lupus erythematosus
		2. Henoch-Schönlein purpura
		3. Systemic necrotizing vasculitis
		4. Relapsing polychondritis
	Drugs	1. Allopurinol
		2. Rifampicin
		3. D-penicillamine
		4. Hydralazine
	Malignancy	Colon, lung, lymphoma
	Miscellaneous	1. IgA nephropathy
		2. MPGN with crescents
		3. Behçet's disease

the initial nonspecific symptoms and features of glomerulonephritis (GN), i.e. glomerular hematuria, proteinuria and edema. Patients with RPGN are often oligoanuric. Proteinuria is in the subnephrotic range and severe hypertension is not a dominant feature. Renal insufficiency is present at diagnosis in almost all cases. Untreated RPGN progresses to end-stage renal disease over a period of weeks or few months. Constitutional features like fever, myalgias and weight loss are common in pauci-immune systemic vasculitis.

Patients with anti-GBM antibody disease may also have pulmonary hemorrhage and hemoptysis at some stage of the disease (Goodpasture's disease). This combination of RPGN and hemoptysis can also be seen in other causes of RPGN, namely Wegener's granulomatosis (GPA) and microscopic polyangiitis (MPA) or in renal failure with associated infection or pulmonary edema.

RPGN also has distinct age preponderance. Children most often have immune complex mediated RPGN. Middle aged and older individuals are more commonly affected with the pauci-immune type of RPGN. Anti-GBM disease has a bimodal presentation affecting young individuals and older men and women.

A preceding upper respiratory or influenza like illness or exposure to hydrocarbon fumes has been observed in anti-GBM disease.

LABORATORY FEATURES

The key to diagnosing RPGN begins with a good urine examination in the appropriate clinical context. The urinalysis reveals variable degree of proteinuria associated with hematuria, red cell and RBC casts. Nephrotic range proteinuria is unusual. Circulating immune complexes with low complement C3 levels are seen in immune complex-mediated crescentic GN. Serum complement levels are usually normal in anti-GBM disease and pauci-immune GN. ANCA and anti-GBM antibodies are often positive in pauci-immmune and Anti-GBM disease respectively. ANCA and anti-GBM antibodies may coexist (double positive) in up to 30% of patients. Other serological investigations like anti-nuclear antibodies (ANA), anti-DNA antibodies and hepatitis B and C serology and cryoglobulins are performed in patients with RPGN with systemic features.

RPGN results from three underlying immunopathogenetic mechanisms. The different immunohistological patterns and their serological and disease associations are given in Table 17.3.

Anti-GBM Antibody-mediated Crescentic Nephritis (Fig. 17.1)

Linear staining with IgG and C3 involving basement membrane of glomerular capillaries, Bowman's capsule and the distal tubules is characteristic of anti-GBM disease. The antibody is directed against non-collagenous globular domain of α3 chain of type IV collagen.

Pauci-immune Crescentic Nephritis

Patients with pauci-immune RPGN have a little or no immunoglobulin deposits. More than 80% of these patients have circulating ANCA. Two types of staining pattern are demonstrated. Cytoplasmic ANCA (cANCA) produces a cytoplasmic staining pattern and pANCA demonstrates a perinuclear staining pattern of alcohol-fixed neutrophils. ANCA specificity is determined by ELISA. cANCA is an antibody directed against antiproteinase 3 (PR3) and pANCA against myeloperoxidase (MPO). Nonspecific pANCA can occur in association with autoimmune diseases such as SLE, inflammatory bowel disease, sclerosing

Table 17.3: Immunopathogenic mechanisms in RPGN

Immunohistology	Serological markers	Disease
1. Linear deposition of antibody along the GBM	Anti-GBM antibodies	Anti-glomerular basement membrane disease
2. Renal microscopic vasculitis with scanty glomerular deposits of immunoglobulin	c-ANCA (anti-PR3) pANCA (anti-MPO)	Wegener's granulomatosis Microscopic polyangiitis
3. Renal microscopic vasculitis with granular deposits of immunoglobulin	ANA, anti-dsDNA antibodies, anti SmAb anti-C1q Ab Cryoglobulinemia Complement reduction	SLE HCV, HIV Crescents complicating pre-existing nephritis, e.g. IgA, mesangiocapillary nephritis, Henoch-Schönlein purpura, rheumatoid arthritis Infective endocarditis Post-streptoccal nephritis

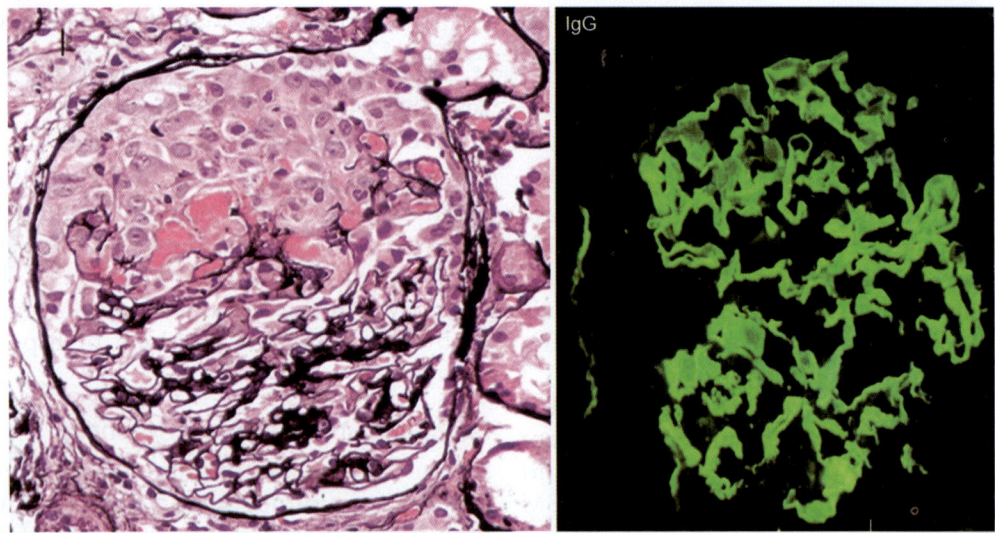

Fig. 17.1: Crescentic GN in anti-GBM disease (left). Silver stain showing proliferation of the parietal cells compressing the underlying glomerular tuft with rupture of Bowman's capsule (right). Linear IgG staining along the glomerular basement membrane suggestive of anti-GBM disease

cholangitis, autoimmune hepatitis, rheumatoid arthritis, and Felty's syndrome.

Immune Complex-mediated Crescentic Nephritis (Fig. 17.2)

Granular deposition of immunoglobulin and complement along the capillary loops and mesangium suggests immune complex-mediated pathogenesis, e.g. post-streptococcal glomerulonephritis. Predominant deposition of IgA suggests the diagnosis of IgA disease or HSP. Predominant C3 deposits with a little or no immunoglobulins are seen in patients with MPGN complement-mediated. Deposits of IgG, IgM and IgA along with complement C3 and C1q (full house pattern) suggest SLE. In

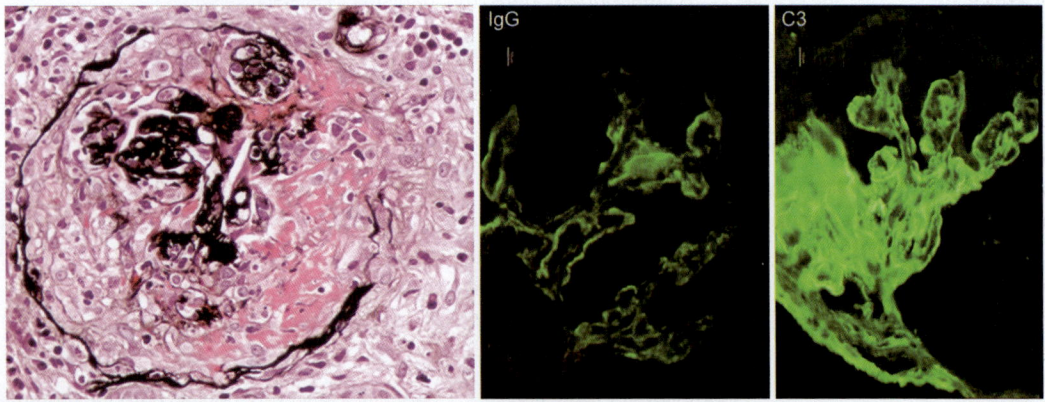

Fig. 17.2: Crescentic GN in immune complex glomerulitis (left). Silver stain showing proliferation of the parietal cells compressing the underlying glomerular tuft with rupture of Bowman's capsule (middle). IgG staining (right) and C3 staining on immunofluorescence suggestive of immune complex-mediated crescentic glomerulonephritis

bacterial endocarditis, IgM is seen prominently.

Pathology

On gross examination the kidneys are usually swollen and the surface is studded with petechial hemorrhages (flea bitten kidneys). Renal biopsy is the gold standard in making the diagnosis of RPGN excluding it from other causes of RPRF. To call it a crescent there should be extracapillary proliferation of parietal cells at least 2 layers thick. The crescent may be localized to one or more lobules and referred to as a 'segmental/partial' crescent. In others, the proliferation of parietal cells is more severe and fills the Bowman's space compresses the underlying glomerular tuft and encases it. This is called 'circumferential' crescent.

The crescent formation follows 5 'stages':
1. *Stage 1:* Accumulation of cells in the glomerular tuft
2. *Stage 2:* Fibrin formation in Bowman's space
3. *Stage 3:* Accumulation of cells in the Bowman's space forming a cellular crescent
4. *Stage 4:* Accumulation of matrix materials to replace damaged glomerular cells (fibrocellular crescent)
5. *Stage 5:* Permanent replacement of the glomerulus by scar (fibrous crescent).

The stages up to stage 4 are potentially reversible with treatment. Crescents may resolve without scarring, especially in children with a post-infectious GN and in patients in whom the glomerular tuft is relatively intact and Bowman's capsule is not ruptured.

If all the crescents are at the same stage of evolution, it would suggest a one-time insult (e.g. PIGN, anti-GBM) and if crescents are seen at different stages of evolution, it may suggest multiple immunological insults over a longer period of time (e.g. pauci-immune GN, lupus nephritis). The underlying glomerular tuft may be normal or show varying degrees of proliferation, necrosis or scarring. The glomerular tuft shows diffuse endocapillary proliferation in post-infectious type, focal and segmental necrosis in vasculitis, systemic lupus erythematosus (SLE) and Henoch-Schönlein purpura (HSP).

Mechanism of Crescent Formation

Crescent formation represents a nonspecific response to severe injury to glomerular capillary tuft resulting in the movement of plasma products into Bowman's space and subsequent fibrin formation, influx of macrophages and T lymphocytes, and the release of proinflammatory cytokines, such as interleukin-1 and tumor necrosis factor-α. The basic stimulus for crescent formation might be the presence of fibrin in Bowman's space. Polymorphonuclear cell and macrophages under the chemotactic influence of fibrin, migrate into Bowman's space, phagocytose fibrin and are transformed into epithelioid cells. Inflammatory macrophages release large amounts of growth factors capable of stimulating parietal epithelial cell division (extracapillary parietal cell proliferation). Rupture of Bowman's capsule allows inward migration of fibroblasts. Monokines released by monocytes also influence fibroblastic behavior and cellular crescent progress to fibrocellular and finally to fibrotic stage.

Outcomes of RPGN

The outcome of RPGN is generally unfavorable with about 20% of patients presenting with dialysis dependency and 50% progressing to end stage by 1 year. Oligoanuria and advanced renal azotemia at presentation carry a poor prognosis. Pauci-immune RPGN has the best prognosis. Immune complex RPGN has better prognosis compared to anti-GBM disease. Patients with more than 80% circumferential fibrous/fibocellular crescents often present with advanced renal failure and do not respond well to therapy. Those with non-circumferential crescents in less than 50% of the glomeruli follow a more indolent course. Associated endocapillary proliferation is a good prognostic factor but glomerular tuft necrosis, global glomerular sclerosis, ruptured Bowman's capsule and interstitial fibrosis are bad prognostic features.

Treatment, Course and Prognosis

A high index of suspicion is necessary for arriving at an early and accurate diagnosis. All patients with suspected RPGN should undergo kidney biopsy urgently to confirm the diagnosis and to prognosticate the reversibility of renal failure. Initiating early treatment is of great importance and patients unable to undergo a kidney biopsy should be considered for empiric therapy with immunosuppressive agents. A variety of immunosuppressive regimens have been tried in idiopathic RPGN. Therapy is most effective if begun early before the patient is oliguric or requires dialysis.

Anti-GBM-mediated Crescentic Glomerulonephritis

Plasma exchange with immunosuppressive therapy is administered to remove circulating anti-GBM antibodies and suppresses the formation of new antibodies. Pulmonary disease responds better than renal disease. When immunosuppression and plasma exchange are started early, the outcomes are more favorable. Plasma exchange should be continued for at least 2 weeks and immuno-suppression with pulse methylprednisolone followed by oral steroids and cyclophosphamide for 8 weeks. Plasma exchange is also indicated when there is severe pulmonary hemorrhage. Plasma exchange is not recommended in anuric patients with more than 85% crescents unless they have pulmonary hemorrhage.

Immune Complex-mediated Crescentic GN

In post-infectious RPGN, 50% recover spontaneously without specific therapy, 20% have partial recovery and 30% develop chronic kidney disease. Outcome can be improved with the use of high doses of pulse methyl-prednisolone in doses of 7–15 mg/kg/day (up to a maximum of 1 gm/day) for 3 days followed by 1 mg/kg/day of oral prednisolone for 1 month, gradually tapering.

Pauci-immune Crescentic GN

Pulse methyl prednisolone therapy is beneficial in dialysis dependent patients and nearly 70% of patients may come off dialysis. Remission is induced using steroids combined with cyclophosphamide/rituximab and maintained by long-term treatment with steroids combined with mycophenolate mofetil/azathioprine. Cyclophosphamide is given orally in a dose of 2 mg/kg/day or monthly doses intravenously starting at 0.5 g/m^2 and increased monthly by 0.25 g/m^2, to a maximum of 1 g/m^2. The dose must be adjusted for renal insufficiency and maintaining leukocyte count over 4000 cells/mm^3. Cyclophosphamide is continued for at least 6 months and later is replaced with azathioprine or mycophenolate. In patients who are ANCA positive, monitoring for relapse with ANCA titres is recommended.

The responders often show improvement in creatinine within 7 to 10 days. Microhematuria resolves over 3 to 6 months. Variable degree of proteinuria may persist because of irreversible glomerular injury and scarring. Renal transplantation should be delayed in anti-GBM-mediated RPGN progressing to ESRD until there are no detectable antibodies in the serum, so as to prevent the recurrence of disease in the allograft. In other types of RPGN, the patients can be transplanted if they do not have clinical evidence of disease activity.

VASCULITIS

Vasculitis is a life-threatening autoimmune disease characterized by inflammatory leukocytes in the vessel walls causing reactive damage. Blood vessels of any size from the aorta to capillaries or small venules may be affected by vasculitis. Based on the size of the affected blood vessel and clinical characteristics, vasculitis is broadly classified as large vessel, medium vessel and small vessel vasculitis (Fig. 17.3). The classification of vasculitis is shown in Table 17.4. The clinical manifestations also depend on the organs affected. Since kidneys are highly vascular, they are involved in most forms of the vasculitis. Renal involvement includes inflammation and narrowing of renal arteries, branches and/or inflammation with necrosis of smaller blood vessels and capillaries. Renal manifestations include hematuria, proteinuria, hypertension, acute glomerulonephritis, or rapidly progressive renal failure. The classification of vasculitis evolved at a consensus conference held at Chapel Hill, USA in 1998.

Takayasu Arteritis or Aortoarteritis

Takayasu arteritis or aortoarteritis is a chronic granulomatous arteritis affecting the large blood vessels. Aortic arch, thoracic or abdominal aorta and its major branches including upper limb vessels, carotids or renal arteries may be affected. Major clinical manifestations include claudication, absent pulsations in the extremities and hypertension. Involvement of renal arteries is an important cause of renovascular hypertension particularly in young individuals.

Giant Cell Arteritis

Giant cell arteritis affects the extracranial branches of carotid artery, especially temporal artery in the elderly females and presents as severe headache, tenderness, nodularity, decreased pulsation of temporal artery, blindness, deafness and jaw claudication. Associated polymyalgia rheumatica is common. Renal artery involvement is rare.

Polyarteritis nodosa is a necrotizing arteritis mainly affecting the medium-sized arteries. The blood vessels supplying the kidneys, liver, heart, eyes, testis, nervous system and skin may be involved. Main renal trunk,

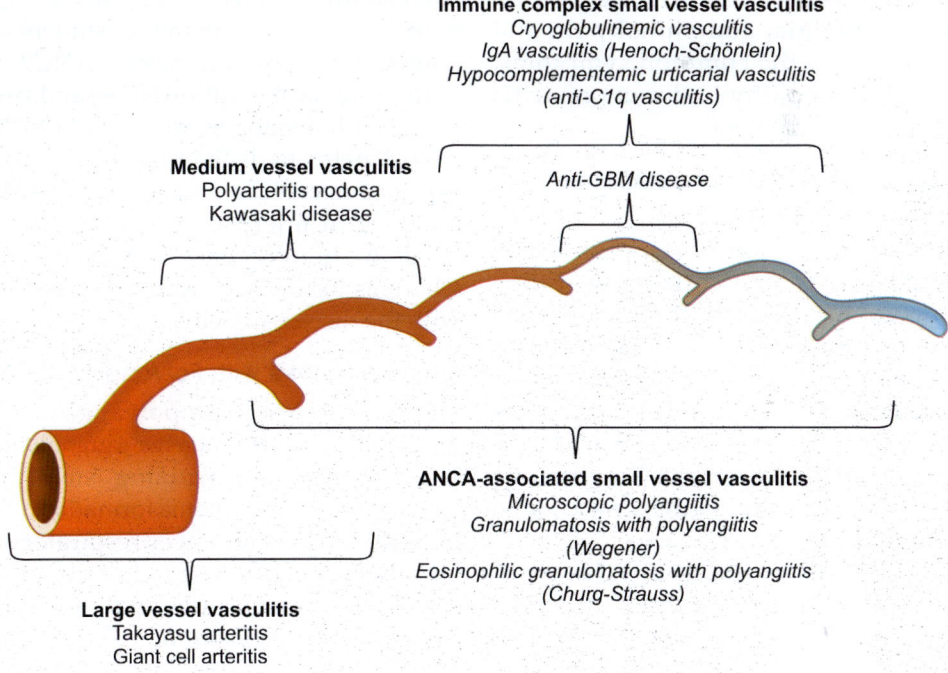

Immune complex small vessel vasculitis
Cryoglobulinemic vasculitis
IgA vasculitis (Henoch-Schönlein)
Hypocomplementemic urticarial vasculitis
(anti-C1q vasculitis)

Medium vessel vasculitis
Polyarteritis nodosa
Kawasaki disease

Anti-GBM disease

ANCA-associated small vessel vasculitis
Microscopic polyangiitis
Granulomatosis with polyangiitis
(Wegener)
Eosinophilic granulomatosis with polyangiitis
(Churg-Strauss)

Large vessel vasculitis
Takayasu arteritis
Giant cell arteritis

Fig. 17.3: Chapel Hill nomenclature for systemic vasculitides

Table 17.4: Classification of renal vasculitis

Immune complex vasculitis	Pauci-immune vasculitis
• Henoch-Schönlein purpura	• Renal limited ANCA GN
• Lupus vasculitis	• Vasculitis with no asthma or granuloma (MPA)
• Rheumatoid vasculitis	• Vasculitis with granuloma but no asthma → granulomatosis with polyangiitis (GPA)—Wegener's granulomatosis
• Cryoglobulinemic vasculitis	• Vasculitis with asthma → granuloma and eosinophilia → eosinophilic granulomatosis with polyangiitis (EGPA)—Churg-Strauss syndrome.
• Serum sickness vasculitis	
• Infection-induced immune complex vasculitis	
– Bacterial	
– Viral (hepatitis B, C)	
• Paraneoplastic vasculitis	
• Drug-induced vasculitis	
• Leukocytoclastic vasculitis	

interlobar, arcuate or interlobular artery may be affected by inflammation, necrosis or aneurysm formation. Hypertension, hemorrhage or infarction may occur. The disease is common in young adults with a male preponderance. There is a strong association with hepatitis B infection. Fever, weight loss, myalgia, arthralgia, abdominal pain and hypertension are the common symptoms. Peripheral neuropathy and mononeuritis multiplex are also common.

Kawasaki Disease or Mucocutaneous Lymph Node Syndrome

Kawasaki disease or mucocutaneous lymph node syndrome is a necrotizing vasculitis affecting young children. It presents with fever, nonsuppurative lymphadenopathy, bulbar conjunctivitis, oropharyngeal conges-tion, 'strawberry tongue', palmar erythema and limb edema followed by desquamation of extremities. Coronary artery aneurysm and thrombosis result in myocardial infarction in children.

Small vessel vasculitis is classified as pauci-immune and immune complex-mediated vasculitis. In pauci-immune vasculitis, there is no significant immune complex deposition in the vessel wall and is usually necrotizing

vasculitis with or without granuloma forma-tion. Anti-neutrophil cytoplasmic antibodies (ANCAs) are often positive. Based on the staining pattern, ANCA is classified into pANCA (perinuclear) and cANCA (cytoplasmic) by indirect immunofluorescence of alcohol fixed neutrophils. The ANCA in these groups of diseases reacts with the constituents of the neutrophils and monocytes. cANCA reacts with proteinase 3 (PR3-ANCA) and pANCA reacts with myeloperoxidase (MPO-ANCA). ANCA helps in differentiating the different types of necrotizing vasculitis. pANCA is positive in microscopic polyangiitis and cANCA in Wegener's granulomatosis. Changes in the ANCA titres correlate well with the disease activity.

Granulomatosis with Polyangiitis (GPA)

Granulomatosis with polyangiitis (GPA), formerly known as 'Wegener's granulomatosis' is a systemic necrotizing small vessel vasculitis with granuloma formation affecting both the upper and lower respiratory tracts and the kidneys. The triad of upper, lower respiratory tract and renal involvement associated with constitutional symptoms like fever, anorexia, weight loss, large and small joint arthritis is the common clinical presentation. Pulmonary involvement is characterized by single or multiple, unilateral or bilateral granulomatous, nodular or cavitary lesions. Sinusitis causes mucosal thickening and destruction of the cartilaginous nasal septum resulting in the characteriztic 'saddle nose' deformity. Skin manifestations include painful subcutaneous nodules, ulcers and palpable purpura.

Eosinophilic Granulomatosis with Polyangiitis (EGPA)

Eosinophilic granulomatosis with poly-angiitis (EGPA), formerly known as 'Churg-Strauss syndrome' is a pauci-immune vasculitis associated with granuloma formation. In addition to renal involvement in the form or rapidly progressive crescentic glomerulo-nephritis, patients have asthma and eosinophilia.

Microscopic Polyangiitis

Microscopic polyangiitis (MPA) is a form of necrotizing vasculitis affecting the small blood vessels including arterioles, venules and capillaries and is not associated with granuloma formation. The clinical manifestations depend on the organs involved. Pauci-immune crescentic glomerulonephritis manifests as hematuria, proteinuria and rapidly progressive renal failure. The general symptoms are fever, malaise, anorexia, weight loss, myalgia and arthralgia. Nodular cutaneous lesions and purpura occur due to dermal vasculitis. Rarely, pancreatitis, hepatitis, mononeuritis multiplex and mesenteric vasculitis are seen. Abdominal vasculitis manifests as severe abdominal pain, intestinal bleeding or perforation.

Pathogenesis

The pathogenesis of ANCA-associated vasculitis (AAV) is multifactorial, with complex interplay between genetic factors, environ-mental exposures, infections, innate and adaptive immune system, and the intensity and duration of the injury. Acute vascular inflammation is induced when resting neutrophils with ANCA autoantigens in cytoplasmic granules are exposed to priming factors, e.g. cytokines or complement activation. This causes the release of ANCA antigens on the surface of neutrophils. ANCA binds to these ANCA antigens, and activates neutrophils. ANCA-activated neutrophils then release factors that activate the alternative complement pathway generating C5a, a chemoattractant for neutrophils; C5a also primes the arriving neutrophils for activation by ANCA. Activated neutrophils adhere to and penetrate vessel walls, and they release toxic oxygen radicals and destructive enzymes that cause apoptosis and necrosis of the adjacent vessel wall cells and matrix.

Diagnosis

The diagnosis is made based on high index of suspicion, clinical clues, laboratory para-meters and renal biopsy study.The laboratory tests usually performed are serum ANCA, antinuclear antibodies (ANA), anti-glomerular basement membrane (anti GBM) antibody and complement C3 and C4. These tests are used in combination with the tissue diagnosis which is the gold standard. Measurement of ANCA by both ELISA and indirect immuno-fluorescence (IIF) ensures optimal sensitivity and specificity. Serial ANCA testing (ELISA and IIF) to monitor disease activity is useful as disappearance of ANCA is associated with disease remission and a lower risk of relapse, reappearance or rising ANCA titre is of greater relevance in the setting of worsening clinical features, and the persistence of anti-proteinase 3 (anti-PR3) antibodies is associated with a higher risk of relapse. Other tests like imaging also contribute to the diagnosis.

Focal or diffuse necrotizing extracapillary glomerulonephritis is the histological hallmark of ANCA-associated vasculitis (Fig. 17.4). Tuft necrosis and extracapillary proliferation (crescents) are variable in intensity and distribution. While some show isolated segmental necrosis of the glomerular tuft

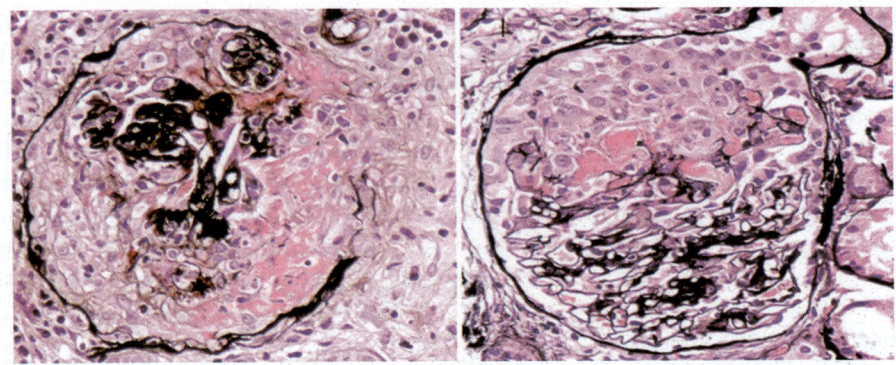

Fig. 17.4: Histopathology of crescentic glomerulonephritis. Extracapillary proliferation of parietal epithelial cells more than 2 cell layers thick with compression of the underlying glomerular tuft and rupture of Bowman's capsule

without extracapillary proliferation (crescents), massive tuft necrosis is usually associated with diffuse circumferential crescents. Periglomerular leukocyte infiltration is another distinctive feature and is seen in close proximity of the necrotizing extracapillary lesion. A rupture of the Bowman's capsule is commonly observed. The massive circumferential leukocyte infiltration gives a picture of 'glomerular granuloma-like lesion'. In active lesions, fibrin deposition is invariably present and focal and segmental forms show fibrin deposition in areas of the tuft. ANCA-associated renal vasculitis by definition are 'pauci-immune' glomerulonephritis. Immunofluorescence can be either negative or characterized by scattered C3 granular deposition. In 20% of cases, a mild mesangial and parietal deposition of IgG and C3 can be observed in low intensity.

Management

The initial step in the management is staging of disease (Table 17.5) and planning the

	Table 17.5: EUVAS/EULAR staging of vasculitis			
Disease stage	*EUVAS/EULAR definition*	*Systemic vasculitis outside ENT or lung*	*Threatened vital organ function*	*Creatinine mg/dl*
Localized	Upper/ lower respiratory tract disease without systemic involvement or constitutional symptoms	No	No	<1.2
Early systemic	Any disease without organ threatening or life-threatening involvement	Yes	No	<1.2
Generalized	Renal or other organ threatening disease	Yes	Yes	<5.7 mg/dl
Severe	Renal or other vital organ failure	Yes	Organ failure	>5.7 mg/dl
Refractory	Progressive disease unresponsive to standard therapy	Yes	Yes	Any

Table 17.6: Regimens for inducing remission

Disease stage	Treatment	Dose
Localized	Cotrimoxazole with /without steroids	Cotrimoxazole 960 mg BD
Localized	Methotrexate with glucocorticoids	Methotrexate 15 mg/week increasing to 20–25 mg/week with folic acid and glucocorticoids
Early systemic	Methotrexate with glucocorticoids	Methotrexate 15 mg/week increasing to 20–25 mg/week with folic acid and glucocorticoids
Generalized	Cyclophosphamide with glucocorticoids	IV pulse cyclophosphamide three pulses of 15 mg/kg every 2 weeks, then every 3 weeks for a total of 6–9 pulses and glucocorticoids or oral cyclophosphamide 2 mg/kg with glucocorticoids, duration 3–6 months
Generalized	Rituximab and glucocorticoids	Infusion of rituximab: 375 mg/m^2 once /week for 4 weeks
Severe	Plasmapheresis as adjunct to cyclophosphamide/rituximab	Seven rounds of plasma exchange 60 ml/kg body weight
Refractory	Rituximab/MMF/ATG /IvIgG/infliximab	

Table 17.7: Regimens for maintaining remission

Disease stage	Treatment	Dose
Localized	Cotrimoxazole	960 mg twice daily
Early systemic	Methotrexate	20–25 mg/week with glucocorticoids
Early systemic with severe upper respiratory tract involvement	Cotrimoxazole	960 mg twice daily or 3 times/week
Generalized	Azathioprine	2 mg/kg for 12 months, thereafter 1.5 mg/kg daily with low dose glucocorticoids
Generalized	Mycophenolate mofetil	30 mg/kg for 12 months followed by taper with low dose glucocorticoids
Generalized	Methotrexate	20–25 mg/week with low dose glucocorticoids
Generalized	Leflunomide	20 mg/day with low dose glucocorticoids
Generalized	Rituximab	375 mg/m^2 or 500 mg or 1 gm infusions every 4–6 months

treatment. The recommendations of the European League Against Rheumatism (EULAR) and the European Vasculitis Society (EUVAS) are generally followed. Treatment is broadly divided into induction phase, maintenance phase, monitoring during remission and disease specific management.

Treatment

Treatment of vasculitis involves two distinct phases. The induction phase involving use of pulse steroids, cyclophosphamide, rituximab or methotrexate (Table 17.6) is aimed at bringing the disease into a quick remission and this if followed by maintenance phase with the use of drugs like mycophenolate mofetil, azathioprine and low dose steroids to sustain remission (Table 17.7).

In summary, vasculitides are a group of inflammatory diseases affecting vessels of various sizes and in different locations. They are classified based on size of vessels involved and on serological markers. The diagnosis is based on clinical, serological, imaging and tissue diagnosis. Treatment involves the disease staging, induction of remission and maintenance therapy. Though some of the vasculitides could be life-threatening, early diagnosis and appropriate treatment could save the involved organ and life of the patient.

Lupus Nephritis

• Sahil Bagai • HS Kohli

INTRODUCTION

Systemic lupus erythematosus (SLE) is a systemic autoimmune disease characterized by chronic inflammation. It can affect predominantly females and any organ may be involved. The clinical course is characterized by remissions and relapses. The predominant age group affected in SLE is 15–45 years with males to female ratio of 1:9. However, this gender predominance is less pronounced in children and older individuals. Lupus nephritis (LN) denotes involvement of kidneys and is a common as well as serious manifestation of SLE. In LN, there is lack of female preponderance. Though males and females are equally involved, the manifestations are more severe in males. Similarly, it is more severe in children as compared to elderly who have a milder form. The diagnosis of SLE was made as per American College of Rheumatology (ACR) criteria till 2012 but because of shortcomings in identifying all lupus nephritis and CNS lupus. Systemic Lupus International Collaborating Clinics (SLICC) criteria was introduced in 2012 (Table 18.1). To diagnose SLE >4 of 17 criteria,

Table 18.1: Systemic Lupus International Collaborating Clinics (SLICC) criteria (2012)

>4 of 17 criteria, including at least one clinical criterion and one immunologic criterion or biopsy-proven lupus nephritis with positive ANA or anti-dsDNA

Clinical criteria	Immunological criteria
Acute cutaneous lupus	ANA
Chronic cutaneous lupus	Anti-dsDNA
Nonscarring alopecia	Anti-Sm
Arthritis	Low C3/C4/CH50
Serositis	Antiphospholipid
Oral or nasal ulcers	Direct Coombs' test (not counted if hemolytic anemia present)
Renal (proteinuria >500 mg/day or RBC cast)	
Neurological	
Hemolytic anemia	
Thrombocytopenia (<1 lakh at least once)	
Leukopenia (<4000/mm^3 at least once)	

including at least one clinical criterion and one immunologic criterion or biopsy-proven lupus nephritis with positive ANA or anti-DNA are required to diagnose SLE. All criteria need not be present at the same time. Even if they are present at different time frames, they may be considered sufficient for diagnosis.

Pathogenesis

Lupus nephritis is an immune complex-mediated glomerulonephritis. First step in pathogenesis is the formation of antibodies. Tolerance to nuclear antigens is lost, antibodies are produced against them and it manifests as presence of antinuclear antibodies. Additionally, apoptotic neutrophils (neutrophils undergoing 'programmed death') release nucleic acids which in turn activate both innate and adaptive immune system through nucleic acid-specific toll-like receptors. There is decreased clearance of these nuclear antigens from extracellular space resulting in increased interaction between antigens and autoantibodies. Dendritic cells, plasma cells, T helper cells and B cells contribute to the aberrant polyclonal auto-immunity. Amongst environmental insults, silica, ultraviolet light, Epstein-Barr (EB) virus and smoking have been incriminated.

The pathogenic mechanisms in kidneys involve:

a. Binding of antinuclear antibodies to multiple intrarenal autoantigens which induce production of proinflammatory substances.

b. Deposition of circulating immune complexes in mesangial, subendothelial or sub-epithelial sites in the glomeruli results in activation of complement cascade and inflammation.

Characteristics of both the antigen and antibody determine the site of immune complex formation.

Negatively charged (anionic) antigens or large intact immune complexes (which cannot cross the anionic charge barrier of the glomerular capillary wall) are deposited in the mesangium and subendothelial space. Severity of the disease is determined by the degree and site of immune deposition. Disease is mild if deposits are limited to the mesangium. If deposits are in subendothelial space, severe forms of focal or diffuse proliferative glomerulonephritis occur. Subepithelial deposits may form when there is a cationic antigen that can cross the GBM or when an autoantibody directed against visceral epithelial cell antigens. Pathogenetic mechanisms of LN are shown in Fig. 18.1.

Clinical Features

Most patients with SLE will have clinical evidence of renal disease. Renal involvement occurs in 20–60% of patients with SLE. In a patient of SLE, the presence of nephritis is suspected by an abnormal urinalysis and/or elevation of the serum creatinine and the diagnosis is confirmed by histopathologic

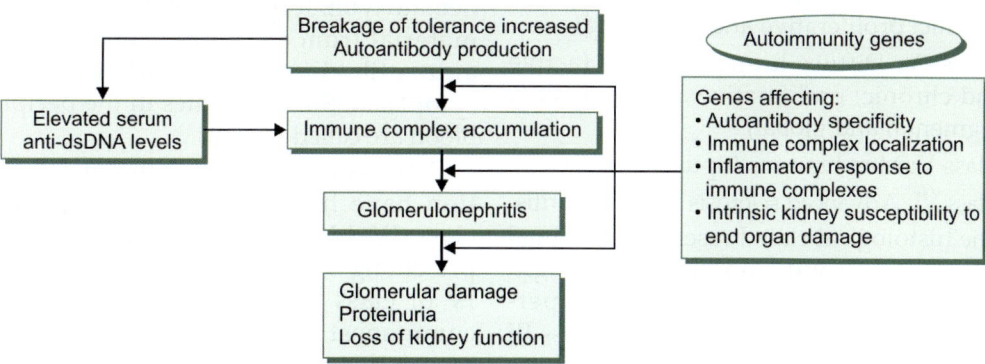

Fig. 18.1: Pathogenesis of lupus nephritis

findings on renal biopsy. African races, younger age, lower socioeconomic status, family history of SLE, longer duration of disease, more systemic features and hypertension predispose patient of SLE to develop LN. The clinical pointers to suspect renal involvement in SLE are:

a. Proteinuria or urine protein to creatinine ratio of >500 : 1
b. 24-hour urine protein >500 mg
c. Presence of RBC cast in urine sediment
d. Elevation of serum creatinine

Almost all patients with renal involvement will have proteinuria. Microscopic hematuria, hypertension and renal dysfunction are the other common renal involvement seen. Extrarenal manifestations may or may not be present in patients with LN. Various clinical features and their relative frequency are listed in Table 18.2.

Histopathology

The type of renal involvement in LN can be made only on study of kidney biopsy which reveals widespread and variable glomerular, vascular and interstitial lesions. The International Society of Nephrology (ISN)/Renal Pathology Society (RPS) has classified lupus nephritis into 6 classes:

1. Class I: Minimal mesangial lupus nephritis
2. Class II: Mesangial proliferative lupus nephritis
3. Class III: Focal lupus nephritis (active and chronic; proliferative and sclerosing)
4. Class IV: Diffuse lupus nephritis (active and chronic; proliferative and sclerosing; segmental and global)
5. Class V: Membranous lupus nephritis
6. Class VI: Advanced sclerosis lupus nephritis

The histological class I resembles minimal change disease with no change on light micoscopy. In class II, mesangial hypercellularity or expansion is present. In class III the lesions are focal and in class IV diffuse. There is proliferation of the cells in the

Table 18.2: Clinical features of lupus nephritis

Clinical feature	Percentage
Proteinuria	100
• Nephrotic syndrome	45–65
Hematuria	
• Micropcopic hematuria	80
• Red cell casts	40–60
• Macroscopic hematuria	1–2
Reduced renal function	40–80
• Rapidly declining kidney function	30
• Acute renal failure	1–2
Hypertension	15–50
Hyperkalemia	15
Tubular abnormalities	60–80

glomerular capillary tuft (endocapillary) or parietal epithelial cells of the Bowman's capsule (extracapillary), along with mesangial changes. 'Wire loop' lesions, segmental necrosis, hematoxylin body, crescents and hyaline thrombi are pathognomonic of lupus nephritis. Wire loop lesions are greatly thickened walls of the glomerular capillaries due to large amounts of immune deposits in the subendothelial region. Since they are arranged circumferentially along the capillary loop, they resemble a 'wire loop' and hence the name. On electron microscopy, tubuloreticular structures (clustered microtubules measuring about 250 nm in diameter) are often found in the cytoplasm of endothelial cells. Hematoxylin body is a dense, homogeneous, basophilic particle, easily stainable with hematoxylin. It consists of degraded nuclear material from an injured cell, along with autoantibodies and a limited amount of cytoplasm. Similar bodies in the peripheral blood are called LE cells.

Patients who present with renal dysfunction have highest probability of having class IV LN in kidney biopsy. Patients presenting with proteinuria may have class III, IV or class V LN. By far, class IV is the commonest form. Immunofluorescence reveals deposits of all classes of immunoglobulins and complement (full house positivity

(IgA, IgG, IgM, kappa, lambda, C3 and C1q positive). Various histopathological changes and important clinical manifestations are shown in Table 18.3. ISN/RPS classification does not consider changes in vascular, interstitial and tubular compartment. These changes are also important for treatment and prognostication.

Diagnosis

A series of preliminary and advanced laboratory tests are necessary to evaluate renal involvement in patients with SLE. They are:

a. Urinalysis to check for protein, red blood cells (RBCs), and cellular casts. The characteristic abnormality associated with LN is

Table 18.3: ISN/RPS classification of lupus nephritis

Class of LN	Light microscopy	Immuno-fluorescence	Electron microscopy	Clinical presentation
1. Minimal mesangial LN	Normal	Mesangial deposits	Mesangial deposits	Normal serum creatinine with no or minimal proteinuria
2. Mesangial proliferative	Mesangial hypercellularity (of any degree) or mesangial matrix expansion	Mesangial deposits++++ subepithelial or subendothelial deposits ±	Mesangial deposits ++++ subepithelial or subendothelial deposits ±	Microscopic hematuria and/or proteinuria HTN/renal insufficiency rare
3. Focal proliferative	Mesangial with endocapillary or extracapillary proliferation involving <50% glomeruli	Mesangial + subendothelial deposits	Mesangial + subendothelial deposits	Hematuria +/proteinuria +/ renal insufficiency +/HTN+
4. Diffuse proliferative	Mesangial with endocapillary or extracapillary proliferation involving >50% glomeruli with global/segmental involvement	Mesangial + subendothelial deposits	Mesangial + subendothelial deposits	Hematuria ++/ proteinuria ++/ renal insufficiency +++/ HTN++
5. Membranous	Diffuse BM thickening + subepithelial deposits	Subepithelial + intramembranous deposits, sub-endothelial if associated with class III/IV	Subepithelial + intramembranous deposits	Nephrotic syndrome
6. Advanced sclerotic	>90% glomeruli sclerosed			ESKD or irreversible renal failure

ISN: International Society of Nephrology
RPS: Renal pathology society
LN: Lupus nephritis
BM: Basement membrane
HTN: Hypertension
ESKD: End-stage kidney disease

called 'Telescoped' urine sediment. The urine deposits under light microscopy will show equal proportion of RBCs, WBCs, RBC and WBC casts. However, similar abnormality of urinary sediments may be seen in crescentic glomerulonephritis, malignant hypertension and some other conditions.

b. Spot urine test for creatinine and protein concentration

c. 24-hour urine test for creatinine clearance and protein excretion

d. Blood urea nitrogen (BUN) testing

e. Serum creatinine assessment

Laboratory tests for SLE disease activity include the following:

a. Antibodies to double-stranded DNA (dsDNA)

b. Complement (C3, C4, and CH50)

c. Erythrocyte sedimentation rate (ESR)

d. C-reactive protein (CRP)

Additional investigations pertaining to any other system involvement due to SLE may also be carried out. Kidney biopsy is considered in any patient with SLE who has clinical or laboratory evidence of active nephritis to know the exact picture. Although the role of renal biopsy for a patient already on treatment with immunosuppression for extrarenal manifestation is debatable, it is mandatory for patient of SLE with rapidly declining kidney function. Kidney biopsy must preferably be done at the initial presentation of LN since it helps to identify the class, activity and chronicity markers. Thus, prognostication and therapeutic decisions can be made with confidence. It will be possible to identify if the worsening is due to the basic illness or a preventable /treatable complication. Markers of activity and chronicity (Table 18.4) help to assess and plan or withhold aggressive treatment.

Management

Treatment of LN is as per KDIGO/ACR guidelines is outlined below.

Table 18.4: Activity and chronicity markers in biopsy

Active lesions	Chronic lesions
Glomeruli Glomerulosclerosis	
• Hypercellularity	Tubular atrophy
• Fibrinoid necrosis	Fibrous crescents
• Karyorrhexis	Interstitial fibrosis
• Crescents (cellular)	
• Wire loops	
• Hyaline thrombi	
• Leukocyte infiltration	
Tubules/interstitium Mononuclear infiltration	

All patients require hydroxychloroquine, angiotensin receptor blockers or angiotensin converting enzyme inhibitors, antihypertensive drugs as per requirement in addition to immunosuppressive drugs.

Class I LN: These do not require any immunosuppressive therapy if not associated with any extrarenal manifestation which warrant this.

Class II LN: Manifestations similar to minimal change disease are present due to the Podocytopathy as a part of class II LN. Management is by using only corticosteroids.

Class III and IV LN: These classes have proliferative patterns in renal histology and may progress to irreversible renal damage. Hence, immunosuppressive therapy is indicated. Treatment is done in 2 phases: Induction/initial phase to achieve remission and maintenance phase to sustain the remission.

Induction/initial phase: Drugs commonly used are cyclophosphamide or mycophenolate a long with corticosteroids 0.5 mg/kg/day. Cyclophosphamide is used either as high dose monthly pulse therapy, i.e. 500–1000 mg/m^2 for 6 months or low dose 500 mg, 6 pulses every 2 weeks. Certain precautions are required before administering intravenous cyclophosphamide, pre-hydration and antiemetics are to be used. Hydration is important

Table 18.5: Side effects of drugs used in lupus nephritis

Drug	Side effect and management
1. Hydroxychloroquine Recommended dose: 5 mg/kg	Retinal toxicity Annual fundus check up is essential
2. ACEI/ARBs	Dizziness, hypotension Contraindicated in pregnancy as can cause oligohydramnios
3. Mycophenolate mofetil	Gastrointestinal intolerance, contraindicated in pregnancy, bone marrow suppression
4. Azathioprine	Bone marrow suppression

5. Cyclophosphamide
   Renal dose and agewise modified doses
   Age <60 years or normal S creat: 15 mg/kg
   Age 60–70 years or S creat 3.4–5.7 mg/dl: 12.5 mg/kg
   Age >70 years or S creat > 5.7 or on RRT: 10 mg/kg
	Bone marrow suppression, gonadal toxicity, hemorrhagic cystitis
	Preventive strategies:gonadotropin-releasing hormone (GnRH) analogue agonists, oocyte and sperm banking

6. Steroids	Peptic ulcer disease, osteoporosis, cataract, glaucoma

S creat: Serum creatinine
RRT: Renal replacement therapy
ACEI: Angiotensin converting enzyme inhibitor
ARB: Angiotensin receptor blocker

as cyclophosphamide can cause hemorrhagic cystitis. Mycophenolate mofetil is used at doses of 2–3 gm in initial phase for around 6 months. Cyclophosphamide is a time tested and well tried drug in the treatment of even severe lupus nephritis but its potential oncogenicity and gonadal toxicity are concerns. Hence, in mild to moderate lupus nephritis in younger individuals and women in particular, mycophenolate mofetil is preferred. In severe cases, cyclophosphamide should be the first choice.

Maintenance phase: Mycophenolate mofetil or azathioprine plus low dose steroids are used for maintaining remission. Mininmum period of maintenance is 1 year after achieving remisission. Mycophenolate mofetil is maintained at doses of 1–2 gm/day and azathioprine 2 mg/kg/day.

Class V LN: Initial treatment is mycophenolate mofetil and steroids for 6 months followed by maintenance phase with azathioprine or mycophenolate mofetil may be tried.

Class VI LN: No immunosuppression required for renal involvement and class VI. Failure of clinical or histological improvement at end of 3 months can be an indication for change of treatment. Mycophenolate mofetil may be switched to cyclophosphamide and vice versa. In case of refractory disease rituximab, plasmapheresis, intravenous immunoglobulins and multi-targeted therapy (tacrolimus, mycophenolate mofetil and steroids) can be offered in specialty departments. Since the drugs used in treatment of LN have significant side effects are listed in Table 18.5, one must be careful while prescribing them.

Prognosis

The long-term prognosis is good if long-lasting complete remission is achieved. In active proliferative LN, even complete or partial response is associated with an improved outcome compared with no response. Patient survival is 95% and 30%, respectively for those that attain complete response vs who do not attain any response.

IgA Nephropathy

• Namrata Rao • Krishan Lal Gupta • Raja Ramachandran

INTRODUCTION

IgA nephropathy (IgAN) is among the most common glomerulonephritis in the world. The disease traces its origin to disordered mucosal immunity, specifically gut-associated mucosal immunity, which leads to defective galactosylation of secretory IgA1 and its recognition as an autoantigen. While it presents commonly with episodic gross hematuria, its natural progression follows a slow, indolent course in many, culminating in chronic kidney disease (CKD) in a proportion of patients. In children, a related systemic vasculitis, Henoch-Schönlein purpura occurs in the first two decades of life, with accompanying skin rash and gut involvement. IgAN is solely diagnosed by immunofluorescence microscopy of the renal biopsy specimen, and recent scoring systems (Oxford-MEST scoring) can help prognosticate and plan therapeutic decisions. While renin-angiotensin system (RAS) blockade has an essential role in ameliorating proteinuria and improving renal survival, results with immunosuppressive drugs are still unclear.

Epidemiology

IgAN is prevalent worldwide, but is more common in the developed countries of the East, and is much rarer in Africa. Since renal biopsy is necessary for the diagnosis. biopsy, the difference in pattern of distribution depends on the local policies for urine screening and the availability of renal biosy with immunofluorescent study. The prevalence pattern is also influenced by other factors since IgA deposition in postmortem biopsies is lower in Finland compared to Japan. Genetic studies have identified several disease-predisposing loci in East Asians. Although it was considered more common in males, recent studies show roughly equal sex distribution. IgAN is commonly a disease of children and young adults.

Certain diseases like alcoholic liver disease, HIV have been associated with IgA nephropathy. In HIV, it is thought that prolonged polyclonal activation of B cells might predispose the formation of abnormally glycated IgA and its corresponding autoantibodies.

Pathophysiology

The most accepted theory for the development of IgAN is the "multi-hit" hypothesis.

a. Hit 1—formation of abnormally glycated IgA.

b. Hit 2—generation of autoantibodies to the abnormally glycated IgA.

c. Hit 3—development of immune complexes and mesangial deposition.

d. Hit 4—mesangial activation and subsequent renal injury.

a. *Hit 1 (formation of abnormally glycated IgA):* IgA is an essential component of mucosal immunity. IgA exists in two isoforms, IgA1 and IgA2. Secretory IgA (SIgA) is the form of IgA released into mucosal secretions. It has a 'J' chain, which links IgA monomers and confers stability to the immunoglobulin against proteolysis. The hinge region of the IgA molecule has 2–6 sites for attachment of peptidoglycans. Defects in glycosyltransferases resulting in galactose deficiency in IgA1 has been observed and may be the initiating step in the chain of events.

b. *Hit 2 (generation of autoantibodies to the abnormally glycated IgA):* Commonly, IgG or IgA1 antibodies are formed in response to galactose-deficient IgA1.

c. *Hit 3 (development of immune complexes and mesangial deposition of nephritogenic immune complexes):* The autoantibodies bind to a transferrin receptor and form immune complexes which activate the complement system.

d. *Hit 4 (mesangial activation and downstream renal injury):* Complement activation results in increased expression of genes encoding pro-inflammatory cytokines, and local release of cytokines. In the acute phase of injury, increased urinary podocalyxin levels are seen, and in the chronic phase, glomerulosclerosis occurs with podocytopenia. Activation of the renin-angiotensin system also contributes to glomerulosclerosis and tubulointerstitial fibrosis. Non-immune factors such as coexistent obesity, hypertension, smoking can aggravate glomerular injury and can lead to faster progression of the disease.

Clinical Features

Episodic gross hematuria: IgAN can have a myriad of clinical manifestations, but the classic presentation is that of macroscopic hematuria in an adolescent/young adult, often following an upper respiratory tract (synpharyngitic), urinary tract or gastro-intestinal infection. Unlike post-streptococcal glomerulonephritis (PSGN), there is no lag period of 1–2 weeks between the episode of pharyngitis and the development of hematuria. Even though gross macroscopic hematuria may occur, the associated proteinuria is usually sub-nephrotic, accelerated hypertension and complement abnormalities are rare and acute kidney injury is uncommon as compared to PSGN.

Asymptomatic urinary abnormalities: In countries where urinary screening programs are actively implemented, the diagnosis is suspected based on asymptomatic urinary abnormalities. Persistent microscopic hematuria after acute episodes of macroscopic hematuria is common in IgAN. The urinary protein excretion usually remains <1 g/day.

Nephrotic syndrome: About 10% patients may present as nephrotic syndrome as evidenced by nephrotic range proteinuria. Minimal change disease may coexist with IgAN. Lesions with diffuse mesangial and endocapillary proliferation may be present. Gross or clinically apparent nephrotic syndrome is seen only in later stages of the disease when podocytopenia and secondary glomerulo-sclerosis occur and cause massive proteinuria.

Acute kidney injury (AKI): IgAN can present as AKI either during episodes of gross hematuria due to formation of erythrocyte casts in tubules or as a result of acute presentation as crescentic IgAN. AKI may also occur secondary to sepsis or use of nephro-toxic drugs in patients with IgAN related chronic kidney disease.

Chronic kidney disease (CKD): Generally, this is a late presentation of IgAN especially patients who never had a history of macro-scopic hematuria or were never screened for hypertension and urinary abnormalities.

Henoch-Schönlein purpura (HSP): IgAN may present in childhood or in later life as palpable purpuric skin rash on the extensor surfaces, along with joint pains and pain abdomen. Microscopic hematuria and subnephrotic proteinuria are the typical renal manifestation. Less frequently, AKI due to crescents or nephrotic syndrome can occur.

Laboratory Diagnosis

Urine examination may be negative or may show variable degree of proteinuria and or hematuria. No specific abnormality may be present in the routine hemogram or biochemical tests. Serum levels of IgA also do not contribute to the diagnosis. While serum levels of the nephritogenic immune complexes (Gd-IgA1) may be elevated, they do not help to predict the severity of disease and are influenced by steroid use.

Pathology

IgAN is a diagnosis made solely by immuno-fluorescence microscopy done on renal biopsy specimens. Light microscopy in IgAN classically reveals segmental or diffuse mesangial proliferative lesions (Fig. 19.1A), along with variable endocapillary cellularity. Extensive lesions may cause extracapillary proliferation and development of crescents. Acute tubular injury and RBC cast formation may be seen in some cases presenting with gross hematuria. Chronic lesions can show focal or global glomerular sclerosis and tubulointerstitial inflammation and fibrosis. Blood vessels may show arteriolar hyalinosis.

Immunofluorescence microscopy shows diffuse mesangial deposition of IgA (Fig. 19.1B) in a dominant or co-dominant fashion. 'κ' chains are more common than 'κ' chains. Electron microscopy reveals the mesangial location of immune deposits. Subepithelial deposits are usually not seen in IgAN, whereas they occur commonly in association with staphylococcal infection related glomerulo-nephritis with IgA deposits. However, in such cases, dominant C3 deposits are also seen.

Once the diagnosis of IgAN has been confirmed based on immunofluorescence microscopy or immunohistochemistry, it is necessary to use the information for assessing the severity, prognosticate and plan the management. The recently introduced scoring system called 'Oxford-MEST score' is useful for the purpose. This classification reduces interobserver variability, correlates better with progression of disease and has reiterated the definite need of renal biopsy for the diagnosis.

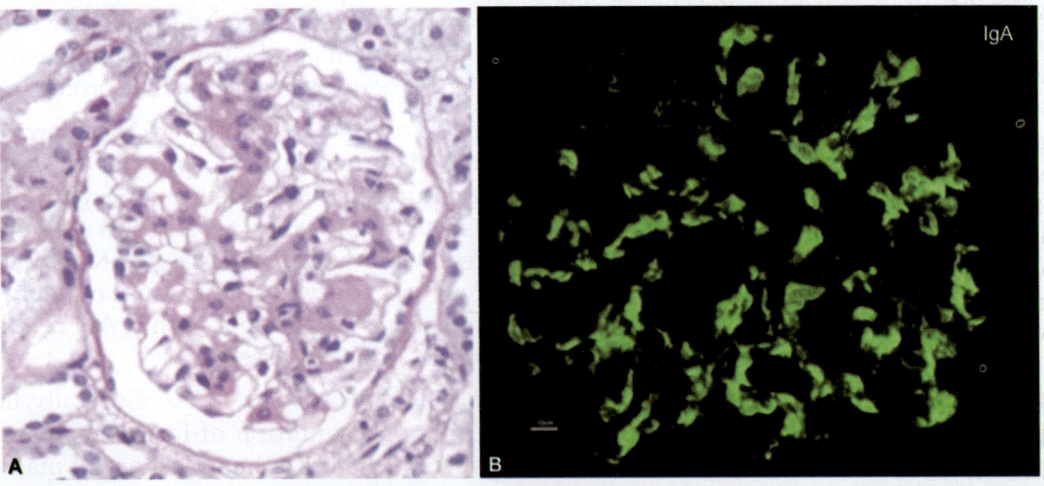

Fig. 19.1A and B: (A) Light microscopy of a glomerulus with mesangial increase. No significant proliferation; (B) Immunofluorescence showing mesangial IgA deposits

In this classification, four pathologic features are scored on light microscopy as follows.

a. Mesangial hypercellularity:
    i. M0 = absent or involving <50% of glomeruli
    ii. M1 = present in >50% of glomeruli.
b. Endocapillary hypercellularity
    i. E0 = no endocapillary hypercellularity
    ii. E1 = any glomeruli showing endo-capillary hypercellularity
c. Segmental glomerulosclerosis
    i. S1 = any segmental glomerulosclerosis)
d. Tubular atrophy and interstitial fibrosis
    i. T0 = involving 1–25% of cortical area affected by fibrosis
    ii. T1 = involving 26–50%
    iii. T2 = involving >50%

More recently, scoring of crescents has also been added to the MEST classification (MEST C score) as follows:
    i. C0 = no cellular or fibrocellular crescents
    ii. C1 = crescents <25% of glomeruli
    iii. C2 = crescents in >25% of glomeruli.

Prognosis

Among the clinical factors, obesity, older age, smoking and male sex have been associated with poorer prognosis. The severity of proteinuria, and inability to achieve remission of proteinuria to <1 g/day are also poor prognostic factors and predict the development of ESRD. Higher cumulative MEST-C scores, podocytopenia and thrombotic microangiopathy on biopsy, and DD genotype of angiotensin-converting enzyme (ACE) predicts poorer renal prognosis.

Treatment

Broadly, the treatment is divided into non-immunosuppressive, immunosuppressive therapies, management of crescentic IgAN and role of renal transplantation.

Nonimmunosuppressive Therapies

a. General measures should be employed as appropriate
    i. Weight reduction
    ii. Smoking cessation
    iii. Blood pressure control
    iv. Salt restriction
    v. Lipid lowering
b. *RAS blockade:* Angiotensin-converting enzyme inhibitors (ACEi) and angiotensin receptor blockers (ARBs) have significant renoprotective effect when used in proteinuric IgAN patients. BP targets of <130/80 mm Hg in those with proteinuria of <1 g/day and <125/75 mm Hg in those with proteinuria >1 g/day is recommended. Recently, aliskiren, a direct renin inhibitor in combination with ACEi or ARBs and has been shown to be beneficial but the risk of hyperkalemia was greater.
c. *Fish oil:* Fish oil containing omega-3 fatty acids can reduce local eicosanoid levels and platelet aggregation and prevent progression of IgAN. Although the evidence for its use is weak, fish oil may be used in doses of 4–12 g/day in patients with persistent proteinuria despite RAS blockade.
d. *Role of tonsillectomy:* Tonsil crypts may harbour pathogenic microbes and tonsillar B lymphocytes can be involved in the production of Gd-IgA1. Although this has been incriminated in the pathogenesis, there is no scientific support now for use of tonsillectomy routinely.

Immunosuppressive Therapies

Since the pathogenesis of IgAN is immune-mediated, immunosuppressive therapies are tried to reduce the production of defective IgA, suppress immune complex formation and subsequent renal injury.

a. *Corticosteroids:* In patients with urinary protein excretion of >1 g/day, dose of >0.5 mg/kg body weight of prednisone for <1 year offered significant renal protection by reducing proteinuria, retarding progression and preserving GFR.

b. *Cyclophosphamide:* Combined with steroids and RAS blockade to target BP <125/75 mm Hg helps to achieve remissions, or death due to kidney failure but caused serious infections.

c. *Mycophenolate mofetil and azathioprine:* While a few randomized trials have shown better response while using mycophenolate mofetil alone or with low dose prednisolone. Such observations have not been fully validated. Azathioprine was also not been found to be beneficial. Numerous trials have been performed in different countries with variable observations and results.

d. *Enteric budesonide:* A relative new idea in the treatment has emerged in the form of budesonide, a drug targeted to be released in the distal ileum where it can suppress mucosal B lymphocytes producing defective IgA1. Since it is metabolized in the liver extensively, it does not reach systemic circulation and the side effects are minimal. When added to baseline RAS blockade, proteinuria reduction and no significant adverse events were observed.

Management of Crescentic IgAN

Steroid and cyclophosphamide based immunosuppressive treatment protocols are advocated in patients of IgAN with >50% crescents, analogous to the treatment used in ANCA vasculitis.

Renal Transplantation in IgAN

Following renal transplantation, histologic recurrence in the form of mesangial IgA deposits occur in around 60% who had IgAN as the basic renal disease. However, graft dysfunction due to recurrence is uncommon in the first 5–10 years after which the chances of accelerated graft loss increases.

IgAN constitutes is very common in India and neighboring countries. It forms 7–10% of total biopsies done in India. Epidemiologic features include onset at 25–32 years, male preponderance, proteinuria over 2 g/day, and variable renal dysfunction. The severity of disease and high rates of CKD progression were observed in those who presented with higher serum creatinine. Many of the so-called 'obscure' renal failure in whom renal biopsy is not performed may in fact be undiagnosed IgAN.

Diabetic Nephropathy

• Mohit Madken • Vijay Kher

INTRODUCTION

Diabetes mellitus is a growing epidemic and is the single most common cause of ESRD worldwide. Diabetic patients account for 25 to 45% of all patients enrolled in ESRD programs. It is the commonest cause of ESRD in India accounting for 44% in a population based study. Diabetic nephropathy (DN) develops in 15 to 35% of patients with diabetes. Early identification and management is critical to prevent development or slow progression of diabetic nephropathy.

Definition and Natural History

Diabetic nephropathy, as a syndrome, has been defined as:

- Persistent albuminuria (>300 mg/d or >200 µg/min) confirmed on at least 2 occasions 3–6 months apart.
- Progressive decline in the glomerular filtration rate (GFR)
- Hypertension
- Additional criteria required for diagnosis include-presence of diabetic retinopathy and absence of clinical or laboratory evidence of other kidney or renal tract disease.

*Diabetic kidney disease (DKD):*A proportion of diabetic patients with renal impairment do not have classical features of diabetic nephropathy including proteinuria and other microvascular complications. These patients have renal impairment due to involvement of tubulointerstitial or vascular compartment and are included under diabetic kidney disease.

Natural History

Natural history (Fig. 20.1) of diabetic nephropathy has been classically described with type 1 diabetes mellitus but is less defined in type 2 diabetes mellitus. The stages in type 2 diabetes mellitus may not be as well characterized. Though the natural history of type 2 disease may be similar, the time of onset of the disease is not apparent. Diabetic nephropathy evolves through different phases such as phase of glomerular hyperfiltration, incipient nephropathy characterized by microalbuminuria, overt nephropathy characterized by macroalbuminuria and end stage renal disease characterized by decrease in GFR to less than 15 ml/min.

There are five stages in the development of diabetic nephropathy:

- *Stage 1* is characterized by hyperfunction and hypertrophy that are present at the time of diagnosis of diabetes. In this stage, GFR is either normal or increased. The size of the kidneys is increased by approxi-

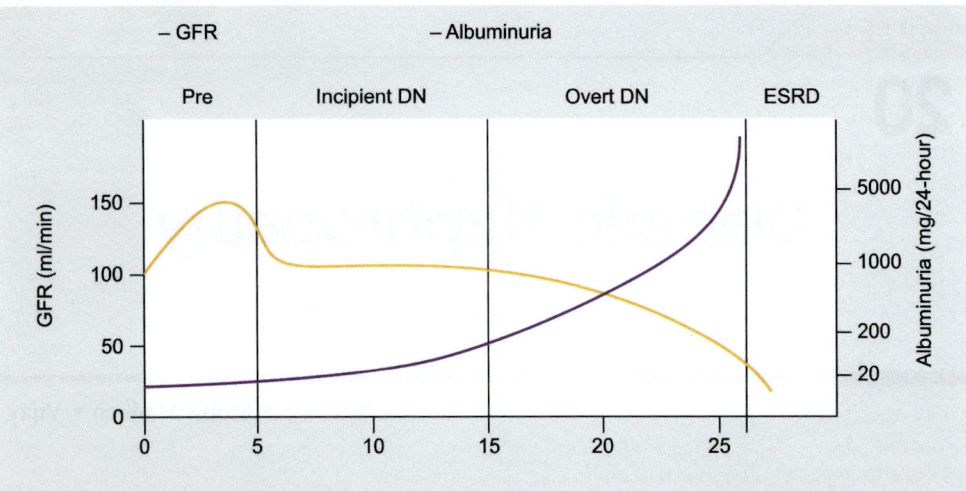

Fig. 20.1: Natural history of diabetic nephropathy. Initial increase followed by steady fall in renal function (yellow line) and progressive increase in urinary protein excretion (blue line)

Stage	Pre	Incipient	Overt
Functional	GFR (25–50%)	Moderately increased albuminuria	Severely increased albuminuria, nephrotic syndrome, GFR
Structural	Renal hypertrophy	Mesangial expansion, GBM thickening, arteriolar hyalinosis	Mesangial nodules (Kimmelstiel-Wilson lesion), tubulointerstitial fibrosis

mately 20% and renal plasma flow is increased by 10–15%, while albuminuria and blood pressure remain within the normal range. Changes are at least partly reversible by intensive glycemic control.

- *Stage 2* develops silently over many years and is characterized by morphologic lesions without signs of clinical disease. This stage is characterized by basement membrane thickening and mesangial proliferation. There are still no clinical signs of the disease.
- *Stage 3* also known as incipient diabetic nephropathy is the forerunner of overt diabetic nephropathy. Patients in this stage develop microalbuminuria (albumin 30–300 mg/day) now termed stage of 'moderately increased albuminuria' and is the first clinically detectable sign of glomerular damage. It usually occurs five to ten years after the onset of the disease. Blood pressure may be increased or normal.

Approximately 40% of patients reach this stage.

- *Stage 4* is overt diabetic nephropathy. This is the classic entity characterized by persistent macro-albuminuria (>300 mg/ 24 hours) now termed 'severely increased albuminuria' associated with hypertension and progressive decline of GFR (at rate greater than 1 ml/min/month).
- *Stage 5* is end-stage disease with uremia due to diabetic nephropathy.

Pathogenesis and Pathology

There are different pathogenetic processes leading to the development and pathologic changes in diabetic nephropathy

a. *Hemodynamic pathways of diabetic nephropathy:* Afferent and efferent arteriolar hyalinosis in diabetic nephropathy leads to loss of renal autoregulation and activation of Renin-angiotensin system (RAS). This leads to increased angiotensin II levels which cause efferent arteriolar vasoconstriction which leads to increased pressure within the glomerular capillaries (intra-glomerular hypertension) and hyper-filtration resulting in glomerular damage, albuminuria and decline in renal function. Renin angiotensin blockade is therefore beneficial in decreasing albuminuria and slowing progression of renal failure.

b. *Metabolic pathways of diabetic nephropathy:* Hyperglycemia and advanced glycation end products (AGEs)—hyperglycemia may directly induce mesangial expansion and injury, perhaps in part via increased matrix production or glycation of matrix proteins. Hyperglycemia leads to increased glycolysis which then upregulates four distinct entities: the polyol pathway, hexosamine pathway, production of AGEs, and activation of protein kinase C (PKC).

c. *Inflammatory pathways of diabetic nephropathy:* Chronic inflammation and upregulation of inflammatory pathways has been observed in patients with diabetic kidney disease. Inflammatory cytokines such as TNF-α and interleukins 1, 6, and 18 are expressed in greater proportions in the kidneys of diabetic models when compared to nondiabetic controls.

Pathology (Fig. 20.2): Light Microscopy

One of the earliest changes in patients with diabetic nephropathy is thickening of glomerular basement membrane (GBM) and is paralleled by thickening of tubular basement membranes (TBM). Classic findings of diabetic nephropathy include mesangial expansion mainly due to increased mesangial matrix, which can be diffuse or nodular. Nodular expansion of mesangial matrix is the Kimmelstiel-Wilson nodule. Afferent and efferent glomerular arteriolar hyalinosis can be present within 3 to 5 years of diabetes onset. Involvement of both vessels is virtually pathognomonic of diabetes.

Microaneurysms of glomerular capillaries are often seen along with mesangiolysis or nodules. Segmental glomerulosclerosis, especially at the tubular outlet (i.e. tip lesion), is common in later stages of diabetic nephropathy. Hyalinosis may be present within the glomerular tuft under the endothelial cells or under the parietal epithelial cells (capsular drop).

In type 1 diabetes, interstitial fibrosis and tubular atrophy follow glomerular lesions and may be less severe or proportional to diabetic glomerulopathy. In type 2 diabetes, in which arteriosclerosis is commonly present, the lesions are more heterogeneous, and chronic tubulointerstitial injury may be more severe than the diabetic glomerulopathy.

Immunofluorescence Microscopy

Diffuse linear accentuation of glomerular and tubular basement membranes with IgG and albumin is typical. Nonspecific segmental staining of hyaline deposits or glomerular sclerotic regions for IgM, C3, and C1q is common in advanced disease.

Nodular glomerulosclerosis can also develop in pathological conditions other than diabetic nephropathy. These are:

a. Dysproteinemias such as amyloidosis and monoclonal immunoglobulin deposition diseases (MIDD).

b. Fibrillary and immunotactoid glomerulonephritis, fibronectin glomerulopathy, and collagen III glomerulopathy.

c. Conditions associated with chronic ischemia (cyanotic congenital heart disease).

d. Chronic membranoproliferative glomerulonephritis.

e. Idiopathic nodular glomerulosclerosis, frequently associated with smoking, hypertension and metabolic syndrome.

Differences between Diabetic Nephropathy and Non-diabetic Renal Disease

Diabetic nephropathy does not occur in all patients who have long-standing diabetes and any renal disease occurring in diabetics is not

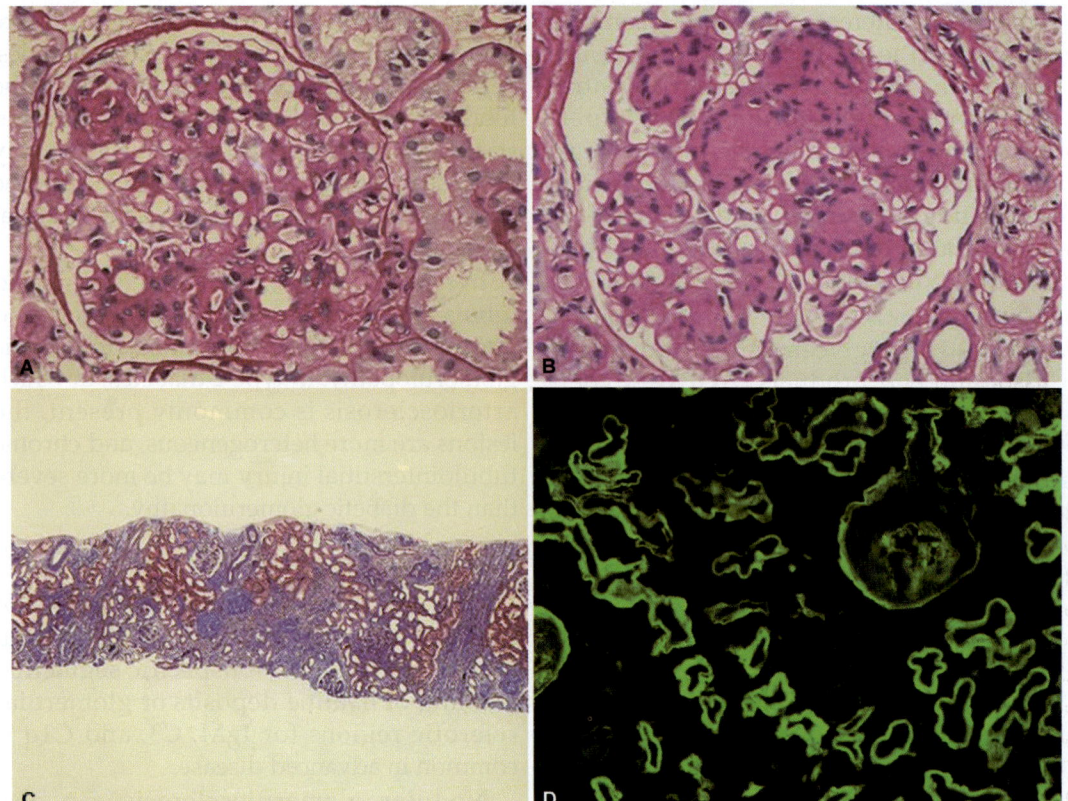

Fig. 20.2A to D: Histopathology of glomerular lesions in diabetic nephropathy. (A) PAS stained section → mild thickening of the glomerular capillary wall with mild mesangial matrix expansion (PAS, original magnification 400X)—early lesion; (B) PAS stained section → nodular glomerulosclerosis (Kimmelstiel-Wilson lesion) (PAS, original magnification 400X)—late lesion; (C) Masson's trichrome (MT) stain → advanced diabetic nephropathy with significant glomerulosclerosis and interstitial fibrosis (original magnification 100X); (D) Direct immunofluorescence → 3+ linear albumin staining along tubular basement membrane common immunofluorescence finding in diabetic nephropathy cases (DIF albumin stain, original magnification 400X)

diabetic nephropathy. Some diabetics can develop other renal diseases as general population. It is necessary to rule out other diseases before labeling as diabetic nephropathy. Proteinuria and/or hematuria occurring in a patient with diabetes mellitus may also be due to a glomerular disease other than diabetic nephropathy. Glomerular disorders like membranous nephropathy, IgA nephropathy, focal segmental glomerulosclerosis, Henoch-Schönlein purpura (IgA vasculitis) and proliferative glomerulonephritis which occur in others can also occur in diabetics. Those diabetics who are suspected to have non-diabetic renal disease will need renal biopsy for confirmation of diagnosis.

Major clinical clues suggesting the presence of non-diabetic glomerular disease occurring in a diabetic patient are:

1. Absence of diabetic retinopathy
2. Sudden and rapid onset of nephrotic range proteinuria
3. Duration of diabetes mellitus (in type 1—less than 5 years)

4. Atypical progression, without transition through the usual stages, e.g. development of nephrotic syndrome without previous microalbuminuria.
5. Macroscopic hematuria or active nephritic sediment—numerous RBCs, many dysmorphic red cells or red cell casts or acanthocytes.
6. Rapid decline in renal function (usual decline in diabetic nephropathy is 0.5–1.5 ml/min/1.73 sq.m/month)
7. Renal dysfunction in presence of other associated systemic diseases.

Risk Factors

Genetic susceptibility: The likelihood of developing diabetic nephropathy is higher in patients with a strong family history of diabetic nephropathy. There is a 14% probability for a child of the parents without proteinuria to develop clinical proteinuria, 23% probability in cases where one of the parents has proteinuria, and 46% probability in case that both parents have proteinuria. This increased risk cannot be explained by the duration of DM, increased blood pressure or glycemic regulation.

Blood pressure: There is association between the development of diabetic nephropathy and higher systemic blood pressure.

Glycemic control: Diabetic nephropathy is more likely to develop in patients with poor glycemic control. The importance of tight glycemic control for protection against microvascular and cardiovascular disease in diabetes was established in numerous studies.

Race: The incidence and severity of diabetic nephropathy are increased 3- to 6-fold in Blacks compared to Caucasians, Mexican-Americans and Pima Indians with type 2 diabetes. The incidence of nephropathy in diabetics of Asiatic origin is also high.

Obesity: High body mass index (BMI) has been associated with an increased risk of chronic kidney disease among patients with diabetes. In addition to control of diabetes, dietary restriction and weight loss may reduce albuminuria and improve kidney function in them.

Smoking: Smoking is associated with a variety of adverse effects like increase in albuminuria, risk of end stage renal disease and decreased survival on dialysis.

Relationship between Diabetic Nephropathy and Retinopathy

Patients with nephropathy and type 1 diabetes almost invariably have other signs of diabetic microvascular disease, such as retinopathy and neuropathy. The retinopathy typically precedes the onset of overt nephropathy in these patients. At the same time, the relationship between diabetic nephropathy and retinopathy is less predictable in type 2 diabetes. Only 50 to 60% of proteinuric type 2 diabetic patients may have retinopathy. The absence of retinopathy should prompt further investigation for nondiabetic glomerulopathies.

Clinical Features

There are no specific clinical features of nephropathy in its early stages. In people with type 1 diabetes a rise in blood pressure is a subtle sign but usually accompanies an increase in albuminuria. The clinical features of established nephropathy are often dictated by concomitant microvascular (retinopathy and neuropathy) or macrovascular complications (disease in the coronary, cerebral or peripheral vasculature). The majority of people entering end-stage renal disease due to diabetic nephropathy will have evidence of microvascular or macrovascular complications of diabetes. Blindness due to severe proliferative retinopathy or maculopathy is approximately five times more frequent in types 1 and 2 diabetic patients with nephropathy than in normoalbuminuric patients. Peripheral neuropathy is present in almost all patients with advanced nephropathy. Foot ulcers leading to sepsis, gangrene and amputation is due to a combination of neuropathy and peripheral vascular disease and is common in diabetic patients. Macrovascular complications like stroke, coronary artery disease, peripheral vascular disease are two to five times more common in patients with diabetic nephropathy. Autonomic neuropathy, diabetic cystopathy and recurrent UTIs are other complications commonly encountered in patients with diabetic nephropathy (Table 20.1).

Anemia due to combination of dietary iron deficiency and erythropoietin deficiency is more common and occurs earlier in people with diabetic nephropathy compared to non-diabetic kidney disease. Symptoms of uremia such as nausea, anorexia, pruritus, tiredness and weight loss develop in advanced CKD. Even the asymptomatic diabetic patient with CKD must be monitored at regular intervals for timely detection of microvascular and macrovascular complications. Planning and initiation of renal replacement therapy (RRT) should be considered earlier in diabetics.

Investigations and Identifying Non-diabetic Renal Disease

Investigations are planned for screening and confirming diagnosis. The following investigations are undertaken depending on the indications usually.

a. Measurements of blood pressure every visit.

b. Urinalysis with urine microscopy. Blood glycemic prolife: Fasting (AC) and post-prandial (PC) blood sugars or GTT and a HbA1c.

c. Urine albumin excretion rate to be done annually in type 1 diabetes mellitus of >5 years and in type 2 diabetes mellitus from the time of diagnosis.

d. Serum creatinine and estimation of GFR annually in all diabetic patients regardless of albuminuria.

e. Ophthalmological evaluation—fundus for evidence of diabetic retinopathy.

f. A renal USG/Doppler to look for bilateral kidney size, echogenecity and patency of the renal arteries.

Prevention, Management and Future Strategies

The natural history of diabetic nephropathy has prolonged course so appropriate measures can be taken to prevent development or to slow the progression of diabetic nephropathy.

a. Lifestyle Modification

All diabetic patients should undergo lifestyle modification to lower risk of progression as well as CVD. The measures include:

- Dietary restriction of salt and saturated fats
- Weight reduction
- Exercise
- Smoking cessation

b. Glycemic Control

Tight glycemic control is one important step in the prevention and management of diabetic nephropathy. Poor glycemic control is a risk factor for both the development of micro-albuminuria and for progression to macro-albuminuria in patients with type 2 diabetes.

Table 20.1: Urinary albumin excretion in different stages of diabetic nephropathy

	Normal	Stage of moderately increased albuminuria (incipient nephropathy)	Stage of severely increased albuminuria (overt nephropathy)
Albumin–creatinine ratio (ACR)—spot (µg/mg creatinine)	<30	30–299	≥300
24-hour urinary albumin excretion (mg/day)	<30	30–299	≥300
Timed collection (µg/ min)	<20	20–199	≥200

Strict glycemic control is recommended in all patients because of its beneficial effects on the microvascular complications. Glycemic goals for optimal glycemic control are: HbA1c <7%, Fasting capillary plasma glucose, 70–120 mg/dl, and postprandial capillary plasma glucose, <180 mg/dl. In individuals with co-morbidities or limited life-expectancy and risk of hypoglycemia, the target HbA1c should be maintained above 7.0% since hypoglycemia is more harmful compared to mild degrees of hyperglycemia.

c. Blood Pressure Control

Treatment of hypertension dramatically reduces the risk of cardiovascular and microvascular events in patients with diabetes. Hypertension is common in diabetic patients, even when renal involvement is not present. It is recommended to achieve a target BP of 140/90 mm Hg or less for all diabetic patients and 130/80 mm Hg or less for patients with moderately increased albuminuria and above. Any drug may be used for control of blood pressure however, ACEI or ARBs are the preferred drugs. In the initial stages, diabetic nephropathy is associated with renal hypertrophy, hyperfunction and glomerular hyperfiltration.

Blocking the renin-angiotensin-aldosterone pathway has significant effect on slowing the progression. Angiotensin II has vasoconstrictor action on afferent and efferent arterioles. The effect on efferent is more and therefore, the pressure in the glomerular capillary is increased leading to hyperfiltration. Blockage of RAAS axis with ACEI or ARBs effectively reduces efferent arterial tone, glomerular pressure and hyperfiltration. If started early in the course of the disease, it may help to arrest or even reversing the progression of diabetic nephropathy.

Treatment of patients with type 2 diabetes mellitus without clinically apparent DN with an ACEI is effective in reducing the development of early nephropathy. In diabetic patients with established DN, RAS blockade with ACE inhibitors or ARBs confer preferential renoprotection, independent of BP reduction.

d. Control of Dyslipidemia

Dyslipidemia is common in patients with diabetes and CKD. Cardiovascular events are a frequent cause of morbidity and mortality in this population. Lowering low density lipoprotein cholesterol (LDL-C) with statin-based therapies reduces risk of major atherosclerotic events, but does not significantly improve mortality. Goal for low-density lipoprotein (LDL) cholesterol is <100 mg/dl (2.57 mmol/L) for diabetic patients in general and <70 mg/dl (1.81 mmol/L) for diabetic patients with cardiovascular disease. Use of LDL-C lowering medicines, such as statins or statin/ezetimibe combination is recommended to reduce risk of major atherosclerotic events. It is recommended for patients with diabetes and CKD and kidney transplant recipients. Statin therapy is not recommended routinely in patients with diabetes who are treated by dialysis.

e. Dietary Advice

Blanket prescription of protein restriction should not be advised since protein energy wasting (PEW) may occur if dietary protein is restricted. It is advisable to advise protein intake of 0.8–1.0 g/kg body wt/day in individuals with diabetes and the earlier stages of DKD and around 0.8 g / kg body wt/day in the later stages of CKD. At least 50% protein should be high quality protein. 'Protein supplements' such as protein shakes or powders are preferably avoided. Low-sodium diet is generally advised in diabetic nephropathy. Diet containing less than 6 g of NaCl (1 teaspoonful)) or 100 mEq/day in patients with diabetes and hypertension or any degree of proteinuria is recommended.

f. Avoidance of Nephrotoxic Drugs/Agents

Nephrotoxic drugs/agents should be avoided. Nonsteroidal anti-inflammatory drugs

(NSAIDs) can cause a significant drop in GFR in patients with diabetic nephropathy, particularly when used with angiotensin-blocking agents. Radiocontrast media is particularly nephrotoxic for diabetics. Even with a normal serum creatinine level, patients with diabetes and proteinuria should be hydrated with saline 12 hours before and after exposure to contrast. Diuretics should be temporarily discontinued, and hyperglycemia should be controlled. Risk benefit assessment should be done before deciding for radio contrast study especially in patients with diabetes and kidney disease due to increased risk for contrast-induced acute kidney injury (CIAKI).

Combination with other potential nephro-toxic drugs like aminoglycosides, acyclovir, amphotericin, cefotaxime should be avoided. Patients should be counceled regarding using 'natural' preparations assuming them to be non-toxic, or powders and 'native' medicines which may contain heavy metals.

g. *Treatment of DN with CKD*

Screening for complications of CKD is indicated when GFR falls below 60 ml/min such as anemia, bone mineral disease. Vaccination against hepatitis B, pneumococcal and annual influenza vaccine should be advised. Timely referral of the patient to nephrologist when GFR falls below 60 ml/min. It will improve quality of care, delay the onset of renal replacement therapy and reduce the cost of treatment in the long-term. The dose of insulin or other short acting oral anti-diabetic drugs will need dose reduction. Since >50% insulin is metabolized in the kidneys, the duration of action of insulin is prolonged and the requirement reduces as the renal failure advances. Metformin should be stopped when GFR falls below 45 ml/min due to increased risk of type B lactic acidosis. Long-acting OHAs should also be discontinued. All OHAs should be discontinued when eGFR is <30 ml/min/1.73 m². Only short-acting insulin

should be used for glycemic control. The patient and relatives should be councelled regarding modalities of further treatment including renal replacement therapies.

h. *Management of End-stage Kidney Disease (ESRD) in Diabetics*

A diabetic patient with ESRD has several options for renal replacement therapy: Continuous ambulatory peritoneal dialysis or its variants, Life-long hemodialysis, or renal transplantation are the main methods of renal replacement therapy. Survival rates of patients on peritoneal dialysis and hemo-dialysis are inferior to renal transplantation. But, between peritoneal dialysis and hemodialysis, they are comparable.

Blindness from proliferative diabetic retinopathy may limit a patient's ability to perform peritoneal dialysis by self. Patients with DM have an accelerated course to peritoneal membrane failure and higher rates of recurrent peritonitis. Systemic glucose absorption from the dialysate may lead to worsening hyperglycemia and increasing insulin requirements.

In patients undergoing hemodialysis, the preponderance of vascular disease in those with diabetes limits the maturity and increases the rate of complications of vascular access. The increased rate of cardiac disease, left ventricular hypertrophy, and autonomic insufficiency observed in patients with diabetes can contribute to intradialytic hypotension, arrhythmias, or even sudden death on hemodialysis.

Currently, there is consensus that survival rates are best after kidney transplantation. Transplantation of only kidney or pancreas and kidney simultaneously or pancreas transplantation after kidney transplantation are the options.

i. *Future Strategies*

Various novel drugs targeted against different steps in diabetic pathophysiology are currently under research and different phases of trials such as:

- Bardoxolone—inflammation modulator
- Sulodexide—glycosaminoglycan
- Pirefenidone—TGF-β inhibitor
- Ruboxistaurine—protein kinase C inhibitor
- Benfotiamine
- Vitamin D receptor activation: Paricalcitol
- Pentoxifylline
- Baricitinib—JAK-STAT pathway inhibition

Conclusion

As diabetes becomes a global epidemic worldwide, incidence and prevalence of diabetic nephropathy is steadily increasing. Early detection of diabetic nephropathy combined with multifactorial interventional approach and use of ACE inhibitors and ARBs hold the key to slowing renal disease progression. For patients reaching ESRD, renal transplantation has definite survival advantage over hemodialysis and peritoneal dialysis.

Courtesy: Dr Rajan Duggal, Associate Director, Renal and Uropathology, Fortis Kidney and Urology Institute, Fortis Escorts Hospital, Okhla Road, New Delhi.

Amyloidosis

• Upal Sengupta

INTRODUCTION

Amyloidosis is a unique disease presenting with wide variety of clinical findings and diagnosis can be confirmed only by noting a characteristic histological finding. The disease is more commonly diagnosed incidentally. High index of clinical suspicion in clinical scenarios where this disease has high probability may help to diagnose it clinically. Since it is a disorder of abnormal protein deposition in various organs, majority of clinical manifestations are explained by the malfunction of the affected organ. Correctly folded proteins are soluble, degraded by proteolysis and the amino acids are recycled during protein turnover. The misfolded proteins on the other hand are insoluble, prone to aggregation, form masses, compress surrounding structures, resist proteolysis and damage the surrounding cells. The uniqueness of this illness is that naturally occurring body proteins gets irreversibly deposited in extracellular spaces inside various organs and cause the manifestations.

History

The word amyloid derived from the Greek word *amylon* (starch). This was coined by famous pathologist Rudolph Virchow in 1854 after noticing iodine staining reactions markedly similar to starch. The pathological uniqueness was further established in 1922 after Congo-red staining and in 1927 when the characteristic apple-green birefringence is noticed in polarized microscopy. However, the exact molecular nature of the entity became clear only after viewing them in electron microscopy in 1959 by Cohen and Calkins.

Epidemiology

Data regarding the incidence of amyloid is sparse. It is a rare disease and the estimated incidence may vary from 5.1 to 12.8 per million inhabitants per year. AL amyloidosis is the most common (65%) followed by AA amyloidosis (18%) and the wild-type and hereditary transthyretin amyloidosis (ATTR) (15%). The median age of diagnosis for AL and AA amyloidosis is between 55 and 60 years. Overall, the prognosis in amyloidosis is unfavorable with median survival of 6 to 12 months for AL amyloidosis and 3 to 4 years for AA amyloidosis. Due to the presence of greater burden of chronic infectious diseases in developing countries, the prevalence of AA amyloid may be more as compared to AL amyloid.

Pathogenesis and Pathology

The following are the characteristics of amyloidosis:

a. It is a disease due to systemic or localized extracellular deposition of amyloid.

b. The deposition does not contain any cellular material.

c. Electron microscopy has demonstrated the nature the deposits to be small protein fibrils 8 to 10 nm, arranged in antiparallel β-pleated sheet conformation.

d. Loss of three-dimensional structure of the parent protein molecule leads to the unstable folding or unfolding of the molecule.

e. These lead to the formation of unstable intermediate forms which self aggregrate to form β-pleated amyloid fibrils.

f. Associated glycosaminoglycans (GAGs) promote fibrinogenesis.

g. Associated GAGs and serum amyloid protein (SAP) prevent proteolysis.

h. Deposition of amorphous material occurs in tissues which are PAS negative.

i. Congo red staining leads to orange-red color in non-polarized light and characteristic apple-green birefringence under polarized light.

j. In the kidney, deposition occurs in the mesangium, capillary loops and interstitium (Fig. 21.1).

It is still not completely clear as to why amyloids are formed. Existing hypothesis suggests point mutations, excessive formation (AL) or proteolytic remodelling of the precursor protein. With the discovery of role of amyloid in various neurodegenerative diseases, it is recognized that some of the precursor proteins become prone to misfolding as age progresses. Once formed, they cannot be removed by the body and deposited amyloid lead to disease process and clinical manifestations in the following way:

a. Tissue deposition leads to mechanical effects of structural and functional distortion leading to organ dysfunction.

b. Deposition in the vascular structures lead to tissue hypoxia in the organs.

c. Direct toxicity by protofibril oligomers has been documented in heart and CNS.

Diagnosis

Often the diagnosis of amyloidosis is by a surprising finding in the biopsy. When clinically suspected, the diagnosis needs to be

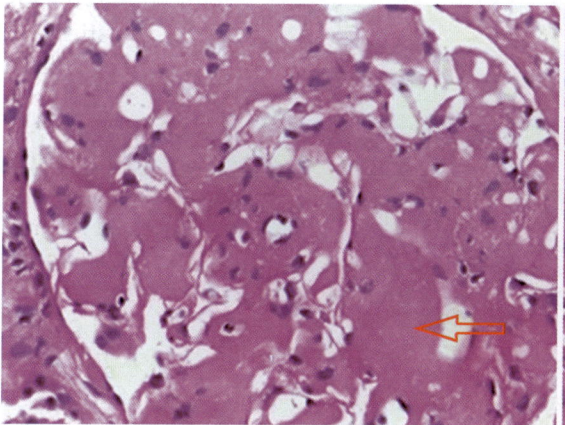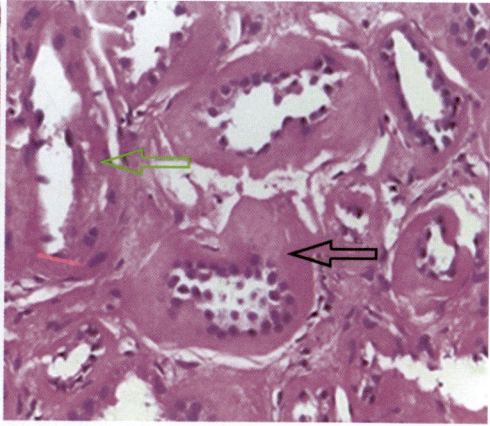

Fig. 21.1: Extensive amyloid deposits in glomeruli and tubules. Left: Glomerular changes: Pale eosinophilic amorphous 'waxy' material in mesangium with matrix thickening (red arrow). Tuft distortion and basement membrane widening. Right: Tubules and interstitium: Faintly eosinophilic uniform extracellular deposition in tubular wall (black arrow), interstitium, blood vessel wall (green arrow)

confirmed by histological examination of the relevant tissue. The biopsy has to be stained by Congo red and examined for 'apple green birefringence' under polarized light. The next step is to identify the type of amyloid by immunofluorescence or immunohistochemistry. The extent of the disease has to be assessed by appropriate tests depending on the organ involved (Fig. 21.1). The 'diagnostic pyramid' for systematic evaluation of amyloidosis is depicted in Fig. 21.2.

Assessment of Extent of Involvement

Since amyloidosis may involve and affect multiple organ systems, a consensus was necessary to uniformly approach the disease. In 2010, the International Society for amyloidosis updated and recommended the criteria for approach to AL amyloidosis (Table 21.1). Isotope studies using iodine-123 labelled serum amyloid protein (^{123}I labelled SAP) are used assess the extent of the distribution of amyloid and its magnitude in a semi-quantitative manner. The ^{123}I labelled SAP distributes and gets attached to the various amyloid deposits throughout the body except in the nervous tissue. This test may be useful to detect disease remission after specific therapy is given.

Classification

Amyloidosis can be classified in three different ways:

1. Depending upon the nature of the parent protein molecule. Thirty different proteins are identified till date.

2. Depending on the site of deposition of the abnormal protein it may be systemic (S) or localized (L) forms of amyloidosis. Almost all forms of major amyloidosis are systemic and only a few are localized. Major forms of non-hereditary amyloidosis with the abnormal precursor protein and organ involvement are given in Table 21.2.

3. Depending on the whether they are inherited and acquired. It should be remembered that even in case of hereditary amyloid, the clinical manifestations does not start from birth. Important hereditary amyloids are listed below in Table 21.3.

Some of the common types of amyloidosis are discussed below.

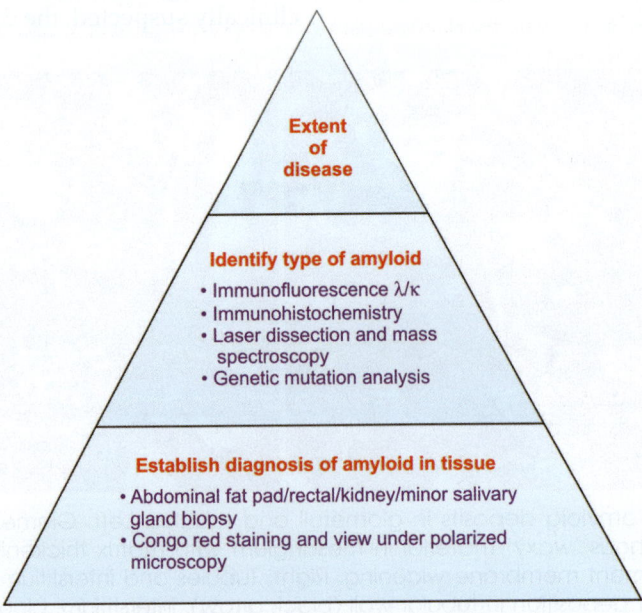

Fig. 21.2: Diagnostic pyramid in amyloidosis

Table 21.1: Consensus criteria, updated in 2010 meeting of the International Society of Amyloidosis in Rome for AL amyloidosis

Involved organ or tissue	Criteria
Kidney	24-hr urine protein > = 0.5 g/day, predominantly albumin
Heart	NT-proBNP >332 ng/L (in the absence of renal failure or atrial fibrillation) or
	mean wall thickness in diastole by echography >12 mm associated with no other cardiac cause
Liver	Total liver span >15 cm in the absence of heart failure, or
	Alkaline phosphatase >1.5 times of institutional upper limit of normal
Nerve	*Peripheral:* Symmetric lower extremity, sensorimotor peripheral neuropathy
	Autonomic: Gastric-emptying disorder, pseudo-obstruction, voiding dysfunction not related to direct organ infiltration.
GI tract	Direct biopsy verification with symptoms
Lung	Direct biopsy verification with symptoms
	Interstitial radiographic pattern
Soft tissues	Tongue enlargement, arthropathy, claudication (presumed vascular amyloid), skin lesions
	Myopathy (by biopsy or pseudohypertrophy)
	Lymph node (may be localized), carpal tunnel syndrome

Table 21.2: Major forms of non-hereditary amyloidosis

Name of the amyloid	Precursor protein	Organ involvement	Systemic (S) or localized (L)
AL	Immunoglobulin light chain	All organs sparing CNS	S > L
AH	Immunoglobulin heavy chain	All organs sparing CNS	S > L
AA	(Apo) serum amyloid A	All organs sparing CNS	S
Aβ2M	β_2 Microglobulin wild type	Musculoskeletal. Dialysis related	S
ATTR	Transthyretin, wild type	Cardiac, musculoskeletal	S, L
AApoAI	Apolipoprotein AI, variants	Heart, liver, kidney, PNS, testis, larynx	S
AApoAII	Apolipoprotein AII, variants	Kidney	S
AApoAIV	Apolipoprotein AIV, variants	Kidney mainly	S
ALect2	Leukocyte chemotactic factor 2	Kidney mainly	S
Aβ	Ab protein precursor, wild type	CNS	L
APrP	Prion protein, wild type	CNS	L
ACal	Procalcitonin	C cell thyroid tumors	L
AIAPP	Islet amyloid polypeptide	Insulinoma	L
AANF	Atrial natriuretic factor	Cardiac atria	L
APro	Prolactin	Pituitary prolactinomas	L
AIns	Insulin	Local insulin injection sites	L

AL Amyloidosis (Earlier known as Primary Amyloidosis)

This is caused by proliferation of plasma cell clones, that produce abnormal monoclonal light chains. These light chains deposited in various organs leading to characteristic clinical manifestations (Table 21.1). The clinical suspicion should be based on the

Table 21.3: Major forms of hereditary amyloidosis

Name of the amyloid	Precursor protein	Organ involvement	Systemic (S) or localized (L)
Fibrinogen Aα amyloidosis	Fibrinogen Aα chain	Kidney, liver, spleen; hypertension is common; kidney involvement is predominantly glomerular	S
Apolipoprotein AII amyloidosis	Apolipoprotein AII	Kidney	L
Apolipoprotein AI amyloidosis	Apolipoprotein AI	Kidney (with predominant medullary deposition), liver, heart, skin, larynx	S
Transthyretin amyloidosis	Transthyretin	Peripheral nervous system, heart, vitreous opacities; kidney involvement is not typical	S
Gelsolin amyloidosis	Gelsolin	Cranial nerves, lattice corneal dystrophy	S>L
Lysozyme amyloidosis	Lysozyme	Kidney, liver, gastrointestinal tract, spleen, lymph nodes, lung, thyroid, salivary glands	S

knowledge of relative frequency of organ involvement in the clinical spectrum. AL amyloid is suspected if following findings are present particularly in combination (Table 21.4).

About 10–15% of patients with AL amyloidosis will have associated plasma cell dyscrasias. Most commonly associated diseases are multiple myeloma or Waldenstrom's macroglobulinemia. When present, patients with AL amyloid will also have clinical manifestations of the associated disease.

The diagnosis consists of the following aspects:

1. Documentation of presence of amyloid in tissue biopsy with characteristic appearance after Congo red staining and polarized microscopy.
2. Documentation of presence of monoclonal serum/urine component
a. Immunofixation electrophoresis is positive in around 85% of the cases
b. Serum free light chain assay positive in 91% cases
c. Both combined sensitivity approaches around 99% cases.
d. There is almost always $\lambda > \kappa$ with a $\kappa:\lambda$ ratio less than 0.26

Table 21.4: Relative frequency of various organs involvement in AL amyloidosis

Organ involved	Frequency of involvement (approx)	Clinical syndrome
Kidney	70%	Asymptomatic proteinuria, nephrotic syndrome
Heart	60%	Diastolic heart failure, restrictive cardiomyopathy
Liver and spleen	70%	Hepatosplenomegaly, hypersplenism
Peripheral nervous system	20%	Sensorimotor neuropathy, carpal tunnel syndrome
Autonomic nervous system	15%	Postural hypotension, erectile dysfunction constipation
Musculoskeletal	15%	Macroglossia
Hematologic	25–50%	Bleeding diathesis

The ideal tissue of choice for biopsy is the involved organ itself. However, abdominal fat pad biopsy in trained hand is highly sensitive (90%) and specific (100%). The advantage of this procedure is that it is the simplest and safest to document amyloid deposits. Rectal biopsy is also highly sensitive (60%). Once a diagnosis of AL amyloid is established, a bone marrow biopsy is mandatory to assess the percentage of the plasma cells. It also helps to rule out multiple myeloma.

AA Amyloidosis (Earlier known as Secondary Amyloidosis)

The precursor protein in this case is serum amyloid A (SAA) protein, which is synthesized from hepatocytes in response to various inflammatory cytokines (IL-1, IL-6, TNF-α).

The most common set of diseases associated with AA amyloid are:

a. Chronic infections like tuberculosis, leprosy.
b. Chronic inflammatory conditions like rheumatoid arthritis, ankylosing spondylitis, juvenile rheumatoid arthritis, inflammatory bowel disease.
c. Surprisingly, AA amyloid is rarely or never seen in SLE patients.

Recently there has been some changes noted in the epidemiology of AA amyloid. With early detection and effective treatment, chronic infections are now less common causes of AA amyloid. Even inflammatory disorders can be diagnosed early and effectively treated with biological agents with good results. So, the incidence of AA amyloid appears to be decreasing now. Obesity is considered a chronic inflammatory disease and obesity related amyloidosis is emerging as a new cause for morbidity and kidney failure. AA amyloidosis is becoming the most common cause of kidney involvement in intravenous drug abusers particularly those associated with active HIV infection.

The clinical manifestation is predominantly due to renal and gastrointestinal involvement with nephrotic state, ascites, pleural effusion and hepatosplenomegaly. Cardiac involvement is less common than seen in AL amyloidosis and neurological and musculoskeletal involvement (macroglossia) is rarely seen. The diagnostic work up is similar to AL amyloid without the requirement to perform bone marrow biopsy.

Dialysis-related Amyloid

Dialysis-related amyloidosis (DRA) is characterized deposition in tissues of amyloid fibrils consisting of β_2-microglobulin which is cleared by the normal kidney. When renal clearance declines, it results in slow tissue deposition. It is mostly seen in patients who has been on long-term hemodialysis, particularly with low-flux dialyzers and cellulose based membranes. Further accumulation and deposition of amyloid occurs in bone, periarticular structures and viscera. With the advent of high-flux biocompatible membranes and convective therapies, the incidence has come down. Clinically it is characterized by following features:

- Symptoms are related to bones and joints. They may present with carpal tunnel syndrome (CTS).
- Scapulohumeral periarthritis, tenosynovitis, destructive spondyloarthropathy or bone cysts.
- Advanced age and low or absent residual renal function are also important risk factors.
- Patients on peritoneal dialysis also have similar incidence as hemodialysis.
- The diagnosis is by tissue biopsy.
- Kidneys are also involved in the hereditary amyloid (fibrinogen Aα, apolipoprotein AI and AII).
- Kidney involvement is rare in wild type of transthyretin (TTR) amyloid (senile amyloid).

Amyloidosis and the Kidney

Kidney involvement is a common clinical manifestations in AL and AA amyloidosis. Nephrotic syndrome is the most common presentation. Progressive worsening of renal function occurs in due course. If tubulo-interstitial involvement predominates, proteinuria may be less pronounced. Though rare, nephrogenic diabetes insipidus and Fanconi's syndrome are the two specific clinical conditions due to renal involvement. Diabetes insipidus occurs is due to amyloid deposition around collecting ducts and Fanconi's syndrome due to proximal tubular involvement.

The important findings in the pathology of amyloid kidney disease are:

a. Contrary to the common perception, kidney size is mostly normal not enlarged.
b. Bleeding is no more common after kidney biopsy compared to other diseases with comparable renal function.
c. The amorphous 'congophilic' deposits in amyloid are PAS negative.
d. In immunofluorescence (IF) microscopy, κ light chain is more common in AL amyloidosis, whereas λ light chain restriction is more common in other types.
e. Light chain IF positivity may not be seen in some cases of AL amyloidosis because of structural alteration immunoglobulin light chains occurring after being deposited as amyloid fibrils.
f. Potassium permanganate treatment of biopsy specimen may alter the affinity to Congo red staining in case of AA amyloid deposits. Immunohistochemical staining with anti-SAA antibody is more sensitive and specific for confirming AA amyloid.
g. 8 to 10 nm sized non branching fibrils although are specific for presence of amyloid, does not give any information regarding the type of amyloid.

Light Chain Deposition Disease (LCDD)

This is another immunoglobulin light chain related disease. LCDD may present similar as AL amyloidosis with proteinuria and renal dysfunction. The salient differences between the two are given in Table 21.5.

Treatment Strategies

Treatment of renal amyloidosis depends on the type of amyloid. Supportive therapy also plays a very important role in these cases. Overall renal prognosis depends on the extent of extrarenal manifestations. Overall outcome is poor in cases of advanced cardiac involvement. Renal response to therapy parallels hematological response in AL amyloid. Prognosis is bad in patients with associated multiple myeloma.

Supportive Treatment

For patients presenting with nephrotic state, fluid restriction and diuretic therapy is the standard treatment strategy. These patients may not tolerate diuretics and the lack of

Table 21.5: Differences between AL amyloid and LCDD in kidney

AL amyloidosis	LCDD
Hypertension uncommon	Hypertension common
Associated multiple myeloma ~10%	Associated multiple myeloma 30%–50%
Bland urinary sediment	Active urinary sediments
Amorphous glomerular deposits	Nodular glomerulosclerosis
PAS negative deposits	PAS positive deposits
'Congophilic'	Non-congophilic
IF: λ >> κ	IF: λ << κ
EM: Organized and fibrillar deposits	EM: non-organized and granular deposits
Recurrence after kidney transplantation leads rarely to graft loss	Graft loss more in recurrence after transplantation

PAS: Periodic acid–Schiff ; IF: Immunofluorescence ; EM: Electron microscopy

Table 21.6: Specific treatment for some types of amyloidosis

AL amyloid	• High dose melphalan/autologous stem cell transplant
	• Bortezomib based therapy
AA amyloid	• Colchicine for familial Mediterranean fever. Immunosuppressive therapy Azathioprine, methotrexate, cyclophosphamide
	• Anti-cytokine therapy (infliximab, etanercept)
β_2 microglobulin amyloid	• High-flux dialysis
	• Nocturnal hemodialysis
	• Short daily dialysis
	• HDF (theoretical advantage, no clinical evidence till date)
	• Renal transplantation

diuretic tolerance may be due to either cardiac involvement or autonomic nervous system involvement. Both lead to episodes of symptomatic postural hypotension. Hemodialysis is not well tolerated and the survival on transplantation is better than dialysis.

Specific treatment is available only for a few types of amyloidosis (Table 21.6).

Patients with AA amyloid tolerate transplant well and their survival is comparable to other matched recipients with CKD. Although recurrence may occur, graft loss seldom occurs due to recurrence of the disease in the transplanted kidney. In AL amyloid two strategies are employed to prevent recurrence:
a. Initially, stem cell transplant is performed to achieve hematological remission followed by renal transplantation (Mayo clinic strategy).
b. Renal transplant followed by autologous stem cell transplant (Boston university strategy).

Summary

Amyloidosis is a often diagnosed based on clinical suspicion or may be diagnosed as an unexpected finding in tissue biopsy. Most of the times, presence of one or two of the diagnostic features will be clinically apparent. Invasive tests for final diagnosis should always be carried out without fearing for the risks of complications. Histopathological diagnosis is mandatory for initiation of therapy. Symptomatic treatment should be given more than equal importance compared to definitive treatment. Multidisciplinary approach, in an experienced center is needed for a better therapeutic outcome.

Renal Failure

Acute Kidney Injury

• V Sivakumar • A Sunnesh

INTRODUCTION AND HISTORY

Acute kidney injury is an important entity not only when it presents as an isolated form but also when it presents as part of multiorgan dysfunction. Early description of acute renal failure dates back to early 19th century. Subsequently, during world war time it was called 'war nephritis'. During Second World War, it was named acute tubular necrosis associated with crush injury, The term 'acute renal failure' was introduced in 1950s and now, term acute kidney injury (AKI) is used to refer to an abrupt decrease in kidney function, resulting in the retention of urea and other nitrogenous waste products and in the dysregulation of extracellular volume and electrolytes. It may be associated with oliguria but not invariably so.

Definition and Classification

The definition for AKI used in clinical and epidemiologic studies is based on specific criteria that have been developed over time. The kidney disease improving global outcomes (KDIGO) definition and staging system is the most recent and preferred definition. The two other recent definitions are the risk, injury, failure, loss of function, end-stage criteria (RIFLE) and the modification proposed by the acute kidney injury network (AKIN).

Recent diagnostic staging criteria for AKI

The **KDIGO criteria** for diagnosing and staging AKI utilizes changes in serum creatinine and urine output but not eGFR except those under 18 years of age. AKI is diagnosed when there is:

i. Increase in serum creatinine by ≥0.3 mg/dl (≥26.5 µmol/L) within 48 hours, **or**

ii. Increase in serum creatinine to ≥1.5–2 times baseline (which is known or presumed to have occurred) within the prior seven days, **or**

iii. Urine volume <0.5 ml/kg/hour for six hours.

Using the same criteria, AKI is staged as follows:

Stage 1: Increase in serum creatinine to 1.5 to 1.9 times baseline, **or**

Increase in serum creatinine by ≥0.3 mg/dl (≥26.5 µmol/L), **or**

Reduction in urine output to <0.5 ml/kg/hour for 6 to 12 hours.

Stage 2: Increase in serum creatinine to 2.0 to 2.9 times baseline, **or**

Reduction in urine output to <0.5 ml/kg/hour for ≥12 hours.

Stage 3: Increase in serum creatinine to 3.0 times baseline, **or**

• Increase in serum creatinine to ≥4.0 mg/dl, **or**

• Reduction in urine output to < 0.3 ml/kg/hour for ≥24 hours, **or**

• Anuria for ≥12 hours, **or**

• Initiation of renal replacement therapy, **or**

• In patients <18 years, decrease in eGFR to <35 ml/min/1.73 m²

In AKIN criteria also, the diagnosis is based on increase in creatinine, rate of increase or urine output. There are 3 stages which are similar to KDIGO but minor differences.

Stage 1
- Increase in serum creatinine of ≥0.3 mg/dl, or
- Increase in creatinine 50–100%
- Urine output of <0.5 ml/kg/hour for 6 to 12 hours

Stage 2
- Increase in creatinine of >100–200%, **or**
- Urine output <0.5 ml/hour for 12 to 24 hours

Stage 3
- Increase in creatinine of >200%, or
- Increase in serum creatinine >0.5 mg/dl or >4 mg/dl
- Urine output <0.3 ml/hour for >24 hours, **or**
- Anuria for 12 hours.

In the **RIFLE** classification, there are 5 stages.

Risk	:	Increase in serum creatinine × 1.5 times, **or**
		Fall in GFR more than 25%, **or**
		Urine output less than 0.5 ml/kg/hour for >6 hours
Injury	:	Increase in creatinine × 2 times, **or**
		Fall in GFR >50%, **or**
		Urine output less than 0.5 ml/kg/hour for >12 hours
Failure	:	Increase in creatinine × 3 times, **or**
		Fall in GFR >75%, **or**
		Serum creatinine >4 mg% ,**or**
		Urine output <0.3 ml/kg/hour for >24 hours, **or**
		Anuria for more than 12 hours
Loss of function	:	Need for renal replacement therapy for >4 weeks
End stage	:	Need for renal replacement therapy for >3 months.

Etiology

The traditional approach to kidney disease has been to categorize the clinical etiology as prerenal, intrinsic renal (involving blood vessels, glomeruli, tubule or interstitium) or postrenal.

Prerenal Causes (Table 22.1)

Conditions that cause reduction in blood volume (loss of blood, plasma, fluids and electrolytes or water) due to blood loss, burns, dehydration or heat stroke) may cause hypovolemia, hypotension, reduced renal perfusion and prerenal AKI. This is a reversible stage of AKI. Renal perfusion may also be low in other hypervolemic states with low effective circulating (arterial) volume, such as heart failure where the ejection fraction is reduced. It may occur in patients with decompensated liver function and portal hypertension (hepatorenal syndrome). Changes in renal vascular autoregulation, such as afferent arteriole vasoconstriction caused by nonsteroidal anti-inflammatory drugs (NSAIDs), and inhibition of efferent vasoconstriction by renin-angiotensin system (RAS) blockade may also cause prerenal AKI. In most of the above conditions, if the causative factor is promptly corrected, the damage to the tubule can be avoided and the urine output and renal functions improve.

Table 22.1: Prerenal causes of AKI

1. Conditions producing reduced blood volume leading to renal hypoperfusion
   a. Loss of blood: External or internal hemorrhage
   b. Loss of plasma: Extensive burns
   c. Loss of electrolytes and water: Diarrhea and other gastrointestinal losses
   d. Loss of water: Heat stroke, untreated polyuric syndromes
2. Conditions producing decrease in cardiac output, hypotension and renal hypoperfusion
   a. All conditions mentioned above if significant and prolonged cause hypotension
   b. Septicemic shock
   c. Cardiogenic shock
   d. Severe congestive heart failure
   e. Massive pulmonary embolism and cardiac tamponade
3. Hepatorenal syndrome

Intrinsic Renal Causes (Table 22.2)

a. *Vascular disease:* Intrinsic renal vascular diseases directly affect both large or small-sized blood vessels within the kidneys. Intrinsic renal vascular diseases that involve larger vessels may lead to renal infarction from aortic dissection, systemic thromboembolism, or renal artery aneurysm/bleeding. Subacute intrinsic diseases that involve small blood vessels include small vessel vasculitides affecting glomerular capillaries and diseases that cause micro-angiopathy and hemolytic anemia (MAHA), e.g. thrombotic thrombocytopenic purpura/hemolytic uremic syndrome (TTP/HUS), scleroderma, and malignant hypertension. Renal vein thrombosis is frequently associated with massive proteinuria in the setting of nephrotic syndrome.

b. Intrinsic glomerular diseases include nephritic illness with relatively abrupt onset of facial puffiness, pedal edema, hypertension, hematuria, proteinuria, dysmorphic red blood cell and RBC casts in urine. Sometimes, nephrotic syndrome may also be associated with AKI.

c. Renal tubule is highly vulnerable to ischemic or toxic injury. When the condition causing prerenal failure is prolonged, tubular damage ensues. In ischemic injury, the tubule cell undergoes necrosis and the cellular debris may block the intrarenal passage and prevent urine formation. Damage to tubular cell due to toxins may damage the cell function and lead to AKI.

d. The renal interstitium is often affected together with the tubular cell. The interstitium is also closely involved in the maintenance of the milieu intérieur in the kidney. It provides a suitable extracellular environment for the optimal functioning of the cell. Certain drugs and infections affect the interstitial compartment, conditions like cast nephropathy in multiple myeloma, acute urate nephropathy in tumor lysis syndrome or acute phosphate nephropathy following a phosphate-containing bowel preparation cause acute tubulointerstitial nephritis and AKI.

Postrenal Causes (Table 22.3)

Obstruction in the urethra, bladder neck, both ureters or ureter in a single functioning kidney leads to AKI. Substantial reduction in glomerular filtration rate (GFR) with normal urine examination and anuria should raise suspicion of urinary tract obstruction. Urethral obstruction can be diagnosed easily by noting a distended bladder. In bilateral ureteric obstruction, the kidney may be

---

Table 22.2: Intrinsic renal causes of AKI

1. Abnormalities in renal circulation
   a. Bilateral renal artery thrombosis or embolism
   b. Vasculitis
   c. Bilateral acute renal vein thrombosis
   d. Malignant hypertension
2. Abnormalities in glomerulus
   a. Acute glomerulonephritis, e.g. poststreptococcal, systemic lupus erythematosus
   b. Rapidly progressive glomerulonephritis
3. Abnormalities in renal tubules and interstitium
   a. Ischemia as a result of the prerenal factors mentioned (ATN)
   b. Toxic
      i. Dose-related nephrotoxicity
      ii. Hypersensitivity allergic interstitial nephritis
      iii. Other toxic agents—methanol, ethylene glycol, carbon tetrachloride, radiographic contrast media, heavy metals, weedicides.
   c. Pigment-induced renal failure—hemoglobin, myoglobin
   d. Infection—leptospirosis, falciparum malaria
   e. Snake bite
   f. Obstetric AKI

Table 22.3: Postrenal causes of AKI

Acute obstruction to the urinary collecting system which may be extrinsic or intrinsic
a. Urethral obstruction
b. Ureteric obstruction of single functioning kidney
c. Bilateral ureteric obstruction

palpably enlarged or minimal distension seen in ultrasonogram.

Relative Frequency of Causes of AKI

Broadly 2 different types of AKI occur. Community acquired (CAAKI) and hospital acquired (HAAKI). In general, patients with CAAKI have shorter hospitalization and better long-term survival in comparision to patients with HAAKI. Since CAAKI often results from prolonged volume depletion or a single insult to the kidney, the response to treatment and prognosis are more favorable. HAAKI occurs as postoperative complication or due to sepsis, radiocontrast-mediated injury, multiple insults and as part of multi organ dysfunction syndrome and the prognosis is less favorable. Acute tubular necrosis is the most common cause and occurs when the prerenal factors are not corrected in a timely fashion. AKI can be superimposed on chronic kidney disease and is also a common presentation. Urinary tract obstruction, glomerulonephritis, vasculitis or interstitial nephritis also account for the causes of AKI.

Pathophysiology of Prerenal Phase

In the prerenal phase, decreased kidney function may occur due to generalized decrease in tissue perfusion or in selective renal ischemia. When systemic hypoperfusion occurs, it is sensed by cardiac and arterial receptors and activation of these receptors result in increased sympathetic tone, release of renin and antidiuretic hormone. These homeostatic mechanisms help to maintain systemic blood pressure, intravascular volume and cardiac output. The arteriolar vasoconstriction occurs primarily in the renal, splanchnic, and musculocutaneous circulations, resulting in the relative preservation of blood flow to the heart and brain. Renal vasoconstriction can diminish renal blood flow and the glomerular filtration rate (GFR). In addition, if the compensatory systemic responses are incomplete, persistent reductions

in cardiac output and/or arterial pressure can contribute to the decline in GFR. In true volume depletion, hypovolemia is caused due to dehydration, hemorrhage, renal loss (diuretics) or gastrointestinal loss (vomiting, diarrhea). Renal perfusion can also be reduced in edematous states such as heart failure and cirrhosis due to 'pump failure' as in myocardial dysfunction and splanchnic venous pooling and systemic vasodilation. In prerenal causes, the GFR is diminished because of decreased renal blood flow. The glomeruli, kidney tubules, and interstitium are intact. The appropriate treatment is to increase renal perfusion, as with volume repletion in patients with true volume depletion reverses the abnormality and the GFR improves promptly.

If the prerenal phase is prolonged, the renal tubules undergo necrosis. The necrotic tubular debris may block the tubule lumen, the filtrate may back-leak into the circulation and the patient develops oliguria and retention of waste products. Various inflammatory mediators released by the damaged tubules contribute to the damage. The distribution of lesions within the kidney may be random.

In toxic damage to the tubule, generally, the same segment of the tubule of all nephrons will be affected. There will be no disruption of the tubular basement membrane. The functional integrity of the tubular cell will be affected.

Clinical Features of AKI

Clinical features are mostly due to the underlying disorder. Symptoms due to renal failure include oliguria, fluid overload, nausea, vomiting or uremic symptoms. In severe cases, metabolic acidosis and hyperkalemia may occur. The clinical course of acute tubular necrosis is broadly divided into:

1. Incipient or initiating phase
2. Phase of established acute tubular necrosis
3. Diuretic phase
4. Phase of functional recovery (post-diuretic phase)

Incipient phase starts from the onset of ischemia or toxic injury to the stage of established of tubular necrosis. There are no specific symptoms relating to renal failure during this stage and a high index of suspicion is necessary to detect renal involvement. If the patient develops oliguria, the clinician often suspects this problem. In presence of high risk factors, periodic blood examination for urea and creatinine must be done to detect renal failure early. During the incipient stage, since the tubules have not undergone necrosis, they continue to reabsorb water, sodium and other substances from the tubular fluid. Therefore the patients may pass smaller volumes of concentrated urine which is high in urea and creatinine content and low in sodium concentration. The specific gravity or osmolality of urine is also high. Identification of patients in this stage is important because correction of the factors responsible for renal hypoperfusion and improvement of blood pressure help to reverse the process promptly and normalise the renal function.

When tubular necrosis has occurred the patient may become oliguric or remain non-oliguric. Accumulation of nitrogenous waste products and water lead to uremic symptoms and fluid overload or pulmonary edema. Retention of potassium and acid ions result in hyperkalemia and metabolic acidosis. These patients are more prone to develop infections, gastrointestinal hemorrhage, paralytic ileus, convulsions or hypertension. The oliguric phase may last for a few days to a few weeks. If appropriate treatment is given and complications prevented, most patients enter diuretic phase in 2–3 weeks. In patients who have crush injury or obstetric accidents, hypercatabolic renal failure characterized by daily rise of urea of more than 100 mg/dl, creatinine of more than 1.5 mg/dl and potassium more than 1 mEq/L may occur. Such patients require aggressive dialysis support.

The onset of diuretic phase is heralded by the doubling of urine output everyday leading to polyuria in most patients. In the early diuretic phase, there may be further rise of urea and creatinine before it starts coming down. This phase signifies recovery of glomerular filtration and partial healing of tubular lesions. During this phase, since the tubular function has not returned to normal completely, the patients may have uncontrolled urinary losses of water and electrolytes leading to dehydration, hyponatremia, hypokalemia and postural hypotension. This phase must be managed with appropriate fluid and electrolyte replacement because failure to do so may result in fatal complications.

During the post-diuretic phase, the renal function and urine output return to normal. The recovery can be considered complete for all practical purposes. However, if the ability of kidney to maximally concentrate, dilute or acidify the urine is challenged by appropriate tests, there may be mild impairment in spite of apparently complete clinical recovery in some cases.

In some patients the oliguric phase may be prolonged for more than 4–6 weeks. In such patients, renal cortical necrosis should be suspected and a renal biopsy is performed to confirm the diagnosis. Once diffuse renal cortical necrosis has occurred, recovery of renal function is unlikely and the patient is managed as a case of irreversible chronic renal failure. In some patients, cortical necrosis may be patchy and recovery of renal function though incomplete permits survival without dialysis.

Poisonous snakes like Russels viper, saw-scaled viper cause renal failure depending on the quantity of venom injected, site of bite, the movement of the limb after the bite and the promptness and effectiveness of treatment with antivenom. The renal failure is often due to acute tubular necrosis, intravascular coagulation and direct toxicity of the venom. Severe cases of envenomation may be associated with hyperviscosity, disseminated intravascular coagulation, hemolysis, myocardial failure and hypotension. In the case of sea snakes, muscle necrosis and myoglobinuria are additional features. Rarely, renal failure with renal cortical necrosis may occur due to envenomation by rattlesnake, green pit viper and sea snakes. This depends on the amount of venom injected, extent of DIC and hypotension that may ensue.

Renal failure is one of the serious manifestations of infection with leptospiral group of organisms. The other manifestations are, abrupt onset of febrile illness, muscle pain, deep jaundice and hemorrhagic tendency. Persons who have risk of exposure to water which is contaminated with infected rat's urine are commonly affected. The disease has an initial leptospiremic phase when fever and myalgia predominate and an immune phase when renal and hepatic failures manifest. This is usually a self-limiting disease and subsides in about 10–14 days. Patients die of intractable hypotension due to myocarditis, intracerebral bleed, acute respiratory distress or complications of renal failure. Treatment with early dialysis improves the survival. The patients are often given benzyl penicillin in doses of 1,000,000 to 2,000,000 units intravenously 4 to 6 times a day for 5–7 days. Doxycycline or any other antibiotic may be used. Infection with Hantavirus closely resembles leptospirosis but hepatic involvement and jaundice does not occur in Hantavirus infection.

During early pregnancy, septic abortion may lead to AKI. In late pregnancy, obstetric complications like pre-elampsia, eclampsia, abruptio placentae, postpartum hemorrhage or sepsis may lead to AKI. The incidence of cortical necrosis is high in obstetric AKI.

In the tropical countries, gastroenteritis, cholera, salmonellosis, malaria, scorpion sting or heat stroke may also lead to AKI. Other conditions include insect bite, poisoning due to paraquat, copper sulfate or formic acid and toxicity of drugs radiocontrast agents or herbal nephrotoxins. Individuals deficient in

the enzyme G6PD may develop severe intravascular hemolysis precipitated by infection or drugs followed by AKI.

Organ Crosstalk in Acute Kidney Injury

It is important to know in brief that AKI mediates a systemic response that can lead to multiorgan failure and often it is described as organ crosstalk or remote organ damage following AKI. It is postulated that pro-inflammatory cytokines, interleukin-1β, interleukin-6 and tumor necrosis factor-α mediates systemic response with the recruitment of pro-inflammatory cells leading to distant organ failure (Fig. 22.1).

Diagnosis

A careful history and examination to rule out urinary infection, structural anomaly or obstruction must be undertaken. All patients with AKI must also undergo a thorough examination of all systems with a view to detect involvement of kidney, systemic diseases affecting kidney, renal hypoperfusion, drug or toxin intoxication. Examination of the respiratory system and sputum may help to suspect conditions like rapidly progressive glomerulonephritis and Wegener's granulomatosis. An examination of the eye for jaundice, band keratopathy, uveitis, hypertensive or diabetic retinopathy and the skin for features of vasulitis or lupus erythematosus help in the diagnosis.

In children, pregnant women and adults, examination of blood smear for microangiopathic hemolytic anemia helps in the diagnosis of hemolytic uremic syndrome. Acute renal failure following febrile illness with myalgia, deep jaundice and subconjunctival hemorrhage suggest leptospirosis. Bleeding tendency, fever and acute renal failure are suggestive of hemorrhagic fever with renal syndrome. When there is history of nephrotoxic drug intake, viperine snakebite envenomation or pregnancy related complication, the diagnosis may be obvious. AKI is

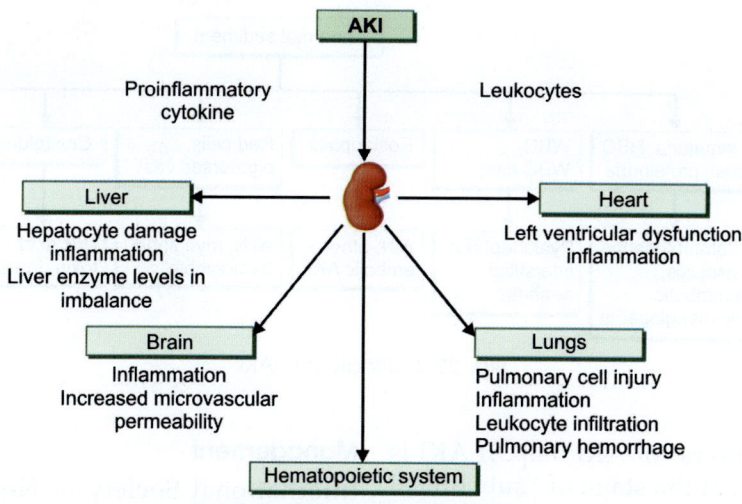

Fig. 22.1: Organ crosstalk in AKI

clinically suspected when a susceptible person has been exposed to one or more of the factors causing acute renal failure or has any of the extrarenal manifestations of renal failure. The clinical diagnosis is confirmed by examination of urine and biochemical examination of blood.

Since it is very important to differentiate between the state of incipient renal failure and established acute tubular necrosis, the main clinical and biochemical features in blood and urine in these conditions are summarised in Table 22.4.

Urinalysis gives useful information about diagnosis and management. The various abnormalities in urinalysis and the corresponding clinical conditions are shown in Fig. 22.2.

AKI in critically ill patients is associated with significant morbidity, mortality, economic impact for the family and is a concern in term of public health. Diagnosis may be delayed when it is based on oliguria and increase in serum creatinine. It is in this context, the newly introduced molecules

Table 22.4: Differentiating features between incipient renal failure (prerenal) and established ATN		
Laboratory test	*Prerenal*	*ATN*
Urinary sediment	Normal	Dirty brown casts/cellular debris
Urine osmolality (mOsm/kg)	>500	<400
Urine sodium (mEq/L)	<20	>40
Fractional excretion of sodium (FENa)	<1	>1
Urine/plasma urea ratio	>8	<3
Urine/plasma creatinine ratio	>40	<20
Renal failure index (RFI)	<1	>1

$$FENa = \frac{Urinary\ sodium}{Serum\ sodium} \times \frac{Serum\ creatinine}{Urinary\ creatinine} \times 100$$

$$RFI = \frac{Urinary\ sodium}{Urinary\ creatinine} \times Serum\ creatinine$$

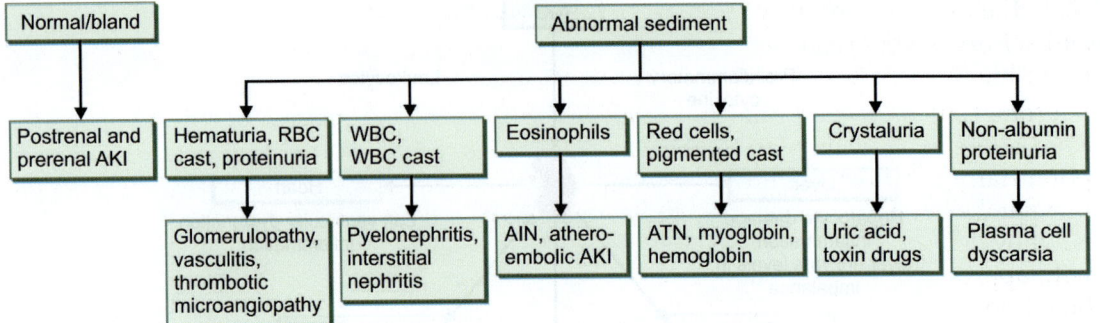

Fig. 22.2: Urinalysis in AKI

called "biomarkers" of AKI help. If AKI is detected early, at the stage of "subclinical acute kidney injury", the morbidity and mortality can be reduced. The available treatment modalities can be used to preserve and protect kidney function or at least promote early recovery. The biomarkers may be classified as follows (Fig. 22.3).

Management

International Society of Nephrology has recognized AKI as major health concerns and it aims to curb down mortality associated with AKI to zero by 2025 (0/25 initative). Prevention is the first and foremost step. Immediate therapy for the management of life-threatening fluid and electrolyte abnormalities due to AKI

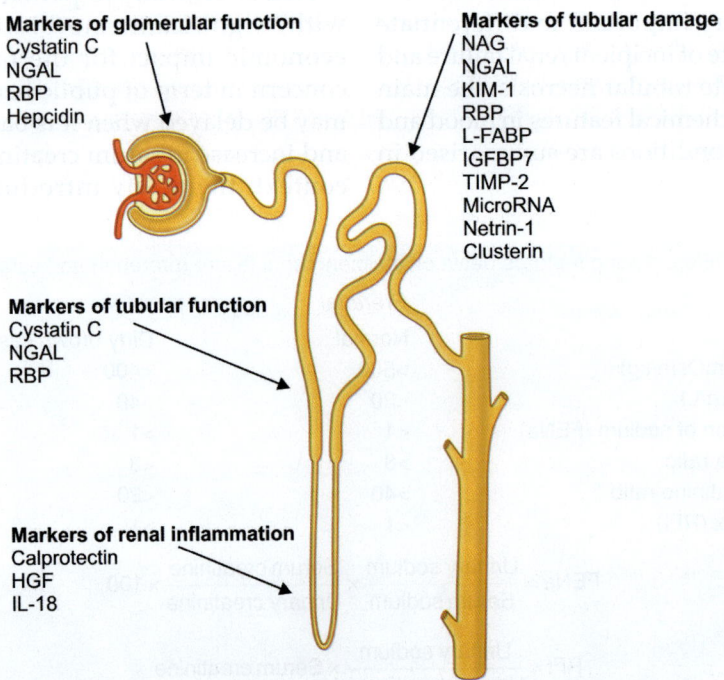

Markers of glomerular function
Cystatin C
NGAL
RBP
Hepcidin

Markers of tubular damage
NAG
NGAL
KIM-1
RBP
L-FABP
IGFBP7
TIMP-2
MicroRNA
Netrin-1
Clusterin

Markers of tubular function
Cystatin C
NGAL
RBP

Markers of renal inflammation
Calprotectin
HGF
IL-18

Fig. 22.3: Biomarkers and the relevant nephron segments

should be started immediately. Fluid, electrolyte and acid-base abnormalities account for the major life-threatening complications in AKI.

Prompt detection and treatment of prerenal causes like hypotension and avoidance of potentially toxic drugs and toxins help to prevent the development of AKI. When there is hypovolemia and shock it must be corrected with appropriate fluid replacement and the blood pressure maintained above 100 mm of Hg. Normal saline should be prefered over 5% dextrose since the intravascular distribution of saline is more compared to dextrose. Patients in prerenal AKI usually respond to correction of hypovolemia and hypotension. Usually the urine output increases up to 30 to 40 ml/hour over the next 2 hours. If the output does not improve, the patient is given frusemide 1 to 2 mg/kg body wt. If the urine output does not improve, it may be assumed that the patient has gone into established acute tubular necrosis. In clinical settings known to predispose to DIC, intravascular hemolysis, hyperuricemia, rhabdomyolysis, cisplatin nephrotoxicity and radiocontrast administration, mannitol may be used prophylactically since it may prevent cell swelling and oxygen-free radical induced injury.

In some oliguric patients not responding to frusemide, administration of dopamine 1 to 2 µg/kg/min as a controlled infusion may help to improve the urine output but not the renal failure. Since it is easier to manage the nonoliguric AKI than an oliguric AKI, low dose dopamine infusion may be tried in some cases. The cardinal principles in management of oliguric phase are to sustain life, to prevent complication and to give time for natural recovery of kidney. To sustain life, the load to the kidney is reduced by appropriate adjustments of diet and fluid intake. The blood chemistry is maintained within acceptable limits till renal function recovers. Careful management and timely dialysis help to prevent the complications and give time for the natural recovery of renal function.

Water Balance

A daily weight recording and fluid intake and output chart are used to decide the volume of fluid to be administered. If facilities are available, monitoring of central venous may be useful. A patient with oliguric AKI should have a restricted fluid intake of approximately 500 ml in addition to actual loss of fluid over the previous 24-hour period so that a daily weight loss of 0.2 to 0.3 kg is achieved. A daily increase in weight at this stage often suggests overhydration and may be tackled with more vigorous fluid restriction. In patients with hypovolemia, fluid administration is guided by clinical parameters like skin turgor, dry mucosa, postural hypotension or central venous pressure. Patients with nonoliguric AKI may be allowed more liberal fluid intake.

Hypervolemia may be present upon initial evaluation or occur due to excessive fluid administration in the setting of impaired ability to excrete sodium and water. This is especially true for patients with sepsis who commonly receive aggressive intravenous fluid resuscitation. Daily fluid balance is commonly positive in critically ill patients with ATN as a result of obligate fluid intake due to the administration of antibiotics, blood products, other intravenous medications, and nutritional support. This may result in progressive volume expansion and pulmonary edema, which may be especially poorly tolerated in patients with acute lung injury and which is associated with poor outcomes. Less commonly, volume overload may result from primary left ventricular dysfunction and cause AKI or type 1 cardiorenal syndrome.

Calories and Proteins

Diet containing 2000 calories with 20 g protein (0.6 gm/kg/day), high in carbohydrate and fat can be used. If the fluid administration can be liberal, patients may take normal food. If the fluid intake is to be restricted to 300 to 500 ml/24 hours, patients must be advised sufficient calories and proteins as semisolid food so that the total fluid intake is within the acceptable limits. Care must be taken to restrict the fluid intake because unrestricted intake leads to fluid overload and pulmonary edema. A diet containing no protein is also detrimental since it favors excessive endogenous protein breakdown. If the patient is on regular dialysis, normal diet may be advised (*see* Section 11 on diet in renal disease).

Electrolyte Balance

The daily sodium intake should be restricted to 2–4 g of sodium chloride. As 'salt-free' diet contains about this amount of sodium, patients must be advised salt-free diet throughout the oliguric phase. Measurement of serum and urine sodium may be undertaken to plan sodium administration in individual cases. Potassium intake must be restricted in the oliguric phase. Potassium accumulation occurs as a result of endogenous muscle breakdown and stored blood transfusion, some drugs, fruits and fruit juices. Since hyperkalemia is asymptomatic, periodic monitoring of serum potassium or ECG is needed for an early diagnosis. Undetected hyperkalemia may lead to cardiac arrythmias or cardiac arrest. The following ECG changes sequentially occur when serum potassium goes above 5.5 mEq/L. Tall peaked T wave, widening of QRS complex, prolongation of PR interval, disappearance of P wave, sine wave, ventricular fibrillation and asystole. If ECG or biochemical evidence of hyperkalemia is present, 20 ml of 10% calcium gluconate is administered to the patient intravenously over 10 minutes. Calcium administration temporarily protects myocardium from the effect of hyperkalemia, without reducing serum potassium levels. Administration of 7.5% sodium bicarbonate 50–100 ml intravenously helps in temporary correction of metabolic acidosis. Such correction also enables the movement of potassium from the extracellular to intracellular compartment. Administration of 200 to 300 ml of 20% glucose

with 10 units of plain insulin temporarily retains the potassium in the intracellular compartment. The actual removal of potassium from the body can be achieved by the use of exchange resins like kayexalate (administered orally or by retention enema) and by dialysis. If metabolic acidosis with acidotic breathing develops in AKI or when serum bicarbonate is less than 15 mEq/L, careful intravenous administration of sodium bicarbonate may be necessary.

Hypertension

Hypertension may occur in AKI as a result of fluid overload. If fluid and salt restriction is not successful in bringing down blood pressure, appropriate antihypertensive drugs may be used.

Routine administration of antibotics as a prophylaxis is not necessary in AKI. Some patients are prone to the development of infective complications. Such patients may be given suitable doses of appropriate antibiotics. Care should be taken to avoid nephrotoxic antibiotics and proper dose modification should be instituted in case such drugs are used. Although anemia may occur in some patients, aggressive management with blood transfusion is advocated only if there is ongoing blood loss or symptoms due to anemia or if the hematocrit is less than 20%. Attempts must be made to identify and prevent infective or metabolic complicatons during oliguric and diuretic phase.

During the diuretic phase, dehydration, postural hypotension, hypokalemia and hyponatremia must be looked for and appropriate correction given. Since the renal tubules are incapable of reabsorbing the glomerular filtrate adequately, patients may go into severe dehydration and shock if appropriate fluid replacement and necessary corrections are not substituted. The intake of protein and potassium may be more liberal during this stage. Since death may occur during the diuretic phase due to dehydration, electrolyte imbalance and infection, proper management with fluid balance chart, weight recording and regulation of fluid and electrolyte intake must be continued during this phase as well.

Dialysis in AKI

In order to give time for the natural recovery of the kidney, peritoneal or hemodialysis is performed in an attempt to maintain the blood chemistry under acceptable limits. Since early dialysis prevents the complications of AKI, prophylactic dialysis is preferred. By starting dialysis early, the chances of further deterioration are minimized. Dialysis is usually given 2 to 3 times per week so as to give time for the recovery of the renal function. The choice of peritoneal or hemodialysis depends on the condition of the patient, cause of renal failure and the available facilities. Since the rate of accumulation of waste products in hypercatabolic renal failure is rapid, peritoneal dialysis may not be effective in improving the blood chemistry. Such patients may even need daily hemodialysis. Patients who are anuric usually require hemodialysis at least on alternate days. More stable patients of AKI are usually dialysed on 2 days a week. For patients with AKI associated with hemodynamic instability or multiorgan failure, procedures like continuous arteriovenous hemodialysis or hemofiltration may be used. The indications for dialysis can be broadly grouped into clinical indications, biochemical indications and emergency indications.

Clinical indications are symptomatic uremia, anuria of more than 24 hours, gastrointestinal symptoms like nausea, vomiting and cardiovascular complications like pericarditis. The biochemical indications are:

a. Blood urea level >200 mg/dl (BUN >100 mg/dl) or daily rise of urea >50 mg/dl (BUN >25 mg/dl)
b. Serum creatinine >5 mg/dl or daily rise of creatinine >1 mg/dl
c. Serum potassium >6.5 mEq/dl or daily rise above 0.5 mEq/dl
d. Metabolic acidosis

The emergency indications include:

a. ECG evidence of hyperkalemia
b. Fluid overload and pulmonary edema refractory to diuretics.
c. Resistant metabolic acidosis pH <7.1 where administration of bicarbonate is not possible (volume overload, lactic acidosis).
d. Neurologic manifestations—convulsions, encephalopathy, recent alteration of mental status
e. Uremic pericarditis.

Continuous arteriovenous hemodialysis can be performed in patients of AKI associated with hemodynamic instability. This procedure can be performed without the help of a dialysis machine in the intensive care unit as a bedside procedure.CRRT may have some advantages compared with IHD but the procedure is more laborious and expensive. It has the advantage of enhanced hemodynamic stability, which is beneficial in hemodynamically unstable patients. Since increased salt and water removal can be achieved, it may permit better management of volume and nutritional status. Clearance of inflammatory mediators can be increased and may provide benefit in septic patients. Continuous therapy may be more useful in acute brain injury or fulminant hepatic failure. Hyperalimentation and cytoprotective therapy may become important modalities of treatment in future.

If obstructive uropathy is present, immediate relief of obstruction is usually associated with a phase of excessive urine output and normalization of renal function.

Course and Prognosis

The mortality in uncomplicated cases of AKI has improved considerably with dialysis. The mortality rate is higher if renal failure is associated with serious infection, multiple injuries, major surgeries or following nephrotoxic insults. Mortality rate can be reduced by the speedy and efficient treatment and institution of timely dialysis.

Stem cell therapy is now undergoing trials. It may help in tissue or organ repair. Bone marrow stem cells after engraftment may help in the recovery of AKI.

Earlier, it was assumed that those who survived AKI would have nearly complete renal recovery. It is observed now that about 20–30% patients may progress to CKD and this depends on the duration, severity and frequency of the episode of AKI. The outcome of AKI may be different when associated conditions like pregnancy, burns, cardiac surgery, trauma, myoglobinuria, snakebite and poisonings are associated. The recovery may be nearly complete except for inability to concentrate or dilute the urine under extreme conditions, partial recovery with slightly lower GFR, recurrent renal injury, dialysis-dependent renal failure or development of progressive worsening of GFR.

Conclusion

Acute kidney injury continues to be a challenge for healthcare providers. In this write up, emphasis was given for early diagnosis, intervention and outcome for the readers benefit. Recent advances were briefly touched upon to broaden the understanding. Importance of HAAKI as a multifaceted problem requiring multidisciplinary management was stressed.

Chronic Kidney Disease

• Dipankar Bhowmik • Vineet Behera

INTRODUCTION

Chronic kidney disease (CKD) is an important cause of long-term morbidity and mortality. It is estimated that nearly 10% of the adult population worldwide has chronic kidney disease. The rising incidence is thought to be due to aging population, higher incidence of diseases such as diabetes mellitus (DM) and hypertension, environmental impact, overuse of drugs and increased incidence of renal diseases. As most patients remain asymptomatic until the disease has significantly progressed, it is necessary to look for, diagnose and manage the condition early.

Definition

CKD is an irreversible, progressive reduction in renal function. The National Kidney Foundation's Kidney Disease Outcomes Quality Initiative (KDOQI) guidelines define CKD as sustained kidney damage as indicated by the presence of structural or functional abnormalities like microalbuminuria/proteinuria, hematuria, histologic or imaging abnormalities, and/or reduced glomerular filtration rate (GFR) to less than 60 ml/min/ 1.73 m^2 for at least 3 months.

Staging and Classification

Based on estimation of glomerular filtration rate (GFR), CKD has been classified into five stages as shown in Fig. 23.1. The ideal method for measurement of GFR (mGFR) is inulin clearance but can be used only in research laboratories. Radionuclide DTPA renogram for assessment of mGFR cannot be used routinely since it is costly and not widely available. Formulae using common clinical and laboratory parameters are the common bedside method used for estimated GFR (eGFR) (Table 23.1). Mobile apps and free online calculators are now available for calculation of eGFR. Presence of evidence of renal involvement for a period of more than 3 months, together with eGFR greater than 90 ml/min is termed CKD stage 1. In CKD stage 2, the eGFR is between 60 and 89 ml/min with other evidence of renal disease. If the eGFR is less than 60 ml/min, the term CKD stage 3 is used irrespective of presence of renal disease. Stage 3 is subdivided into 3a, if eGFR is between 59 to 45 ml/min and 3b when eGFR is between 44 and 30 ml/min. In stage 4, eGFR is between 29 and 15 ml/min and in stage 5 is eGFR less than 15 ml/min or the patient is receiving renal replacement therapy (Fig. 23.1). Suffix 'A' is added to any stage to denote degree of proteinuria 'A1' if albuminuria is <30 mg/g of creatinine, 'A2' if albuminuria is 30–300 mg/g and 'A3' if albuminuria is >300 mg/g. The suffix 'D' is used if patient is receiving dialysis and 'T' if

				Persistent albuminuria categories description and range		
				A1	**A2**	**A3**
				Normally mildly increased	Moderately increased	Severely increased
				<30 mg/g <3 mg/mmol	30–300 mg/g 3–30 mg/mmol	>300 mg/g >30 mg/mmol
GFR categories (ml/min/1.73 m²) description and range	**G1**	Normal of high	≥90		Monitor	Refer*
	G2	Mildly decreased	60–89		Monitor	Refer*
	G3a	Mildly to moderately decreased	45–59	Monitor	Monitor	Refer*
	G3b	Moderately to severely decreased	30–44	Monitor	Monitor	Refer*
	G4	Severely decreased	15–29	Refer*	Refer*	Refer*
	G5	Kindly failure	<15	Refer*	Monitor	Refer*

*Refer to nephrology center for planning further treatment

Fig. 23.1: Classification and staging of CKD. Adapted from KDIGO 2012 clinical practice guideline for the evaluation and management of chronic kidney disease.

Table 23.1: Commonly used methods for calculating eGFR

$$\text{Cockcroft} - \text{Gault formula (ml/min)} = \frac{[140 - \text{age in years}] \times \text{weight in kg}}{72 \times \text{serum creatinine in mg\%}}$$

(multiply by 0.85 if female)

MDRD equation (ml/min/1.73 m²) = 186 × (SCr$^{-1.154}$) × (age$^{-0.203}$) × #

\# Multiply by 0.742 if female
\# Multiply by 1.212 if African American

CKD EPI formula (ml/min/1.73 m²) = **141 × min (S$_{Cr}$/κ, 1)$^{\alpha}$ × max (S$_{Cr}$/κ, 1)$^{-1.209}$ × 0.993^{age}**

• × 1.018 (if female)
• × 1.159 (if black)
• κ = 0.7 (females) or 0.9 (males)
• α = −0.329 (females) or −0.411 (males)

the subject has undergone renal transplantation.

Etiology

The common causes of CKD are diabetes mellitus (DM) (22–45%), glomerulonephritis (10–23%), hypertension (5–25%), chronic pyelonephritis (0.5 to 7%), adult polycystic kidney disease (2–7%), renal vascular disease (2–7%), other recognized conditions like vesicoureteral reflux, obstructive nephropathy, lupus nephritis or vasculitis (2–5%) and unknown causes (4–26%). The most common cause in the adult population is DM, accounting for approximately 40% of patients on renal replacement therapy. It is estimated that one-third of patients with DM will develop nephropathy within 5 to 10 years after the diagnosis of diabetes and progress to ESRD. Hypertension is also a common cause, accounting for one-third of patients. The risk factors for CKD are given in Table 23.2.

Pathophysiology

The pathophysiology is complex. Regardless of the method of renal injury, once renal damage has occurred, a cascade of events ensues. In response to renal injury, there may be nephron loss and increase in intraglomerular pressure with glomerular hypertrophy occurs in the surviving nephrons, as the kidney attempts to maintain constant glomerular filtration. Increase in glomerular permeability to macromolecules and protein leak occurs and the damage is mediated through cytokines, transforming growth factor-β (TGF-β), fatty acids and oxidative stress. Thus, toxicity to the mesangial matrix, mesangial cell expansion, inflammation, fibrosis, and glomerular scarring occurs. Renal injury also results in an increase in angiotensin II production, causing an upregulation of TGF-β, contributing to collagen synthesis and renal scarring within the glomerulus. Both the structural alterations and accompanying biochemical, cellular, and molecular changes account for progressive renal scarring and loss of kidney function. All forms of CKD are associated with tubulointerstitial changes of varying degree. Although the exact mechanism is not known, interstitial fibrosis and tubular atrophy may be secondary to a reduction in blood supply, infiltration of lymphocytes and inflammatory mediators and the severity of tubulointerstitial damage correlates with poorer prognosis.

Several pathophysiological changes occur as the renal functions decline progressively.

a. Concentration and/or dilution of the urine—impaired

Table 23.2: Risk factors of CKD	
Non-modifiable factors	• Age
	• Gender
	• History of pre-eclampsia
	• Ethnicity
	• Genetics (family history—renal and cardiovascular)
	• Type of renal disease
	• Prenatal programming (e.g. malnutrition, low birth weight)
Modifiable factors	• Elevated blood pressure
	• Activation of renin–angiotensin system
	• Proteinuria
	• Smoking
	• Salt intake
	• Obesity/metabolic syndrome

b. Excretory function—impaired (accumulation of uremic toxins)

c. Conservation of sodium—impaired

d. Excretion of potassium—impaired (life-threatening hyperkalemia)

e. Excretion of acid—impaired, result in metabolic acidosis

f. Calcium/phosphate/vitamin D/bone homeostasis—impaired

g. Erythropoietin production—impaired (normocytic normocytochromic anemia)

h. Endocrine functions—impaired

Clinical Presentation

Patients remain asymptomatic till their GFR declines well below 50 ml/min, and remain unaware. They may be diagnosed during a routine medical examination, or not until they become unwell with advanced stages of CKD. However, depending on the cause, some have symptoms like edema, anemia, nocturia or hypertension. As CKD progresses, and kidney function becomes less effective, various substances known collectively as uremic retention solutes accumulate in the body. Those that exert adverse biological effects are called the 'uremic toxins'. Uremia affects nearly all body systems and organs (Table 23.3).

Investigations in CKD

The investigations for diagnosis of CKD are simple. The basic tests are urine routine examination including microscopy and serum creatinine. Urine for microalbumin would be indicated in patients with diabetes if there was no evidence of proteinuria on urine dipstick. Blood urea is not used to diagnose CKD, since it does not directly reflect changes in GFR. At the same time, serum creatinine is a useful investigation since it reflects the changes in glomerular filtration more accurately compared to other markers and is easily available. The estimated GFR can be calculated from serum creatinine and other parameters by simple formulae. Blood urea may be increased in

---

Table 23.3: Symptoms and signs in CKD stages 3, 4 and 5

- *Urinary abnormalities:* Oliguria, nocturia, frothing, hematuria
- *Anemia*
- *Hypertension*—due to renin mediated or volume overload
- *Edema:* Peripheral, periorbital
- *Gastrointestinal:* Anorexia, nausea, vomiting
- *Dermatological:* Sallow appearance (deposition of pigment 'urochrome' and due to anemia), itching, 'uremic frost', prurigo nodularis, Kyrle's disease
- *Nails:* Burrowing, brittleness and 'half and half' nails
- *Tongue:* Macroglossia, cracked lips
- *Eyes:* Red eye and 'band keratopathy' (rare)
- *Musculoskeletal:* Aches, cramps, 'restless leg syndrome'
- *CKD–mineral bone disease:* Disorders of serum calcium, phosphate, iPTH; renal osteodystrophy, vascular calcifications
- *Pulmonary:* Pleurisy, shortness of breath (due to pulmonary edema or metabolic acidosis—'Kussmaul's breathing' or acidotic breathing), 'flash' pulmonary edema, 'uremic lung' (non-cardiogenic accumulation of proteinaceous fluid in the alveoli with hilar butterfly shadow in X-ray chest)
- *Neurological:* Cognitive impairment, drowsiness, seizures, peripheral neuropathy, dementia, 'dialysis disequilibrium' syndrome
- *Cardiovascular:* Congestive cardiac failure, uremic pericarditis, effusion or tamponade, cardiomyopathy, generalized atherosclerosis, ischemic heart disease
- *Sexual dysfunction:* Decreased libido, infertility
- *Immunological dysregulation:* Predisposition to infections—bacterial, tuberculosis

several non-renal conditions like dehydration, gastrointestinal hemorrhage and steroid therapy. Defective conversion of vitamin D to its active form by the kidney, combined with bone lesions, changes in calcium, phosphorus and vitamin D are collectively called mineral and bone disease (MBD). CKD-MBD includes osteitis fibrosa, osteomalacia, adynamic bone disease and osteopenia. Pathogenesis is complex. Progressive worsening of renal function is associated with retention of phosphates, which leads to a chain of biochemical changes. Hyperphosphatemia leads to hypocalcemia, stimulation of parathyroid, secondary and later tertiary hyperparathyroidism.

The inability of the kidney to excrete 'acid' from the body results in acidosis. Blood urea, serum creatinine, uric acid, phosphorus, calcium, alkaline phosphatase, parathyroid hormone, magnesium, bicarbonate, sodium, potassium and chloride are the usual tests performed to assess the biochemical melieu in stage 3 of CKD onwards.

A renal ultrasound is done to evaluate for kidney size, echotexture, mass lesions and evidence of urinary tract obstruction is done to rule out reversible factors and confirm chronicity. In selective cases a duplex examination for assessment of renal arterial blood flow may be done. Certain infections, such as hepatitis B and C, and HIV are associated with chronic glomerulonephritis. Hence, serological tests for these conditions are also done. A renal biopsy to determine a pathological diagnosis is indicated if a glomerular nephrotic or nephritic syndrome is suspected, or in people with diabetes with atypical presentations such as rapidly progressive kidney failure. Imaging of the genitourinary tract may be helpful in the evaluation of a patient with CKD. Plain abdominal X-ray is a non-specific test that may aid in the detection of calcium-containing kidney stones. It is also useful to detect aortic calcification, which may occur in CKD. Other radiological tests, such as an abdominal CT, are reserved for evaluation of stone disease and further characterization of renal cystic or mass lesions.

Management of CKD

Once the presence of CKD and the disease stage have been established, the following stage-specific clinical action plan is recommended. During stages 1 and 2, the focus should be on treating co-morbid conditions, addressing reduction of cardiovascular risk factors and instituting measures to slow the progression of kidney disease. During these early stages, aggressive blood pressure control is the mainstay of therapy. The primary systemic or renal disease causing CKD should be controlled. In stage 3, in addition to continuing with the measures described, the focus shifts to evaluating and treating complications of CKD, such as anemia and the effects of abnormal mineral metabolism on bone and overall health. By stage 4, preparations for renal replacement therapy (dialysis, transplantation, or both) should begin. When stage 5 is reached, or when symptoms of the uremic syndrome ensue, renal replacement therapy is started.

The management of CKD may be considered under the following three heads:

1. Nephroprotection
2. Treatment of complications of CKD
3. Preparation for renal replacement therapy

Nephroprotection

All attempts should be made to protect the function of the native kidneys. This entails a two-pronged approach, namely trying to reverse the renal impairment by treating the underlying disease, and steps to retard the progression of renal disease. All steps must be taken to find the etiology of renal disease. Appropriate treatment of primary glomerulonephritis, lupus nephritis vasculitis and obstructive nephropathy can often reverse so-called 'CKD'. Since diabetic nephropathy is an important cause of CKD, good control of diabetes with a view to delay renal and systemic complications are important.

Slowing Progression CKD

Given the progressive nature of most forms of CKD, with a continued decrease in the GFR over time, it is important to address factors known to contribute to loss of renal function. Strategies for limiting the progression of CKD are presented in Table 23.4.

Hypertension

The progression of CKD is strongly linked to hypertension control. Elevated blood pressure is associated with a faster decline in GFR in diabetic and non-diabetic kidney disease. Reduction in systemic hypertension slows or prevents progression and the target BP should be 130/85 mm Hg in the absence of proteinuria, and 125/75 mm Hg when proteinuria >1 g/day is present. Treating isolated systolic hypertension in older patients also helps to slow the progression of CKD. Although most antihypertensive medications can be used in CKD, ACE inhibitors are more protective, particularly in proteinuric disease. In patients who cannot tolerate ACE inhibitors, an angiotensin receptor blocker (ARB) may be prescribed.

Proteinuria

Microalbuminuria and proteinuria are well-recognized prognostic factors for the development and progression of CKD. If proteinuria is more than 3 g/day, irrespective of whether the renal disease is glomerular or non-glomerular, faster decline in GFR may occur. By reducing proteinuria by dietary modifications and using ACE inhibitors, better outcomes are obtained in CKD patients. Proteinuria can initiate and cause tubulo-interstitial inflammation and toxicity from filtered proteinaceous compounds like transferrin-iron, albumin-bound fatty acids, inflammatory cytokines and eventually lead to interstitial fibrosis.

Diabetes

Strict blood sugar control with HbA1c <6.5 is advisable in CKD stages 1, 2 and possibly 3a as well. In CKD stages 3b, 4 and 5, the role of tight blood sugar is unclear and may even be detrimental. It is advisable to maintain the HbA1c around 7. Metformin is contraindicated when eGFR <45 ml/min (3b, 4 and 5). SGLT2 inhibitors are contraindicated when eGFR <30 ml/min (CKD 4–5). Self-blood sugar monitoring by the patient at home is very important. Only short acting oral anti-diabetic drugs or insulins are used. As the renal function worsens, the metabolism of endogenously produced insulin is impaired and the duration of action is prolonged. Reduction in oral drug or insulin requirement or development of repeated episodes of hypoglycemia suggest further reduction in GFR.

Table 23.4: Renoprotective strategies for slowing progression of CKD		
Parameter	*Goal*	*Intervention*
Blood pressure control (mm Hg)	<130/80 if proteinuria <1 g/day; <125/75 if proteinuria >1 g/day	ACE inhibitors, ARBs, sodium, restriction, diuretics
Reduction in proteinuria	<0.5 g/day	ACE inhibitors, ARBs
Glycemic control	HbA1c <7%	Dietary counselling, oral hypoglycemic agents, insulin
Dietary protein intake	Minimum of 0.6–0.8 g/kg/day	Dietary counselling
Lipid lowering	LDL <100 mg/dl	Dietary counselling, statins
Lifestyle modifications	Smoking cessation, achieving ideal body weight, regularly exercising	Counselling, exercise program

Treatment of Complications of CKD

Dietary Recommendations

The typical dietary recommendations are shown in Table 23.5. It is important to see that the patient gets adequate dietary counselling.

Sodium and Water Imbalance

Sodium and intravascular volume balance are usually well maintained until the GFR falls below 15 ml/min/1.73 m^2. This is caused by an increase in the fractional excretion of salt and water by the remaining nephrons. The optimal level of daily salt intake varies from patient to patient. Less than 6 g/day of sodium chloride (<2 g/day of sodium) is the typical initial recommendation. Patients with a GFR below 20 ml/min/1.73 m^2 in whom, despite sodium restriction, edema ensues, respond well to diuretic therapy, usually a loop diuretic. Since the ability to concentrate or dilute the urine maximally becomes progressively impaired as GFR declines, patients with stage 4 or 5 CKD tend to be isosthenuric. If the patient has no edema, total fluid intake should be approximately equal to volume of urine output plus an additional volume to account for insensible losses. The insensible loss may vary greatly from region to region depending on factors like atmospheric temperature, body temperature and physical activity.

Potassium Imbalance

Ability of the kidney to excrete potassium is preserved at near-normal levels in patients with CKD as long as both the renin-angiotensin-aldosterone system (RAAS) and distal nephron flow are maintained. Therefore, hyperkalemia develops in oliguric patients, those with GFR lower than 20 ml/min/1.73 m^2, those in whom intake is increased or due to medications causing hyperkalemia (e.g. ACE inhibitors, ARBs, nonsteroidal anti-inflammatory drugs, β-blockers and potassium sparing diuretics). Fatal hyperkalemia may occur when the above factors are combined. Patients with tubulo-interstitial disease are more prone for hyperkalemia. Dietary potassium restriction to <40–70 mEq/day is the mainstay of management of chronic hyperkalemia. If it persists, the next step is the addition of a loop diuretic particularly if hypertension or volume overload is present. Loop diuretics promote urinary potassium loss by increasing sodium delivery to the distal nephron. Smaller doses of potassium-binding resins such as sodium polystyrene sulfonate (Kayexalate) than those typically used for the treatment of acute hyperkalemia, may be given for a short period. The powder is combined with sorbitol (to avoid constipation), if given by oral route. It can also be administered as retention enema in hospitalized patients for acute hyperkalemia. The resin binds with potassium in the bowel lumen and helps to eliminate it through stools. Newer antikalemics like patiromer and zirconium may be given safely for prolonged periods.

Anemia

Anemia is almost a universal finding in patients with stages 3 to 5 CKD and should be looked for when the estimated GFR is lower than 60 ml/min/1.73 m^2. The anemia may be

Table 23.5: Typical dietary recommendations for CKD patients	
Protein	Minimum of 0.6–0.8 g/kg/day (preferably first class protein)
Sodium	<2 g/day (<6 g/day of salt)
Potassium	40–70 mEq/day (restrict in advanced stages of CKD)
Phosphate	600–800 mg/day
Calcium	1400–1600 mg/day (not to exceed 2000 mg/day)
Free water (in excess of urine output)	1–1.5 L/day (achieve output around 2400 ml if possible)

multifactorial. Iron deficiency is common. Typically, anemia due to CKD is normochromic and normocytic and is primarily due to decrease in erythropoietin production by the damaged kidney. Hemoglobin level is maintained around 12 g/dl in women and 13.5 g/dl in men. If a patient with chronic kidney disease has hemoglobin of less than 11 g/dl and symptoms attributable to anemia, treatment to restore hemoglobin to the range 11 to 12 g/dl is warranted. Before the initiation of treatment with erythropoiesis-stimulating agents (ESAs) or by erythropoietin, other common causes of anemia like iron or vitamin B_{12} or folic acid deficiency should be excluded. Treatment involves optimization of iron status, usually using intravenous iron, correction of B12 and folate deficiency and nutritional support. Subsequently, treatment with ESAs is started with periodic monitoring of hemoglobin to achieve target in the range 11 to 12 g/d. Even partial correction of anemia improves physical, physiological, clinical status and offers better 'quality of life' to the patient. However, overcorrection of anemia should be avoided since this is associated with poorer patient outcomes.

Metabolic Acidosis

The ability of the kidneys to buffering the daily net acid production and regenerate bicarbonate diminishes as nephron mass decreases. This occurs because of a defect in a combination of factors involved in acid excretion. The kidneys have to regenerate at least 1 mEq/kg body weight of HCO_3 to excrete the acid which enters the body through diet. In advanced stages of CKD, reduced production of ammonia, decreased filtration of titratable acids (e.g. sulfates, phosphates, urates, hippurates), decreased proximal tubular bicarbonate reabsorption, and decreased renal tubular hydrogen ion secretion occur. The result is the development of non-anion gap metabolic acidosis initially. As the GFR declines further, the anion gap widens due to accumulation of uremic waste products and the serum bicarbonate concentration comes down. The goal of therapy is to maintain the serum bicarbonate concentration at or above 22 mEq/L to avoid the deleterious effects of acidosis on bone histology and protein catabolism. The first-line agent is sodium bicarbonate, 0.5 to 1 mEq/kg/day; a typical starting dosage is 500 mg twice daily, which may be increased cautiously to a maximum of 1 gm thrice daily.

Renal Osteodystrophy and Calcium and Phosphorus Imbalance

The impact of MBD in CKD extends beyond the bones to cardiovascular structure and function, which increases cardiac and vascular complications. Prevention of secondary hyperparathyroidism starts with the control of hyperphosphatemia.

a. Dietary phosphate restriction-regulated use of milk and meat products.

b. Reducing GI absorption by using phosphate binders.

c. If hyperphosphatemia is associated with hypocalcemia, calcium carbonate (as calcium-based phosphate binder) 0.5 to 1.0 g is administered with each meal.

d. If hyperphosphatemia is associated with normal or high serum calcium, calcium-free phosphate binder like sevelamer 400–800 mg with each meal is administered. Lanthanum carbonate in doses of 500–1000 mg with each meal is used to prevent secondary hyperparathyroidism. Cholecalciferol 1000 IU/day is given if the serum 25(OH) D level is low.

e. If iPTH is high and serum calcium and phosphorus are normal, calcitriol 0.125 to 0.25 µg/day/equivalent doses of α-calcidol/other active vitamin D analogues (α-calcidiol, paricalcitol, doxercalciferol) are used. Alternatively, cinacalcet, is used 30 mg OD initially, which may gradually be increased to 60 mg TDS. (Cinacalcit is calcimimetic which renders the calcium receptor more sensitive to calcium.)

f. If iPTH remains high and hypercalcemia/ hyperphosphatemia persist and fail to respond to cinacalcit, consider parathyroidectomy.

g. If patient is already started on dialysis, increase in dialysis frequency, changes in dialysis membrane, reducing dialysate calcium concentration can be tried.

Immunizations

Patients with CKD are prone to develop a variety of infections. Therefore, all patients should be immunized as per the recommendations as under:

- *Hepatitis B vaccine:* Dose is usually twice as compared to individuals who have normal renal function. In CKD, 20 µg (1 ml) each is injected into both deltoid intramuscularly (total 40 µg every dose). A total of four doses at 0, 1, 2 and 6 months are administered for adequate antibody response.

- *Pneumococcal vaccine:* Inj pneumococcal conjugate vaccine is administered intramuscularly once followed at 8–12 weeks by inj pneumococcal polysaccharide vaccine intramuscularly. The pneumococcal polysaccharide vaccine is to be repeated every five years.

- Influenza vaccine is administered yearly.

- Chickenpox vaccine (if the patient did not have the disease earlier)

- In young females human papillomavirus (HPV) vaccine may also be given.

Preparation for Renal Replacement Therapy

Since CKD is a progressive condition, every patient of CKD should be counselled early so that the individual is mentally prepared to accept renal replacement therapy (RRT) when he reaches stage 5. The creation of a vascular access, namely arteriovenous fistula (AVF) should be discussed and planned even during stage 4, since it may take 2–6 months for the AVF to mature. Also, financial arrangements have to be organized before undertaking this expensive therapy. Renal replacement therapy involves a modality of dialysis or a renal transplant (*see* section V, Chapters 24 to 26).

Conclusion

Since CKD is associated with significantly high morbidity and mortality, the management requires a multifaceted approach. Close monitoring of GFR, timely institution of measures to slow progression of the disease, controlling comorbidities like hypertension, diabetes, hyperlipidemia and primary renal disease should be started in the early stages. These initial measures and developing a clinical action plan are best instituted by the primary care provider, with assistance from the nephrologist. As the disease progresses, the roles of the nephrologist increases with steps to determine the cause, initiate specific therapies, to slow down progression, manage complications and later, prepare and execute renal replacement therapy. Special attention should be given to patient education, counselling regarding renal replacement therapy and timely creation of vascular access for those opting for hemodialysis. For those who plan to undergo kidney transplantation, donor evaluation should be done early so that the period on dialysis can be minimized to the minimum.

Renal Replacement Therapies

Peritoneal Dialysis

• K Sampath Kumar

INTRODUCTION

Peritoneal dialysis (PD) as a therapy utilizes transport properties of peritoneum as a semipermeable membrane. It enables removal of water-soluble toxins from the body and normalizes the fluid, electrolyte balance in patients with renal failure. PD can be successfully carried in clinical settings of both AKI and CKD stage 5. In AKI, the main advantages of PD are that the procedure is technically simple, yet efficacious and it can be successfully employed in varied clinical settings without the need for sophisticated machinery. As for chronic PD therapy for end stage renal failure it offers a choice of home-based management which is preferred by those who value their independence from machines. Some of the other advantages over hemodialysis include the absence of post-dialysis fatigue, lower blood loss leading to lesser iron and erythropoietin requirements, lower blood pressure and left ventricular hypertrophy. However, patients require adequate manual dexterity and eyesight to carry on the exchanges by themselves. Else, a dedicated caregiver is necessary.

Anatomy of Peritoneal Membrane

Peritoneal cavity is a large potential serosal sac inside abdomen which is lined by thin mesothelial membrane whose surface area is $1.5–2 \, m^2$ approximating to the body surface area. It has a parietal and visceral layer. The visceral layer of peritoneal membrane covers the bowel forming 80% of surface area of Peritoneum but plays a minor part in peritoneal dialysis. Arterial supply is through the mesenteric arteries while the venous drainage is into portal venous system. The parietal layer of peritoneum lines the inside of anterior abdominal wall and diaphragmatic surface of abdomen. Though forming only 20% of total surface area of peritoneum, it is involved as the primary layer for dialysis in PD. It is supplied by the arteries of the abdominal wall and venous drainage occurs through the IVC. Posteriorly, the peritoneum covers the retroperitoneal structures. The blood flow to the peritoneum varies between 50–100 ml/min. In addition to venous outflow, lymphatic absorption ensures flow of fluid from the peritoneal cavity back into the circulation. Three anatomic areas offer barriers for diffusion: The capillary wall, the interstitium and the mesothelial cell layer. The capillary endothelium contains three different-sized pores which are size selective in restricting solute transport as shown in Fig. 24.1. They are small pores (20–50 Å) which constitute 80% of membrane pores, large pores

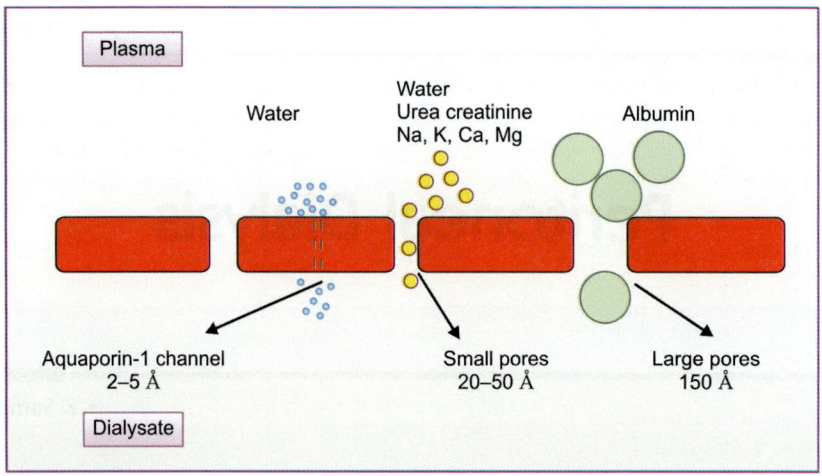

Fig. 24.1: Three-pore model of peritoneal membrane transport in PD

(150Å) which transport macromolecules such as proteins and ultra-small pores of aquaporin-1 which are transcellular water channels of the endothelial cell (2–5 Å).

Principles of Peritoneal Dialysis (Fig. 24.2)

Three transport processes, namely diffusion, ultrafiltration and lymphatic absorption occur simultaneously. Peritoneal membrane is a

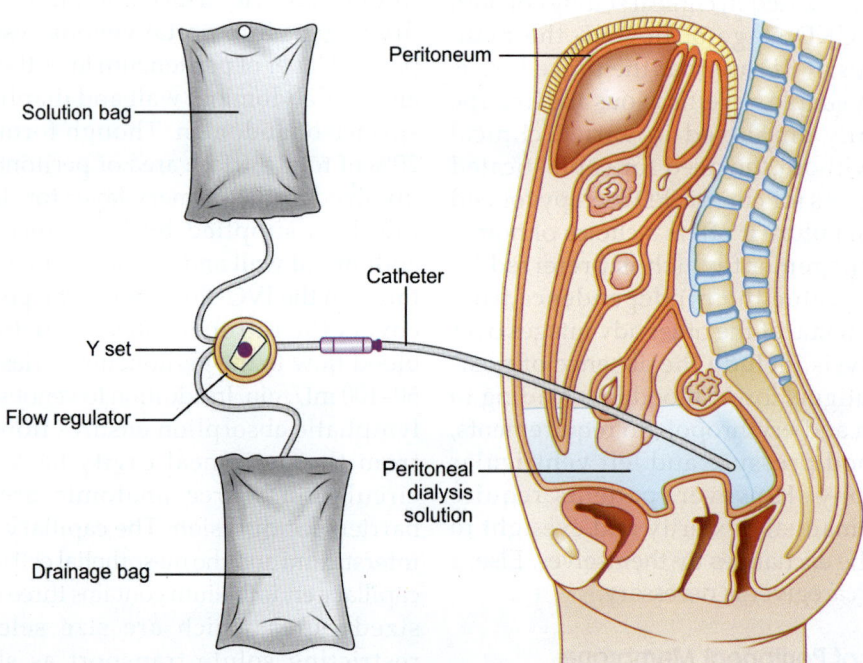

Fig. 24.2: Peritoneal dialysis using double bag system. Note: Flow from solution bag to the peritoneal cavity and drainage from peritoneum to drainage bag are regulated by the flow regulator

semipermeable membrane through which molecules can be transported. The electrolytes and solutes with lower molecular weight like potassium, urea (molecular wt. 60 D), move from the blood to dialysis fluid by diffusion because of the concentration difference. Glucose concentration in regular dialysis fluid ranges from 1.5 to 2.5%. It moves from the dialysis fluid in the peritoneum to the blood by diffusion. Since the tonicity of the peritoneal fluid is high, the osmotic forces draw the water from the blood to the peritoneal fluid. The process by which a solvent moves from an area of lower solute concentration to an area of higher solute concentration through a semipermeable membrane is called osmosis. If the concentration of glucose in dialysis fluid is increased, more osmotic action results in more fluid removal from blood. Ultrafiltration is the process by which the water/solvent moves based on hydrostatic pressure difference between the two sides of the membrane. In peritoneal dialysis, fluid removal occurs mainly by osmosis. This is in contrast to hemodialysis where hydraulic pressure difference ensures ultrafiltration. Since the semipermeable membrane does not permit passage of high molecular weight substances, proteins are not freely filtered. If the membrane is damaged because of infection, more protein leak may occur. If the membrane is grossly thickened, it will not be able to transport water by osmosis resulting in 'ultrafiltration failure'. The flow can be in opposite directions simultaneously if the concentration of different solutes is different on either side. In the above example, simultaneous movement of glucose from peritoneum to blood and urea from blood to peritoneal fluid can occur.

A sterile dialysis fluid containing hypertonic solution of glucose is introduced into the peritoneal cavity through a percutaneous catheter under sterile precautions. The solution comes into contact with capillaries perfusing the peritoneum and viscera. Diffusion of urea and other low molecular substances including other waste products occurs towards the dialysate. A transmembrane osmotic gradient develops because of glucose molecules resulting in ultrafiltration of water from the capillaries into the dialysate. After allowing for an optimal time for these transport processes to occur (dwell time), the fluid is drained out and discarded and the peritoneal cavity is filled again. The diffusion is highest during the first hour and lessens over time. 90% of equilibration for urea and 60% for creatinine occur by 4 hours. Even if the dwell time is increased, further small solute clearance does not occur significantly. However, larger molecular weight solutes can be better removed by longer dwells. The process of inflow, dwell, and outflow constitute one exchange. The end result and efficiency depend on composition and quantity of dialyzed PD fluid. This depends on factors such as the initial composition of the PD fluid, membrane characteristics, duration of dwell time and patient's hemodynamic status. The composition of dialysis fluid varies by glucose concentration as shown in Table 24.1.

Table 24.1: Composition of peritoneal dialysis fluid

pH	5.2
Glucose	1.5% or 2.5% or 4.25%
Sodium	132 mEq/L
Chloride	101 mmol/L
Calcium	3.25 mg%
Magnesium	1.5 mg%
Lactate	32 mmol/L

Patient Selection and Catheter Placement

A patient with ESRD who is not obese and has significant residual urine output can be considered for CAPD catheter placement in preparation for long-term dialysis. This is not the treatment of choice for emergencies. In those with previous laparotomy scars and extensive adhesions or multiple abdominal surgeries, hemodialysis may be preferred. After adequate patient counselling, and informed consent, the patient is prepared for catheter insertion. Meticulous skin care is essential. A silastic double-cuffed catheter with pre-curved swan-neck design (Tenckhoff catheter) is commonly used. This catheter has a straight intra-abdominal portion with multiple side holes of 1 mm size to permit quick inflow and outflow of PD fluid. The 2 cuffs are positioned as follows. The cuff near the peritoneal end is positioned extra-peritoneally on the anterior abdominal wall and the second cuff subcutaneously about 2 cm from the exit site. The catheter is placed by surgical dissection, percutaneously—by Seldinger technique or under vision through laparoscopy. A titanium adapter is attached to the external end of the catheter which in turn is fitted onto a transfer set with Luer lock connection. The system is closed with a secure 'mini-cap' as shown in Fig. 24.3. The implanted catheter is ready for use after 2 weeks.

In CAPD, the manual exchanges are carried out in a clean room with proper hand hygiene. Double bag system with attached tubings made of 'Y' set design have reduced the rates of peritonitis. After secure connections are made a 'flush before fill' technique is employed where the initial fluid which runs in from the suspended PD bag is drained out into the empty bag by clamping the stem of Y set. This ensures that potentially infectious fluid containing bacteria introduced by touch contamination during manual connection are safely drained off. After intra-abdominal infusion of two liters of PD fluid, the twin bags are disconnected and patient is allowed to ambulate for 4–6 hours. In a given day, multiple such two-liter exchanges (commonly three daytime and one long night time) are carried out continuously thereby ensuring a smooth steady state of less severe azotemia. This is in contrast to the saw-tooth pattern of plasma levels of uremic retention solutes seen in a hemodialysis patient. Adequate bowel action enhances the efficiency and constipation should be avoided.

Cycler assisted PD delivers three to six exchanges at night time with a 12-hour exchange at daytime. Thus, its time course of PD exchanges is a mirror image of that with CAPD. Both CAPD and cycler assisted PD have been shown to be equally efficacious and the choice is made by the patient based on preference and cost considerations.

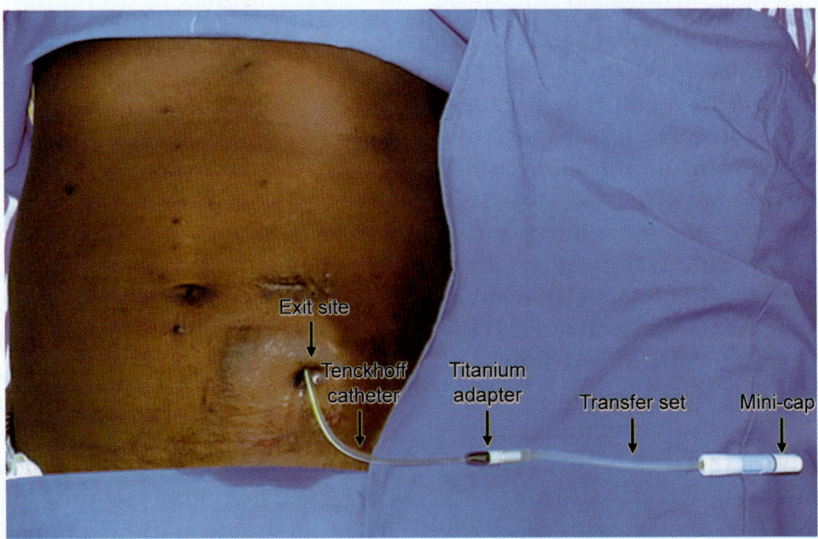

Fig. 24.3: PD catheter with transfer set connection and mini-cap. Note the exit site of PD catheter, titanium adapter, transfer set and mini-cap during 'dwell time'

The transport characteristics of peritoneal membrane are variable and determine the efficiency of peritoneal dialysis. It is determined by studying the time taken for transport of solutes such as dextrose and creatinine across the PD membrane to achieve equilibrium. A standardized peritoneal equilibration test (PET) is done to plan the type of peritoneal dialysis offered. In PET, 2 liters of 2.5% PD fluid is infused and the composition of dialysate drained is studied after second and fourth hours. A rapid transporter is one in whom the membrane transports small solutes rapidly with osmotic equilibration attained within 2–3 hours. Such patients are at a higher risk of fluid overload since higher permeability of PD membrane results in rapid dissipation of osmotic forces. These patients may have difficulty in achieving adequate clearance of uremic solutes by standard CAPD exchanges. Cycler assisted PD is indicated for rapid transporters. On the other hand, slow transporter is one, in whom the glucose absorption is delayed and the osmotic ultrafiltration continues for 6–8 hours resulting in adequate fluid removal from blood. However, solute removal will be limited if the dwell time is short.

Complications of PD

Optimal function of PD catheter is ensured if the catheter tip is placed in the pelvis in the recto-/uterovesical pouch. Liberal use of lactulose and senna is advised to prevent constipation and subsequent mechanical complications and catheter dysfunction. Migration of catheter can occur due to omental entrapment and it acts like a 'one way valve' permitting inflow of PD fluid but blocking/retarding outflow. Since the catheter has a radiopaque line, identification of the position by X-ray will be easy. Repositioning and omentectomy can be performed successfully by surgery or laparoscopy. Back pain is common and is due to increased mechanical stress on the lumbar spine due to lordotic position. Underlying osteoporosis and disc disease will further aggravate the pain. Decreasing dialysate volume is useful but the efficiency of PD comes down. Abdominal pain after PD fluid infusion is due to low pH of fluid. It can be alleviated by injection of 3–5 ml/L of local anesthetic, lignocaine 1% into the dialysate bag. In long-term patients, inguinal, femoral or umbilical hernias may develop in 15% of patients and surgical correction is indicated. Rarely, congenital diaphragmatic defects will lead to rapid onset right-sided pleural effusion soon after instillation of fluid intraperitoneally. If it occurs, fluid is drained immediately. Recurrence is prevented by chemical pleurodesis (with talc, autologous blood or tetracycline) before resuming PD. Other mechanical complication in the form of scrotal leak may be suspected when the patient develops sudden onset hydrocele. Treatment is surgical drainage and closure of patent processus vaginalis. Gastroesophageal reflux, delayed gastric emptying and gastroparesis are relatively common in diabetic patients treated on CAPD. The treatment involves judicious use of oral metoclopramide or erythromycin.

PD solution contains unphysiologically high glucose concentration which results in both hyperglycemia and hyperinsulinemia. This is especially common in diabetic patients initiated on PD. Use of non-glucose polymer in the form of icodextrin reduces the risk of hyperglycemia. Hypokalemia is common in one-third of PD patients which can be treated with oral potassium replacement. If other electrolyte abnormalities like hypernatremia and hypomagnesemia occur, they are managed appropriately.

Protein energy wasting is common in more than two-thirds of CAPD patient population. It is characterized by loss of weight, anorexia and hypoalbuminemia. In a patient who is on 3 exchanges of 1.5% dextrose and one overnight exchange of 2.5% dextrose as much as 332 kcal of glucose is absorbed into plasma per day. The resultant appetite suppression leads to reduced protein intake in the long run. In addition, 6–8 g of albumin is lost daily in peritoneal dialysis . The albumin losses may substantially increase during a peritonitis episode. Hypercatabolism of uremic inflammation also contributes to low albumin levels in PD patients. Elevated ESR and CRP levels in these patients suggest that uremic inflammation also contributes to the overall clinical picture. Management is by increasing protein intake to >1.2 g/Kg per day, ensuring adequacy of PD, increasing the dialysis dose or transfer to hemodialysis either temporarily or permanently.

PD peritonitis is the dreaded complication which threatens both the technique and patient survival. The commonest reason is due to touch contamination of PD fluid by pathogenic skin bacteria during exchanges. Exit site or tunnel infection also may extend to peritoneum. The patient develops abdominal pain which is associated with cloudy effluent dialysate. Diffuse abdominal tenderness is elicited on physical examination. Analysis of PD fluid with total and differential count, gram stain and culture should be done immediately.

An aliquot of 50 ml of PD fluid is centrifuged at 3000 g for 15 minutes. The supernatant is decanted and the sediment is resuspended 5 ml of sterile saline. If the peritoneal dialysis fluid WBC count is more than 100 cells/mm^3 with the differential showing >50% neutrophils, a diagnosis of peritonitis is made and empiric intraperitoneal antibiotic therapy started. The fluid is cultured using both plate and broth media and antibiotics are changed according to culture and sensitivity results subsequently.

In a suspected PD peritonitis empiric intraperitoneal antibiotic therapy covering both gram-positive and gram-negative bacteria should be started with due consideration for the commonly encountered organisms and local sensitivity pattern. A popular initial combination therapy includes either vancomycin or a first-generation cephalosporin for gram-positive coverage and a third-generation cephalosporin or aminoglycoside for gram- negative coverage. Once the culture reports are received the antibiotics are modified according to sensitivity pattern of the organism. Multi-drug resistant bacteria are increasingly encountered mandating use of carbapenems. Table 24.2 describes the pathogenesis and treatment of commonly encountered organisms in PD peritonitis.

Once prompt antibiotic therapy is started, the usual clinical course is characterized by a reduction of abdominal pain along with clearing of effluent PD fluid signifying resolution of peritonitis. But if symptoms persist even after five days of antibiotic therapy and the dialysate remains cloudy, catheter is removed and patient transferred to hemodialysis at least temporarily. Fungal peritonitis is usually managed by prompt catheter removal and antifungal therapy. Rarely, a patient who is treated for recurrent peritonitis ends up with encapsulating sclerosing peritonitis which is a life-threatening condition. Approach to prevention of peritonitis is crucial for the long-term success of peritoneal dialysis. A multipronged strategy is required including use of double cuffed catheters, double bag systems, titanium adapter and adequate and fool-proof connectology. Adequate training, proper hand hygiene, performing flush before fill technique and periodic surveillance while performing the exchanges help to prevent infective episodes in CAPD.

PD for AKI

PD offers many advantages in the setting of AKI since it is technically easy to perform, requires far less complex logistics for set up than HD, provides adequate clearances of solutes and the final outcomes are almost equal to HD. It can be successfully employed to treat patients who are hemodynamically unstable and in children with AKI. PD can be successfully carried out for AKI due to rhabdomyolysis occurring in natural disasters in the field settings. Snake bite, poisonings, diarrhea, sepsis, cardiorenal and hepato-renal syndromes are some of the commonest indications for PD. Systemic anticoagulation is not required which makes it a viable option in AKI associated with bleeding diathesis.

In AKI, PD can be initiated by percutaneous insertion of a stiff temporary catheter at the midline below the umbilicus after filling up the abdomen with PD fluid via 16 gauge needle. The stiff plastic catheter with stylet is introduced into the peritoneal cavity, the stylet removed and the catheter with perforations stationed in intra-abdominal portion. The catheter is fixed to the skin at the exit site. Exchanges can be started immediately with 1–2 liters of PD fluid which is drained after variable dwell time. Usually 30 minutes to 2 hours of dwell time is allowed for equilibration between blood and peritoneal fluid before draining to external collecting bag. About 20 such exchanges are given, one after the other over 48–72 hours. Heparin in a dose of 500 units/L is added to dialysis fluid to prevent fibrin clot formation. Since heparin is not absorbed through the peritoneum it is not contraindicated even in systemic bleeding diathesis with AKI. Although the fluid removal and clearance of waste products is not as rapid as hemodialysis, the removal is adequate for management of usual types of AKI.

Complications of PD in AKI include bowel or bladder injury during insertion of catheter and risk of infection which escalates after 3 days of acute peritoneal dialysis. Newer techniques involving insertion of soft cuffed catheters have resulted in reduced rates of infection and better outcomes comparable to hemodialysis. However, PD is relatively contraindicated in recent laparotomy, florid acute pulmonary edema, severe hyperkalemia with impending cardiac arrest and in states of hypercatabolism. In hypercatabolic types of AKI, rapid rise of urea, creatinine and potassium levels occur and PD cannot achieve adequate clearance. Such patients should be treated by hemodialysis.

Table 24.2: Common organisms, source and drugs used in PD peritonitis

Organism	Pathogenesis	Antibiotic dose
Staphyloccoccus epidermidis	Touch contamination	IP* vancomycin 15–30 mg /kg q 5–7 days or cefazolin 500 mg/L loading dose followed by 125 mg/L on all bags for 14 days
Staphylococcus aureus	Skin, nasal colonization	IP vancomycin 15–30 mg/kg q5–7 days for 21 days along with oral rifampicin 300 mg 5 days for nasal carriers. Consider catheter removal
Enteric gram-negative organisms (E. coli, Klebsiella)	Bowel, urinary tract	IP amikacin 2 mg/kg on a single exchange per day or cefepime 500 mg/L as loading dose followed by 125 mg/L in all bags Imipenem—cilastatin at loading dose of 250 mg/L followed by 50 mg/L in all bags in ESBL producing gram-negative bacteria
Pseudomonas species	Skin and bowel colonization, tunnel infection	Ceftazidime 500 mg/L followed by 125 mg/L in all bags for 21 days. Consider catheter removal
Candida, Aspergillus	Repeated antibiotic use	Prompt catheter removal

*IP: Intraperitoneal

Outcomes of PD

Patients starting on PD have survival rates which are equal or superior to hemodialysis especially in the first two years. Residual renal function is crucial for the success of PD. In later years emotional burn out both of the patient and caregiver may pose a problem for long- term continuation of PD. Adequate and periodic counselling of the patient and care-giver should be undertaken. These patients can be taken up for renal transplantation safely and the PD catheter removed after ensuring optimal graft function. In summary, peritoneal dialysis is an excellent form of renal replacement therapy providing the patient with an option of home dialysis. Peritonitis free clinical course is crucial for its long-term viability. The outcomes of PD are almost equal to and not inferior to hemodialysis especially in the first few years of its inception. It should be included as modality choice during the counselling sessions for patients in the predialysis period.

Hemodialysis, CRRT and Other Extracorporeal Therapies

• Ravi Shankar Bonu

INTRODUCTION

Hemodialysis (HD) is purification blood outside the body (extracorporeal), and involves circulation of blood through a hemodialyzer also known as artificial kidney. The blood is passed through the dialyzer made which is up with a semisynthetic membrane. The nitrogenous toxins are removed from blood through this membrane and the cleansed blood is returned to the body. The process is controlled by a dialysis machine, which pumps the blood through the extracorporeal circuit and regulates the cleaning process.

Continuous renal replacement therapy (CRRT) also known as slow continuous therapy is a form of extracorporeal blood purification often done in patients who are critically ill. Critically ill patients often have multiorgan dysfunction often associated with acute kidney injury (AKI) and many such patients need dialysis support. CRRT is usually done for 24 to 96 hours with lower blood flow and dialysis flow rates. This principle make this modality a better option for critically ill and who have very low blood pressure and tolerated well. Adequate solute, fluid removal, better correction of acidosis and maintenance of blood pressure can be achieved.

In this chapter, the following sections are covered:

1. Basic principles of dialysis treatment
2. Requirements for hemodialysis treatment
3. Hemodialysis procedure
4. Indications for hemodialysis
5. Complications of hemodialysis
6. Continuous renal replacement therapy (CRRT).
7. Other extracorporeal therapies
   a. Plasmaphresis/plasma exchange (PLEX)
   b. Hemoperfusion
   c. Extracorporeal membrane oxygenation (ECMO)
   d. Molecular absorbant recirculating system (MARS)

BASIC PHYSICAL PRINCIPLES OF DIALYSIS TREATMENT

The basic principle of hemodialysis involves the following physical principles, convection, diffusion, ultrafiltration and osmosis. Based on these principles dialysis helps to remove accumulated nitrogenous products like urea, creatinine, potassium and fluid from the blood. It also helps to provide the body with missing electrolytes by using dialysate or dialysis fluid during the process of dialysis.

Diffusion is a process by which solute particles move from an area of higher solute concentration to lower solute concentration across a semipermeable membrane. In patient with renal failure, hemodialysis enables solute particles in higher concentration in blood like urea, creatinine and potassium move from blood compartment to dialysate. The other electrolytes in the blood also move across the membrane and normalize the blood levels since the composition of dialysate is nearly the same as normal plasma.

Convection is the process which allows movement of water (solvent) across the semipermeable membrane based on pressure gradient. The movement of water is from an area of higher hydrostatic pressure to lower hydrostatic pressure. The dialysis machine can regulate the pressure gradient across the membrane and the fluid removal can be regulated by the operator by adjusting the machine. The removal of fluid from patient blood by convection also called ultrafiltration which depends not only on the pressure gradient but also the characteristics of the membrane.

Osmosis is the process in which the solvent moves from an area of lower solute concentration to higher solute concentration across a semipermeable membrane. Osmosis and osmotic pressure are applicable more in peritoneal dialysis.

Reverse osmosis (RO) is the process opposite of osmosis wherein the fluid is made to move using pressure pump to achieve high hydrostatic pressure from higher solute concentration to an area of lower solute concentration (against the normal osmotic forces). This principle is used in water treatment to supply pure water needed for dialysis. Regular water filter, carbon filter, water softener, deionizer RO and ultraviolet irradiation are used to procure adequate water quality for dialysis.

REQUIREMENTS FOR HEMODIALYSIS TREATMENT

There are three basic requirements for performing hemodialysis.
a. Vascular access

b. Artificial kidney
c. Dialysis monitor.

a. Vascular Access

Vascular access is the lifeline for a patient on hemodialysis treatment. It can enable removal of blood from patient body with the help of a hemodialysis machine for circulation through extracorporeal circuit consisting of blood artificial kidney and return purified blood to the body after. It can be either temporary or permanent access.

The temporary vascular access is usually obtained by inserting double lumen dialysis catheters into one of major veins such as internal jugular, femoral or subclavian veins. It is most often done for patients with acute kidney injury and are often removed after a few days to a few weeks (Fig. 25.1).

Permanent vascular access is usually:
  i. Arteriovenous fistula (AVF)
 ii. Arteriovenous graft (AVG)
iii. Permanent catheter

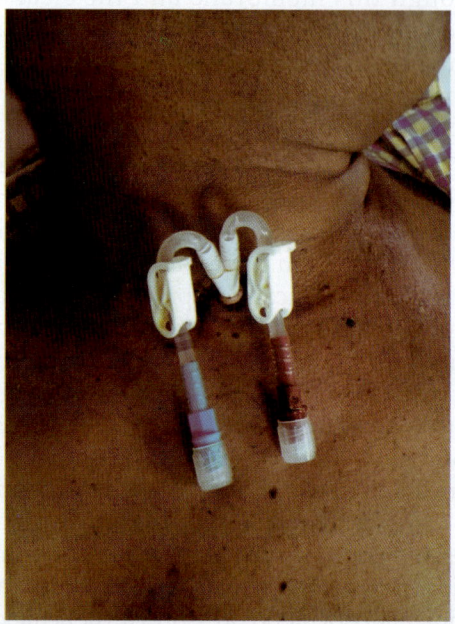

Fig. 25.1: Non-cuffed double lumen (temporary) dialysis catheter inserted into right internal jugular vein in the neck

i. Arteriovenous fistula (AVF) is created by surgically anastomosing radial artery to cephalic vein at the wrist (radiocephalic AV fistula) (Fig. 25.2) or brachial artery to basilic vein or cephalic vein at the elbow (brachiobasilic or brachiocephalic AV fistula) in the arm. AVF is more biological, less expensive and function longer and is the other accesses and is the accesses of choice for patient on maintenance hemodialysis. It should be done electively, few weeks to months before the anticipated time of initiating dialysis. Once the blood

from the artery flows directly through the vein, the vein enlarges, the muscle layer hypertrophies and the wall thickens. This process is known as 'arterialization of the vein'. This will enable smooth dialysis with optimal blood flow and smooth venous return. The usual time to counsel, plan and create AVF is before the patient reaches stage CKD 5, the recommended time for AVF is at stage 4 CKD when the eGFR is 15–30 ml/min.

ii. Arteriovenous graft (AVG) is created by anastomosing one end of the graft to

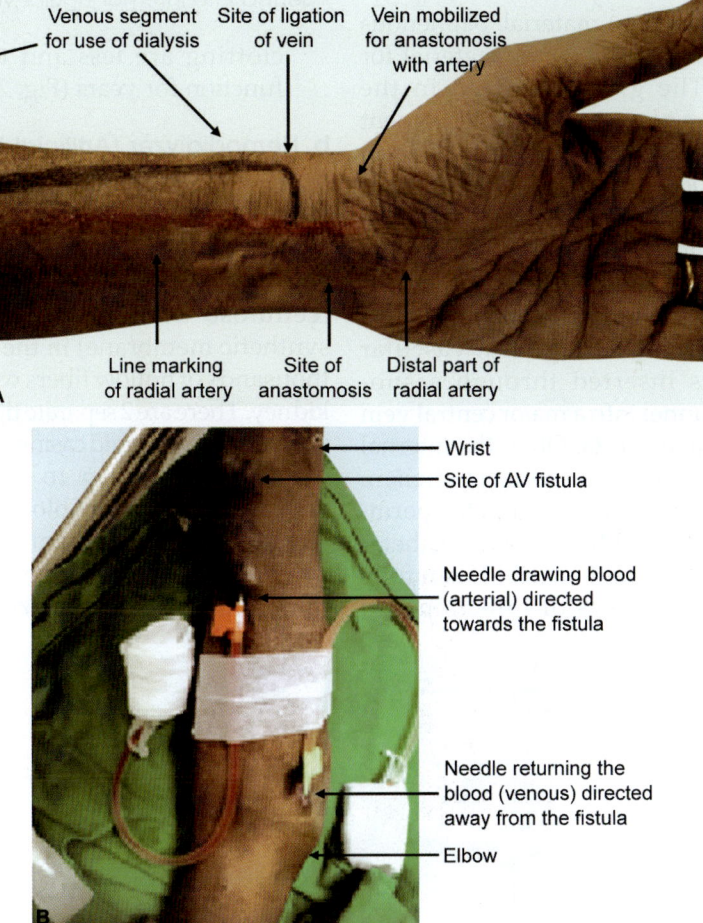

Fig. 25.2A and B: AV fistula: Created at wrist by anastomosing cephalic vein to radial artery. (A) Diagram of left radiocephalic AV fistula; (B) Photo of radiocephalic fistula cannulation by 'buttonhole' technique

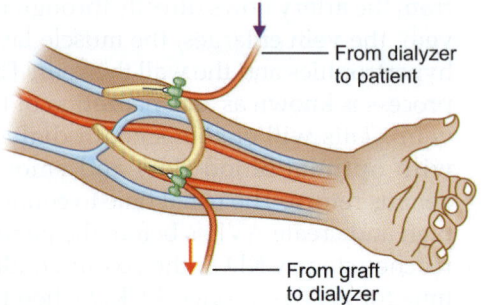

Fig. 25.3: U-shaped AV graft in forearm

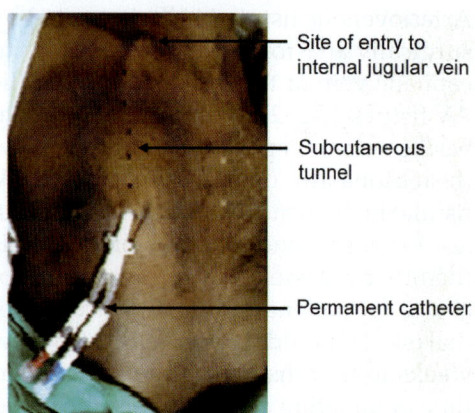

Fig. 25.4: A tunneled double-cuffed permcath inserted into internal jugular vein

radial or brachial artery and the other end to the basilica/cephalic vein at the elbow. The graft is often a synthetic PTFE (poly-tetrafluoroethylene) material. Saphenous vein can also be used as the material for AV graft. The graft is placed in the subcutaneous plane as a straight segment from wrist to elbow or like an 'U' from elbow to elbow (Fig. 25.3). The time for maturing of AVG is lesser than AVF but chances of thrombosis are higher.

iii. *Permanent central venous catheter (permcath):* It is a cuffed double lumen vascular catheter used as a long-term vascular access. It is inserted through a subcutaneous tunnel into a major central vein under local anesthesia. Often the internal jugular or subclavian vein is chosen. Compared to temporary catheter permcatheter is long and the tip of the catheter is usually in the right atrium. If carefully handled the chances of infection and clotting are less and the catheter can function for years (Fig. 25.4).

b. Hemodialyzer (Artificial Kidney)

Earlier, dialysis membranes in the form of cuprophane sheets in the configuration of parallel plates were used. The artificial kidney used now consists of the dialysis membrane (cellulose acetate or polysulfone semi-synthetic membrane) in the configuration of thousands of hollow fibers within the artificial kidney. There are 2 separate tight compartments surrounded by a rigid casing. One compartment through the lumen to the hollow fibers permits movement of blood in one direction. The second compartment outside the hollow fibers enables movement of dialysis fluid (Figs 25.5 and 25.6). Dialyzer is the important

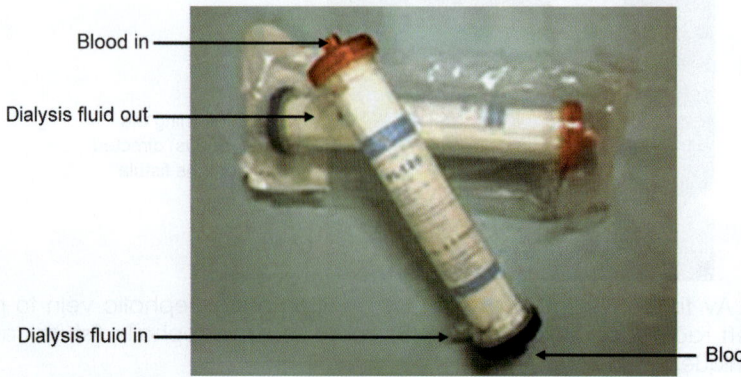

Fig. 25.5: Hollow fiber artificial kidney

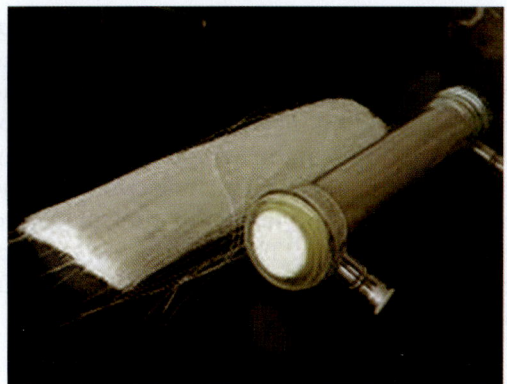

Fig. 25.6: Hollow fiber. Hemodialyzer shows the fibers removed from the casing

component of dialysis where the actual removal of waste products and water from the blood and gain of substances like bicarbonate, calcium, sodium, glucose useful for the body occurs.

c. Hemodialysis Machine/Monitor

The hemodialysis machine is an ultramodern mobile unit with various monitoring systems (Fig. 25.7). Essentially, it takes in treated water provided by the water treatment system, mixes the optimum amount of hemodialysis concentrate from the concentrate container and prepares the fluid. The mixed fluid is checked online for temperature and concentra-

tion. If suitable, the dialysis fluid is circulated through the artificial kidney and returned to the machine. The usual dialysate flow rate is 500–800 ml/min. The dialysate leaving the artificial kidney is checked for blood leak, quantity of fluid removed from the body and the used dialysis fluid is discarded. The machine has inbuilt blood pumps to propel the blood through the blood tubings, syringe pumps to add prescribed doses of heparin into the blood lines, monitor the pressures in the extracorporeal circuit, detect foam or air in the blood and shut off the blood circuit in case of any alarm situation. The knobs or touch screen in the machine will enable the technologist/nurse to set the parameters as prescribed.

Dialysis machine works with electric power and has an inbuilt battery backup system as another important safety feature. Some features of dialysis machine can also be used for other procedures like hemofiltration, hemoperfusion and plasmaphresis. Separate and more sophisticated similar machines are available for continuous renal replacement therapy (CRRT).

Other requirements for hemodialysis.

Anticoagulation

Anticoagulation of blood is very essential to prevent clotting of the blood while the blood is

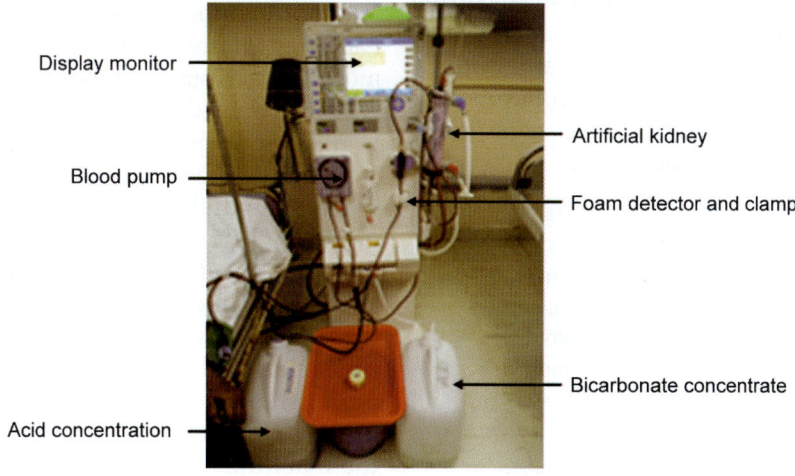

Fig. 25.7: HD monitor

circulated in the extracorporeal circuit. A proper anticoagulation will allow adequate removal of solutes and water during the treatment. Clotting of the extracorporeal circuit will result interruption of treatment and needs changing of the dialyzer and blood tubings. The dose of heparin used can be decided earlier and administered as an initial bolus followed by constant infusion. The adequacy of anticoagulation is monitored by testing blood for activated partial thromboplastin time (APTT) during the dialysis session. It is also possible to neutralize the excess of heparin by using protamine sulphate injection. In some circumstances, when heparin or anticoagulation is contraindicated, it will be possible to offer 'heparin free' dialysis in which, saline rinses are given periodically during dialysis and the excess saline given is removed by increasing ultrafiltration. Other anticoagulation methods like 'citrate anticoagulation' are also coming into vogue.

Dialysis Fluid Concentrate

Since each session of 4 hours of dialysis require 120 liters of dialysate fluid or dialysate. This is prepared by the machine from 34 volumes of water and 1 volume of concentrate. Thus, about one liter of dialysis concentrate per hour will be used by the machine for each 4-hour session of hemodialysis. The dialysis fluid delivered to the artificial kidney will have composition almost identical with normal plasma and contain glucose, sodium, potassium, calcium, bicarbonate with pH close to normal. The concentration of electrolytes in the dialysis fluid is:

a.	Glucose	0–200 mg%*
b.	Sodium	135–145 mmol/L**
c.	Chloride	98–124 mmol/L
d.	Potassium	0–4 mmol/L
e.	Calcium	2.5–3.5 mmol/L
f.	Magnesium	0.5–0.75 mmol/L
g.	Bicarbonate	30–45 mmol/L
h.	pH	7.1–7.4

*Concentration can be adjusted in the concentrate
**Minor changes can be set in the machine

Since the dialysate is made to run in an opposite direction (countercurrent) to the blood flow through the hemodialyzer, the efficiency is enhanced. The composition of dialysate fluid can be adjusted by changing concentration of a particular electrolyte in the concentrate depending on the need and clinical situation. The facility for sodium profiling will enable automatic variation in sodium concentration during hemodialysis.

Water Supply

Water treatment plant with facilities for pretreatment of regular water supply by filtration, softening, carbon filter and deionizing (if needed) followed by reverse osmosis is an integral part of any hemodialysis treatment facility. The success and the quality of hemodialysis facility depend on good quality of water used for dialysis. The water treatment unit usually placed in the proximity of the dialysis facility as this water will be fed to the machine throughout the procedure.

Infrastructure and Manpower

The dialysis facility or unit is a specified area in a hospital or satellite unit where the dialysis equipment is placed with dialysis chairs or the cots for the patients to have the treatment. It is usually segregated area with restrictions of entry of people to prevent cross infection. Facilities for entertainment are provided in most dialysis rooms for the benefit of patients. A team of trained dialysis nurses or technicians is needed to perform and supervise the dialysis treatment. The role of dialysis nurse is to start the dialysis treatment, monitor the patient while the dialysis treatment is in the process and the end of the treatment. The dialysis nurse carries out the dialysis prescription given by a nephrologist or renal physician and also gives feedback of any patient complications that occur during dialysis treatments. The technical aspects of the machine are generally handled by the technician.

HEMODIALYSIS PROCEDURE

The patient is received in dialysis room, vital signs recorded, predialysis weight is taken, weight gained after the previous dialysis recorded, target weight loss calculated and the patient is moved to the couch or bed. Sterile artificial kidney with blood lines are primed with heparinized saline are assembled in the machine for the extracorporeal blood circuit (Fig. 25.8). After cleaning the access site, the veins are cannulated in the case of AV fistula and the lines connected to the extracorporeal blood circuit and hemodialysis started (Fig. 25.9). The vital signs are monitored over

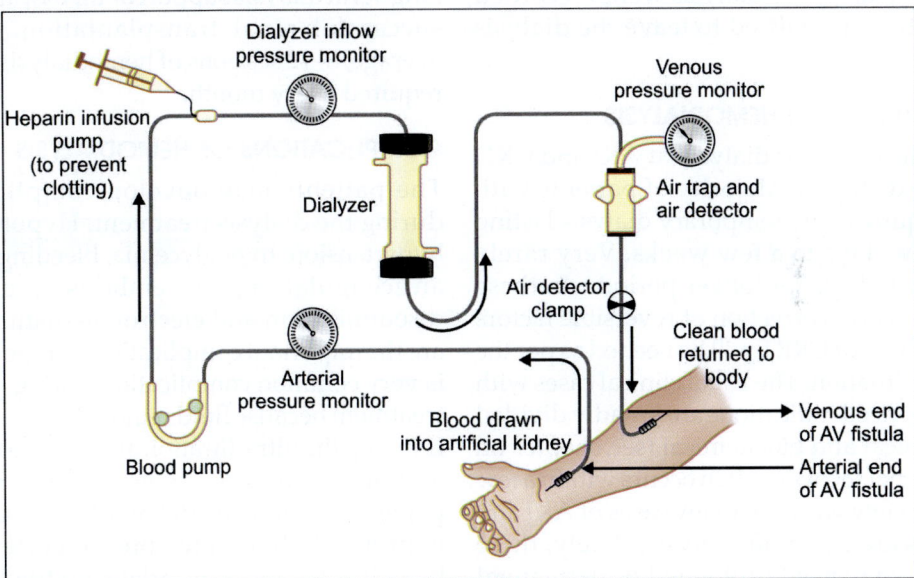

Fig. 25.8: Hemodialysis extracorporeal circuit. Patient's blood is drawn from 'arterial' end of the AV fistula (the dilated 'arterialized' vein), circulated through the arterial pressure monitor, blood pump, heparin infusion site, dialyzer, air trap, venous pressure monitor, air bubble detector and clamp and returned to patient through the venous end of AV fistula

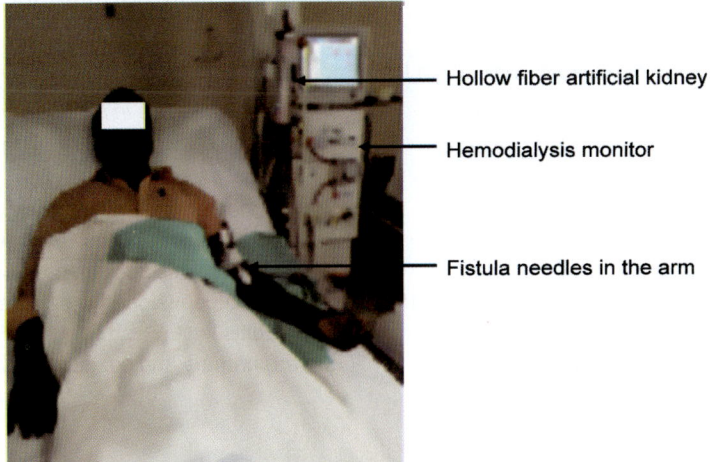

Fig. 25.9: Hemodialysis in progress. Patient undergoing dialysis through left high radial AV fistula

the next 4 hours. Blood sample is taken after 2 hours for APTT test to confirm adequacy of anticoagulation. At the end of dialysis, the blood is returned, the artificial kidney and tubing's prepared for reuse or discarded as per the hospital protocol. After achieving homeostasis, the patient is observed for some time, BP rechecked, post-dialysis weigh recorded and patient permitted to leave the dialysis room.

INDICATIONS FOR HEMODIALYSIS

The indications for dialysis in AKI and CKD may be different. Majority of patients with AKI requires only temporary dialysis lasting for a few days to a few weeks. Very rarely require dialysis for longer periods. In these patients, early correction of reversible factors and dialysis or CRRT will be needed as per the clinical situation. The usual clinical cases with AKI that need indications are broadly divided into clinical and biochemical (see chapter on AKI). Renal recovery often occurs within a few days to a few weeks in many cases of AKI and patients are taken off dialysis. Rarely, these patients may need prolonged or permanent dialysis. The emergency clinical indications in AKI and CKD are fluid overload, acute pulmonary edema and hyperkalemia, uremic symptoms, pericarditis and severe acidosis (Table 25.1).

Chronic or longstanding diseases like diabetes, hypertension, glomerular and interstitial diseases progress gradually to kidney damage with progressively decrease in glomerular filtration. A patient usually needs dialysis at CKD stage 5 when the GFR is less than 15/ml/minute. Such patients require long-term dialysis support or till they undergo successful renal transplantation. On an average, 8–12 sessions of hemodialysis will be required every month.

COMPLICATIONS OF HEMODIALYSIS

The patients may develop complications during the dialysis treatment. Hypotension, hypertension, hypoglycemia, bleeding due to anticoagulation, air embolism, dialysis disequilibrium and electrolyte disturbances are the important complications. Hypotension is very common complication during dialysis treatment because fluid removal. The first step is to stop the ultrafiltration and elevate the foot end of bed to improve venous return. If it persists, infusion of 100 ml of normal saline improves the blood pressure. Reccurrence can be prevented by appropriate modification of fluid removal and weight adjustments. Hypotension may occur rarely due to dialyzer reactions that occur when patient's blood is exposed to dialyzer membrane. Most patients who have near normal blood pressures on

Table 25.1: Indications for hemodialysis in AKI and CKD*	
Indications for dialysis in patients with AKI	*Indications for dialysis in patients with CKD*
• Volume expansion that cannot be managed with diuretics.	• Hyperkalemia >7.0 mmol/L and refractory to medical therapy.
• Hyperkalemia refractory to medical therapy (>6.5 mmol/L).	• Severe metabolic acidosis pH <7.2
• Correction of severe acid–base disturbances that are refractory to medical therapy HCO_3 <12	• Fluid overload unresponsive to diuretics
• Severe azotemia (BUN >80–100)	• Uremic symptoms such as nausea, vomiting, poor appetite, encephalopathy, seizures
• Daily rise of BUN >25 mg/dl	• Pericarditis
• Daily rise of creatinine >1 mg/dl	• Severe pruritus and coagulopathy
• Daily fall in HCO_3 >5 mmol/L	
• Urine output <5 ml/ hour for 12 hours	

* The indications may vary depending on clinical circumstances.

antihypertensive drugs, are advised to hold the immediate 'pre-dialysis dose' of the antihypertensive drug to prevent hypotension during dialysis.

Dialysis disequilibrium is a common complication which may occur during the first hour of dialysis treatment particularly when dialysis is initiated for the first time. It is more common in patients who have been uremic for a long time and is due to rapid removal of urea resulting in development of cerebral edema. When dialysis clears urea from the blood rapidly, the serum osmolality decreases suddenly. The urea in the tissues remains high. The osmotic difference will drive the fluid from intravascular to interstitial compartment. The resultant cerebral edema and raised intra-cranial pressure lead to altered sensorium, seizures and even 'coning' of medulla oblongata. Identification of dialysis disequlibrium is important as it needs intravenous hypertonic saline to maintain the serum osmolality to prevent cerebral edema. It is for this reason that the patient is given short courses of relatively ineffective dialysis for slow urea removal. This is done by permitting co-current flow within the dialyzer and reduction in blood flow rate aimed to reduce the efficiency of urea removal.

Electrolyte imbalances may occur rarely during dialysis. Most common are hypo-kalemia, hyponatremia, hypercalcemia. They can be managed by appropriate modification in the dialysis concentrate. Patients with hypokalemia needing dialysis can be dialyzed by increasing the potassium concentration in the dialysis concentrate to provide 4 mmol instead of the usual 2 mmol/L concentration. Minor changes in dialysis sodium can be made by adjusting the sodium profiling in most of the modern machines. Since electrolyte abnormality may result in cardiac arrhythmias leading to cardiac arrest, they must be looked for and corrected. Cardiac arrest may occur during hemodialysis and the incidence is nearly 100 times greater than the chances in general population.

Air embolism, though rare, can occur due to sucking of air due to breach in connections of the extracorporeal circuit. This causes entry of air into the venous system and even the lungs resulting in low cardiac output and cardiac arrest. Air embolism is a medical emergency and needs appropriate measures to remove the air from the circulation.

Pericardial tamponade is another rare but a serious complication which can cause severe hypotension and cardiac arrest. An echocardio-graphy should be done in any patient who has prior pericardial effusion with unexplained hypotension. If a patient diagnosed to have pericardial tamponade needs immediate pericardiocentesis.

With the recent developments, refinements in the methods, modern technology used in dialysis machines, hemodialysis has become a relatively smooth procedure and the complica-tions are minimized with timely appropriate monitoring.

CONTINUOUS RENAL REPLACEMENT THERAPY (CRRT)

CRRT has some advantages over conventional HD in critically ill patients and the procedure requires a different machine and adequate replacement fluid. The blood and dialysis parameters are also different from HD (Table 25.2).

CRRT machine has a display monitor and other safety features with different pumps to run the blood, dialysate fluid, replacement fluid. The vascular access is usually a temporary double lumen internal jugular, subclavian or femoral vein catheter. As the blood is withdrawn from patient, heparin is infused with help of an inbuilt heparin pump to prevent clotting of blood. The blood then enters the hemofilter. A commercially prepared replacement fluid with the composition similar to normal plasma is added to the blood line either before or after the hemofilter. The dialysis fluid will be run through the hemofilter opposite direction blood flow as in

Table 25.2: Parameters for CRRT as compared to HD

Parameter	CRRT	HD
1 Dialysate flow	50–200 ml/min	200–350 ml/min
2 Blood flow rate	16–20 ml/min	500–800 ml/min
3 Replacement fluid	Yes	No
4 Anticoagulation	Heparin	Heparin
5 Vascular access	Temporary (central line, femoral, internal jugular)	Permanent (AVF or AVG or perm catheter)
5 Duration of therapy	24 to 72 hours	3–4 hours

hemodialysis. The hemofilter filters the blood and the ultrafiltrate which come from the out port of the hemofilter is collected into the effluent bag. The total effluent or filtrate is measured and replaced continuously as replacement fluid. The purified blood is returned to the patient (Fig. 25.10). As in hemodialysis, there are pressure monitors and controllers in the control panel to regulate the volumes removed and added.

CRRT works on the principles of solute removal (diffusion) and fluid removal (convection) similar to HD, but the process is slow and continuous. There are four important modalities of CRRT.

a. *Slow continuous ultrafiltration (SCUF):* This modality of CRRT is primarily used only when volume overload is the problem and there are no electrolyte and acid–base problems. There is neither dialysate nor replacement fluid used in this modality. Generally low flux dialysis membrane filters which remove fluid slowly are used to remove fluid at the rate of 2–5 ml/min or about 3 to 5 liters per day. The urea clearance rate is only 1.5 to 2.0 ml/min.

b. *Continuous venovenous hemofiltration (CVV-HF):* In this modality, principle of convection is employed. Generally high flux membranes capable of higher ultrafiltra-

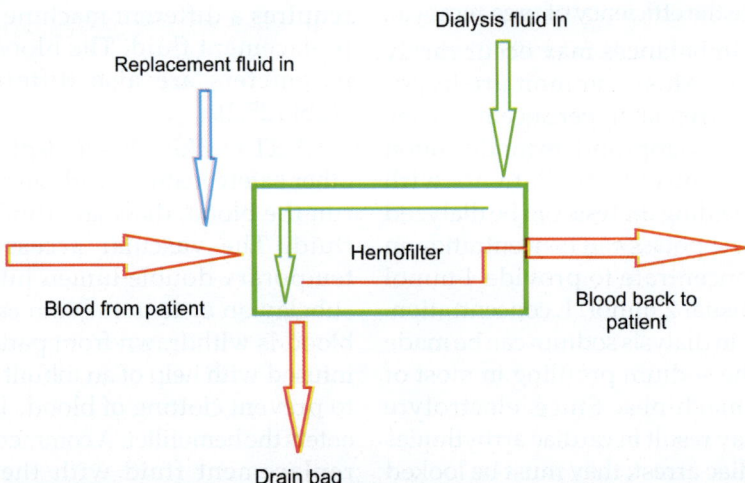

Fig. 25.10: The CRRT extracorporeal circuit is a closed loop by which blood is delivered to hemofilter and retuned back patient after purification. Replacement fluid is added to blood and dialysis fluid is added to hemofilter. The effluent fluid and dialysis fluid are drained, measured and appropriate volume replaced

tion rate are used and can remove fluid at the rate of 10–30 ml/min (15 to 50 liters per day). The urea clearance is between 20 to 70 ml/min and it increases with higher rate of fluid removal. As the rate of fluid removal is high, there is need to replace of 85 to 90% of the fluid removed depending on the volume status of the patient so as to prevent volume depletion and hypotension. As the replacement fluids contain bicarbonate, acidosis also corrected. The cost of the procedure including large volumes of sterile replacement fluid is very high.

c. *Continuous venovenous hemodialysis (CVV-HD):* This modality of CRRT works on the principle diffusion. Here, the dialysate is used as in hemodialysis but the procedure is done at a slow rate for a longer duration. The urea clearance is between 20–25 ml/min and the fluid removal is 3–5 liters a day. Therefore, large volumes of replacement fluid are not necessary.

d. *Continuous venovenous hemodiafiltration (CVV-HDF):* This modality works by principle of both diffusion and convection. As the name implies, in hemodiafiltration, both dialysis and fluid removal are combined at slower rate compared to CVV-HD and CVV-HF. So, this procedure also needs both replacement and dialysis fluids. The urea clearance is 30 to 60 ml/min and the fluid removal is 10–30 ml/min or 15 to 50 liters per day.

The main indication for CRRT is AKI in critically ill, unstable patients with multiple clinical and biochemical abnormalities. In addition to renal indications, there are some non-renal indications for CRRT in critically ill patients (Table 25.3).

e. *Slow continuous therapies:* The type of modality depends on the clinical circumstances and laboratory parameters. Patients with gross fluid overload, minimal acid–base abnormalities, nearly normal potassium and mild elevation of renal parameters in whom, fluid removal is the main concern,

Table 25.3: Renal and non-renal indications for CRRT

Renal	Non-renal
Severe form of AKI	Septic shock
Oliguria >24 hours	ARDS
Severe acidosis	Liver failure
Volume overload	Poisonings
Hyperkalemia	Septic shock
Uremic encephalopathy	

are managed with slow continuous ultra-filtration (SCUF). Patients with fluid over load, severe metabolic acidosis, and mild elevations of BUN/creatinine, where fluid removal and correction of acidosis are necessary, are treated by CVV-HF. If a patient has fluid overload, severe acidosis, uremia and hyperkalemia who needs fluid removal, correction of acidosis, control of uremia and hyperkalemia are subjected to CVV-HDF (Fig. 25.11).

Urea removal is higher with hemodialysis treatment (180–240 ml/min) whereas, it is lower in CRRT (20–70 ml /min). The lower efficiency is compensated by continuous treatment for done for 48–72 hours. CRRT has

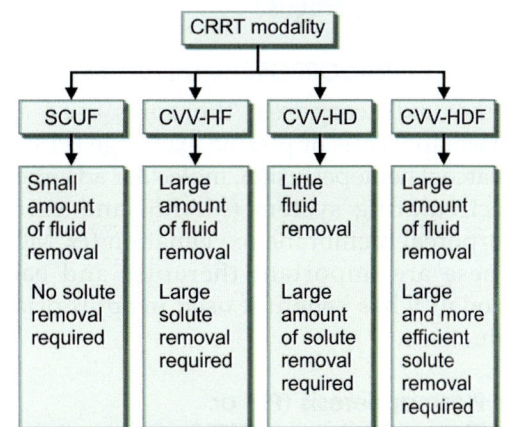

Fig. 25.11: Different CRRT modalities and their clearances. Slow continuous ultrafiltration (SCUF), continuous venovenous hemofiltration (CVV-HF), continuous venovenous hemodialysis (CVV-HD), continuous venovenous hemodiafiltration (CVV-HDF)

advantages over hemodialysis in patients who have compromised hemodynamic status and multi organ dysfunction. It achieves many goals with maintaining hemodynamic stability (Table 25.4).

Table 25.4: Advantages of CRRT in critically ill patients with AKI

a. Better hemodynamic stability
b. Better volume control
c. Better correction of acidosis
d. Better removal of uremic toxins
e. Removal larger molecules such cytokines in sepsis with improvement of organ function
f. Allow supplementation additional nutrition by parenteral nutrition
g. Better removal of drugs in intoxications

The high cost of therapy, need for sophisticated equipment, close monitoring and trained manpower are the limitations. The sterile replacement fluid, the disposable items used and the need for 'ultrapure' water in some situations add to the cost of treatment. The most frequent complications associated with CRRT are electrolyte disturbances such as hypokalemia, hyponatremia, hypophosphatemia. Bleeding is another complication due to prolonged heparin use.

OTHER EXTRACORPOREAL THERAPIES

Other extracorporeal therapies used are plasmapheresis or plasma exchange (PLEX), charcoal hemoperfusion, molecular adsorbent recirculating system (MARS) and extracorporeal membrane oxygenation (ECMO). These are important therapies and each modality has benefit if used in appropriate situations.

a. Plasmapheresis (PP) or Plasma Exchange (PLEX)

Plasmapheresis is a process in which certain volume of plasma is removed from the patient blood with the use of a plasma filter. The volume of plasma removed is replaced with fresh plasma or albumin simultaneously in

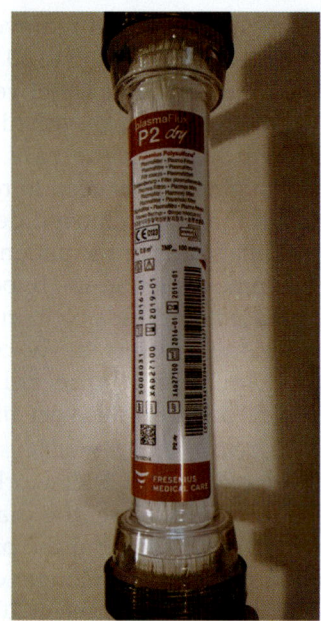

Fig. 25.12: Plasma filter made of hollow fiber with larger pores than hemodialyzer

equal quantities to the volume removed. Plasma exchange can be performed by a machine which uses centrifugal force to separate the plasma or using plasma filters. The plasma filters are similar to hemodialyzer and made up hollow fiber membrane with have bigger pore size which enable removal of larger protein molecules including immunoglobulins (Fig. 25.12).

The amount of plasma to be removed on each plasma exchange is about 35–40 ml/kg and same volume in the form of fresh frozen plasma or albumin diluted in saline is replaced on each session. This is called one volume exchange or volume to volume or 1:1 replacement. Blood circuit of the regular hemodialysis machine can be used for the treatment. Plasmapheresis is primarily offered to remove abnormal levels of circulating antibodies, immune complexes, monoclonal proteins, drugs and toxins (Table 25.5).

Antiglomerular basement membrane antibody disease and thrombotic microangiopathy (hemolytic uremic syndrome and

Table 25.5: Indications for plasmapheresis

1. Removal of circulating antibodies
   a. Renal diseases
      i. Anti-GBM antibody disease
      ii. Thrombotic thrombocytopenic purpura (TTP)
   b. Non-renal diseases.
      i. Guillain-Barré syndrome
      ii. Myasthenia gravis (crisis)
2. Removal circulating immune complexes
      i. Cryoglobulinemia
      ii. Systemic lupus erythematosus
3. Removal of circulating monoclonal protein
      i. Waldenström macroglobulinemia
      ii. Multiple myeloma
4. Removal circulating drugs and toxins
      i. Protein bound drugs
      ii. Paraquat
      iii. Parathion

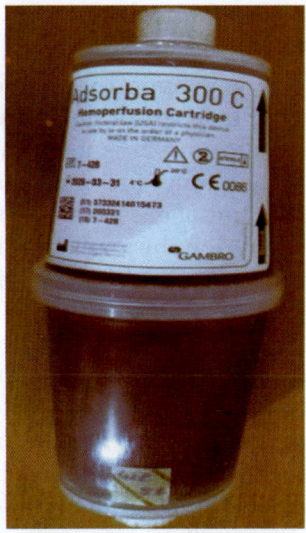

Fig. 25.13: Charcoal cartridge. The cartridge contains 'albumin-coated activated charcoal' and a built in sieve-like mechanism to prevent charcoal embolism in an airtight housing

thrombotic thrombocytopenic purpura) are the two important diseases which cause severe renal failure and are treated by PLEX. Plasma exchange therapy is also offered to renal transplant recipients when they have recurrence of focal segmental glomerulosclerosis or hemolytic uremic syndrome and those who develop antibody-mediated acute rejections after kidney transplantation. Adequate removal antibodies usually require. Usually 6–10 sessions PLEX. The usual complications are mild allergic reactions, hypotension due to plasma infusion and bleeding due to depletion coagulation factors.

b. Charcoal Hemoperfusion

When the blood is circulated through the charcoal filter or cartridge (Fig. 25.13). The toxins are adsorbed onto charcoal. Sterile, albumin-coated activated charcoal filled cartridges are used and the blood flows between the charcoal particles thereby facilitating contact between the charcoal and the toxin. These filters are designed to prevent charcoal from the cartridge entering the body and cause 'charcoal embolism'. Most common indication for hemoperfusion is drug intoxication and poisoning by non dialyzable or highly protein bound drugs (e.g. glutethimide, methaqualone, paraquat, meprobamate, carbamazepine and other phenothiazines group of drugs). The treatment is usually performed using only the blood circuit in the hemodialysis machine. The duration of therapy is about 3–4 hours. Single treatment session can remove 70–80% of the drug from the blood compartment. Once the charcoal gets saturated with toxins, the filter is discarded. Few sessions of treatment may be required to bring down the drug levels. The response depends on the amount consumed, blood level and timing of the treatment. The usual complications of hemoperfusion are bleeding, thrombocytopenia, hypotension and rarely charcoal embolism. In contrast to hemodialysis, hemoperfusion can remove protein bound drugs and toxins as well. Overall, charcoal hemoperfusion is a cost effective treatment and prevents deaths in these intoxications if performed at the appropriate time. The usual limitation is the availability of cartridges.

c. Extracorporeal Membrane Oxygenation (ECMO)

ECMO is a recent supportive extracorporeal therapy which to provides cardiac and respiratory support. It is used in patients whose heart and lungs are unable to provide adequate amount of gas exchange to sustain life. It is usually done by jugular or subclavian vein cannulation and blood is circulated through the ECMO machine which has membrane oxygenator. There are two types of ECMO, one is VA-ECMO when artery and vein are cannulated which is performed in patients with heart–lung failure and second type is VV-ECMO which done only by venous cannulation and often offered patients with only lung failure. ECMO is usually continued for 3 to 10 days till adequate lung and heart function is recovered.

d. Molecular Adsorbent Recirculating System (MARS)

MARS is a detoxification treatment offered to patient with fulminant hepatic failure and decompensated chronic liver disease. It is mainly a 'bridge therapy' till liver transplantation. Albumin enriched dialysate is being used in MARS treatment which facilitate removal of albumin bound toxins. First the patient blood circulated through hemodialyzer and albumin enriched dialysate in opposite direction, therefore protein bound toxins and water-soluble substances diffuse into albumin solution. The next step the albumin solution which comes from hemodialyzer recycled through another dialyzer coated with carbon which will adsorb all protein bound toxins. The final step is passage of the albumin solution comes out carbon-coated dialyzer through an anion exchange resin dialyzer with countercurrent flow of standard dialysis solution by which diffusive clearance of all water-soluble toxins occur. MARS is an expensive therapy and its benefits are equivocal.

Summary

HD is an extracorporeal blood purification therapy for both chronic and acute renal failures. Hemodialysis works by removal of excess uremic toxins, and regulates electrolytes in the blood by the process diffusion, convection and ultrafiltration. Most patients with CKD stage 5 require HD 2 to 3 times week lifelong. Patients with AKI often require dialysis support for a few days to a few weeks. In future, portable and wearable artificial kidneys will be available for the benefit of patients.

CRRT is the renal replacement therapy of choice in critically ill unstable patients with renal failure. The main advantages of CRRT are better hemodynamic stability, better fluid removal and better correction of acidosis. The CRRT is a continuous therapy lasting for more than 24 to 72 hours. CRRT is done for patients who has non-renal condition such liver failure with hyperammonemia, sepsis with ARDS, congestive heart failure and poisonings. CRRT is expensive and needs expert and trained staff.

Extracorporeal therapies other than CRRT are plasmapheresis, charcoal hemoperfusion, MARS and ECMO. Charcoal hemoperfusion therapy is short, relatively less expensive and rapid improvement can be noticed. Procedures like MARS, ECMO and plasmapheresis therapies are expensive and time consuming.

Renal Transplantation

• Georgy K Nainan

Kidney transplantation is a boon to the patients with end stage renal disease. Dr Joseph Edward Murray, a renowned American Plastic Surgeon did the first successful renal transplantation between identical twins at Peter Bent Brigham Hospital, Boston, USA in 1954. The recipient lived for 8 years and the donor died at the age of 84 years in 2010. Dr Murray was helped by Dr J Hartwell Harrison and Dr John P Merril. For his contribution in the field of renal transplantation Dr Murray was honored with Nobel Prize in Physiology in 1990.

Patients Selection Criteria

All patients with CKD stage V, who can undergo immunosuppressive therapy and general anesthesia are fit to be considered for transplantation. A child with 15 to 20 kg and adults below 65 can be considered under normal circumstances. Even elderly patients are considered for renal transplantation provided they have no macrovascular disease, coronary artery disease is corrected, good flow is present in the iliac vessels and there is no bladder outlet obstruction. Patients can be considered for transplant if otherwise fit, 3 months after CABG or 6 months after coronary stenting. Absolute contraindications are presence of infection, systemic neoplastic disease, active immunological disease/vasculitis. Such patients are considered only after the primary disease has been successfully treated or has reaches a stage of quiescence.

Evaluation of a Recipient

Evaluation consists of medical fitness, cardiac fitness, vascular status, status of the immune system, presence of chronic infection like hepatotropic viruses, HIV and tuberculosis. Coronary disease should be excluded in longstanding diabetes and patients over the age of 50 years especially if they are smokers. Cytomegalovirus (CMV) infections are more common in India. Most of the recipients are CMV IgG positive. If they are negative they should receive CMVprophylaxis treatment after renal transplantation. Children with history of urinary tract infection should have a cystoscopy or micturating cystourethrogram (MCU). Basic immunological evaluation consists of ABO grouping, HLA typing (HLA-A, B and DR), screening for cytotoxic antibodies against donor lymphocyte with flow cytometry and donor specific antibodies (DSA). If donor specific antibodies or crossmatch is positive they will need more immunosuppressives to suppress the antibody production and plasmapheresis to remove antibodies in pre-transplant workup.

They also may need immunosuppressive medications like low dose IV anti-thymocyte globulin (ATG), immunoglubulin (IG) or rituximab as induction agents. It is advisable to repeat crossmatch and DSA after the antibody suppression and removal of antibodies. In case of graft dysfunction, DSA titers may be helpful in modifying the therapy.

Donors: In 1994, the Human Organ Transplant Act was passed. There are different types of kidney donors.

1. Live Related Donors (LRD)

First degree relatives—children, siblings, parents, spouse, grandparents and grandchildren are included as first degree relatives. Second degree relatives have been included by the Govt of India as per a recent amendment. A living donor in this group with matching ABO blood group is selected and if found fit can be considered. Routine evaluation (Table 26.1) followed by special tests like ultrasound of the abdomen, isotope scan for split function of the kidneys, CT angiogram with 3D reconstituted picture will give detailed evaluation of the renal arteries and veins. Donors with multiple arteries and veins are discarded if the vessels are not of sufficient size. Angiogram gives vascular supply and number, branching and anatomy of renal vessels. Immunological suitability is confirmed with flow cytometry and identification of donor specific antibodies (DSA).

Table 26.1: List of usual donor investigations

Blood group	HIV/HBsAg / HCV—IgM, ELISA
CBC	VDRL, CMV, IgG, IgM
RFT	Ultrasound scan of abdomen
TFT	DTPA isotope scan
LFT	DSA/CT renal angiogram/
Na / K+	MR angiogram
Urine routine	Crossmatch
24 hours urine protein CXR	Donor specific antibodies (DSA)
ECG	

2. Live Unrelated Donors (LUD) and Altruistic Kidney Donors

Live unrelated donors could be distant relatives, friends, well-wishers or truly altruistic donors. Live unrelated donors or those where the relationship as per 'Human organ transplant Act (HOTA)' of 1994 cannot be proved have to be approved by the state authorization committee and orders passed by the 'appropriate authority' for each state. There are increasing numbers of truly altruistic donors who come forward to donate a kidney for self-satisfaction and as a humanitarian service.

3. Marginal Donors

Willing donors with minor abnormalities like donors with renal stone which can be removed intraoperatively, persons above the age of 60, those with mild hypertension well controlled with one drug and having good renal function are considered if they are in the LR category and if there is no other suitable donors in the family.

4. Swapping

Combination of A group recipient and B group donor and the reverse situation is not ideal for transplant. Swapping is an exchange donation between 2 donor-recipient pairs. For example, if an A group recipient has only a B group related donor and vice versa, the donors can be exchanged so that the A group recipient receives an A group kidney and the B group recipient receives B group kidney. Domino kidney paired exchange starts with a non- directed or altruistic donor. Instead of just one person benefiting from donation, this donor can allow many incompatible pairs to be transplanted. This allows continuation of ABO compatable kidney donation by the relative of the recipient benefitted in this exchange. Johns Hopkins hospital performed the first six-way donor kidney swap among 12 individuals.

5. ABO Incompatible Donors

Now, it is possible to perform transplantation across blood group barrier. The results are improving but the procedure needs more heavy and expensive immunosuppression, removal of antibodies by repeated plasma-phresis and more meticulous postoperative monitoring. The overall cost is very high and results may not be the same as LR donor with matching group.

6. Cadaver Transplantation (Cd Tx)

Two kidneys can be harvested from the deceased donor after brain death with beating heart. While the donor is maintained on ventilation and ionotropes, brain death is declared after examination by 4 independent doctors twice at 6-hour intervals under video recording as per the HOTA. These donors should not have any major medical illness, with good renal function, viral markers negative and free of active infections or malignancy. Organ sharing networks are present in some states and are responsible for co-ordinating the deceased donor sharing program. Organs harvested are distributed as per the waiting list with transparency. A deceased donor can provide kidneys, lung, heart, pancreas, liver, hand in addition to corneas for transplantation.

7. Non-heartbeating Cadaver Transplantation

In some countries like Japan, non-heart-beating donors are also considered. Viable critically ill donors, when they have non-revivable cardiac arrest, organs are immediately harvested and transplanted to suitable recipients.

Procedure of Live Donor Transplant Surgery

The donor and recipient are subjected to surgery almost simultaneously. The donor kidney is removed together with an adequate length of renal artery, renal vein and ureter. The kidney is perfused with a special ice cold solution. The solution is introduced into the renal artery with the help of a cannula and the ice cold solution drains the blood in the vascular systems, prevents clotting and vascular spasm. The perfusion solution exits through the severed end of the vein and perfusion of the kidney removed is continued till the effluent from the renal vein is clear and core of the kidney is cooled. The donor kidney covered with sterile iced saline slush placed in a bowl for external cooling and taken to the recipient side.

The donor kidney is placed in the iliac fossa in the extraperitoneal space. Usually, if the left kidney is removed, it is placed in the right iliac fossa of the recipient and vice versa. The Donor renal artery is anastamosed either to the internal iliac artery end to end or to external iliac artery end to side. Renal vein is anastamosed end to side to the external iliac vein. Ureter is implanted as a submucosal tunnel into the bladder wall (Fig. 26.1). A DJ stent is placed and is removed 4–6 weeks later. When the vascular clamp is released after vascular anastomosis is complete, the kidney turns pink and turgid. Urine flow resumes within minutes and usually, the hourly urine output may be very high. Close monitoring is required in the postoperative phase regarding fluid electrolyte and acid–base management.

Various immunosuppressive protocols are used. Induction is done with interleukin-2 (IL-2) receptor antagonist—basiliximab or anti thymocyte globulin (ATG). This is given before transplantation. Anti-thymocyte Globulin (ATG), a polyclonal immunosuppressive agent is used in patients at high risk of acute rejection. Basiliximab is used for regular patients at low risk. Risk factors for acute rejection are younger recipient and older donor age, positive panel reactive antibody (PRA), presence of donor specific antibody (DSA) delayed graft function, prolonged cold ischemia time and HLA mismatch or ABO incompatibility.

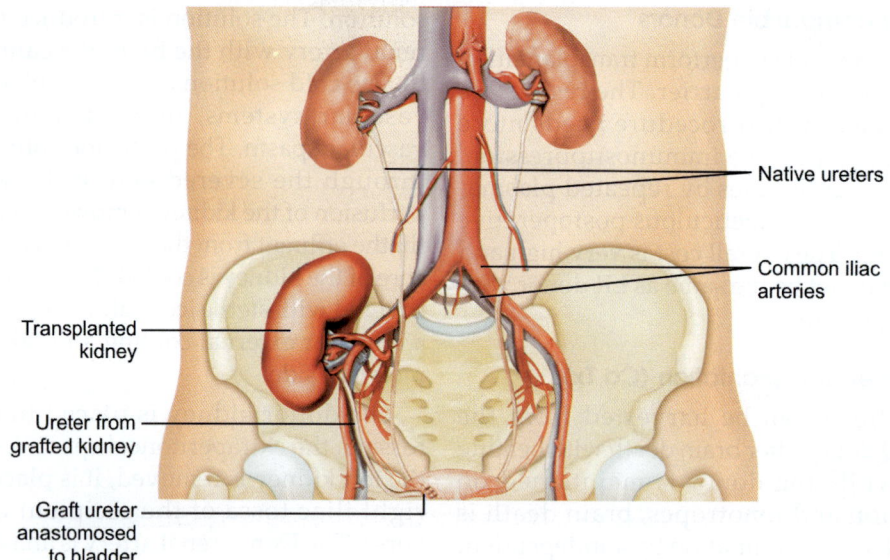

Native ureters

Common iliac arteries

Transplanted kidney

Ureter from grafted kidney

Graft ureter anastomosed to bladder

Fig. 26.1: Native kidneys remain *in situ*. Transplanted kidney in iliac fossa (extraperitoneal), renal artery anastamosed with internal iliac (end to end), renal vein with external iliac vein (end to side) and ureter implanted into bladder

Regular initial immunosuppressive medication following induction consists of IV methylprednisolone 500 mg daily for 5 days, starting on the morning of transplant surgery with an additional dose before release of vascular clamps during surgery. Mycophenolate mofetil, 2 gm per day and tacrolimus in doses of 1 mg/kg body weight are started two days before the surgery. After 5 days, IV methyl prednisolone is replaced with oral prednisolone 20 mg per day which is tapered to 5 mg by 14th day. There are some differences between centers regarding the immunosuppressive protocol used. Some centers use steroid sparing regime, although most use a small dose of steroid for its long-term beneficial effect. Calcinurin inhibitor (CNI), cyclosporine was used as the main medication in the immunosuppressive protocol since the mid-1980s. Because of the renal toxicity following long-term use, newer CNIs like tacrolimus (Tac) is used commonly now. Periodic therapeutic drug monitoring of Tac level guides the dosage. The dose of tacrolimus, starting at 0.1 mg per kg body

weight per day is adjusted subsequently to maintain Tac blood level of at 8–12 µg/L initially and maintain at 5–8 µg/L from 6 months. Everolimus is a newer immunosuppressive medication which acts at a different site of immune activation pathway and can effectively reduce rejection. It is free from nephrotoxicity and has an additional advantage of being an inhibitor of proliferation of fibroblasts. Belatacept is a newer drug which is being used in developed countries. Belatacept has the advantage that it has no nephrotoxicity like cyclosporin/tacrolimus (CNI). As this is administered parenterally, drug compliance is good.

The most important immunological complication of renal transplantation is rejection. Rejection is suspected if there is an increase in creatinine, decrease in the urine output, fever, graft tenderness or sonologically reduced perfusion with increased refractory index (RI). Whenever rejection is suspected, ultrasound-guided needle biopsy from the renal allograft is performed and subjected for light microscopy and immunofluorescence (IF) studies. If there is a suspicion of rejection, treatment consists of IV pulse methylprednisolone 1 g per day for 3 days. Further treatment depends on the type of rejection (*see* acute rejection below).

Immunosuppressive therapy consists of oral prednisolone 5 mg, mycophenolate 1.5 to 2 g/day and tacrolimus 3–4 mg/day to keep a tough level of about 6 µg/L. Economic consideration is crucial in a long-term success of the transplant program. It has to be individualized in such a manner that their chances of rejection are reduced or nullified. With the new surgical techniques and newer immunosuppressive medications the graft survival at 1, 5 and 10 years are 95, 90 and 80% respectively.

Causes of Graft Loss

Many events and complications in the post-transplantation period can result in loss of function of the graft. Early identification and timely intervention may help to reverse at least some of these complications. The important ones are given as follows.

1. Rejection

This is most common cause for the graft loss and can occur within minutes of transplantation or over many years.

a. Hyperacute rejection occurs within minutes or hours of transplantation and is mediated by antibodies against the donor antigens already circulating in the recipient. It is becoming less common because screening with newer immunologic tests and lowering the donor specific antibodies before transplant is performed now. If it occurs, the antibodies circulating in the recipient will attack the donor kidney as soon as vascularity is re-established and the kidney turns flaccid, bluish and does not produce any urine. If it occurs, immediate removal of transplant kidney is the only option.

b. Acute rejection usually occurs within weeks to months after a successful trans-

plantation. There are two types of rejection—acute cellular rejection and acute vascular rejection/antibody-mediated rejection (AMR). Acute allograft rejection should be suspected if there is no expected decrease in serum creatinine in the postoperative period, or an increase by ≥25% from baseline occurs. If the serum creatinine is higher than expected, one of the causes could be rejectioin. Rejection should be anticipated in patients who are at increased risk like ABO incompatibility, sensitized recipients with positive DSA or when immuno-suppression is inadequate or patient non-compliant. Development of oliguria, edema, worsening of hypertension or protienuria are the usual clinical pointers.

Diagnosis is always with biopsy. High index of suspicion and an early biopsy is needed to detect rejection. Histopathological examination can differentiate between T cell-mediated rejection (TCMR) and antibody mediated rejection (ABMR), and determine the degree of irreversible kidney damage (interstitial fibrosis/tubular atrophy (IF/TA). Biopsy of the renal allograft can also reveal other causes of renal inflammation and injury, including cytomegalovirus (CMV) disease, BK (polyomavirus) nephropathy, interstitial nephritis, pyelonephritis, *de novo* or recurrent glomerular disease, and post-transplant lymphopoliferative disease (PTLD).

Cellular rejection to a great extent can be treated with pulse methylprednisolone and ATG. In patients who are diagnosed with acute ABMR within the first year post-transplant, treatment with a combination of glucocorticoids, plasmapheresis and intra-venous immunoglobulin (IVIg) is advised. In some patients rituximab (a monoclonal antibody against CD20 in B lymphocytes) or bortezomib (a therapeutic proteasome inhibitor) may be used in refractory ABMR.

c. Chronic rejection may occur beyond 6–12 months. It is insidious in onset characterized by gradually increasing serum creatinine level. Renal biopsy is mandatory to diagnose this type of rejection. At times, it may manifest as proteinuria and only the histopathology of renal tissue will help to differentiate it from recurrence of the basic disease or *de novo* glomerulopathies.

Chronic ABMR, the most common cause of graft failure and is more difficult to treat compared to acute ABMR since, irreversible tissue damage has already occurred in the renal allograft by this time. Although the treatment of antibody-mediated injury is by combining inhibition of B cells (development, maturation, and activity), it is not clear which combination therapy is safe and effective in patients with chronic ABMR. These patients are usually treated using a combination of glucocorticoids and intravenous immunoglobulin (IVIg) and retuximab/bortezomib (if there is evidence of active microvascular inflammation on renal biopsy).

2. *Recurrence of Disease*

Recurrence of original disease in the transplant occurs in some types of glomerular disease and is another cause of graft loss. 15–20% of IgA nephropathy, FSGS and type II MPGN (20–40%) do recur in the newly transplanted kidney. Anti-GBM disease, hyperoxaluria recurrent in a large proportion of transplants and lead to graft failure. Long-standing diabetes can have recurrence of the disease but do not cause graft loss usually.

3. *Vascular Thrombosis*

This is an uncommon complication and occurs in patients with thrombotic disorders like anti-thrombin III deficiency, factor V Leyden mutation, protein C or protein S deficiency.

4. *Accelerated Hypertension and Malignant Hypertension*

This complication may occur in 60–70% renal transplant recipients especially while on cyclosporin. Now, hypertensive episodes are less frequent because cyclosporin is not used and alternative drugs like evorolimus are available for immunosuppression. Renin secretion from the native kidneys may also cause accelerated hypertension. If blood pressure remains uncontrolled, these patients may have to be subjected to bilateral native kidney nephrectomy. Graft renal artery stenosis is another important cause of post-transplant hypertension. CT Angiogram or arteriogram of graft renal artery can be considered if renal functions are normal. More recently, 3 Tesla MR angiography can identify the lesion easily and it can be corrected with stenting or angioplasty.

Other Complications

5. *Infections*

Since the patients are immunosuppressed, infections are common after renal transplantation commonly. They may lead to sepsis, multi-organ dysfunction (MOD) and even death. It is an important cause of mortality in patients with a functioning graft. In spectrum of the infections, the chronological occurrence and the risk factors are different from that of developed countries. High index of suspicion and search for occult infection before it becomes obvious is necessary. Tuberculosis is seen in a number of allograft recipients and the risk increases in patients diabetes, chronic liver disease, or those who have latent tuberculosis. Post-transplant tuberculosis may present as pyrexia of unknown origin (PUO) or pyuria. Primary drug resistance of the organism can pose problems in management.

Fungal infections with aspergillosis or mucormycosis may be seen in people with poor personal hygiene. They may be progressive despite therapy with potent antifungals like amphoterocin B.

Carini (PCP) or *Pneumocystis jirovecii* pneumonia (PJP) is a common respiratory infection in immunosuppressed transplant recipients. They may present with lower respiratory infection and can progress to fulminant bilateral bronchopneumonia with acute respiratory distress syndrome (ARDS) which may require ventilator support. Chemoprophylaxis with cotrimoxazole is used as prophylaxis.

With active hepatitis B vaccination, in the pre-transplant period and seroprotection attained, protects the transplant recipients from getting hepatitis B. Presently, the incidence of hepatitis C and related chronic liver disease (CLD) have come down. Newer anti-viral treatments for achieving sustained remission of viremia are available. CLD is a common cause of morbidity and mortality.

Cytomegalovirus (CMV) disease occurs in many patients in the first 6 months after transplantation. The infection can trigger a rejection episode. CMV infection is associated with infections like tuberculosis, systemic mycosis and opportunistic infections. CMV can affect the graft, intestine or lung. In the context of renal transplantation, whether the donor or recipient is seropositive or seronegative for CMV is denoted by D+ or D– and R+ or R–. D suggests donor and R suggests recipient. + and – signify seropositivity or negativity. If the status pre-transplant is CMV D–/ R–, it means that both donor and recipient are negative for CMV antibody and do not have infection. Therefore, no specific CMV prevention strategies are recommended. In CMV D+/ R– prophylaxis for the recipient in the post-transplant period is preferred. In D–/R+ situation, pre emptive treatment is advised in the post transplant period. In any situation of R+, CMV prophylaxis is preferred. Valganciclovir is the drug of choice in prophylaxis and treatment. Valganciclovir prophylaxis helps to reduce incidence of immediate post-transplant CMV infection. Intravenous ganciclovir is used in sick patients with CMV disease. Dose of valganciclovir is 450 to 900 mg. The dose is reduced to 450 mg daily if eGFR is between 20 ml and 40 ml/min.

Molecular assays, using polymerase chain reaction (PCR) is a quantitative real-time test to assess the viral load and is useful for monitoring patients at risk for cytomegalovirus (CMV) disease, diagnosing active CMV disease and monitoring response to therapy. Serologic tests measure the presence of anti-CMV immunoglobulin IgM and IgG. In recent or acute CMV infection, CMV-IgM antibodies are detectable. In the case of CMV-IgG titers, a fourfold or greater increase in paired specimens obtained at least two to four weeks apart is necessary for confirmation of active infection.

Post-transplant diabetes mellitus (PTDM): Development of diabetes for the first time after renal transplantation is on the increase. Tacrolimus used as immunosuppressive drug during the last decade has resulted in more cases of post-transplant diabetes. Intitial use of high dose of cyclosporin followed by switching over to tacrolimus by 2nd or 3rd month can reduce the chance of post-transplant hyperglycemia in these patients. Steroids sparing regimes may also help. Irrespective of the cause, the blood sugar should be controlled with oral hypoglycemic agents if renal functions are normal and insulin used if renal functions are compromised.

6. Post-transplant Malignancies

Post-transplant lymphoproliferative disorder (PTLD) is a common complication which occurs many years after renal transplantation. Non-Hodking's lymphoma (NHL) is triggred by the oncogenic integration of Epstein-Barr (EB) virus into the host genome. In addition to NHL, other cancers are also common in transplant recipients. The other malignancies observed in transplant recipients are, carcinomas of skin (basal cell carcinoma, malignant melanoma), oral cavity, female and male genital tract, colorectal, lung, brain, breast and non-Hodgkin lymphoma.

7. Post-transplantation Dyslipidemia

All fractions of lipids that are considered to be 'atherogenic' are increased in transplant recipients. Both immunosuppressive drugs rapamycin and everolimus can cause or aggravate dyslipidemia. Long-term use of prednisolone and tacrolimus also cause lipid anomalies. Diet control along with statin therapy is recommended routinely to all transplant recipients in the same fashion as in cardiovascular risk prevention.

8. Bone Disease

Renal osteodystrophy continues to be a problem in many transplant recipients. Supplementation with vitamin D, bisphosphonates, calcium and steroid-free immunosuppression help to prevent osteoporosis. Some may develop avascular necrosis of the head of femur leading to pain and limping following long-term use of steroids.

There is a huge gap between demand for the kidneys and availability of donors. In order to prevent 'organ trade' and other unethical practices, strict laws are formulated and implemented. Since successful renal transplantation can offer good quality of life for a patient with CKD stage V compared to dialysis, promoting cadaver transplantation is the need of the hour. This requires sensitizing the public on the benefits to patients with renal, hepatic or cardiac failure. Other organs like lung, pancreas, intestine, skin and even hand can be transplanted from brain dead, beating heart cadaver donors. Corneas can be removed within hours of clinical death (stoppage of heart). To encourage availability of cadaver organs for transplantation, many state governments have started implementing regulations for harvesting organs from patients after brain death and streamlined the procedures.

Tubular Diseases

Tubulointerstitial Nephritis (Acute and Chronic)

• Raj Kumar Sharma • Sonia Mehrothra

INTRODUCTION

Tubulointerstitial nephritis is due to injury to renal tubules and interstitium and is an important cause for renal diseases. It can be divided into acute and chronic types. The acute form of interstitial nephritis (AIN) manifests over short period with sudden onset and clinical manifestations. AIN usually recovers once acute insult disappears, but the residual renal damage persists or progresses even after initial insult subsides. In AIN, the glomerular filtration rate (GFR) recovers if patient is not having any pre-existing kidney disease. Chronic interstitial nephritis (CIN) manifests at times slowly and insidiously and it can cause permanent fibrosis of interstitium and decrease the number of functioning nephrons. Sometimes the two can overlap and differentiation may be difficult. CIN may progress to end-stage kidney disease. Primary tubulointerstitial nephritis can be caused by toxic, hematologic, metabolic, and various infectious diseases. Tubulointerstitial injury can also occur in patients who have predominantly glomerular disease, cystic disease, diabetic kidney disease or collagen vascular disease. Kidney biopsy in these patients would show changes of chronic or acute interstitial nephritis besides the histopathological changes of the primary renal disease.

Clinical Features

Tubulointerstitial damage (Table 27.1), may present clinically as acute kidney injury (AKI) due to acute interstitial nephritis (AIN) or chronic kidney disease (CKD) presenting as chronic interstitial nephritis (CIN). Patients frequently present with renal damage, dysfunction and fluid overload. Extrarenal features such as arthralgia, fever and skin rash may be present. Tests of renal dysfunction (blood urea and serum creatinine) estimates

Table 27.1: Clinical features of tubulointerstitial diseases

- Tubulointerstitial diseases are an important cause of acute or chronic kidney disease
- Drugs are the most common cause of acute tubulointerstitial nephritis; other causes include autoimmune diseases, systemic disorders, infections and metabolic diseases
- Chronic tubulointerstitial nephritis may develop following the development of acute tubulo-interstitial nephritis or may be the initial manifestation of an autoimmune or systemic disease process
- Clinical and laboratory findings (blood, urine and radiologic studies) may suggest possibility of tubulointerstitial disease but kidney biopsy is generally required to make a definitive diagnosis
- NSAIDs can cause both acute interstitial nephritis and chronic analgesic nephropathy resulting in CIN

the degree of renal failure. Serological tests help in the diagnosis of systemic diseases causing interstitial nephritis. CIN is often diagnosed during investigations for CKD. Albuminuria is common but not large in amount, and is generally not associated with the nephrotic syndrome. Low-molecular weight proteinuria is common. There may be discrepancy between total proteinuria and albuminuria. Microscopic hematuria is variable and gross hematuria is uncommon. There may be defective tubular handling of water, sodium and hydrogen ions resulting in nephrogenic diabetes and renal tubular acidosis (RTA). Hypertension is seen in some cases only.

Classification and Pathology

Tubulointerstitial disorders are classified according to the basic cause or according to histological changes as AIN or CIN (Figs 27.1 and 27.2). In AIN, the renal injury is characterized by an accumulation of inflammatory infiltrate in the kidney interstitium. It is commonly induced by drugs. AIN can also be caused by autoimmune disorders and systemic diseases (systemic lupus erythematosus (SLE), Sjögren's syndrome, sarcoidosis), various infections (legionella, leptospirosis and streptococcal organisms), and tubulo-interstitial nephritis with uveitis (TINU) syndrome (Table 27.2).

Table 27.2: Causes of acute tubulointerstitial nephritis

Medications/toxins: Beta-lactam antibiotics/rifampin/NSAIDs/proton pump inhibitors (PPIs)/quinine/H_2-antagonists/anticonvulsants/allopurinol/diuretics/sulfonamides/acute radiation nephritis

Infection: Viruses/bacteria/fungi/parasites/spirochetes

Autoimmune diseases: Sjögren's syndrome/sarcoidosis/IgG4 TIN, systemic lupus erythematosus/ vasculitis/tubulointerstitial nephritis with uveitis (TINU)

Systemic diseases: Lymphoproliferative diseases/paraproteinemias/inflammatory/bowel disease/atheroembolic disease

Metabolic disorders: Acute oxalate nephropathy/acute uric acid nephropathy/acute nephrocalcinosis

CIN can occur due to tubulointerstitial damage from direct drug toxicity, local ischemia, inherited disorders of tubular proteins or primary tubulointerstitial inflammation. The TIN may be the result of impaired activation of innate immune mechanisms resulting in continuous chronic damage.

Pathology (Figs 27.1 and 27.2)

Inflammatory cells (macrophages, lymphocytes) play important role in tubulointerstitial nephritis. The pathology involves immune mediated infiltration of the renal interstitium.

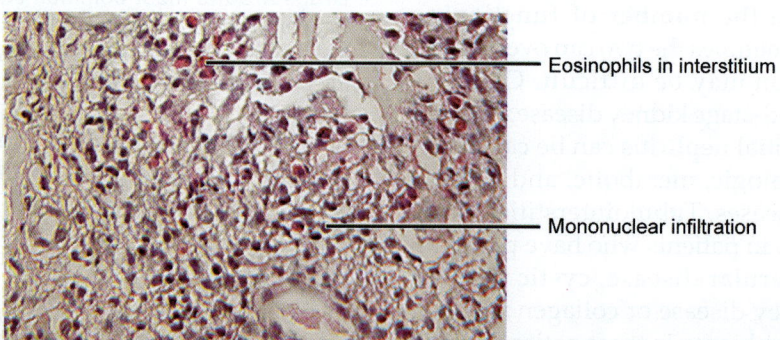

Eosinophils in interstitium

Mononuclear infiltration

Fig. 27.1: Acute interstitial nephritis. Renal biopsy high power. Showing interstitial edema with infiltration by mononuclear cells and eosinophils in acute interstitial nephritis. (Eosinophils are seen mainly in allergic interstitial nephritis)

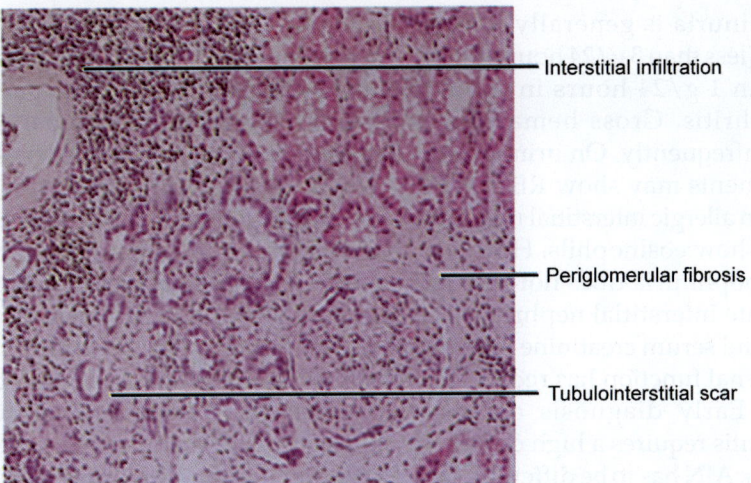

Interstitial infiltration

Periglomerular fibrosis

Tubulointerstitial scar

Fig. 27.2: Chronic interstitial nephritis showing interstitial infiltration, tubular atrophy, tubular interstitial scarring and periglomerular fibrosis. Renal biopsy high power showing one glomerulus with periglomerular fibrosis, interstitial infiltration and tubular atrophy

Injury to renal cells leads to inflammatory cell infiltration and activation of pro-inflammatory cytokines. These cytokines are produced by infiltrating inflammatory cells and also by other renal cells like proximal tubule, vascular endothelial cells, interstitial cells and fibroblasts. This can result in acute or chronic interstitial damage. Depending on the severity of the damage to the tubular epithelium, the renal dysfunction may or may not be generally reversible, possibly reflecting the repairing capacity of tubules which has conserved basement membrane. The main mechanism of allergic acute tubulointerstitial nephritis is hypersensitivity reaction to drugs such as penicillins, nonsteroidal anti-inflammatory drugs (NSAIDs) and sulfa drugs. NSAIDs can also cause 'minimal-change' glomerular lesion resulting in nephrotic syndrome in addition to AIN. The acute tubulointerstitial injury can also result from cellular injury caused by infections (viral or bacterial). Chronic tubulointerstitial nephritis results from interstitial scarring, fibrosis, and tubular atrophy, resulting in advanced chronic kidney disease.

Investigations

Investigations may show the biochemical effects of tubular damage. Eosinophiluria and eosinophilia in peripheral blood smear indicate allergic interstitial nephritis. Anti-neutrophil cytoplasmic antibody (ANCA), anti-nuclear antibody (ANA), extractable nuclear antigens (ENAs), immunoglobulin levels help to suspect and confirm autoimmune etiology. Chest X-ray and other additional imaging studies depending on the indications, screening for mycobacterial and other causative organisms can establish the presence of associated infections. Renal ultrasonography is generally normal in AIN. In CIN however bipolar length of kidneys is often reduced. Depending on cause of CIN, the renal outline may be smooth or irregular suggesting scarring of the kidney. The diagnosis of AIN or CIN may need to be confirmed by renal biopsy (Tables 27.1 and 27.2).

Diagnosis of Acute Tubulointerstitial Nephritis (AIN)

Urine analysis shows mild-to-moderate proteinuria and hematuria in most cases of

AIN. The proteinuria is generally in non-nephrotic range (less than 3 g/24 hours) and is mostly less than 1 g/24 hours in tubulo-interstitial nephritis. Gross hematuria is observed only infrequently. On urine micro-scopy, the sediments may show RBC, WBC and WBC casts. In allergic interstitial nephritis, urinalysis may show eosinophils. However, absence of eosinophiluria does not rule out diagnosis of acute interstitial nephritis. The estimated GFR and serum creatinine may rise only when the renal function has reduced by 50% or more. Early diagnosis of acute interstitial nephritis requires a high degree of clinical suspicion. AIN has to be differentiated from other causes of acute kidney injury, such as acute tubular necrosis or rapidly progressive glomerulonephritis. Since the clinical assessment, laboratory investigations, and imaging tests may not confirm the diagnosis of AIN, kidney biopsy (Fig. 27.1) is often required. This not only helps to confirm the diagnosis but also guides management (Table 27.3).

Treatment of Acute Interstitial Nephritis (AIN)

The initial treatment for AIN is to discontinue the causative drug or treat the infection. If the serum creatinine levels do not decrease after a week, steroids can be started. The optimal dose and duration of therapy are not clear. A

Table 27.3: Clinical manifestations of acute interstitial nephritis (AIN)

- History of drug hypersensitivity or taking anti-biotics and or recent infection
- Fever lasting several days to weeks
- Hypertension
- Rise in creatinine with fractional excretion of sodium (FENa) >1.0
- No expected cause of acute tubular necrosis or glomerulonephritis
- Kidney size increased/normal
- Mild proteinuria (<1.0 g) with microscopic/macroscopic hematuria
- *Urinalysis:* Presence of white blood cells and WBC casts or rarely eosinophils

common approach is to administer prednisone at a dose of 1 mg/kg per day (to a maximum of 40 to 60 mg) for a minimum period of one to two weeks followed by gradual tapering of the dose once serum creatinine levels have come down. Total duration of treatment with steroids is generally for a maximum of two to three months. Most patients start to improve within first one to two weeks. In patients with severe acute kidney injury (AKI), therapy may be initiated with IV bolus infusion of methylprednisolone (0.5 to 1 g/day for three days followed by oral steroids. The duration of glucocorticoid therapy varies widely (from a few days up to 12 weeks). Once the agent inciting allergic interstitial nephritis has been discontinued and the kidney function starts improving, the duration of therapy may be shortened. If patient shows no improvement with steroids, treatment with cyclophospha-mide (1 to 2 mg/kg/day orally) or myco-phenolate mofetil (MMF up to 1 g twice daily), can be added to steroids and continued for a period of further few weeks.

Chemotherapeutic agents are injurious to the kidneys. They can induce AIN and their timely discontinuation can improve renal injury. Drug-induced acute interstitial nephritis should always be considered in the differential diagnosis of acute kidney injury.

Inflammatory diseases can also induce TIN. Several non-infectious inflammatory diseases cause AIN or CIN. They frequently respond to corticosteroids.

Sarcoidosis is associated with renal granulo-matous tubulointerstitial lesions in about 20% of patients, but these do not always clinically manifest TIN.

Sjögren's syndrome is associated with TIN and may manifest as acute renal impairment or renal tubular acidosis. A sicca syndrome with abnormal ocular tests and lymphocyte infiltration in salivary glands biopsy may occur. Thus, loss of lacrimation and salivation, typical of this disease occurs.

Treatment with prednisone (1 mg / kg/day up to 60 mg/day) followed by tapering doses may be prescribed in patients with severe active interstitial nephritis. Azathioprine (1 to 2 mg/kg/day) may be used as a steroid-sparing agent. Patients with Sjögren's syndrome should be screened for hepatitis C virus. Patients with immunoglobulin G4 (IgG4) related disease may also have salivary and lacrimal gland involvement, besides interstitial nephritis. Autoantibodies, anti-Ro (SSA) and anti-La (SSB) are specific for Sjögren's syndrome and if present can help confirm the diagnosis in the proper clinical setting.

Systemic lupus erythematosus and granulomatous microscopic polyangiitis (Wegener's granulomatosis) are systemic diseases that are rarely associated with isolated TIN without glomerular involvement. In such cases there may be significant tubular dysfunction such as renal tubular acidosis. Systemic lupus erythematosus (SLE) is associated with various immunologic abnormalities, like production of antinuclear antibodies (ANA), which is an important feature of this disease .

TIN with uveitis (TINU): The diagnosis of TINU syndrome is suggested by the combination of uveitis associated with renal biopsy consistent with acute interstitial nephritis. TINU commonly presents in childhood, but has been reported in late adulthood. The pathogenesis of TINU syndrome is unknown. An auto-antigen to modified C-reactive protein (CRP) may play a pathogenic role. Delayed-type hypersensitivity and suppressed cell-mediated immunity play a role in pathogenesis. Possible risk factors of TINU syndrome, include infections (Chlamydia and Epstein-Barr virus infections, use of specific drugs [antibiotics, non-steroidal anti-inflammatory drugs (NSAIDs), or use of Chinese herb, "goreisan"]. TINU syndrome has also been reported with various auto-immune diseases like hypoparathyroidism, thyroiditis, immunoglobulin G4 (IgG4)-related autoimmune disease and rheumatoid arthritis.

IgG4-related disease may cause AIN. It is characterized by an elevated concentration of serum IgG4 and infiltration with IgG4-positive plasma cells in the renal interstitium. This is often associated with autoimmune pancreatitis. There can be widespread organ involvement with inflammatory masses, sialadenitis, sclerosing cholangitis, aortitis and retroperitoneal fibrosis. IgG4-related disease causing interstitial nephritis is characterized by 'expansile' interstitial fibrosis described as 'bird's eye'. IgG4 positive plasma cells are detected on immunostaining in the interstitium. Steroid therapy in IgG4-related disease often improves renal function and serum IgG4 levels. High index of suspicion and awareness of this entity is necessary for early diagnosis and prompt treatment.

Chronic Interstitial Nephritis (CIN)

Various disorders of the renal vasculature, glomeruli or urinary tract can result in secondary chronic tubulointerstitial injury. The histological features of CIN correlates well with progression of chronic kidney disease (Fig. 27.2). Sometimes the tubulo-interstitium is the primary site of damage and inflammation (Table 27.4).

In patient with signs of chronic tubulo-interstitial renal injury, the assessment should include history, physical examination and laboratory tests to look for probable causes. These tests include blood urea levels, serum creatinine, electrolytes, bicarbonate, calcium, phosphate, uric acid, total protein, albumin and urine electrophoresis. Urinalysis occasionally shows glycosuria, proteinuria (often <1 g/L), red cells, white cells, and granular casts. Blood cultures, serologic tests for autoimmune diseases (cryoglobulin level, ANA, ANCA, and anti-GBM antibody levels), markers of various viral infections are other important tests to identify the causative factors. Proximal tubular dysfunction such as Fanconi syndrome,

Table 27.4: Chronic tubulointerstitial nephritis

Medications/toxins: NSAIDs, analgesic combinations, lithium, PPIs, calcineurin inhibitors, chemotherapeutic agents, lead, cadmium, aristolochic acid, chronic radiation nephritis

Infections: Chronic pyelonephritis, malakoplakia, xanthogranulomatous pyelonephritis

Autoimmune diseases: Sjögren's syndrome, sarcoidosis, SLE, TINU, IgG4 TIN, hypocomplementemic TIN, vasculitis

Systemic diseases: Lymphoproliferative diseases, sickle cell disease, paraproteinemias, inflammatory bowel disease, cystinosis, Dent disease, atheroembolic disease

Metabolic disorders: Chronic oxalate nephropathy, chronic uric acid nephropathy, nephrocalcinosis, hypokalemic nephropathy, progression of acute TIN, urinary obstruction

aminoaciduria, phosphate wasting, uricosuria, and glycosuria or distal tubular dysfunction with type 1 RTA can be seen occasionally in chronic interstitial nephritis. Patients with Fanconi syndrome may have acidosis with alkaline urine.

TREATMENT OF CHRONIC INTERSTITIAL NEPHRITIS (CIN)

Inciting factors such as obstruction, infections, drugs or toxins should be identified and discontinued as early as possible. Chronic interstitial nephritis is less likely to resolve spontaneously. The treatment is similar to other causes of chronic kidney disease (CKD). Angiotensin-converting enzyme inhibitors or angiotensin II receptor blockers are used early (except when hyperkalemia limits their use) to slow disease progression, with systolic blood pressure goal of less than 140 mm Hg. Systemic acidosis should be treated early with sodium bicarbonate, starting at 600 mg orally three times daily. Anemia is treated with erythropoiesis stimulating agents, hyperphosphatemia with oral phosphate binders and hyperparathyroidism with active vitamin D: calcitriol (starting at 0.25 µg/day). There

may be need to supplement calcirol D_2 to correct vitamin D deficiency. There is no clear role for immunosuppressive drugs in the treatment of CIN, except in early stages of sarcoidosis.

Lithium toxicity: Use of lithium as a therapeutic agent may result in nephrogenic diabetes insipidus, AIN and on long-term use may result in CIN. Long-term lithium use is associated with early chronic kidney disease due to chronic interstitial nephritis in up to 15 to 20% of patients. Major risk factors for chronic nephrotoxicity appear to be the duration of lithium exposure, the increasing dose and advancing age. Lithium therapy may also be associated with distal renal tubular acidosis, minimal change disease, focal segmental glomerulosclerosis (FSGS) and edema during episodes of maniac psychiatric manifestations.

Analgesic nephropathy is characterized by renal papillary necrosis and calcification resulting in chronic interstitial nephritis. It is caused by prolonged and excessive consumption of analgesic medications in various combinations. Individual analgesic agents may also cause chronic kidney disease (CKD), although the associated histologic and clinical features are less well defined than for analgesic nephropathy associated with both phenacetin-containing and non-phenacetin-containing analgesic mixtures. Aspirin alone (in therapeutic doses) does not appear to induce renal injury but may potentiate the toxicity of phenacetin and acetaminophen. Although it is clear that non-steroidal anti-inflammatory drugs (NSAIDs) cause acute kidney injury (AKI), their role in the development of CKD is uncertain.

Aristolochic acid nephropathy, Balkan nephropathy and Chinese herbal nephropathy: There is evidence that contamination of food with impurities like aristolochic acid can result in chronic interstitial nephropathy, although environmental and genetic factors may also contribute to the pathogenesis. Chinese herbal nephropathy was identified in 1992, in Belgian women in whom the causal agent was clearly identified as aristolochic acid, used as a skin lighting agent. There was progressive renal failure, and uroepithelial malignancy with use of these Chinese herbs.

Heavy-metal intoxication due to environmental or industrial exposure results in heavy metal intoxication leading to CIN. Heavy metals may also be present in out-dated medicines. *Radiation nephritis* may cause acute thrombotic microangiopathy and in the long-term CIN.

Chemotherapeutic drugs have nephrotoxic potential as they also get concentrated in kidneys and can cause tubulointerstitial injury. They can be the cause of acute kidney injury due to AIN. Chemotherapy drugs also result in tubulopathy, crystal nephropathy and CIN.

Anorexia nervosa may also be associated with CIN, which causes renal impairment and contributes to the complex electrolyte disturbances. Long-standing hypovolemia and hypokalemia may contribute to development of CIN, with local changes in renal blood flow and tubular metabolism. Anorexia nervosa can affect the kidney in many ways, including increased rates of acute kidney injury and chronic kidney disease, electrolyte abnormalities and nephrolithiasis.

Meso-American nephropathy: Mesoamerican nephropathy (MeN), formerly called chronic kidney disease of unknown cause (CKDu), refers to non-proteinuric CKD that presents in young, agricultural workers predominantly in Central America in the absence of any clear etiology for CKD. MeN is highly prevalent in low-altitude, coastal regions of El Salvador and Nicaragua and possibly Guatemala and Costa Rica. A similar pathology may contribute to the high prevalence of non-proteinuric CKD in Sri Lanka, although this has not been proven. The major risk factor for MeN is agricultural work in a hot climate, which causes dehydration and volume depletion resulting in recurrent acute kidney injury. Other risk factors include exposure to pesticides, excessive use of nonsteroidal anti-inflammatory agents, older age, male sex, low body mass, and consumption of sugar-containing rehydration drinks.

Summary

Acute interstitial nephritis (AIN) is generally diagnosed by renal biopsy. There are many causes and careful clinical assessment with

Table 27.5: Medications associated with interstitial nephritis
• *Antibiotics:* Penicillins, piperacillin/tazobactam, fluroquinolones, cephalosporins, sulfonamides, macrolides, chloramphenicol, clindamycin, colistin, doxycyclin, ethambutol, gentamicin, griseofulvin, imipenem, isoniazid, linezolid, nitrofurantoin, polymyxin B, rifampin, teicoplanin, vancomycin.
• *Anti-retrovirals:* Abacavir, acyclovir, atazanavir, foscarnet, indinavir, interferon-α
• *NSAIDs:* COX-2 inhibitors, aceclofenac, diclofenac, etodolac, ibuprofen, indomethacin, ketoprofen, mefenamate, meloxicam, naproxen, nimesulide, phenylbutazone, piroxicam, sulindac.
• *Aminosalicylates:* Sulfasalazine
• *GI protective drugs: Proton pump inhibitors:* H_2-blockers
• *Chemotherapeutic agents:* Immune checkpoint inhibitors, tyrosine kinase inhibitors, adriamycin, alendronate, azathioprine, BCG, bevacizumab, bortezomib, carboplatin, interleukin-2, interferon, ifosfamide, lenalidomide, methotrexate
• *Diuretics:* Thiazides, indapamide, metolazone, chlorthalidone, loop diuretics, potassium sparing diuretics
• *Antihypertensives:* ACE inhibitors, angiotensin receptor blockers, calcium channel blockers
• *Anticonvulsants:* Carbamazepine, diazepam, lamotrigine, levetiracetam, phenobarbital, phenytoin, valproic acid
• *Others:* Allopurinol, atorvastatin, carbimazole, chlorporpamide, exenatide, febuxostat, gemfibrozil, leflunomide, metamizole, propranolol, propylthiouracil, sildenafil

respect to the medication history is important. Some drugs may present with evidence of multi-organ involvement. If a drug is implicated it must then be withdrawn and further exposure avoided. Corticosteroids may be of benefit in AIN.

Drug-induced AIN is a common cause of acute kidney injury and important differential diagnosis of acute tubular necrosis. It should be considered when recovery of renal function is delayed following an episode of acute tubular necrosis. AKI is common in hospitalized patients who are given multiple drugs capable of causing AIN (Table 27.5).

Chronic interstitial nephritis (CIN) may be primary or due to a recognized disease or therapy. At times there may be extensive chronic tubule interstitial renal damage at presentation itself because manifestations and symptoms can occur insidiously and late.

Cystic Diseases of the Kidney

• OP Kalra • Deepak Jain

INTRODUCTION

Cystic diseases of the kidney include a broad range of disorders, presenting in infants, children and adults with numerous phenotypic expressions. These account for around 10% of patients with end-stage renal disease (ESRD) and are prevalent worldwide irrespective of gender, race or ethnicity. Usually their clinical diagnosis is aided by the age of presentation, clinical features, renal imaging studies including cyst location and distribution and extra-renal manifestations.

Classification

In simple terms, a cyst is described as a cavity lined by epithelium and filled with liquid or semisolid material. There may be single or multiple cysts in one or both kidneys. They may be small, non-enlarging, and clinically insignificant, or large, enlarging and harmful. Classification of cystic kidney diseases is shown in Table 28.1. Cystic disease of the kidney can also be classified based on the pattern of inheritance, as given in Table 28.2.

Out of these, mainly four types of cysts commonly encountered in adults are discussed in this chapter. Autosomal dominant poly-cystic kidney disease (ADPKD) is a hereditary disease and may lead to progressive renal failure. Long-standing renal failure of unknown

Table 28.1: Classification of cystic kidney disorders

Autosomal dominant polycystic kidney disease (ADPKD)

Autosomal recessive polycystic kidney disease (ARPKD)

- Tuberous sclerosis complex
- von Hippel-Lindau syndrome

Autosomal dominant medullary cystic kidney disease

Hereditary recessive ciliopathies with interstitial nephritis, cysts or both

- Nephronophthisis
- Bardet-Biedl syndrome

Renal cystic dysplasias

- Multicystic kidney dysplasia

Other cystic kidney disorders

- Simple cysts
- Medullary sponge kidney
- Acquired cystic kidney disease

Renal cystic neoplasms

- Cystic renal cell carcinoma

Cysts of nontubular origin

- Cystic disease of the renal sinus
- Perirenal lymphangiomas

Pyelocalyceal cysts

etiology may be associated with acquired cystic kidney disease (ACKD). Sporadic presence of simple cysts may be documented in the absence of specific kidney pathology, and these are of a little detrimental clinical consequence. Lastly, medullary sponge

Table 28.2: Classification of cystic diseases of the kidney based on inheritance

Genetic	Nongenetic
1. Autosomal dominant polycystic kidney disease (ADPKD)	1. Multicystic kidney
2. Autosomal recessive polycystic kidney disease (ARPKD)	2. Multilocular cyst
3. Juvenile nephronophthisis—medullary cystic complex	3. Simple cysts—solitary or multiple
4. Cysts associated with multiple malformation syndromes: Tuberous sclerosis, von Hippel-Lindau's disease, Meckel's syndrome, Orofacial syndrome and chromosome disorders like trisomy 21,13,18 and trisomy C	4. Multiple parapelvic cysts
	5. Medullary sponge kidney
	6. Acquired renal cystic disease

kidney is another common cystic kidney disease found in day-to-day clinical practice. The remaining forms of renal cysts are relatively rare.

Autosomal Dominant Polycystic Kidney Disease

ADPKD is one of the most common genetic disorders in humans affecting all ethnic groups worldwide with an incidence of 1 in 400 to 1000 births. It accounts for more than 5% of cases of ESRD in Europe and North America. There are two genetic mutations that have been linked with ADPKD. Mutation of PKD1 gene which is located on chromosome 16 and encodes polycystin-1 and PKD2 gene located on chromosome 4 which encodes polycystin-2 can lead to ADPKD. Around 85% cases are caused by PKD1 mutations. Both polycystin-1 and polycystin-2 are responsible for intracellular calcium signalling and localization of primary cilia of renal epithelium.

Mechanisms of Cyst Formation

None of the several mechanisms proposed to explain the cyst formation has been able to conclusively support the cyst development. Furthermore, the fact that only human PKD cells, and not normal renal cells can form cysts when grown in culture, suggests the presence of a genetic defect directly causing cyst formation. Translocation of basolateral membrane Na-K ATPase pump to the luminal membrane could be responsible for the abnormalities in tubular sodium reabsorption. This in turn would favor sodium and water

secretion into the cyst during early stages in cyst development and cyst growth. This occurs early and may reflect de-differentiation of the cyst-lining cells as a secondary event. The cystic fibrosis transmembrane conductance regulator (CFTR) is present in the apical membrane of ADPKD cells. This channel functions as a cyclic AMP (cAMP)-dependent chloride channel and contributes to cyst growth. Activation of the mammalian target of rapamycin (mTOR) pathway has been implicated in the cyst growth in ADPKD. Alteration in metabolism of blood glucose has been linked with renal cyst formation. The renal cells preferentially shift to aerobic glycolysis, which leads to cyst formation. Lastly, angiogenesis may play a role in cyst growth and disease progression in ADPKD.

Clinical Features

ADPKD usually presents in adults during third or fourth decade of life. Nearly two-thirds of the patients are diagnosed by the age of 55 years. Initial presentation may vary from asymptomatic state to hypertension, hematuria, mild proteinuria, or renal insufficiency. While about half of the younger patients have palpable kidneys, incidence of palpable kidney is much more in older patients. Patient may have cysts of variable sizes scattered throughout the renal tissue (Figs 28.1 and 28.2). Flank pain is one of the most common symptoms of ADPKD and is mainly due to renal calculi, hemorrhage or urinary tract infection. Polycythemia may be found due to increased production of erythro-

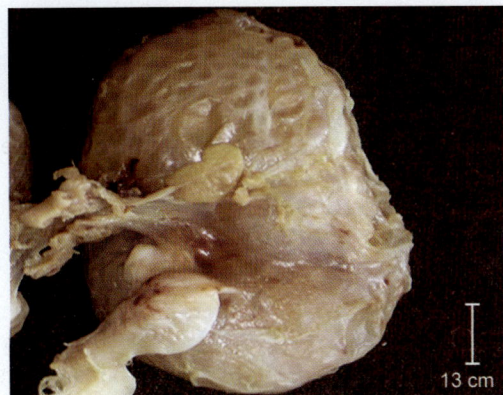

Fig. 28.1: Autosomal dominant polycystic kidney disease—external surface showing multiple cysts with variable sizes

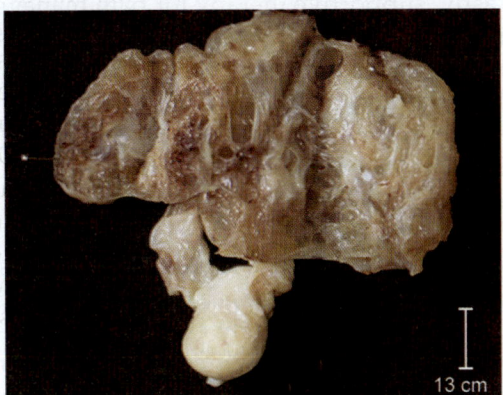

Fig. 28.2: Autosomal dominant polycystic kidney disease—cut surface showing multiple cysts with variable sizes

poietin by the ischemic parenchyma of the kidney. Even if ESRD ensues, anemia is uncommon in ADPKD. Infection of the cysts may lead to fever, pain in the loin and discoloration of the cyst contents. Hemorrhage into a cyst communicating with the drainage system may lead to hematuria. Renal stone formation occurs in about 20% of patients, mainly due to urinary stasis secondary to distorted renal anatomy. Development of malignancy in a cyst occurs rarely. Renal failure may develop as the cysts may become larger and compress the remaining renal parenchyma. Often the renal failure sets in gradually and progresses steadily to ESRD. Polyuria, polydipsia and salt losing state may also develop because of associated tubulo-interstitial damage.

Polycystic liver disease is the most common extrarenal manifestation of ADPKD. It should be suspected when four or more cysts are present in the hepatic parenchyma. Mostly it is asymptomatic but symptoms may be caused by massive enlargement of the liver or by mass effect from cysts. Intracranial aneurysms occur in about 8% of patients with ADPKD. The risk of rupture is related to the size of the aneurysm and is usually extremely small in these patients. Mitral valve prolapse is the most common valvular abnormality seen in around one-fourth of the ADPKD patients demonstrated by echocardiography. Primary dilatation of aortic root and cardiac valvular incompetence are the other important associated features. Cyst formation has also been described in pancreas, spleen, thyroid, ovary, arachnoid membrane, etc. Colonic diverticulosis, horseshoe kidney, immotile sperms and corneal dystrophy are the other associations.

Diagnosis

The diagnosis of ADPKD in patients with positive family history relies on imaging techniques. The plain X-ray of the KUB region often shows large size of the kidneys. The excretory urogram shows the characteristic 'spider leg' deformity. The most commonly used imaging modality for diagnosis of ADPKD is ultrasonography which confirms enlarged kidneys. Revised criteria have been proposed to improve the diagnostic accuracy of ultrasonography in ADPKD and are given in Table 28.3. An ultrasonographic finding of normal kidneys or one renal cyst in an individual aged 40 years or more has a negative predictive value of 100%. CT scan is the 'gold standard' for diagnosis especially in less obvious cases, in children and young

Table 28.3: Sonographic criteria for diagnosis or exclusion of ADPKD

Age (yr)	Criteria for positive diagnosis	PPV(%)	Sensitivity (%)
15–29	≥3 cysts, unilateral or bilateral	100	81.7
30–39	≥3 cysts, unilateral or bilateral	100	95.5
40–59	≥2 cysts in each kidney	100	90.0
≥60	≥4 cysts in each kidney	100	100
	Revised criteria for diagnosis exclusion	*NPV (%)*	*Specificity (%)*
15–29	≥1 cyst	90.8	97.1
30–39	≥1 cyst	98.3	94.8
40–59	≥2 cysts	100	98.2

PPV: Positive predictive value; NPV: Negative predictive value

adults. Further, it can detect malignant change and cysts in other abdominal organs, if present.

Prognosis

Most patients with ADPKD have normal renal function up to 4th decade of life. Beyond that, the glomerular filtration rate begins to decline at the rate of 4.4 to 5.9 ml/minute per year. The risk factors that have been implicated in poor prognosis and progression to ESRD with ADPKD are: Genetic factors (PKD1 has relatively poorer prognosis compared to PKD2), hypertension, early onset of symptoms including proteinuria and hematuria, male gender, increased kidney size (kidney size is greater with PKD1 mutations), increased left ventricular mass index and low birth weight.

Treatment

There is no specific treatment to prevent or delay progression of renal structural disease in ADPKD. Treatment of ADPKD includes non-specific measures, such as dietary protein regulation, low-salt diet, increased fluid intake, strict management of hypertension preferably with angiotensin converting enzyme inhibitors (ACEIs) or angiotensin receptor blockers (ARBs) and use of statins, which may prevent the progression of disease and reduce cardiovascular mortality. During the last decade, new promising therapies being considered include maximal inhibition of the renin-angiotensin-aldosterone system, somatostatin analogues, vasopressin receptor antagonists (tolvaptans) and mTOR inhibitors. Lastly, supportive therapy for pain management, complete bed rest during gross hematuria, and treatment of cyst infection are the key points in treatment of ADPKD.

Patients with ADPKD who progress to ESRD require renal replacement therapy with either dialysis or renal transplantation. Peritoneal dialysis is less preferred than hemodialysis, because it is difficult to infuse large volumes of peritoneal dialysate fluid in the setting of massively enlarged kidneys. Also, it is associated with an increased risk of peritonitis secondary to cyst infection or complications of diverticular disease. Nephrectomy is avoided whenever possible in ADPKD. Rarely, patients require nephrectomy of one or both cystic kidney(s) in order to better accommodate the allograft or for recurrent urinary tract infection, chronic pain, renal cell carcinoma or chronic hematuria requiring repeated blood transfusion. Renal transplantation is the treatment of choice for ESRD in patients with ADPKD.

Genetic counselling is of paramount importance but is often neglected in the management of patients with ADPKD. The newly diagnosed patients should be told about the nature of the disease and the inheritance pattern. Initial screening followed by regular monitoring of blood pressure and periodic ultrasonographic assessment is must in asymptomatic family members. Patients at risk for ADPKD have to be screened before participating in strenuous exercise or sports activities.

Autosomal Recessive Polycystic Kidney Disease

Autosomal recessive polycystic kidney disease (ARPKD) is a cystic kidney disorder usually affecting children. This is a recessively inherited disorder, therefore, it may occur in siblings but not in parents. Earlier called 'infantile polycystic kidney disease', it is characterized by cystic dilatations of the renal collecting ducts and developmental defects of hepatobiliary system resulting in varying degrees of congenital hepatic fibrosis. The incidence of ARPKD is around 1 per 20000 live births.

Pathogenesis

This disorder is caused by the mutation in the PKHD1 gene located on chromosome 6p21 which encodes for the gene fibrocystin, which is found in the cortical and medullary collecting ducts and the thick ascending limb of loop of Henle, and in the epithelial cells of the hepatic bile duct. In this disorder, defective fibrocystin leads to disruption in normal functioning of renal cilia, leading to cyst formation.

Kidneys in patients with ARPKD are usually laden with microcysts (usually less than 2 mm in size). These radiate from medullary junction to the cortex and are grossly visible as pinpoint dots on the kidney surface. Histopathologic examination of renal biopsies demonstrates bilateral cystic dilatations of the collecting ducts; however, the urinary flow in these ducts is not obstructed. The severity of renal manifestations of ARPKD varies directly with the percentage of nephrons affected by cysts. Over time, renal cysts up to 1 cm diameter and interstitial fibrosis develop. This results in progressive deterioration of renal function in children who survive the neonatal period.

ARPKD is almost always associated with developmental defects of the biliary system. This often presents with massive dilatation and biliary dysgenesis, leading to varying degrees of congenital hepatic fibrosis and dilatation of the intrahepatic bile ducts (Caroli disease), which may result in hepatomegaly and portal hypertension.

Clinical Features

The clinical profile of ARPKD varies with the age of onset. Patients present predominantly with either renal involvement or hepatic findings. Patients diagnosed as adolescents or adults typically present with symptoms related to congenital hepatic fibrosis (hepatomegaly, portal hypertension). ARPKD has been classified into following forms based on their presenting features:

1. *Prenatal form:* ARPKD is often detected prenatally during routine ultrasonography. Usually, it is considered in presence of characteristic findings of markedly enlarged echogenic kidneys accompanied by oligohydramnios and the absence of urine in the fetal bladder.
2. *Neonatal form:* Neonatal ARPKD presents with respiratory distress in a newborn due to pulmonary insufficiency resulting from pulmonary hypoplasia. A subset of patients may also have features of skeletal deformities. Renal insufficiency or hypertension may develop during the first few weeks of life.
3. *Infantile and childhood form:* This is the least severe form of ARPKD and over time there is gradual deterioration of renal function, eventually culminating in ESRD. A subset of older patients may present with signs and symptoms due to liver disease, with a little evidence of renal involvement.

Diagnosis

In most cases, diagnosis of ARPKD is made by characteristic renal and hepatic findings on ultrasonography. In cases, in which the diagnosis is uncertain, other imaging modalities, such as MRI or genetic testing may be useful in making the diagnosis.

Management and Outcome

Currently, there is no definitive cure available for ARPKD. The management consists of supportive intervention for respiratory symptoms in neonates and renal replacement therapy, including hemodialysis and kidney transplant in patients who progress to ESRD. Counseling also includes prenatal genetic testing for family members and for siblings of affected patients who may be carriers of a PKHD1 mutation. The outcome of ARPKD is governed by the age of presentation and the degree of renal and hepatic fibrosis and pulmonary hypoplasia.

Medullary Cystic Kidney Disease/Nephronophthisis

Nephronophthisis (NPH)/medullary cystic kidney disease (MCKD) is a group of genetic disorders characterized by small to normal sized cysts at the corticomedullary junction. The mode of inheritance is autosomal recessive NPH and autosomal dominant MCKD. Other distinguishing features are the age of onset of ESRD, and the type of extrarenal organ involvement.

NPH accounts for 10 to 20% of cases of renal failure in childhood. In approximately 15% of the families, it is associated with retinitis pigmentosa, cerebellar involvement or congenital hepatic fibrosis. Defects in NPHP1 gene account for most of NPH cases. Three distinct forms of NPHP have been described based on the age of onset of ESRD—infantile, juvenile, and adolescent.

MCKD is a chronic, progressive kidney disease characterized by bilateral, multiple medullary cysts and tubulointerstitial nephropathy with preserved or reduced kidney size. There are two types of MCKD— type 1 and type 2.

Type 1 MCKD is caused by mutations of the MCKD1 gene which is located at chromosome 1q21, and type 2 disease is associated with mutations of the MCKD2 gene, located on chromosome 16p12. Presenting features of MCKD include polyuria, polydipsia, hyper-uricemia, and gradually progressive renal parenchymal disease leading to ESRD. The family history, clinical features, hyper-uricemia and gout and adjuvant imaging studies are the mainstay of diagnosis. The imaging findings include a preserved or reduced renal size with numerous cysts at medulla/corticomedullary junction bilaterally. The only definitive therapy described in patients of NPH/MCKD is renal replacement therapy with kidney transplantation. MCKD in not known to recur in transplanted kidneys.

von Hippel-Lindau Disease

von Hippel-Lindau (vHL) disease is an autosomal dominant inherited disorder. It is a 'multisystem tumor syndrome' which involves development of benign and malignant neoplasms affecting multiple organs. Mutations of the vHL tumor-suppressor gene, which is located at chromosome 3p25 is responsibe for this disorder. Around 65% of cases diagnosed with vHL have renal involvement which may include simple and complex cysts and multiple, bilateral clear cell renal cell carcinomas. Common extrarenal tumors include central nervous system heman-gioblastomas, retinal angiomas, pancreatic cysts and tumors, and pheochromocytomas. Renal cell carcinoma associated with VHL develops at a much younger age as opposed to its sporadic variants.

Tuberous Sclerosis Complex

Tuberous sclerosis complex (TSC) is an autosomal dominant disorder comprising of both renal and extrarenal manifestations. Renal involvement is seen in about 50–60% of patients, which includes renal cysts (14–32%) and angiomyolipomas (30–40%). The extrarenal manifestations of TSC include central nervous system lesions including multiple cortical tubers, subependymal nodules and astrocytomas. Inactivating mutations of TSC1 gene which is located at chromosome 9q34 is involved in the pathogenesis.

Medullary Sponge Kidney

Medullary sponge kidney (MSK) is a diffuse or focal ectasia and cystic dilatation of the collecting ducts and cyst formation confined strictly to medullary pyramids. It is hypothesized to result from disruption of the interface between the developing ureteral bud and metanephric blastema during embryogenesis. A majority of patients with MSK are asymptomatic; however, some patients may present with renal colic, hematuria, or recurrent urinary tract infections. For diagnosis of MSK, intravenous urography reveals the characteristic 'paint brush' appearance, contrast accumulation and linear radiation from the calyces. On ultrasound, the medullary pyramids appear uniformly hyperechoic due to the deposition of calcium in the affected tubules. On CT examination, presence of medullary nephrocalcinosis is commonly identified and CT urography demonstrates 'papillary brush' morphology and stones within the dilated collecting ducts. The long-term outcome of MSK is favorable and involves less morbidity as opposed to other cystic kidney diseases; however, the complications of recurrent urinary tract obstruction and infections may cause progressive renal failure and ESRD.

Simple Cysts

Simple renal cysts are the most commonly acquired renal cystic lesion, occur twice as frequently in men as in women. They may be solitary or multiple and are filled with fluid. They are very rare in children, but the frequency increases with age. For simple renal cysts the pathogenic mechanisms are unknown but most likely they originate from the diverticula of distal convoluted and collecting tubules.

Simple cysts are typically asymptomatic. Patients may present with polycythemia, hematuria, flank pain, urinary tract infection or obstruction of the collecting system. The kidneys are not enlarged but cysts may be large with no adjacent smaller cysts. Cysts in other organs are absent. These cysts do not impair renal function and are of a little consequence to patient survival. Differentiation of simple cyst from renal cell carcinoma is a common problem because the appearance of a renal mass on the excretory urogram alone never excludes a malignancy. Ultrasonography, computerized tomography or magnetic resonance is commonly required to characterize the lesion. The primary clinical concern is to distinguish simple renal cyst from complex renal cyst which is associated with an increased risk of malignancy.

Treatment is indicated only for symptomatic cysts or for cysts causing obstruction. Intermediate-sized cysts can be aspirated percutaneously. Laparoscopic cyst unroofing may be more appropriate for large cysts greater than 500 ml volume.

Acquired Cystic Kidney Disease

Acquired cystic kidney disease (ACKD) is non-hereditary developmental disorder presenting with three or more renal cysts in both kidneys and is characterized by small cysts distributed throughout the renal cortex and medulla of patients with chronic renal failure unrelated to inherited renal cystic diseases. These cysts are usually small, 0.5 to 2.5 cm in diameter. Though the association between hemodialysis and development of ACKD has been well demonstrated but at least 8–13% of patients develop cysts before the initiation of dialysis. The initial insult in development of ACKD is compensatory hypertrophy of the functioning nephrons in ESRD patients leading to secretion of mitogens that cause renal tubular epithelial hyperplasia and may result in the development of renal cell carcinoma.

The disease is usually asymptomatic and discovered accidentally during abdominal imaging procedures. The complications associated with ACKD include cyst hemorrhage, spontaneous rupture leading to pericystic hematoma, infection of cyst, development of ureteric stone and renal cell carcinoma. ACKD can be easily distinguished from ADPKD with absence of family history of ADPKD and small- or normal-sized kidneys with smooth contour. The cysts may stabilize or regress following successful kidney transplantation.

To summarize, cystic diseases of the kidney may result from various genetic or non-genetic conditions and occur in a variety of diseases in adults and children. Early detection and targeted management may result in preservation of renal function or slowing the progression of kidney disease. In cystic diseases due to genetic causes, antenatal counseling and fetal ultrasonography are of paramount importance.

Acknowledgments

The authors would like to acknowledge the generous help of Dr Amit K Dinda, MD, PhD, Professor, Department of Pathology, All India Institute of Medical Sciences, New Delhi, for providing the figures.

Disorders of Renal Tubular Function

• Rajesh Rajasekharan Nair

The renal tubule performs many functions and helps to maintain the milieu intérieur end excrete the metabolic waste and excess water. In times of diminished intake, it conserves the water and electrolytes. The common functions and disorders of tubular function are summarized in Table 29.1.

In this chapter, disorders of renal tubular function with particular reference to renal tubular acidosis (RTA) is discussed (*see* Section 10, Chapter 47 on inherited renal diseases).

Role of Kidneys in Acid–Base Balance

Every day, the diet and body metabolism result in generation of about 1 mmol H^+/kg body weight in adults. The range varies from 0.4 to 1.6 mmol/kg depending on the diet and is between 1 and 3 mmol/kg in children. Non-vegetarian diets contains more sulfur-containing amino acids and contribute to greater acid load whereas, the vegetarian diet is more alkaline. The lungs and the kidneys are mainly responsible for the maintenance of acid–base balance within the body. They maintain the bicarbonate level in the plasma within the narrow range of 24–26 mmol/L by eliminating carbonic acid as carbon dioxide in the breath and H^+ ions as titratable acid and ammonia in urine. The kidneys also perform the function of reclaiming the filtered bicarbonate (HCO_3) completely.

Table 29.1: Functions of tubule segments and disorders of tubular functions

Tubule segment	Function	Disorder
Proximal tubule	Phosphate, glucose, amino acid and bicarbonate transport	Hypophosphatemic rickets (isolated) renal glucosuria (isolated), phosphaturia Generalized aminoaciduria Proximal RTA
Ascending limb of Henle	Sodium, potassium, chloride transport	Bartter syndrome
Distal tubule	Proton (H^+) secretion Sodium, chloride transport Distal RTA	Gitelman syndrome
Collecting duct	Sodium, potassium transport	Pseudohypoaldosteronism Liddle syndrome
	Water transport	Nephrogenic diabetes insipidus

Reabsorption of bicarbonate: Most of the bicarbonate that is filtered by the glomerulus returns to the circulation, predominantly as a result of Na–H exchange by the proximal tubules. Approximately 85 to 90% of the filtered load is reclaimed at this site (Fig. 29.1). The remaining 10 percent is reclaimed in the distal nephron through hydrogen secretion by proton pumps (H+ATPase and H-K ATPase).

Acid excretion: The excretion of the daily hydrogen ion load is primarily a function of the collecting tubules. Free H+ ions cannot be excreted and should be buffered. The principal buffers in the urine are ammonia and phosphate buffer. Ammonia is synthesized in the kidney and since it is freely diffusible, reaches the lumen of the tubule. The H+ ions are actively transported into the tubular lumen by the H+ ATPase and H-K ATPase. In the lumen, they combine with NH_3 to form NH_4 (ammonium) which cannot diffuse back into the tubule (Fig. 29.2).

Thus, it is excreted in the urine. Similarly, disodium hydrogen phosphate (Na_2HPO_4) is converted to sodium dihydrogen phosphate (NaH_2PO_4) in the tubule thereby facilitating elimination of the H+. When the acid load is high, the homeostasis is maintained by increased ammonia production and excretion. Failure to excrete sufficient ammonium often leads to the net retention of hydrogen ions and the development of metabolic acidosis. The clinical and laboratory features suggesting RTA are summarized in Table 29.2.

The term "renal tubular acidosis" (RTA) refers to a heterogenous group of disorders characterized by relatively well-preserved glomerular filtration rate associated with metabolic acidosis and is mainly due to inability of the renal tubules to perform the normal functions required to maintain acid–base balance. All forms of RTA are characterized by a normal anion gap (hyperchloremic) metabolic acidosis.

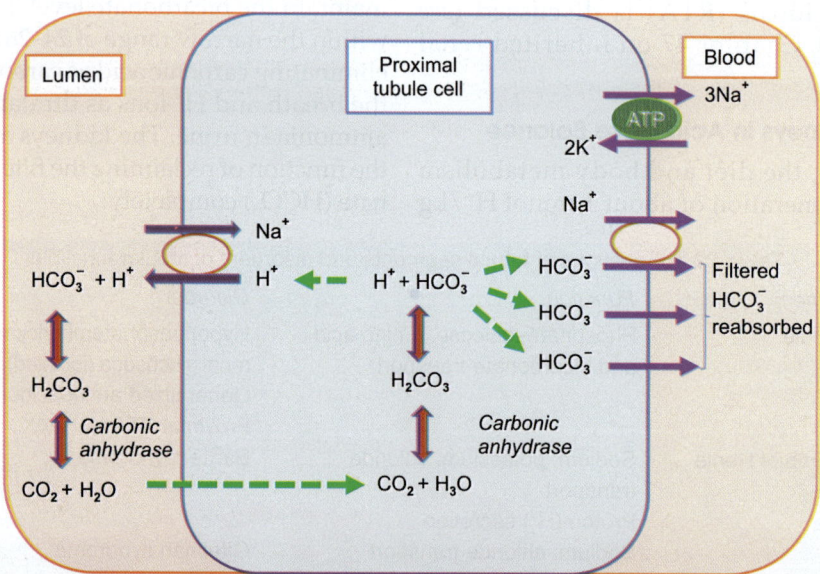

Fig. 29.1: Bicarbonate reabsorption in the proximal tubule. Filtered HCO_3^- combines with secreted H+ (via Na+–H+ antiporter) to produce CO_2 and H_2O. The CO_2 diffuses into the cytoplasm and combines with OH- to produce bicarbonate. The HCO_3^- crosses the basolateral membrane via the Na–HCO_3^- symporter (3 HCO_3^- for 1 Na+) and the Na+–K+ ATPase transports 3 Na+ out per 2 K+

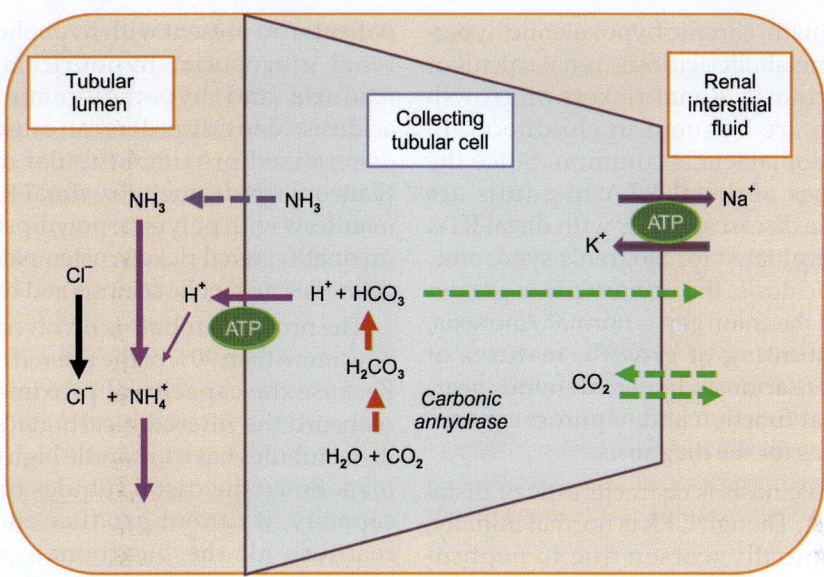

Fig. 29.2: Buffering of hydrogen ion secretion by ammonia (NH$_3$) in the collecting tubules. NH$_3$ reacts with secreted H$^+$ ions to form NH$_4^-$ which is then excreted. For each NH$_4^-$ excreted a new HCO$_3^-$ is formed and returned to the blood

Table 29.2: Features suggestive of renal tubular disorders	
Clinical	*Laboratory*
Growth retardation, failure to thrive	Hyperchloremic metabolic acidosis
Polyuria, polydipsia	Metabolic alkalosis with or without hypokalemia
Refractory rickets, unexplained hypertension	Hyponatremia with hyperkalemia
Renal calculi, nephrocalcinosis	Hypercalciuria with normal serum calcium

Classification of Renal Tubular Acidosis (RTA)

Broadly, RTA can be grouped into two categories:

a. Hypokalemic RTA
   i. Distal/classic/type 1 RTA
   ii. Proximal/type 2 RTA.
b. Hyperkalemic RTA
   i. Hypoaldosteronism/type 4 RTA
   ii. Voltage-dependent RTA (considered a subtype of distal RTA)

Distal (Type 1) RTA

Type 1 RTA can be primary or secondary. Primary disorder may be hereditary or sporadic. Hereditary RTA is autosomal dominant and may present in childhood or adult life or as a part of genetically transmitted systemic disease like Ehlers-Danlos syndrome, hereditary elliptocytosis, osteopetrosis, carbonic anhydrase deficiency and Marfan's syndrome. Secondary or acquired type could be part of autoimmune disorders (Sjögren's syndrome/SLE), hyperglobulinemia, primary cirrhosis, hypercalciuria and hyperparathyroidism. Drugs like NSAIDs, amphotericin B, lithium or cyclosporin may also lead to acquired type 1 RTA.

The primary defect is impaired distal acidification and may be hereditary or acquired. Hereditary distal RTA is most common in children. The manifestations are weakness due to hypokalemia, retarded physical growth, chronic hypokalemic hyper-chloremic metabolic acidosis, renal calculi or nephrocalcinosis. Renal rickets or growth retardation are frequent in childhood. In adults, osteomalacia is common. Since the major causes of distal RTA in adults are autoimmune diseases, adults with distal RTA should be evaluated for Sjögren's syndrome. In spite of acidosis, the urinary pH is greater than 5.5 and the anion gap is normal. Anorexia, lethargy, stunting of growth, features of rickets, severe acidosis, hyperchloremia, near-normal renal function and nephrocalcinosis, provide clues for the diagnosis.

Nephrocalcinosis is characterestic of distal (classic) RTA. Though GFR is normal initially, it may eventually worsen due to nephro-calcinosis, urinary tract obstruction and development of UTI. Under normal circum-stances, when acid is added to the body, the bicarbonate level comes down and the kidneys excrete the acid load by acidifying the urine. Failure to acidify the urine inspite of the plasma HCO_3 being less than 15 mmol/L is the characteristic finding in distal RTA and distinguishes it from other types.

If the patient has no acidosis, the diagnosis can be confirmed by 'ammonium chloride loading' test. In this test, ammonium chloride is given as encapsulated powder at the dose of 0.1 g/kg body weight and the urinary pH is measured every hour for the next five hours. Normally, the urine pH will reduce to less than 5.5 in at least one of the samples. If the urine pH of less than 5.5 is not achieved, the diagnosis of distal RTA can be confirmed.

Proximal (Type 2) RTA

The defect in proximal (type 2) RTA is either an isolated defect in proximal bicarbonate reabsorption or in association with other defects in proximal tubular function. Genera-lized dysfunction of proximal tubule is associated with impaired reabsorption of other solutes such as phosphate, glucose, uric acid, amino acids and bicarbonate. These patients can present with hypophosphatemia, renal glucosuria, hypouricemia, amino-aciduria and hyperchloremic metabolic acidosis. Many disorders can cause isolated or generalized proximal tubular dysfunction (Fanconi syndrome). Proximal RTA usually manifests with polyuria, polydipsia, proximal myopathy, renal rickets, osteomalacia, hyper-chloremic metabolic acidosis and hypokalemia.

The proximal tubule is involved in reabsor-bing more than 90% of the filtered bicarbonate. Because the capacity of proximal tubule to reabsorb the filtered bicarbonate is limited, distal tubules have to handle high bicarbonate load. Since the distal tubules have limited capacity, it cannot produce enough H^+ to reabsorb all the bicarbonate and hence, bicarbonate wasting occurs in urine. The acidosis in type 2 RTA is due to the loss of bicarbonate. In early stages, the urine pH is alkaline even though the blood pH is <7.35. Eventually, when more severe acidosis develops, the filtered load of bicarbonate comes down and the proximal tubule reabsorbs most of the filtered bicarbonate and the distal tubule is now able to acidify the urine. Thus, when blood pH is lower, the urine pH will be <5.5 in proximal RTA whereas, it will be >5.5 in distal RTA.

There is associated urinary sodium wastage and secondary aldosteronism, resulting in hyponatremia and hypokalemia respectively. Polyuria is due to defective concentrating mechanism. The common causes of acquired type 2 RTA are vitamin D deficiency, lead poisoning, multiple myeloma, hyperpara-thyroidism, and nephrotic syndrome.

Mixed (Type 3) RTA

This term was used initially to describe a transient severe form of distal RTA in infants, the term is most often applied to a rare autosomal recessive syndrome (resulting from carbonic anhydrase II deficiency) with features of both proximal and distal RTA. In addition to RTA, affected patients suffer from osteopetrosis, cerebral calcification, and mental retardation.

Type 4 RTA

This type of RTA is characterized by hyperkalemia whereas, the other types are associated with hypokalemia. Aldosterone deficiency is the key factor and occurs in Addison's disease and inborn errors of steroid biosynthesis. Conditions causing destruction of juxtaglomerular apparatus due to chronic tubulointerstitial disesase and diabetic nephropathy causes deficient renin production and is associated with type IV RTA. In diabetic nephropathy, there is also defective conversion of inactive renin precursor to its active form. Type 4 RTA occurs in patients receiving NSAIDs, aldosterone antagonists and in infants with hypoaldosteronism. Renal insensitivity to the action of aldosterone may also be responsible in some cases. Hyperkalemia is related to mineralocorticoid deficiency and has additional effect of suppressing the renal production of NH_4^+. In RTA-4, if the acidosis is severe or hyperkalemia is serious, treatment with mineralocorticoid, fludrocortisone in doses of 0.05–0.15 mg daily improves NH_4^+ excretion and corrects hyperkalemia and acidosis.

Diagnosis

Renal tubular acidosis (RTA) should be considered in any patient who has an otherwise unexplained normal anion gap (hyperchloremic) metabolic acidosis. The different mechanisms involved in the different types of normal anion gap metabolic acidosis are as outlined in Table 29.3.

The following tests are useful in diagnosis and characterization of RTA.

1. *Plasma anion gap:* Anion gap represents the difference of unmeasured anions and cations in the plasma, and is measured as follows:

Plasma anion gap = $Na^+ - (Cl^- + HCO_3^-)$

The normal value of the plasma anion gap is 10–12 mEq/L. Accumulation of organic acids like lactate and acetoacetate, as in diabetic ketoacidosis, uremic toxins as in uremia and poisoning due to ethylene glycol are characteristically associated with metabolic acidosis and an increased anion gap. Normal anion gap in the presence of acidosis (hyperchloremic metabolic acidosis) suggests increased urinary (proximal RTA) or gastrointestinal loss (diarrhea) of bicarbonate or impaired excretion of H+ ions (distal RTA).

2. *Urine anion gap:* Urine anion gap (net charge) also represents the difference between anions and cations in urine. It is calculated by:

$$UAG = Na^+ + K^+ - Cl^-$$

Since urine contains no bicarbonate and higher potassium the formula is appropriately modified. It provides an estimate of urinary ammonium (NH_4^+) excretion and is important in the evaluation of hyperchloremic acidosis. Under normal circumstances, urine anion gap is positive due to the presence of dissolved anions like sulfates and phosphates. Metabolic acidosis is associated with a compensatory rise in NH_4^+ production, resulting in a negative urine anion gap. Patients with RTA typically show impaired renal NH_4^+ excretion and a positive urine anion gap.

Table 29.3: Causes of normal anion gap metabolic acidosis	
Mechanism	*Cause*
Loss of bicarbonate or bicarbonate precursors	Diarrhea/intestinal losses, type 2 RTA, following correction of ketoacidosis, carbonic anhydrase inhibitors, ureteral diversion
Decreased renal acid excretion	Chronic kidney disease and tubular dysfunction, type 1 and type 4 RTA

3. *Urine pH:* Urine pH is an estimate of the number of free H^+ ions in the urine which are secreted in response to metabolic acidosis. The presence of alkaline urine during metabolic acidosis suggests defective renal acidification, as in distal RTA and early stages of proximal RTA. However, alkaline urine may also be found in patients with metabolic acidosis due to extrarenal disorders, as in acute or chronic diarrhea.

HYPERCHLOREMIC (NORMAL ANION GAP) METABOLIC ACIDOSIS

The first step in the evaluation of a patient with hypokalemia and metabolic acidosis (Fig. 29.3) is to differentiate gastrointestinal bicarbonate loss from RTA. The presence of polyuria, failure to thrive and rickets, are suggestive of RTA. Gastrointestinal bicarbonate losses can be differentiated from RTA by estimating the urine anion gap (urine net charge). Negative urine anion gap indicates increased renal NH_4^+ production (tubules functioning normally, therefore, usually extrarenal cause for metabolic acidosis). If the urine anion gap is positive, NH_4 production is defective suggesting the diagnosis of RTA.

Children with proximal (type 2) RTA need to undergo estimation of fractional excretion

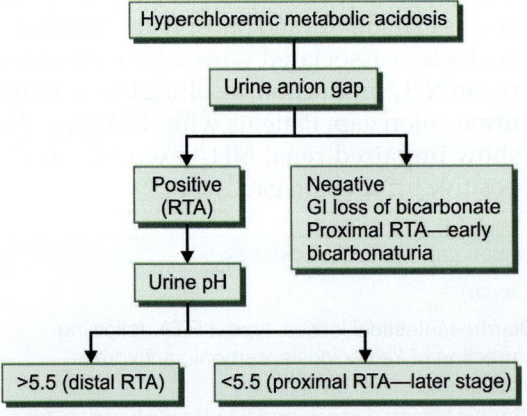

Fig. 29.3: Approach to a patient with metabolic acidosis and hypokalemia

of bicarbonate and evaluation for other proximal tubule functions like phosphate, electrolytes, glucose and amino acid excretion. They should also be screened for an underlying etiology like Wilson disease or cystinosis. Investigations in children with distal (type 1) RTA should include estimation of urine calcium excretion, ultrasound for renal calcification and work-up for secondary causes like, obstructive uropathy, reflux nephropathy, chronic tubulointerstitial nephritis.

Management

If acidosis is associated with moderate to severe hypokalemia, the serum potassium must be corrected before correcting acidosis. If acidosis is corrected first, movement of K^+ to the intracellular compartment occur leading to further lowering of plasma K^+ and cardiac complications. If severe muscular weakness occurs due to hypokalemia, artificial ventilation may be necessary for respiratory failure. In chronic stages, alkali therapy usually combined with potassium replacement are given to avoid severe hypokalemia. Potassium supplements are usually administered as citrate salts. Oral bicarbonate with potassium replacements can be given in the form of Shohl's solution with potassium. This therapy maintains serum bicarbonate and potassium levels, diminishes hypercalciuria, prevents acidosis, renal rickets, osteomalacia and growth retardation. In addition, progression of nephrocalcinosis and renal damage may be halted. One milliliter of Shohl's solution provides equivalent of one millimol of bicarbonate. Bicarbonate requirement is more in patients with proximal RTA (5–6 mmol/kg/day) compared to distal RTA (1–2 mmol/kg/day). Patients with proximal RTA often require supplementation of phosphate in the form of Joule's solution, neutral phosphate solution combined with small doses of vitamin D. In severe cases, hydrochlorothiazide is added since it increases the proximal tubular reabsorption of bicarbonate and stimulate H⁺ secretion.

These patients are followed up to monitor growth, blood levels of electrolytes, pH and bicarbonate. Subjects with distal RTA are at risk for nephrocalcinosis, which should be screened for by ultrasound. Early recognition of RTA, prompt treatment and lifelong follow up are important.

METABOLIC ALKALOSIS AND HYPOKALEMIA

Renal tubular causes of hypokalemia with alkalosis include a spectrum of conditions involving reduced electrolyte reabsorption (Bartter syndrome, Gitelman syndrome) or increased mineralocorticoid action (Liddle syndrome, syndrome of apparent mineralocorticoid excess and glucocorticoid remediable aldosteronism) (Fig. 29.4).

Initial evaluation should include history to rule out upper gastrointestinal loss (vomiting and nasogastric drainage), chronic diuretic or laxative use and measurement of blood pressure. Urine chloride level <10 mEq/L suggests nonrenal causes and >20 mEq/L, renal cause for hypokalemic alkalosis.

Elevated blood pressure suggests hyperaldosteronism, congenital adrenal hyperplasia. Syndromes of apparent mineralocorticoid excess and Liddle syndrome are also associated with hypertension, hypokalemia and metabolic alkalosis. These disorders can befurther classified based on blood levels of aldosterone, renin and response to treatment with corticosteroid and/or spironolactone. Low blood levels of aldosterone and lack of response to glucocorticoid and spironolactone is suggestive of Liddle syndrome. Bartter syndrome can be differentiated from Gitelman syndrome by presence of hypercalciuria in the former and hypomagnesemia in the latter.

Management

Treatment of Bartter syndrome consists of ensuring adequate hydration and potassium supplementation (as chloride salts) along with indomethacin (2–4 mg/kg/day). Specific therapy with magnesium (50–100 mg/kg/day) is indicated in Gitelman syndrome and amiloride in Liddle syndrome so as to ameliorate the biochemical features of the respective diseases.

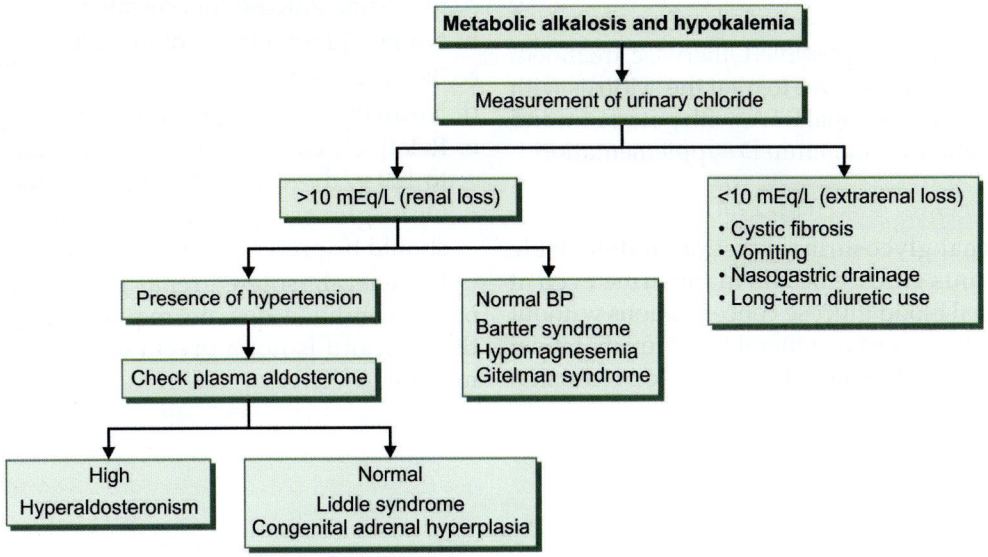

Fig. 29.4: Approach to a patient with metabolic alkalosis and hypokalemia

Table 29.4: Causes of Fanconi syndrome

Inherited causes	Acquired causes
Cystinosis	Drugs: Cisplatin/ifosfamide/tenofovir/cidofovir/adefovir/gentamicin/azathioprine
Galactosemia	Dysproteinemias: Multiple myeloma/Sjögren's syndrome/light-chain proteinuria/amyloidosis
Wilson's disease, hereditary fructose intolerance, tyrosinemia, mitochondrial cytopathies, idiopathic	Heavy metal poisoning: Lead/cadmium/Chinese herbal medicine/glue sniffing/diachrome/nephrotic syndrome/renal transplantation

Heritable Disorders of Proximal Tubular Function

A number of mainly heritable disorders, affects proximal tubule functions. The common ones are described below.

Fanconi Syndrome (Table 29.4)

In the 1930s, Fanconi and others described several children with the combination of renal rickets, glycosuria, and hypophosphatemia. 'Fanconi syndrome' can be considered to be a dysfunction of the proximal tubule leading to excessive urinary excretion of amino acids, glucose, phosphate, bicarbonate, and other solutes handled by this nephron segment.

Causes of Fanconi syndrome: Therapy should be directed towards treating the underlying cause. In such patients, at least resolution of the syndrome is possible. Otherwise, treatment would be supportive to treat the acidosis with alkali as in proximal RTA, with potassium and phosphate and vitamin D supplementation.

Renal Glycosuria (Fig. 29.4)

In renal glycosuria, excretion of detectable amounts glucose occurs in the urine even at normal blood glucose concentrations without any other signs of generalized proximal renal tubular dysfunction. This is due to a reduction in the capacity of proximal renal tubule to reabsorb glucose. The inherited form of this disorder is called familial renal glucosuria (FRG). This is a rare disorder inherited as a codominant trait with variable penetrance. Mutations in the SLC5A2 gene that codes for the SGLT2 glucose transporter is responsible. This transporter found in the early portion of the proximal tubule transports sodium and glucose from the lumen to the tubular cell. (The SGLT2 inhibitors introduced recently as oral antidiabetic drugs inhibit this transporter, promotes more glucose loss in the urine to maintain the blood sugar level.)

The revised criteria for diagnosis of renal glycosuria include:
a. Normal oral glucose tolerance test in regard to plasma glucose concentration
b. Normal plasma levels of insulin
c. Normal free fatty acids level
d. Normal glycosylated hemoglobin
e. Relatively constant levels of glycosuria (10 to 100 g/d)—except during pregnancy
f. Only glucose (no other carbohydrate) should be present in all urine samples.

In general, isolated renal glycosuria is a benign condition, does not require any specific therapy and is not a precursor of diabetes mellitus.

Section

VII

Infections of
the Urinary Tract

Urinary Tract Infection (UTI): Defense Mechanisms and Predisposing Factors

• S Gomathy

DEFENSE MECHANISMS AGAINST UTI

Several factors operate at each anatomical level in the urinary system and prevent the development of urinary infection. The incidence and pattern of urinary infection is different between males and females of different age groups. When urinary infection occurs in a young male child it usually indicates an underlying structural anomaly. Urinary tract infection is common in girls and young adult females. It may occur rarely in young adult males. However, in the elderly it is more common in males than in females. Bacteria usually invade the urinary tract by ascending from the perineum. It may rarely gain entry through lymphatics or blood stream. The factors in the host and characteristics of the urinary pathogens, especially the adhesion of the bacteria to the urinary tract, contribute to the development and persistence of infection.

The host defense mechanisms (for prevention of UTI) are summarised in Table 30.1.

The constituents of normal urine themselves provide an important antimicrobial defense mechanism. The high or low osmolality of urine, high concentration of urea, presence of organic acids and acidic pH inhibit bacterial growth. Since the urine of women have a more favorable pH and osmolality for the growth of

E. coli, urinary infections are more common in females. The short female urethra and its close proximity to the perianal region generally predisposes women to UTI. The urethral trauma and massage which occurs during sexual intercourse is another precipitating factor. The uropathogens, predominantly *E.coli* have easy access to periurethral region from the fecal reservoir and perianal area. This is why persons with relatively poor perineal or perianal hygiene have more chance of developing UTI in conditions of lowered host resistance and increased susceptibility. The presence of glucose in the urine provides a better medium for bacterial growth and so, UTI is more common and difficult to eradicate in uncontrolled diabetic subjects. The small quantity of prostatic secretions containing zinc and other antibacterial substances in the urethra at the end of micturition, prevent the colonization of the urethra and prevent infection in males. Tamm-Horsfall protein (uromucoid), a constituent of normal urine, acts as a urinary defense mechanism by aggregating *E. coli* to it thereby preventing adherence of bacteria to the mucosa. The normal periurethral, introital and vaginal flora contains lactobacilli, coagulase negative staphylococci, corynebacteria, streptococci and anaerobic bacteria. Bacterial multiplication

Table 30.1: Host defense mechanisms

Mechanism

1. Natural defenses in the urinary tract:

  a. Urine
     a. Osmolality, urea concentration, organic acid concentration, pH, absence of glucose, prostatic secretion, uromucoid (Tamm-Horsfall protein), antibacterial constituents of urine.

  b. Urethral length
     b. Short urethral length in females predispose to infection in them

  c. Vaginal pH
     c. Acidic pH of vagina helps to prevent bacterial colonization

  d. Bladder
     d. Flushing effect of micturition, absence of residual urine, uromucoid preventing adhesion of pathogens, superficial mucopolysaccharide layer of bladder mucosa, antibacterial activity of mucosa and mucosal phagocytosis

  e. Prostate
     e. Prostatic secretions contain bactericidal zinc

  f. Normal vesicoureteric junction
     f. Intramural length of the distal ureter acts as an antireflux mechanism preventing the entry of urine back into ureter from bladder at the beginning of micturition and this helps to prevent UTI

  g. Kidney cortex
     g. Blood flow rate, osmolality and pH prevent bacterial colonization in the cortex

2. Immune mechanisms
     2. (a) *Native immunity:* Toll-like receptor (TLR) 4 is upregulated during inflammation. They are capable of recognizing bacterial endotoxins and cause local release of cytokines. Thus, polymorphs and other inflammatory cells extravasate into the tissue. The polymorphs phagocytose the bacteria with or without opsonization. Immunoglobulin either IgA or IgG or antibacterial peptides are needed as the main opsonins for opsonization

     (b) *Antibodies:* IgA, IgG, IgM in the urine are protective. They either opsonize, or target bacterial adhesins or trigger agglutination of bacteria, thereby promoting bacterial clearance by voiding

     (c) Cell-mediated immunity (T and B cells) plays an important role in chronic and recurrent infections

3. Antimicrobial proteins and peptides
     3. Epithelial derived antimicrobial proteins:
     (a) Tamm-Horsfall protein (THP) is a potent activator of innate and adaptive immune response which can lead to interstitial nephritis. Other antimicrobial peptides:
     (b) Beta defensins—from renal epithelium
     (c) Alpha defensins—infiltrating neutrophils
     (d) Cathelcidins (LL-37)—direct bactericidal action (from renal tubular cells and from urothelium)
     (e) Lactoferrin and lipocalins—bactericidal activity by restricting the availability of iron for bacteria

4. Genetic variability in the hosts
     4. (a) Patients of P1 blood group possess a high density of cell surface receptors for P fimbriae and are prone to recurrent UTI
     (b) TLR4 (see above)
     (c) CXCR1 (see notes below)—associated with recurrent UTI

of pathogenic bacteria in the normal urethra is inhibited by the resident normal flora. The low vaginal pH (<5) also prevents the introital colonization of the pathogenic bacteria. Antibiotic chemotherapy, by altering the normal flora may predispose to colonization by pathogenic bacteria and lead to infection in certain individuals. Certain genetic factors may be responsible for controlling the bacterial adherence in periurethral and urethral cells.

The normal bladder seems inherently resistant to UTI. The inoculation of urethral organisms into the bladder after sexual intercourse produces a state of low level bladder bacteriuria. In most instances, these organisms are completely eliminated within 24 hours. The bladder has a superficial layer of mucopolysaccharide which prevents the adhesion of uropathogens. The organisms are probably removed by a combination of:

a. Efficient urination without residual urine

b. Inhibition of multiplication of bacteria within the urine

c. Failure of adherence of bacteria to the bladder mucosa

d. Effectiveness of antibacterial property of intact mucosa

e. Efficiency of mucosal phagocytosis.

A competent and anti-refluxing vesico-ureteric junction prevents the spread of any bladder infection to the upper urinary tract. The susceptibility of various parts of the kidney to infection is not uniform. Because of the high blood flow rate, low osmolality and near-normal pH, the renal cortex appears less susceptible to infection than the renal medulla and pyramids. The physiological peculiarities of renal medulla like the countercurrent multiplier system and low blood flow rate makes this area easily susceptible to infection by impeding the humoral and cellular defenses. The high ammonia concentration inhibits the leukocyte chemotaxis and suppresses the complement system.

No natural barrier or defense mechanism against bacterial adherence has been identified in the kidney. However, the steady flow of urine helps in flushing down the bacteria. Infiltration by inflammatory cells itself may produce local tissue damage, scarring and bacterial adhesion.

Immune mechanisms: The genitourinary tract forms part of the secretory immune system where IgA is secreted in the urine. The presence of IgA seems to offer some protection against development of UTI.

Genetic variability in the host: Patients prone to UTIs tend to be blood group P1 and possess high density of cell surface receptors for P fimbriae. Two other host factors are associated with UTI. Chemokine (CXC motif) receptor 1 (CXCR1) is an interleukin-1 receptor and its deficiency is associated with acute pyelo-nephritis. Toll-like receptor (TLR) 4 deficiency results in a carrier state.

BACTERIAL VIRULENCE FACTORS

Ability of bacteria to adhere to mucosal or urothelial cells is an important factor in determining bacterial virulence. Some urinary pathogens are relatively avirulent and opportunistic. These organisms induce urinary infection only when the natural host defenses are compromised. Others are capable of causing upper and lower tract infections even in the absence of structural abnormalities. Certain virulence factors of pathogenic microorganism predispose to UTI. They are:

a. Fimbriae

b. Adhesins

c. Flagella

d. Hemolysins

e. Siderophores

f. Proteases (ureases)

g. 'L' forms

h. Exotoxins

i. Lipopolysaccharide capsule

a. Fimbriae

Fimbriae or pili are proteinaceous structures involved in the adhesion of uropathogenic E. coli (UPEC) to urothelium and help the bacteria to withstand the stress of the flow of filtrate or urine. The different types of fimbriae are P fimbria, type 1 fimbria F1C, S, Afa/Dr adhesins. Each strain of UPEC expresses one type of fimbria at a time. Type I fimbriae in E. coli increase the inflammatory response to infection, inhibits the ureteric motility and favor ascend of bacteria from the bladder to kidneys. Fimbriae also regulates the synthesis of flagellum, that mediates bacterial mobility. Type 1 fimbriae is made up of 500–3000 repeat subunits of FimA protein and a tip adhesion protein FimH. This tip adhesion FimH are able to bind to mannose containing glycoproteins present in the urothelium. Thus, bacterial adhesion and colonization occurs. The type 1 fimbriae also mediate inter-bacterial contact resulting in formation of a biofilm which provides a means for bacteria to withstand the stress and survive. In the bladder uroplakins on the surface of the bladder epithelium containing monomannose moieties bind to FimH adhesins. It is likely that chemoprophylaxis of recurrent UTI with low (non-bactericidal) dose antibiotic reduces the frequency of relapses because of diminished fimbrial adhesion.

Bacteria adhere to the uroepithelial cells with the help of structures called pili or fimbriae. Two types of pili have been identified. Type 1 pili help in the adhesion to the cells of the lower urinary tract leading to lower urinary tract infection. Bacteria possessing type II or 'P' pili commonly lead to upper urinary tract infection or pyelonephritis.

P fimbriae also promote the renal tropism, prevent the clearance of infection and act as a virulence factor by promoting persistence of the infection. They were first isolated in patients with acute pyelonephritis. They facilitate colonization of the UPEC the renal tubule in the face of shear stress from renal filtrate flow. They were designated 'P' because of their ability to agglutinate red blood cells of the P blood group. It was also demonstrated that P fimbriae act in synergy with type I fimbriae to facilitate renal tubule colonization. P fimbriae mediates bacterial binding to the epithelium whereas, type I fimbriae mediate interbacterial binding as the colony expanded into the tubule and away from the epithelium.

F1 C fimbriae are implicated in both upper and lower UTI. The fimbriae help to bind to distal tubular and collecting tubule epithelial cell as well as renal vascular endothelial cells.

S fimbriae play only minor role in the causation of UTI.

b. Adhesins

There are 2 types of adhesins, fimbrial and non-fimbrial. Adhesins found at the tip of fimbriae are the fimbrial adhesins also called pili (explained above) and those found on the bacterial surface are called non-fimbrial adhesins. These are a family of proteins found on the extracellular surface of E. coli which bind to 'Dr' blood group antigens. Dr adhesins mediate binding of E. coli to the bladder epithelium has been correlated with recurrent UTI in young adults and pyelonephritis in pregnant women.

The net negative charge of the epithelial cells and small electronegative surface charge of the UPEC repel each other and prevent bacterial adhesin. Presence of fimbriae or other surface adhesin systems and the hydrophobic nature promote adhesin between bacteria and urothelium. The fimbriae allow irreversible attachment to the uroepithelial cell membrane via adhesins. Adhesin is particularly important when infection occurs in an anatomically normal urinary tract. In cases of recurrent cystitis and infection complicating indwelling bladder catheters, minor trauma will cause disruption of the protective mucosal coat.

Non-fimbrial adhesins [afimbrial adhesins—(AFA)]: Dr blood group antigen is a cell membrane protein in RBCs (also called decay accelerating factor) as their receptor. Some Dr family adhesins are afimbrial adhesins. Afa-I and Afa-III are the other non-fimbrial adhesins.

c. Flagella

The bacterial flagella are tube-like helical filaments made up of the protein flagellin. The arrangement of proteins enable the bacterium to turn clockwise and anticlockwise thus enabling bacterial motility.

d. Hemolysin

Hemolysins produced by the bacteria are cytotoxic to a number of cells and causes cell lysis. In sublytic concentration, they elicit the Ca signaling in proximal tubular cells and mediate a proinflammatory response via activation of NFkB (nuclear factor kappa B). The α-hemolysin is a virulence factor and is expressed in more than 50% of of pyelone-phritogenic strain of *E. coli*.

e. Siderophores

These are proteins which scavenge free iron within the host. Since low iron availability limits bacterial viability, iron deprivation is a host defence mechanism in the face of UTI. UPEC also expresses siderophore associated receptors. Bacterial strains with impaired iron acquisition capability have decreased virulence, colonization and growth.

f. Ureases

These are urea splitting enzymes secreted by uropathogenic organisms like *Proteus mirabilis*. Ammonia which is liberated when urea is split, turns the pH of urine alkaline. The alkaline urine, favors formation of stones which contains proteinaceous matrix, leuko-cytes, struvite (magnesium ammonium phosphate) and bacteria. Such stones act as permanent sources of bacteria within the urinary system.

g. 'L' Forms

Certain types of bacteria lose their cell wall during adverse conditions in the host in order to survive. These are called 'L' forms. Since they have no cell wall, antibiotics like penicillin or cephalexin which act on the bacterial cell wall are ineffective. When the conditions are more favorable, these bacteria resynthesize the cell wall, multiply and turn pathogenic resulting in relapses of UTI.

h. Exotoxin

Secreted autotransporter toxin is a 107 KDa protein isolated from pyelonephritogenic *E. coli*. It has serine protease activity and shows cytopathic effects on human bladder and kidney cell lines. Originally isolated from UPEC strain CFT073, sat was found to share homology with various virulence-related proteins from a range of *E. coli* pathotypes.

i. Lipopolysaccharide Capsule

The serotyping of *E. coli* strain is based on 3 determinants: The somatic antigen O, the capsular antigen K and the flagella antigen H. This classification system identified more than 50,000 serotypes. Studies show that some O serogroups are more frequent in isolates from symptomatic UTI. However, clear experimental evidence correlating a particular O type with a pathogenic tendency is lacking.

Entry into urothelial cells: When UPEC enters into bladder epithelial cells, these cells provide a protected niche, where the bacteria can persist, remain quiescent for long periods protected from antibiotics and host defences, serving as sources of recurrent infection.

HOST CONDITIONS PREDISPOSING TO UTI

Any condition or abnormality which interferes with urinary tract defenses or favors bacterial adhesion can result in urinary infection.

a. Obstruction anywhere along the urinary tract inhibits normal flow of urine and cause stasis. Since the flushing action is lost, bacteria can colonise and perpetuate an infection. Congenital anomalies like posterior urethral or other valves, bands, stenosis/strictures, calculi, compression of ureter, polycystic kidney and vesicoureteric reflux result in stasis or accumulation of urine.

b. Calculi predispose to urinary infection and difficulty in eradicating the infection due to partial or complete urinary stasis or irritation and injury to the urothelium. The calculi due to calcium or magnesium ammonium phosphate may be the result of long-standing urinary infection with urea splitting organisms like Proteus or Klebsiella.

c. Vesicoureteric reflux is a condition which leads to easy spread of infection from the lower urinary tract to the upper urinary tract. It also leads to functional obstruction to the normal urinary flow in the upper urinary tract and residual urine in the bladder.

d. Incomplete emptying of bladder due to mechanical or neurological causes predisposes to stasis, secondary stone formation and persistence of urinary infection.

e. Diabetics who have neurological complications involving the urinary bladder are at an increased risk of developing UTI. However, factors like sugar in urine, underlying nephrosclerosis, sluggishness of renal medullary circulation and leukocyte dysfunction may contribute to renal parenchymal destruction and scarring.

f. Ascending infection is the commonest mode of entry of bacteria from lower tract. The organisms are usually derived from the bowel, which may colonise in the peri-urethral tissue before entering the bladder through urethra. This is more commonly seen in females in whom the combination of short urethral length and anal to urethral distance (<4.5 cm), favor the easy entry of the organism into the urinary tract. These anatomical risks can be worsened further by sexual intercourse, use of spermicidal jellies, fecal contamination of perineum and use of urethral catheters.

g. Aging in males and females is associated with increased prevalence of UTI because of obstructive uropathy. Poor emptying of the bladder may occur in older women because of uterine prolapse, cystocele or urethral stricture. In elderly males, loss of bactericidal activity of prostatic secretion, prostatic obstruction and its effects on the urinary tract may predispose to UTI.

Various structural and functional characteristics make urinary tract inherently resistant to infection. Along with anti bacterial peptides and proteins elaborated in the urinary tract, innate and adaptive immunity are also essential for protection from UTI. Bacteria elaborate several virulence factors like fimbrie and pili which help them not only to colonise and cause infection but can result in persistent infection. There are many host conditions which predispose to infection like obstruction, calculi, vesicoureteric reflux, incomplete bladder evacuation, etc. Genetic variation in the natural defense mechanisms also make some patients more prone to UTI. So, any breakdown in the natural defense mechanisms and presence of virulent bacteria lead to establishment of infection.

Urinary Tract Infection in Adults

• M Sreelatha

INTRODUCTION

Urinary tract infection (UTI) is the 3rd most common infection in humans, after respiratory and gastrointestinal infections. Any site in the urinary tract can be affected. The site of infection determines the pattern of symptoms. The infection can vary in severity from asymptomatic colonization to life-threatening sepsis. Infecting organisms are usually bacteria. Fungal infections are common in immuno-suppressed individuals. Infection is caused by viruses or parasites are relatively rare.

Definitions

It is important to know and understand various definitions and terminologies used in relation to urinary tract infection.

Urinary tract infection is the presence of bacteria or other micro-organisms in the urine or genitourinary tissue, which are normally sterile.

Pyuria is the presence of white blood cells (WBCs) in the urine and is generally indicative of an inflammatory response of the urothelium to microbial invasion.

Bacteriuria is the presence of bacteria in the urine, which is normally free of bacteria.

Significant bacteriuria is the presence of ≥1,00,000 (10^5) or more colony forming units

(CFU) of same organism per milliliter of urine in culture (Kass criteria).

Asymptomatic bacteriuria is defined as significant bacteriuria (10^5 cfu/ml) without any symptoms or signs attributed to local or systemic urinary tract infection.

Symptomatic UTI is significant bacteriuria along with signs and symptoms depending on the site of infection (kidney, collecting system, bladder, urethra or prostate).

Upper urinary tract infection: Infection of the kidney (also called pyelonephritis).

Lower urinary tract infection: Infection involving urinary bladder (cystitis), prostate (prostatitis) or urethra (urethritis).

Uncomplicated UTI: Documented UTI in an otherwise healthy person with structurally normal urinary tract.

Complicated UTI: Documented UTI in a patient with structurally and functionally abnormal urinary tract or in patients susceptible to infection like diabetics or immunocompromised.

Catheter-associated UTI (CA-UTI): It is defined by the presence of symptoms or signs compatible with UTI, along with ≥10^3 CFU/ml of one or more bacterial species in a new single catheter urine sample or in MSU sample within 48 hours of catheter removal.

According to the criteria laid by the European Association of Urology (EAU) in 2011, complicated UTI is a condition where a patient has positive urine culture associated with one or more of the following features:

a. Presence of indwelling catheter, stent or the use of intermittent bladder catheterization
b. Post-void residual urine >100 ml
c. Obstructive uropathy of any etiology (e.g. bladder outlet obstruction, neurogenic bladder, stones, tumor)
d. Vesicoureteric reflux (VUR)
e. Urinary tract modifications like ileal loop or pouch
f. Chemical or radiation injuries of urothelium
g. Perioperative and postoperative UTI
h. Renal insufficiency, post-transplantation, diabetes mellitus, or immunodeficiency.

Recurrent infection is defined as at least 3 episodes of UTI in the preceding 12 months or 2 episodes in last 6 months.

Relapse of infection: UTI with same organism within 3 weeks after successful completion of treatment of previous episode.

Reinfection: Occurrence of UTI with a different organism within 3 weeks after treatment of previous episode.

Resistant infection: Pathogens which fail to respond to effective antibiotics within 48 to 72 hours.

UTI is common in women, with a peak incidence between 20 and 40 years of age. During their lifetime, about 40% of women will have a UTI and 20 to 30% will suffer recurrent UTI. In most cases, the second attack occurs within 3 to 6 months after the first episode. Symptomatic UTI affects 30% of women between the age of 20 and 40 years and is 30 times more than in men in the same age group. With increasing age, ratio of female to male with bacteriuria progressively decreases. By age 60 years, at least 20% of women and 10% of men have bacteriuria. Overall prevalence of bacteriuria is 3.5%.

Symptoms

The common symptoms of lower urinary tract infection are dysuria (painful micturition), increased frequency, urgency and strangury (painful desire to pass urine even though the bladder is empty). These symptoms are common in acute urethritis and prostatitis. Most of these patients will have pyuria, but only <50% will have bacteriuria. Gross hematuria may also be present. Suprapubic pain and gross hematuria along with dysuria and frequency and urgency indicate cystitis.

Symptoms due to upper urinary tract infection are fever with rigor and chills, nausea and vomiting, flank pain and renal angle tenderness. Since they have constitutional symptoms and may be toxic, they usually get hospitalized. They may have burning sensation in urethra but other symptoms of lower UTI are usually absent. Numerous risk factors contribute to development of UTI in males and females in different age groups (Table 31.1).

Microbiology

Most common organism producing uncomplicated UTI is *E. coli* (70–95%). *Staphylococcus saprophyticus* may be responsible for 5–20% of cases with cystitis. Other organisms identified are Proteus, Klebsiella, Pseudomonas, Entero-

Table 31.1: Risk factors of urinary tract infections

1. Age
2. Female sex
3. Pregnancy and postmenopausal status
4. Atrophic vaginitis
5. Sexual intercourse
6. Presence of catheter
7. Neurogenic bladder
8. Urinary incontinence
9. Diabetes mellitus
10. Immunosuppressed persons
11. Poor personal hygiene
12. Increased post-voidal residual urine

Table 31.2: Bacteria causing UTI		
Organism	Uncomplicated UTI (%)	Complicated UTI (%)
Gram negative:		
E. coli	70–95	21–54
Proteus	1–2	1–10
Klebsiella	1–2	2–17
Pseudomonas	<1	2–19
Enterobacter	<1	2–10
Other	<1	6–20
Gram positive:		
S. saprophyticus (CoNS)	≥5–20	1–4
Group B streptococci	<1	1–4
Enterococci	1–2	1–23
S. aureus	<1	1–2

bacter, Streptococcus, enterococci and *Staph. aureus* and tend to cause complicated UTI (Table 31.2). In 95% cases, the infection is caused by a single organism and in only 5%, it is due to two or more organisms. Polymicrobial infections are more common in immunosuppressed individuals, or those with retained foreign bodies, or on long-standing indwelling urinary catheters.

Infection occurs most commonly via ascending route from gut flora that colonizes in the vagina or periurethral area. Mere presence of bacteria in the urinary tract does not cause infection. Adhesion of bacteria to the uroepithelium is necessary for establishing urinary infection. Production of FimH, an adhesin enables attachment to receptor on uroepithelial cells. Other virulent factors have been described with *E. coli* like characteristic pili which enhances their adherence to bladder wall, biofilm related factors, iron uptake, etc. Some of the host factors are also important in the pathogenesis of UTI like genetic propensity, nonsecretors of ABH blood group antigens, sexual intercourse, use of spermicidal jelly and estrogen deficiency in postmenopausal females. Trauma to the uroepithelial cell and shedding of the mucous coat enables attachment of the bacteria to the cell and initiates infection.

Diagnosis

Testing of urine is the first and fundamental test for the diagnosis of UTI. The best sample is cleanly collected midstream urine (MSU) sample. The commonly done tests are the following.

1. Urine Dipstick Tests

These tests provide rapid results, do not require microscopy and are ready to use. This method can be used for routine assessment which includes leukocyte esterase test (as a surrogate marker for pyuria) and nitrite reaction (for gram-negative enteric bacteria) for bacteriuria.

2. Urine Microscopy

Urine microscopy is done with a centrifuged MSU sample. Pyuria is defined as >10 WBC/HPF. A gram-stained smear aids in identifying the likely pathogen.

3. Urine Culture and Sensitivity

This is the gold standard diagnostic test in UTI. It is required for confirmation of diagnosis, identification of organisms and the sensitivity to antibiotics, thereby guiding treatment.

How to collect urine for culture in different situations?

a. 'Clean-catch' midstream urine after washing and drying the external genitalia.
b. Sterile needle aspiration of urine from the catheter port if the patient is catheterized.
c. Suprapubic needle aspiration of urine directly from bladder.
d. Urine obtained by single catheterization.

Urine specimen should be cultured within two hours. In case of anticipated delay, it is preserved either by refrigeration at 4°C or by adding boric acid 1.5%, sodium formate 0.5%. The laboratory reports the urine culture as no growth, or quantifies the growth as colony forming units (CFU). The interpretation varies depending on the type of collection. Even a single bacterial colony in a properly performed sterile suprapubic aspiration sample is significant whereas, if the sample is (wrongly) collected from stored urine from a urine bag it has no value (Table 31.3) summarizes the diagnostic significance of CFU in different clinical situations.

4. Total Leukocyte Count (TLC), C-Reactive Protein (CRP) and Serum Procalcitonin (PCT)

These tests are done to confirm the diagnosis of infection. C-reactive protein (CRP) and serum procalcitonin (PCT) are markers for systemic inflammatory response. CRP, is an acute-phase reactant synthesized by the liver and CRP level measurements are used frequently to aid in the diagnosis and assess improvement in bacterial infections. PCT is produced by the liver and peripheral blood mononuclear cells, modulated by lipopolysaccharides and sepsis-related cytokines. Procalcitonin can be used as reliable serum marker for early prediction of renal parenchymal inflammation in patients with febrile UTI. They are usually elevated in bacterial infections in the upper urinary tract. These follow-up tests can be used to monitor response to therapy. Serum creatinine may be elevated in a small percentage of patients with acute pyelonephritis with acute kidney injury.

5. Imaging Studies

Imaging of urinary tract is not routinely indicated in cases of uncomplicated UTI that respond promptly to antibiotic therapy. Indications for diagnostic imaging are severe clinical presentation, resistance to initial treatment, early recurrence after antibiotic treatment, to rule out obstruction, infected calculi or abscesses. This is usually done 3 to 6 weeks after cure of an acute infection. The commonly done studies are:

a. USG—KUB will help to identify congenital anomalies, obstructions in the urinary tract, stones, air or presence of pyonephrosis. In infants with febrile UTI, USG-KUB is recommended within 24 hours to exclude obstruction of upper or lower urinary tract.

b. Intravenous pyelogram (IVP) also called intravenous urogram is helpful to provide anatomical details of calyces, renal pelvis, ureters, shape of bladder, radiopaque or radiolucent calculi in the urinary tract.

c. CT abdomen—best investigation for renal stone. It is also a sensitive indicator of

Table 31.3: Diagnostic significance of bacterial colony count (CFU/ml) in different clinical scenarios

Collection method	Quantitative criteria (CFU/ml)
Voided specimen	
Symptomatic cystitis in women	$\geq 10^3$
Acute pyelonephritis in women	$\geq 10^4$
Symptomatic UTI in male	$\geq 10^3$
UTI in children	$\geq 10^5$
External condom collection	$\geq 10^5$
Catheterized sample	
In-and-out catheter	$\geq 10^2$
Indwelling catheter—asymptomatic	$\geq 10^5$
Indwelling catheter—symptomatic	$\geq 10^2$
Suprapubic bladder puncture specimen	Any bacterial count is significant
Complicated UTI	$\geq 10^5$ females and $\geq 10^4$ in males
Asymptomatic bacteriuria	Two cultures taken more than 24 hours apart should grow the same bacterial strain $\geq 10^5$ in women
	Growth in only one specimen is required for diagnosis in males

pelvicalyceal dilatation, renal abscesses, perinephric collections. Because of better definition and ability to diagnose radio-lucent stones, contrast CT urogram is replacing the conventional IVP.

d. Voiding cystourethrogram (VCUG) is mandatory in boys who develop documented UTI since posterior urethral valve and/or associated vesicoureteric reflux are the commonest causes of UTI in them. In others, the indications are recurrent UTI, residual urine in bladder or renal scars in USG.

6. Blood Culture

Although blood culture may grow the same organism as urine in about 25% of cases of UTI, it does not give additional information. The bacteremia is most often due to spread from lower urinary tract and hence blood culture and sensitivity will be usually the same as urine culture report. Rarely the reverse may occur. Bloodstream infection with *Staphylococcus aureus* may spread to kidneys by hematogenous seedling and result in micro-abscesses and staphylococcal bacteriuria.

Asymptomatic Bacteriuria

Asymptomatic bacteriuria (ABU) is defined as significant bacteriuria (10^5 CFU/ml) without any symptoms or signs attributed to local or systemic urinary tract infection. The incidence of ABU in sexually active premenopausal women is around 5% and it increases up to 10% in postmenopausal women. Prevalence is higher in the elderly, diabetics, during pregnancy and in patients with spinal cord injuries. It is rare in men <65 years. Incidence of ABU is nearly 100% in patients with chronic indwelling catheter. In the case of an indwelling catheter, a biological membrane ('biofilm') forms in the lumen and organisms colonize the 'biofilm' within hours. Therefore, the urine sample for culture, taken through an indwelling bladder catheter is not reliable. To avoid this

fallacy, if and when urine culture sample is required from a catheterized individual, the existing catheter is removed, a new catheter put in and urine sample taken for culture immediately.

In women, the diagnosis ABU is confirmed by midstream urine culture showing bacterial growth of ≥10^5 CFU/ml in two consecutive urine samples 24 hours apart. In men, only a single sample is required for diagnosis. In a freshly catheterized sample in a person not on indwelling catheter earlier, bacterial growth of ≥10^2 CFU/ml is sufficient for diagnosis of bacteriuria. The spectrum of organisms causing asymptomatic bacteriuria is similar to that causing uncomplicated UTI, with *E. coli* responsible for >80% of cases. In men older than 65 years coagulase negative staphylo-cocci was found to be the most common causative organism followed by *E. coli* and Enterococcus.

Since there is no difference in the rate of symptomatic UTIs and there is no added benefit of treatment in patients with asymptomatic bacteriuria and the current guidelines does not recommend screening and treatment of ABU in patients without risk factors. Screening and treatment for ABU is recommended in the following situations:

1. Pregnancy
2. Poorly controlled diabetes
3. Prior to catheter placement/exchange
4. Prior to urological surgery.

The choice of antibiotics and treatment duration is as in symptomatic UTI. Treatment should be tailored and should not be empirical.

Catheter Associated UTI (CA-UTI)

CA-UTI is defined by the presence of symptoms or signs compatible with UTI, along with ≥10^3 CFU/ml of one or more bacterial species in a new single catheter urine sample or in MSU sample within 48 hours of catheter removal. The uropathogens are acquired extraluminally from perineal area in most of the cases. In a catheterized patient, presence of pus cells, cloudy or odorous urine is not diagnostic of CA-UTI and is not an indication for urine culture or antimicrobial therapy.

Catheter associated asymptomatic bacteriuria requires $\geq 10^5$ CFU/ml of one or more bacterial species for diagnosis. Catheter associated bacteriuria is the most common healthcare associated infection worldwide accounting for up to 40% of hospital acquired infections. About 10% of all hospital admissions and >80% of ICU admissions would have been subjected to urinary catheter insertion during their stay. The duration of catheterization is the most important risk factor for the development of CA-UTI. Most common organism associated with CA-UTI is *E. coli*.

Other common organisms are Klebsiella, Serratia, Citrobacter, Enterobacter, Pseudomonas and coagulase negative *S. aureus*. Candiduria is seen in 3–32% of patients. Treatment of asymptomatic candiduria is not indicated. Please see the section on treatment of fungal UTI below. The current guidelines to reduce CA-UTI are described in Table 31.4.

Treatment of Urinary Tract Infections

The choice of route of administration between oral and parenteral therapy should be based on patient age, clinical suspicion of urosepsis, refusal of fluids, vomiting, diarrhea and non-adherence. As a result of increased incidence of urosepsis and severe pyelonephritis in new

Table 31.4: Do's and Don'ts to reduce CA-UTI

	Do's	Don'ts
1.	Use only when indicated	Prophylactic antibiotic before insertion
2.	Remove as soon as it is no longer indicated.	Bedside catheterization. No 'procedure room' for catheterization
3.	Proper education and training of staff about aseptic technique and sterile equipment during catheter insertion	Drainage bag should not be above the level of bladder
4.	Condom catheterization wherever possible	Don'ts screen or treat catheter associated asymptomatic bacteriuria
5.	Intermittent catheterization should be preferred	No long-term catheterization if possible
6.	Clean catheterization technique sufficient	Sterile technique not mandatory
7.	CIC with multiple use catheter permitted	No prophylactic systemic antibiotics prior to catheterization
8.	Use closed catheter drainage system with ports in the distal catheter for needle aspiration of urine	Don'ts use methenamine salt or cranberry juice to reduce CA-UTI
9.	Minimize disconnection of the catheter junction with urinary collection bag	No recommendation on daily external urethral meatal cleansing with povidone-iodine solution, silver sulfadiazine or polyantibiotic ointment
10.	Silver alloy or antibiotic-coated catheters may be used	Catheter irrigation or bladder irrigation with antimicrobials or normal saline should not be routinely used
11.	Treatment of CA-UTI should be only as per urine culture and sensitivity report	Don'ts add antimicrobials or antiseptics to the drainage bag of catheterized patients
12.	Replace the catheter if it is in place for >2 weeks, during an episode of CA-UTI Give treatment of CA-UTI at least 7 days	No recommendation on routine catheter change every 2–4 weeks in patients with long-term catheters No prophylactic antibiotic before catheter placement, removal or during catheter change

born and infants aged <2 months, parenteral antibiotic therapy is recommended. The choice of antibiotic is based on local antimicrobial sensitivity patterns and availability of antibiotics. Prompt and adequate treatment can prevent the spread of infection and renal scaring.

1. Uncomplicated Cystitis

For uncomplicated cystitis, only short course or single dose treatment is required. The commonest clinical scenario is 'honeymoon cystitis' in young women and the commonest organism is *E. coli*. Usually clinical and microbiological resolution occurs within a few days or a few weeks. Antimicrobial therapy is recommended because clinical success is significantly more likely in women treated with antimicrobial. The treatments recommended are:

   i. Nitrofurantoin 100 mg twice per day for 5 days
   ii. Cotrimoxazole (160/800 mg) twice per day for 3 days
   iii. Amoxicillin clavulanic acid 625 mg thrice per day for 3 days
   iv. Fluroquinolones for 3 days
   v. Fosfomycin 3 gm as a single dose

   In men, since associated prostatic infection is common, duration of treatment of at least 7 days is recommended. Antibiotics with better tissue penetration like cotrimoxazole or fluroquinolone is prefered.

2. Uncomplicated Pyelonephritis

a. Oral ciprofloxacin 500 mg twice daily for 7 days or levofloxacin 750 mg as single daily dose for 5 days.
b. Cotrimoxazole (160/800 mg) twice daily for 14 days
c. Ceftriaxone 1 gm
d. Single daily dose of aminoglycoside.

3. Severe Infection with Urosepsis

For more serious infections, patients are hospitalized and given parenteral antibiotics.

Treatment should for at least two weeks is usually recommended with ceftriaxone, cefpodoxime, cefoperazone sulbactam, gentamicin, fluoroquinolones or carbapenem group (Table 31.5). Carbapenems are reserved for treatment of infections with organisms known or suspected to be multidrug resistant strains. The antibiotic should be changed to milder one if culture and sensitivity permits.

4. Prostatitis

The best drugs for treatment of prostatitis are cotrimoxazole and fluoroquinolones. The duration of treatment should be at least one month.

5. Chemoprophylaxis

Chemoprophylaxis is indicated in females with 2 or more uncomplicated UTIs per year and also during pregnancy. Prophylactic antibiotics are usually given for 6 to 12 months. Most commonly used antibiotics for prophylaxis are bed time dose of nitrofurantoin and cotrimoxazole.

   The following prophylactic measures are also helpful in preventing infection:
a. Good perineal hygiene
b. Emptying of the urinary bladder before and after intercourse.
c. Single dose of cotrimoxazole immediately after intercourse.

Table 31.5: Commonly used antibiotics in the treatment of UTI and their dose

Drug	Dose (mg)	Interval
Cefepime	1000–2000	q 12 h
Ciprofloxacin	250–500	q 24 h
Levofloxacin	250–750	q 12 h
Gentamicin	3–5 mg/kg/d	q 24 h
Cotrimoxazole	160/800	q 12 h
Piperacillin–tazobactam	3375	q 6–8 h
Imipenem–cilastatin	250–500	q 6–8 h
Aztreonam	1000	q 8–12 h
Vancomycin	1000	q 12 h

d. Adequate fluid intake and frequent voiding of the bladder.

e. Vaginal estrogen cream daily for 2 weeks, followed by twice per week for 8 months in postmenopausal women.

Monitoring of UTI

With successful treatment, urine usually becomes sterile after 24 hours, and leukocyturia normally disappears within 3–4 days. Normalization of body temperature can be expected within 24–48 hours after the start of therapy in 90% of cases. In patients with prolonged fever and failing recovery, treatment-resistant uropathogens or the presence of congenital uropathy or acute urinary obstruction should be considered.

Fungal UTI

The most common form of fungal infection of urinary tract is that caused by Candida species. Such infections are usually seen in diabetic patients with indwelling bladder catheters, who are exposed to multiple broad spectrum antibiotics. Most of the Candida UTI remain limited to bladder and is responsible only for 10% of episodes of candidemia. Candiduria is usually identified in patients who are seriously ill with multiple comorbid conditions. Clinical manifestations are asymptomatic candiduria, cystitis, and pyelonephritis. Bladder or renal fungus balls and systemic fungemia are rare complications. *Candida albicans* is isolated from more than 50% of episodes. Treatment of asymptomatic candiduria is not beneficial and is currently recommended only for selected patients with neutropenia or

before an urologic procedure. Indwelling devices should be removed wherever possible.

Fluconazole is the treatment of choice for candidal urinary tract infection because it is excreted in the urine in active form and high urinary levels are at achieved. A two-week course fluconazole, 200–400 mg daily, is recommended. Amphotericin B is alternative treatment recommended for fluconazole resistant strains (Table 31.6). Echynocandins such as caspofungin, micafungin and other azoles such as itraconazole, voriconazole, which are not excreted into the urine, are not recommended for treatment of urinary tract infection.

In patient with catheter associated candidal UTI, catheter should be changed. Infusion of amphotericin rinse for a period of 3–5 days eradicates >50% infections. Patient should also be treated with fluconazole 200–400 mg/day for 10–14 days.

Hematogenous spread to kidney may be seen if any fungal systemic fungal infection, but this particularly occurs in coccidioidomycosis and blastomycosis. Disseminated cryptococcal infection can produce appearance of this organism in urine.

Viral Infections of Urinary Tract

Viral urinary tract infections are uncommon in adults and occur largely in immuno compromised patients. Clinical manifestations generally follow reactivation of latent infections, although *de novo* infection may occur. The usual clinical manifestation is hemorrhagic cystitis. The most common viruses are adenovirus, parvovirus B19, and cytomegalo-

Table 31.6: Recommended treatment of candiduria		
Drug	Cystitis	Pyelonephritis
Fluconazole	200–400 mg/day for 14 days	200–400 mg/day for 14 days
Amphotericin B	0.3–0.6 mg/kg/day for 7 days	0.5–0.7 mg/kg/day for 14 days
Amphotericin bladder irrigation	5–50 mg/L continuous irrigation for 2–7 days	
Flucytosine	25 mg/kg qid: 7–10 days	25 mg/kg qid, 14 days

virus (CMV). The diagnosis is by viral culture or identification by polymerase chain reaction (PCR) of the urine. Management includes minimization of immunosuppressive therapy along with appropriate antiviral drugs. CMV infection responds to ganciclovir or foscarnet. Treatment of adenovirus infection employs cidofovir.

In summary, urinary tract infection is one of the most common human infections. Infecting organisms are usually bacteria. Urine culture is the gold standard for diagnosis. Most of the other investigations are required only in specific situations. Appropriate diagnosis and treatment as per guidelines will improve the quality of life and is sometimes lifesaving. Recurrent infections and drug resistance are most commonly due to inadequate dose and duration of the treatment.

Genitourinary Tuberculosis

• Prem Prakash Varma • Venkat Siva Tez Pinnmaneni

INTRODUCTION

India accounts for one-fourth of the world burden of tuberculosis (TB). In 2016, there were 28 lakh fresh cases of TB with a mortality of 4.23 lakh. In recent years with emergence of HIV and other immunocompromised states, there has been a rising trend in incidence of tuberculosis. Pulmonary involvement remains the commonest site. Extrapulmonary involvement is seen in 15–20% of HIV negative and 40% of HIV positive cases. Low immune status of dialysis and renal transplant recipients makes them 10 times more susceptible to develop fresh infection/reactivation of latent infection.

GUTB is the commonest form of extrapulmonary TB accounting for about 20% of all cases in developing countries and is generally encountered in the age group of 20–40 years. 20–25% patients of these may have past history of TB and another one quarter may have radiological evidence of past TB. Usually there is long gap of 5–20 years between initial infection and development of GUTB. As the symptoms related to GUTB are non-specific, the diagnosis usually gets delayed and it is not uncommon to find putty/destroyed kidney even at initial presentation. Multi-drug resistant (MDR) tuberculosis in new cases/previously treated cases is the result of inappropriate, inadequate, incomplete and irregular treatment practices. Drug resistance to isoniazid and rifampicin is encountered commonly. Ambitious national plan titled 'National Strategic Plan 2017–2025', has been setup to achieve the the goal of elimination of TB in India by 2025.

Pathogenesis

GUTB occurs by hematogenous spread. *Mycobacterium tuberculosis* is the offending organism in majority though atypical mycobacteria like *M. kansasii, M. fortuitum, M. bovis* or *M. avium intracellulare* may be responsible in a few patients. This organism is aerobic with thick lipid-rich hydrophobic cell wall which is acid and alcohol fast, hence the organism is commonly called acid-fast bacillus. It multiplies once in 24 hours. Initial infection is the primary complex ('Ghon' focus) which may involve, the tonsil, lung or GI tract. The primary complex consists of the focus of entry, regional lymphatic and an enlarged regional lymph gland. As part of body's defence mechanism, the organisms are trapped by macrophages and remain dormant for a long time within the primary focus. When the body resistance is low, these organisms multiply, travel via thoracic duct and enter the systemic circulation. By hematogenous spread, organisms reach different areas of the body like bones, renal cortex and epididymis. Though organisms reach both the kidneys but usually lesions develop in one kidney or involvement may be asymmetrical. In the kidney, they are trapped within the glomeruli initially where they form a granuloma. From the cortical granuloma, the organisms spill into proximal tubule and get entrapped at the medullary pyramids in the loop of Henle. They multiply here and form granulomas, ulcers, cavities, caseation necrosis or abscesses. The abscesses enlarge, become confluent and result in pyonephrosis, perinephric abscess with destruction of renal parenchyma. Dystrophic calcification containing viable organisms occurs and the kidney is completely destroyed. This stage of calcified kidney is commonly called putty/cement kidney. Vascular involvement can result in papillary necrosis. Caseous material can spill and erode calyx and enter the urinary system, travel down to pelvis, ureters, bladder and urethra. In calyces they cause calycitis with mucosal ulceration, deformation, stricture formation, amputation or dilatation. Ureteric involvement (ureteritis) may be panureteritis (hard pipe-like ureter) but usually UV junction is common site affected. Ureter can develop strictures and hydronephrosis. Almost half of patients with renal tuberculosis develop ureteral TB. The commonest site of bladder involvement is ureterovesical junction. Bacteria lodge around ureteric openings in bladder. This area gets inflamed, granulomas form and later fibrosis develops. The normal opening becomes depressed like 'golf hole'. This becomes incompetent junction and result is development of secondary vesicoureteric reflux. If whole bladder wall gets involved then subsequent fibrosis results in thick walled, small capacity bladder also called 'thimble bladder'. Epididymitis and prostatitis can result due to contiguous or hematogenous spread. Epididymis becomes inflamed, thickened, beaded and can suppurate with sinus formation. Adjoining vas deferens and seminal vesicles also get involved which may lead to sterility. Prostate involvement is unusual but there can be abscess formation and cavitation. Tuberculosis can affect any part of the female genital tract also but more commonly fallopian tubes are the preferred sites. Hydrosalpinx and pyosalpinx usually appear as soft tissue masses on plain abdominal radiographs and infertility is not uncommon. Urethritis occurs rarely due to spread from contiguous organs.

Clinical Features

Since the symptoms are vague, non-specific in nature or absent, the diagnosis gets delayed. High index of suspicion in susceptible individuals is necessary for early diagnosis. Persistent pyuria with repeatedly negative conventional urine culture should raise the suspicion of tuberculosis in the urinary tract. Patients may present with features of UTI which does not respond to conventional treatment with antibiotics. Increased frequency, flank pain, suprapubic pain, dysuria, hematuria and fever are some of the presentations. Hypertension may be present in some cases. Heavy proteinuria may be the presenting feature if renal amyloidosis or mesangioproliferative glomerulonephritis is present. Gross and relatively painless hematuria occurs due to ureteric ulceration, rupture of a blood vessel within a caseous focus in the kidney or papillary necrosis. Hematuria should be differentiated from other causes like stone disease, malignancy and IgA nephropathy. Loss of renal function can be due to extensive necrosis or granulomatous interstitial nephritis or obstruction and back pressure effects.

Patients with epididymitis present with scrotal pain, swelling or discharge which does not respond to conventional antibiotics. Prostatic TB presents with perineal discomfort/pain. Likewise females can present with lower abdominal discomfort or the disease is suspected or confirmed during evaluation for infertility.

Diagnosis

Urine is acidic and microscopy may show numerous WBCs and RBCs. However, the conventional urine cultures are usually negative. This combination is called 'acid sterile pyuria' and is an important pointer towards urinary tract TB. Though ESR is raised, it is a non-specific finding. Mantoux test may be positive in 30–35% patients therefore negative Mantoux does not exclude TB. Centrifuged sample from fully voided early morning urine subjected to Ziehl-Neelsen staining for acid-fast bacilli has poor yield and has low sensitivity and specificity. Non-tuberculous mycobacteria colonising the anterior urethra (*M. smegmatis*) often may give rise to false positive results. As bacteriuria is intermittent, repeated urine cultures for *M. tuberculosis* are suggested. Early morning whole voided urine cultures for consecutive 3–6 days may give positivity of 60–70% only. Two special culture medias are used: (i) Solid media: The Lowenstein-Jensen medium which yields results in more than 4 weeks; (ii) Radiometric media: The BACTEC 460 medium yields result in 2–3 days. Polymerase chain reaction (PCR) for *M. tuberculosis* and Gene Xpert on urinary samples are helpful in confirming the diagnosis and has sensitivity of 80–90% and specificity of 100%. Polymerase chain reaction as line probe assays (2 hours) and cartridge-based nucleic acid amplification techniques (72 hours) have helped to shorten the time to diagnosis. One has to keep in mind that false negative results due to inhibitors of the polymerase reaction in the urine and false positive results due to excretion of dead bacilli.

Radiology is helpful in diagnosing GUTB. X-ray chest may show evidence of old healed lesion in around one-fourth of patients. X-ray abdomen may show calcification in renal area. Ultrasonography is nonspecific and identifies hydronephrosis, areas of scarring and calcification. High resolution ultrasonography can identify calyceal ulcers and medullary granulomas. Characteristic changes on intravenous urography are calyceal destruction, stricture, dilatation, involvement of pelvi-ureteral junction, sharp angulation and pulled up pelvis. Ureter may show multiple strictures along the course with hydronephrosis. Uretero-vesical junction stenosis with proximal dilation and shrunken bladder are common findings.

CT scanning is useful not only in the diagnosis of renal tuberculosis but also in the assessment of renal function and the extent of parenchymal destruction. It may also detect the involvement of other abdominal organs. CT can demonstrate prostatic sloughing, cavitation or calcification. MRI is useful when fistulae or tuberculous tracts are formed. Hysterosalpingographic images may suggest female genital tuberculosis by demonstrating abnormal findings within the uterus and fallopian tubes.

Management

Management is aimed to treat active disease, make patient non-infective as early as possible, preserve as much renal tissue as possible and avoid drug resistance. Once diagnosed treatment is with conventional four drugs anti-tubercular therapy (ATT): Isoniazid (H), Rifampicin (R), pyrazinamide (P) and ethambutol (E). Initial induction treatment is for 2 months with four drugs, followed by INH and rifampicin for next 4 months. Since excretion of drugs is through kidneys and adequate drug levels are achieved, therefore short-term therapy for 6 months is often adequate. DOTS regimen can also be advocated. There are four populations of *Mycobacterium tuberculosis*. Rapid multipliers are susceptible to all anti-tuberculous drugs. Rifampicin based regimens are needed for Intermittent multipliers. For bacteria in acidic environment like intracellular locations or within caseous material, regimens including pyrazinamide are necessary. Dormant population is not affected by any drug and can result in reactivation at later stage. There is no dose modification for INH and rifampicin in patients with renal dysfunction. However, dose of pyrazinamide and ethambutol are reduced by half in dialysis patients (GFR <10 ml/min). Either full dose is given on alternate days or 50% of dose can be taken daily. Streptomycin and ethambutol are best avoided in renal failure for fear of ototoxicity and optic toxicity respectively. The dose of INH is 300 mg/day and rifampicin 450 mg (if weight <60 kg) and 600 mg (for body weight 60 kg and above). The dose of pyrizinamide is 25 mg/kg body weight and ethambutol, 15 mg/kg body weight.

In renal transplant recipients, interaction of calcineurin inhibitors and steroids with rifampicin and in HIV patients interaction of antiretroviral drugs and rifampicin should be kept in mind. Duration of therapy is extended to 9–12 months when using non-rifampicin based therapies.

Resistance to isoniazid and rifampicin is termed multi-drug resistance (MDR). Six drugs regimen is used in such cases. Kanamycin, levofloxacin, ethionamide, pyrazinamide, ethambutol and cycloserine during 6–9 months of the intensive phase and four drugs—levofloxacin, ethionamide, ethambutol and cycloserine during the 18 months of the continuation phase.

Extensively drug resistant (XDR) bacilli are those that are resistant to INH, rifampicin, fluoroquinolones (ofloxacin, levofloxacin, moxifloxacin) and the injectable second line drugs (kanamycin, amikacin, capreomycin). In XDR tuberculosis, the "intensive phase" of treatment will consist of seven drugs—capreomycin (Cm), para-aminosalicylic acid (PAS), moxifloxacin (Mfx), high-dose INH, clofazimine, linezolid and amoxicillin clavula-nate combination. The "continuation phase" will consist of six drugs—PAS, Mfx, high-dose INH, clofazimine, linezolid and amoxicillin clavulanate combination. The treatment of XDR tuberculosis should be given as 6–12 months of intensive phase and another 18 months of continuation phase.

Every effort should be made to give appropriate and regular ATT. It is wise to involve family members also so that compliance is achieved and discontinuation of drugs is avoided.

Surgery

In the era of modern medical therapy, indications for surgery are limited to relief of obstruction, drainage of pus, reconstruction of upper and lower urinary tracts. Nephrectomy is limited to poorly functioning kidney with hypertension or malignancy. In patients with thimble bladder augmentation cystoplasty is generally needed. Up to 50% patients reporting late to tertiary care center may need surgical intervention.

Conclusion

GUTB is the commonest form of extra-pulmonary TB. Incidence of TB is almost 10 times higher in immunocompromised patients on dialysis and following transplantation. Due to vague and non-specific symptoms, the diagnosis usually gets delayed. Any part of urinary tract can get affected though kidney, ureters and bladder are common sites. As presentation is non-specific, high index of suspicion is necessary for timely diagnosis. Radiology is useful in pointing to diagnosis. PCR for MTB and gene Xpert help in clinching the diagnosis early. Once diagnosed short course of ATT is adequate in majority of patients.

Urinary Tract Infections in Special Situations

• M Thomas Mathew • Jayanth Thomas Mathew

UTI IN DIABETES MELLITUS

Lack of proper control of blood glucose levels, presence of glucose in urine, diabetic neuropathy with neurogenic bladder, recurrent vaginitis and vulvitis of females, diabetic microangiopathy, leukocyte dysfunction and large vessel renal vascular disease are the factors responsible for the high incidence of UTI in diabetics. Among diabetics, older age and female sex are additional risk factors. UTI may precipitate ketoacidosis in diabetics. Nosocomial UTIs are also more common among diabetics following catheterization or instrumentation. Diabetics tend to develop asymptomatic UTI and infection of the upper tract more commonly compared to non-diabetic population. The higher incidence of parenchymal damage in diabetics is probably due to underlying vascular disease and leukocyte dysfunction. They are more prone to develop bacteremia, papillary necrosis, perinephric abscesses and fungal infections. Papillary necrosis occurs commonly in diabetics with UTI. In this condition, the necrotic pyramids may get sloughed off and may block the collecting system or passed in urine. Following episodes of papillary necrosis, calyceal deformities may be demonstrated on intravenous urogram (IVU). Emphysematous cystitis and emphysematous pyelonephritis

characterized by gas production are common in diabetics. If aggressive antibiotic therapy fails, surgical management may be required in these patients. Diabetics are more prone to develop Candida infection particularly following instrumentation. Deep seated candidiasis and fungal balls in the renal pelvis and ureters may result in oliguria, anuria or obstructive uropathy. Systemic amphotericin B, flucytosine or fluconazole combined with surgical measures may be necessary. As in the case of children, any diabetic developing fever, abdominal pain or vague abdominal symptoms must be investigated for UTI.

Patients with diabetes may also develop fulminant emphysematous pyelonephritis and xanthogranulomatous pyelonephritis.

EMPHYSEMATOUS PYELONEPHRITIS

Emphysematous pyelonephritis is a fulminant, necrotizing, life-threatening variant of acute pyelonephritis caused by gas-forming organisms, including *E. coli*, Klebsiella, *P. aeruginosa* and *P. mirabilis*. Nearly 80% of cases occur in diabetic patients and obstruction may be present. Symptoms are suggestive of pyelonephritis and there may be a flank mass. Gas within the renal shadow is usually detected by plain X-ray KUB or USG of the abdomen. However, CT is the diagnostic modality. Powerful parenteral antibiotic therapy and percutaneous catheter drainage with relief of obstruction may be adequate in the majority. However, nephrectomy is warranted in those who are severely ill who do not respond to medical treatment. The mortality is very high.

XANTHOMATOUS PYELONEPHRITIS

Xanthomatous pyelonephritis is relatively uncommon, is a severe chronic destructive granulomatous inflammation of the renal parenchyma associated with obstruction and severe infection. The renal parenchyma is replaced with diffuse or segmental cellular infiltration of lipid laden foam cells. The process may extend beyond the renal capsule to the retroperitoneum as well. The infecting organisms are often *E. coli*, other gram negative bacilli or *S. aureus*. Kidney becomes non-functioning, response to medical treatment is poor. Since it is usually unilateral, total or partial nephrectomy may be necessary.

RENAL ABSCESSES

Renal corticomedullary abscesses are usually associated with vesicoureteric reflux or urinary tract obstruction and the usual organisms include *E. coli*, Klebsiella and Proteus species. Clinical syndromes include acute focal bacterial nephritis, acute multifocal bacterial nephritis or the finding of 'focal nephronia' in the ultrasound scan. These cases will need parenteral antibiotics as per urine culture reports.

Renal cortical abscesses or renal carbuncles, usually result from hematogenous spread of bacteria. Primary sources of infection include skin infection, osteomyelitis and endovascular infection. The most common organism isolated is *S. aureus*. Ten percent of cortical abscesses may rupture through the renal capsule and form perinephric abscesses.

A perinephric abscess is defined as collection of purulent material between the renal capsule and Gerota's fascia. It may develop secondary to an intrarenal abscess, renal cortical abscess, recurrent pyelonephritis, chronic pyelonephritis or following hematogenous dissemination of infection. Culture specific parenteral antibiotics are required and in severe cases, aspiration of large single abscess or surgical drainage of abscess may be need.

UTI IN PREGNANCY

In normal pregnancy, mild dilatation of collecting systems occurs and there is some stasis of urine. The ureter may be kinked at the site of crossing the pelvic brim. Factors like relative obstruction of ureters secondary to the enlarging uterus, smooth muscle relaxation of the ureter and bladder secondary to progesterone and amino-aciduria and glycosuria associated with pregnancy increase the risk of developing asymptomatic bacteriuria or UTI during pregnancy. It has been found that 20–30% of pregnant women with asymptomatic bacteriuria will develop pyelonephritis. Hence, asymptomatic bacteriuria in pregnancy should also be treated as a case of UTI. Fourteen-day course of culture specific oral antibiotic suitable for use in pregnancy is the treatment of choice. Drugs belonging to quinolone group and aminoglycosides have to be avoided. In case of severe infection, parenteral antibiotics and hospitalization will be necessary. Women with urinary infection are more prone to develop pre-eclampsia, preterm labor and low birth weight babies.

UTI IN PATIENTS WITH NEPHROLITHIASIS

UTI can be both a causative and complicating factor in nephrolithiasis. A calculus can get secondarily colonized with bacteria and can act as a nidus for bacterial growth leading to pyelonephritis. If obstruction sets in, the situation may worsen leading to renal abscess formation or urosepsis with septicemia. Symptoms are usually variable with flank pain, dysuria, hematuria, pyuria, nausea, vomiting, chills and rigors. Culture specific parenteral antibiotics and relief of the obstruction are lifesaving.

UTI IN NEUROGENIC BLADDER

Patients with neurogenic bladder secondary to central nervous disease or spinal cord diseases have markedly increased incidence of UTI because of urinary stasis, frequent asymptomatic bacteriuria, reflux and catheterization. Patients usually presents with leakage of urine, malodorus urine, fever, abdominal or flank pains. Freshly passed normal urine is nearly odourless. Malodour of freshly passed urine indicates infection with urease producing organisms. The chances of developing pyelonephritis, renal abscess and urosepsis with septicemia are very high. Proper urinary drainage and culture specific antibiotics are necessary to control the infection.

CANDIDIASIS

Risk factors for candidiasis include diabetes mellitus, indwelling catheters and antibiotic use. The presence of Candida species in the urine represents colonization and not infection, and as such require no treatment. However, if there are features of active infection, culture-specific antifungal agents have to be given.

UTI IN CHRONIC RENAL FAILURE

Patients with CRF are more prone to develop UTI. And the higher incidence is due to infrequent voiding, low urine flow rates, impaired concentrating capacity and low level of immunity. Frequent instrumentation, infection of vascular access in patients on dialysis, underlying diseases such as chronic pyelonephritis, polycystic disease or diabetic nephropathy are other important aggravating factors. Though any organism can cause UTI in patients with renal failure, E. coli and enterococci are the most frequently isolated organisms.

UTI IN ELDERLY

Bacteriuria is more common in elderly compared to younger adults. Above the age of 65 years, the incidence of bacteriuria is more in men compared to women. In the elderly, ascending route of infection is the most common. Poor perineal hygiene and lowering of estrogen levels favor colonization of vulva and distal urethra with pathogenic organisms in females. Uterine prolapse with cystocele results in residual urine in the bladder and contributes to the development of infection. Acute and chronic prostatis, benign prostatic hypertrophy, and urinary retention account for the increased incidence or relapses of UTI in men. Decreased amounts of prostatic secretion and Tamm-Horsfall protein also favor bacterial colonization. Organisms other than E. coli like *Staphylococcus saprophyticus*, Proteus, Klebsiella, Pseudomonas and even gram-positive organisms may cause UTI in the elderly. Multiple organisms are also isolated frequently. The greater frequency of hospitalization, instrumentation and concurrent medications for other diseases may contribute to infection by rare organisms.

The elderly patients may present with usual clinical features of dysuria, fever and back pain or atypical symptoms like vomiting, abdominal tenderness or respiratory distress. They may not have any febrile response and may even have hypothermia and normal leukocyte count. An elderly person with pyuria and symptoms of UTI should be treated empirically. If there is suspicion of upper UTI, failure of clinical response or recurrence of symptoms, an underlying abnormality must be looked for. All elderly men with UTI and women with recurrent UTI should be investigated in detail. Presence of residual urine must be determined. In view of the emergence of resistance of E. coli, norfloxacin or trimoxazol is preferred. These drugs have high level of activity against the uropathogens and relatively low toxicity. In males with frequent relapses, chronic bacterial prostatitis must be looked for and treated with long-term therapy with quinolones for more than a month at least. Postmenopausal women with relapsing UTI or troublesome lower urinary symptoms may be put on low-dose oral or intravaginal estrogens.

UTI IN IMMUNODEFICIENCY

UTI ccurs in renal transplant recipients and other immunosuppressed individuals. During the first three weeks after renal transplantation, UTI is very common and it requires 3–6 weeks course of treatment with appropriate antimicrobials. The sulfonamide derived drugs must be used with caution along with cyclosporine for fear of added nephrotoxicity.

Neutropenia occurs with acute leukemia, aplastic anemia, following therapy with antimalignant drugs or following bone marrow transplantation. Such patients are also vulnerable to UTI. Duration of neutropenia is a major determinant. Other factors that predispose to UTI are breakdown in mucosal barriers, breakdown of cutaneous defences, or other foci of infection in the body. Instrumentations, changes in microbial flora induced by illness or therapy and emergence of resistant bacteria are also important considerations. *Pseudomonas aeruginosa, Staphylococcus aureus,* Salmonella, Candida, Cryptococcus and mycobacteria are implicated in UTI in immunodeficient persons. Most of the organisms can be isolated from the patients. In patients with severe granulocytopenia, symptoms of UTI and pyuria are absent, whereas flank pain is usually present. The chances of fungal infection increases if the duration of granulocytopenia and antibiotic therapy increases. Fungal infections occur by hematogenous dissemination from vascular access for dialysis, respiratory tract or gastrointestinal tract. Treatment of neutropenic patients with UTI requires prompt empiric therapy with broad-spectrum antibiotics covering gram-negative organisms and avoiding hepatotoxicity for 4–6 weeks.

UTI IN ACQUIRED IMMUNODEFICIENCY SYNDROME (AIDS)

Primary renal involvement with HIV leads to AIDS nephropathy. Opportunistic infections are the hallmark of AIDS. Among the bacteria, Pseudomonas, E. *coli,* Salmonella and Klebsiella are the common organisms. This probably is due to the acquisition of infection as a nosocomial infection. Asymptomatic persistent bacteriuria is more commonly seen than overt UTI. Infection with cytomegalovirus, *Mycobacterium tuberculosis* and atypical mycobacteria may also be associated. Urinary and systemic fungal infections require therapy with amphotericin B alone or combined with other antifungal agents.

NOSOCOMIAL URINARY TRACT INFECTIONS

UTI is the commonest hospital acquired infection. About 75% of this is associated with urethral catheterization and 10% with genitourinary manipulations. Each year, millions of catheters are used in patients with acute or chronic problems and for rehabilitation in patients with neurogenic bladder. The open catheter system which was previously practiced was associated with significant bacteriuria. The closed catheter system is a major advance and has significantly delayed or avoided infection by limiting the exposure to the contaminated environment. However, the closed catheter system is associated with occurrence of bacteriuria. The catheter may favor bacterial colonization due to the following reasons:

a. The cathether may carry the organisms during insertion.
b. The lumen and external surface of the catheter act as conduits for entry of microorganisms.
c. The outer coating of the catheter by biological materials like mucus and mucosal cellular products (biofilm) forms a good environment for the organism to grow.
d. The catheter may cause chemical and mechanical injury and inflammation which will weaken the protective mechanisms.

e. The urease producing organisms may elicit crystallization on the tip or lumen of the catheter with resulting obstruction that can lead onto increased intravesical pressure and vesicoureteric reflux.

The bacteria may reach the urinary from patients' own colonic flora, organisms in the perineum and urethra, from contaminated instruments, containers or from the hands of health personnel.

Frequent opening of the catheter and container junction or the drainage tube of the container may facilitate bacterial entry. The thin film of urine remaining in the bag may act as the medium for bacterial growth. The major risk factors for bacteriuria can be summarized as follows:

a. Duration of indwelling catheter
b. Female patient
c. Diabetes mellitus
d. Antibiotic abuse
e. Abnormal renal function.

Most of the catheterized patients will develop bacteriuria. *E. coli* is the most common organism in patients on short-term catheterization. *Pseudomonas aeruginosa, Klebsiella pneumoniae, Proteus mirabilis, S. epidermidis* and enterococci are the other organisms. Among long-term catheter users, *E. coli*, Psuedomonas and Proteus are the major organisms. Gram-positive organisms and fungi are uncommonly encountered.

Some simple measures can prevent or delay bacteriuria following catheterization.

1. Use of external collection devices like condom drainage in men is preferred when possible.
2. Intermittent catheterization is advisable in many acute situations. In patients with neurological disorders, intermittent self-catheterization with a clean catheter is advised.

3. Suprapubic catheterization is encouraged because of the lower bacterial density in the anterior abdominal wall. Besides, clamping the suprapubic catheter obviously makes assessment of urethral voiding easy. Complications like cellulitis, hematoma and leakage through the abdominal wall may occur.

4. The closed system drainage is advocated in all patients in whom indwelling urinary catheters are to be used.

5. Use of systemic antibiotics. Most of the patients on catheter will be receiving antibiotics in connection with the treatment of the underlying disease. Antibiotics appear to delay the onset of bacteriuria but favor emergence of resistant organisms and is a potential risk. Routine use of antibiotics in all catheterized patients to prevent bacteriuria is not recommended. A prophylactic regimen with 2 or 3 doses of cephalosporins or ampicillin around the time of catheterization may be considered only in the high-risk group.

Patient-to-patient transmission is also important in the hospital environment. The periurethral bacterial flora, collection containers, fecal matter and skin of patients are sources of contamination of hands of medical personnel. Clusters of nosocomial bacteria with Serratia, Pseudomonas and *E. coli* may occur particularly in the ICUS and calls for enforcement of meticulous hand washing discipline. Transfer of plasmids encoding antibiotic resistance between microorganisms also occurs inside the hospital. UTI in children and during pregnancy are covered in appropriate sections.

Hypertension

Control of Blood Pressure and Essential Hypertension

• Anuradha Raman • Rajeev R

INTRODUCTION

Hypertension is the most common chronic disease of the human race, affecting more than one billion people worldwide. Regulation of blood pressure is a complex integrated response involving the central nervous system (CNS), cardiovascular system (CVS), kidneys and adrenals. The causes of essential (primary) hypertension are multifactorial, involving genetics, environmental and behavioral factors. It contributes to substantial morbidity and mortality by causing cardiac hypertrophy, heart failure, stroke and kidney disease.

CLASSIFICATION

Blood pressure has been classified for adults equal to or more than 18 years old by the Joint National Committee on prevention, detection, evaluation, and treatment of high blood pressure (JNC 7) in 2003, which has later been endorsed by JNC 8 (Fig. 34.1 and Table 34.1).

Guidelines in JNC 8, in contrast to JNC 7, were driven purely by clinical trial evidence. The guidelines relaxed the threshold for initiating pharmacologic therapy for hypertension to a systolic BP is ≥150 mm Hg and/or diastolic BP is ≥90 mm Hg and treat to a goal of <150/90 mm Hg in the general population aged 60 years and older. Initial treatment of hypertension in non-blacks could be chosen

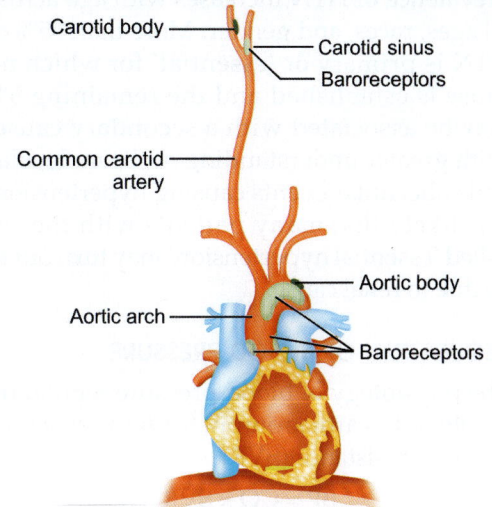

Fig. 34.1: Location of baroreceptors. *Note:* The location of baroreceptors in the aortic arch and carotid sinus close to the bifurcation of the carotid

from thiazide-type diuretic, CCB, ACE inhibitor, or ARB, whereas thiazides and CCBs were to be preferred in people of African American descent. The guidelines suggest ACEIs and ARBs as the cornerstone of treatment of HTN in CKD and diabetes mellitus.

EPIDEMIOLOGY

In the year 2000, more than one billion adults (>25% of world population) had hypertension

Table 34.1: JNC 8 and ACC/AHA classifications of HTN

Category	JNC 8 (2014)		Category	ACC/AHA (2017)	
	Systolic BP (mm Hg)	Diastolic BP (mm Hg)		Systolic BP (mm Hg)	Diastolic BP (mm Hg)
Normal	<120	<80	Normal	<120	<80
Pre-hypertension	120–139	80–89	Elevated	120–129	<80
Stage 1 hypertension	140–159	90–99	Stage 1	130–139	80–89
Stage 2 hypertension	>160	>100	Stage 2	≥140	≥90

(HTN) which is expected to increase to 1.56 billion by 2025. The incidence is very high in most countries including India. Although exact figures are not available, about 25% of all adults over the age of 25 may be hypertensive. Prevalence of HTN increases with age across all ages, races, and gender. More than 95% of HTN is primary or 'essential' for which no cause is established and the remaining 5% may be associated with a secondary cause. With greater understanding of the molecular and subcellular events causing hypertension, it is likely that many patients with the so-called 'essential hypertension' may turn out to be due to renal cause.

REGULATION OF BLOOD PRESSURE

The physiology of blood pressure regulation involves the cardiac output (CO) and systemic vascular resistance (SVR)

$$BP = CO \times SVR$$

CO = Total blood flow through systemic and pulmonary circulation per minute. Changes in cardiac output cause short-lived BP

$$CO = SV \times HR$$

SV = Stroke volume is the amount of blood pumped out of left ventricle per beat.
HR = Heart rate is number of heartbeats per minute.
SVR = Systemic vascular resistance is the force opposing the movement of blood in vessels and is determined by the radius of small arteries and arterioles. Changes in SVR produce a sustained increase in BP.

When the blood pressure increases suddenly, the baroreceptors (Fig. 34.1) in the aortic arch and carotid sinus are activated sending impulses to the vasomotor center in the brain, which in turn activates the parasympathetic system and inhibits the sympathetic system. The resulting fall in heart rate and dilatation of blood vessels decreases cardiac output and systemic vascular resistance, thus normalizing the blood pressure (Flowchart 34.1).

Over long-term, the regulation of high blood pressure involves:

a. Pressure natriuresis
b. Tubuloglomerular feedback
c. Renin-angiotensin-aldosterone (Flowchart 34.2)
d. Vasopressin system
e. Atrial natriuretic peptide
f. Capillary fluid shift (in response to increased hydrostatic pressure)
g. Myogenic vascular relaxation (in response to pressure stress on vasculature).

Flowchart 34.1: Short-term control of BP

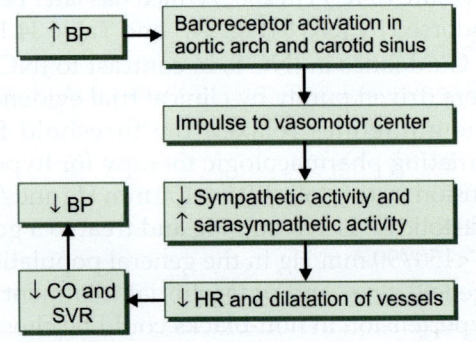

Flowchart 34.2: Long-term control of BP: Renin-angiotensin-aldosterone system (RAAS)

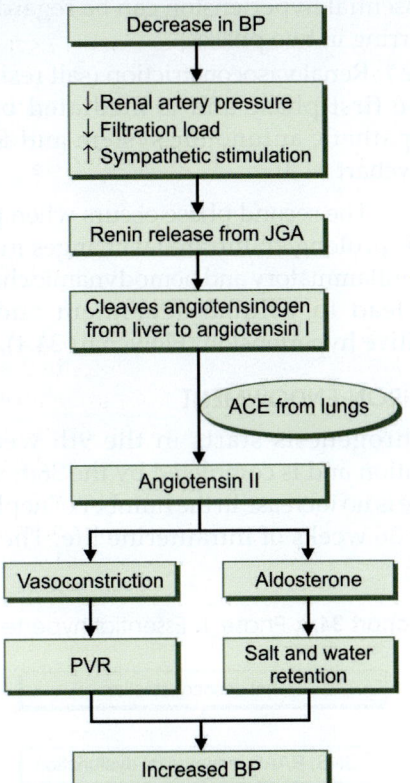

ACE: Angiotensin-converting enzyme
JGA: Juxtaglomerular apparatus

Together, these mechanisms increase excretion of sodium and water and decrease systemic vascular resistance, thereby normalizing intravascular volume and blood pressure.

NATRIURETIC PEPTIDES

Pathophysiology of Essential Hypertension

By definition, hypertension is termed "essential" when no cause can be found. Evidence suggests that kidney is the 'culprit' rather than the victim even in 'essential' hypertension since most patients have an impaired ability to excrete salt.

Factors responsible
• Salt and water

• Renin-angiotensin-aldosterone system (RAAS)
• Nephron endowment
• Genetics
• Obesity and insulin resistance
• Hyperuricemia
• Arterial stiffness

SALT AND HYPERTENSION

Salt is essential for life. Many mechanisms work in concert in the body for tight regulation of body sodium. This is essential for maintaining circulatory volume. Sodium chloride (NaCl) is the primary determinant of BP and extracellular volume (ECV).

Guyton's Pressure Natriuresis

In early 1970s, Arthur Guyton, Coleman and co-workers hypothesized that kidney regulates ECV and governs the level of BP. An increase in BP causes an increase in renal perfusion pressure which causes increased salt and water excretion. This normalizes the BP. However, in chronic hypertension, there is a shift of the equilibrium point for salt and water excretion to a higher level of arterial BP, i.e. shift of pressure natriuresis curve to the right (Fig. 34.2). Impaired sodium excretion, is the hallmark of every form of HTN. Although this hypothesis is largely accepted, there are recent

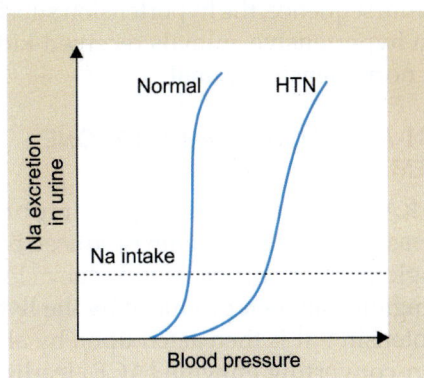

Fig. 34.2: Pressure natriuresis and hypertension. Pressure natriuresis curve shifts to the right in hypertension

suggestions of independent control of BP by neural and vascular pathways.

Salt Sensitivity

In the 1960s Dahl et al selectively bred rats for susceptibility (DS rats) or resistance (DR rats) to the hypertensive effect of a high-salt diet (8% NaCl). When salt was administered to the DS line of (salt sensitive) rats, hypertension resulted whereas, there was no hypertension when administered to DR line of (salt resistant) rats. The Dahl rats showed how an environment factor (salt intake) could interact with a genotype to produce a phenotype of hypertension.

Salt sensitivity in humans manifests as acute BP responsiveness to variation in salt intake. It varies considerably among individuals. The prevalence increases with age, is more in African Americans, in obesity, and with potassium deficiency. Salt-sensitive patients have low renin levels, high ANP levels, microalbuminuria, absent nocturnal BP dip in ambulatory BP monitoring and have altered LDL, HDL and cholesterol levels.

Cross Transplantation Experiments

When kidneys from hypertensive animals were transplanted to non-hypertensive animals, it resulted in hypertension in them. When the experiment was done in the opposite sequence, the hypertension subsided when hypertensive animals received kidney from normotensive animal.

RENIN-ANGIOTENSIN-ALDOSTERONE SYSTEM (RAAS)

The RAAS is one of the most important systems regulating BP. Renin produced by the juxtaglomerular apparatus in kidney cleaves the angiotensinogen produced by the liver to angiotensin I. It is then acted upon by angiotensin-converting enzyme (ACE) leading to the formation of angiotensin II. Angiotensin II acts via angiotensin receptors and causes vasoconstriction. It also causes aldosterone

release from adrenals, which act on the kidney to stimulate the reabsorption of salt and water.

Essential hypertension can be regarded as occurring in two phases:

Phase 1: Renal vasoconstriction (salt resistant) is the first phase and is mediated by the sympathetic autonomic system and RAAS (Flowchart 34.3).

Phase 2: The second phase occurs when phase one is prolonged. Intrarenal changes include both inflammatory and hemodynamic changes and lead to volume dependent and salt sensitive hypertension (Flowchart 34.4).

NEPHRON ENDOWMENT

Nephrogenesis starts in the 9th week of gestation and is completed by the 36th week. There is no increase in the number of nephrons after 36 weeks of intrauterine life. The total

Flowchart 34.3: Phase 1: Essential hypertension

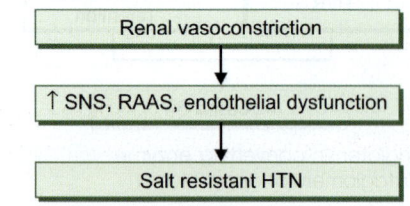

SNS: Sympathetic nervous system

Flowchart 34.4: Phase 2: Essential hypertension

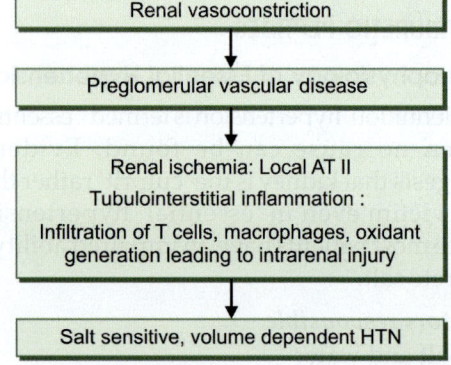

Flowchart 34.5: Nephron number and hypertension

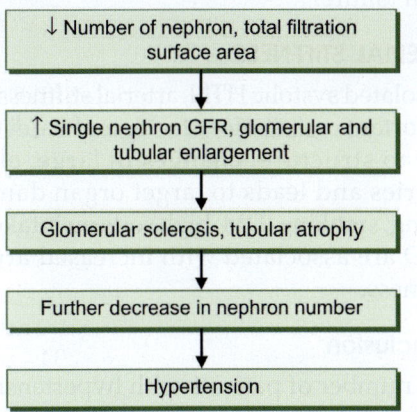

number of nephrons per kidney is variable and the number of nephrons one is born with is the 'nephron endowment for the person. The number of nephrons at birth varies from 200,000 to 2,700,000. In 1988 Prof Barry Brenner hypothesized that lower nephron number predisposes to hypertension (Flowchart 34.5). Adverse intrauterine environment increases the risk of HTN, cardiovascular and renal risk due to decreased nephron endowment. The causes of decreased nephron endowment are:
a. Low birth weight
b. Nutritional deficiency—protein, vitamin A, Zn and iron.
c. Race or ethnicity
d. Exposure to teratogens—chronic ethanol intake, smoking.
e. Drugs—NSAIDs, steroids use in pregnancy.

Low birth weight is directly related to nephron number. There is an inverse relationship between glomerular volume and nephron number. One kilogram increase in birth weight causes an increase of more than 250,000 nephrons. Babies born to Australian aborigines are twice as likely to have lower birth weight, 400,000 fewer glomeruli, and increased glomerular volume.

GENETICS AND HYPERTENSION

Mutations in at least 10 genes have been shown to raise or lower BP by altering salt and water reabsorption by the kidney. The BP variability due to genetic factors varies from 25 to 65%. Gene mutations in three rare forms of mendelian hypertensive disorders have been identified.
a. *Liddle's syndrome:* Autosomal dominant. Activation of amiloride-sensitive epithelial sodium channels (ENAC) in the collecting ducts.
b. *Syndrome of apparent mineralocorticoid excess:* Autosomal recessive. Mutation of renal specific isoform 11β-hydroxysteroid dehydrogenase.
c. *Glucocorticoid-remediable aldosteronism:* Autosomal dominant.
d. Autosomal dominant hypertension with brachydactyly.
e. *Inherited essential HTN:* High sodium-lithium countertransporter, low urinary kallikrein excretion, and high fasting plasma insulin.
f. Polymorphism in the angiotensinogen gene.

OBESITY AND INSULIN RESISTANCE

It has been proved that there is a clear-cut association between obesity and hypertension. Abdominal obesity is a risk factor for hypertension. It causes insulin resistance, adult onset diabetes mellitus, left ventricular hypertrophy, hyperlipidemias, and atherosclerotic disease. There is direct association between body mass index (BMI) and HTN. Bosy mass index (BMI) of 26–28 increases the risk of HTN by 180% and insulin resistance by more than 100%. Increased BMI causes an increase in plasma volume and cardiac output. BP in an obese individual is salt sensitive. Fasting plasma insulin is the best predictor of salt sensitivity in obesity. Insulin increases both sympathetic activity and sodium and water retention. Recently insulin-like growth factor and leptin have been implicated in obesity-related HTN. The mechanism for increased susceptibility to renal disease are activation of sympathetic, RAAS and deposition of lipids in the renal parenchyma resulting in increased interstitial pressure.

HYPERURICEMIA AND HTN

Majority of patients with gout have hypertension and histologic evidence of chronic renal injury. The primary histologic lesion is a pre-glomerular vascular disease. Hyperuricemia causes hypertension and renal injury by a mechanism, which involves renal vasoconstriction and RAAS activation. It is not dependent on deposition of crystal in the kidney or urinary system. In experimental hyperuricemia, there are pre-glomerular vascular lesions resulting in reduced blood flow and glomerular hypertension which then results in glomerular hypertrophy and sclerosis. The mechanism involves entry of uric acid into both endothelial and vascular smooth muscle cells, causing local inhibition of endothelial nitric oxide, stimulation of vascular smooth muscles, vasoactive and inflammatory mediators. Hyperuricemia is almost always associated with the obesity-associated metabolic syndrome. In hypertensive subjects, even low dose diuretics can be associated with hyperuricemia which may

lead to a vicious cycle of events culminating renal failure.

ARTERIAL STIFFNESS

In isolated systolic HTN, arterial stiffness is an important contributory factor and it develops due to structural changes in large, elastic arteries and leads to target organ damage. Aging, smoking, DM, high sodium intake and CKD are associated with increased arterial stiffness.

Conclusion

The number of patients with hypertension is increasing in the general population worldwide. Poorly controlled hypertension leads to higher morbidity and mortality. Essential hypertension is multifactorial and occurs in two phases. The basic pathophysiologic abnormality in all forms of essential hypertension is the inability to excrete salt. Essential hypertension is therefore, a form of renal disease. It is preventable. Modifiable factors include restriction of salt intake and obesity. Changes in diet and lifestyle can have profound changes in the morbidity and mortality related to essential hypertension.

Secondary Hypertension

• Girish Narayen

Hypertension is the single most important cause of premature death especially in developed countries. Nearly 30% of the population over 18 years of age is diagnosed to have hypertension and more than half of the cases do not take regular medication. Even among those who are on treatment, hypertension remains uncontrolled in nearly half of the cases. As a result hypertension remains a significant risk factor for cardiovascular (CV) events.

In general, patients with essential hypertension present between 30 and 55 years with mild or no target organ damage. In these patients, extensive laboratory evaluation with a view to identify secondary causes is of low yield and cost prohibitive. If the clinical features are not typical of essential hypertension, it is imperative to look for possible secondary causes (Table 35.1). A variety of conditions can cause secondary hypertension and in a given patient efforts should be made to identify these, as in some of them hypertension is potentially curable (Table 35.2). Patients with hypertension first detected before 30 years or after 60 years of age, 'resistant hypertension' in a drug-compliant patient, hypertensive urgency, target organ involvement and/or the following clinical manifestations should be specifically screened for secondary causes (Table 35.3).

Table 35.1: Atypical features of essential hypertension

a. Age of onset—<30 or >60 years
b. Abrupt onset /severe /'resistant' hypertension
c. Target organ damage
   i. Left ventricular hypertrophy
   ii. Neuroretinopathy
   iii. Acute renal dysfunction.
d. Features suggestive of secondary hypertension
   i. Diffuse atherosclerosis
   ii. Abdominal bruit
   iii. Paroxysmal hypertension
   iv. Sweating, headache, palpitation
   v. Unexplained hypokalemia

Renal Parenchymal Hypertension (due to Renal Parenchymal Diseases)

Kidney diseases are the commonest causes for secondary hypertension. Both primary renal diseases and renal involvement secondary to systemic diseases result in hypertension. Presence of kidney disease is suggested by early morning puffiness of face, pedal edema especially late in the evening, proteinuria, abnormalities in urinary sediment and elevated serum creatinine. Acute post-infectious glomerulonephritis is an immune mediated acute inflammatory lesion in the glomerulus and is common in children. They present with acute nephritic illness characterized by acute onset of facial puffiness,

Table 35.2: Causes of secondary hypertension

Renal
a. Renal parenchymal diseases
   i. Acute/chronic glomerulonephritis
   ii. Tubulointerstitial diseases
   iii. Vesicoureteric reflux
   iv. Polycystic kidney disease
   v. Obstructive uropathy
b. Renovascular diseases
   i. Atherosclerotic
   ii. Fibromuscular dysplasia
   iii. Takayasu's arteritis
c. Renin producing tumors
d. Genetic-tubular transport abnormality—Liddle's syndrome (rare)

Endocrine
a. Oral contraceptives
b. Adrenal
   i. Primary aldosteronism
   ii. Cushing's syndrome
   iii. Pheochromocytoma
   iv. Apparent mineralocorticoid excess
   v. Congenital adrenal hyperplasia
c. Thyroid (hyper- or hypothyroidism)
d. Hyperparathyroidism
e. Hypercalcemia
f. Ectopic ACTH production
g. Exogenous mineralocorticoids (pseudohyper-aldosteronism, fludrocortisones)

Pregnancy-induced hypertension

Neurogenic

Miscellaneous
a. Alcohol,
b. Drugs (NSAIDs, cyclosporine, erythropoietin)
c. Obstructive sleep apnea
d. Coarctation of aorta

Table 35.3: Manifestations of target organ disease

Organ	Manifestation
Cardiac	Clinical, ECG, radiological evidence of coronary artery disease
	LVH, left ventricular dysfunction or cardiac failure
Cerebrovascular	Transient ischemic attack or stroke
Peripheral vascular	Absence of one or more pulses in extremities with or without claudication
Renal	Serum creatinine >1.5 mg/dl, proteinuria 1+ or more, microalbuminuria
Retinopathy	Hemorrhages, exudates, with or without papilledema

developmental and structural abnormalities may also be responsible for hypertension in children. In young adults in the 3rd and 4th decades hypertension could be the only presenting feature of underlying renal disease like polycystic disease. History of nephritic or nephrotic illness in the past, proteinuria and smaller kidneys on ultrasound scan may give clue to underlying chronic renal parenchymal disease, especially chronic glomerulonephritis. Of the various glomerular diseases chronic immunoglobulin A (IgA) nephropathy may sometimes present as hypertensive urgency. Presence of rash, purpura, arthralgias, fever and systemic features may suggest conditions like vasculitis, Henoch-Schönlein disease or systemic lupus erythematosus (SLE).

Hypertension in patients with renal parenchymal disease is multifactorial. It could be volume mediated due to expanded extracellular volume and disproportionate increase in renin-angiotensin-aldosterone system (RAAS) activity (Fig. 35.1). Enhanced sympathetic activity, endothelial dysfunction, increased vascular reactivity and concomitant use of drugs like erythropoietin could also contribute to development of hypertension in these patients.

oliguria, hematuria, hypertension and varying degree of renal failure. Sometimes the severe and rapidly oncoming hypertension may progress to hypertensive encephalopathy. In first decade and adolescent age, history of recurrent urinary infections, pain in lumbar area while voiding, double voiding, persistent nocturia and enuresis may point to a possibility of underlying reflux nephropathy which may account for nearly 50% of cases of hypertension in 1st decade of life. Other

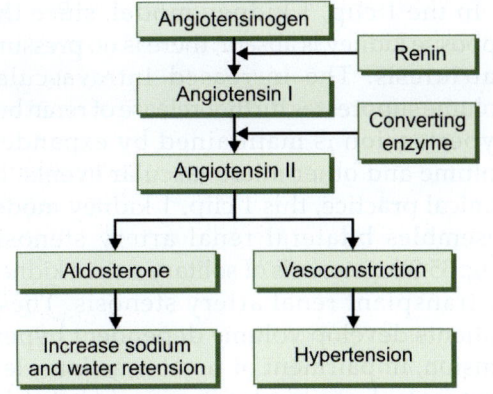

Fig. 35.1: Effect of activation of renin-angiotensin-aldosterone system

Renovascular Hypertension

Renal artery stenosis (RAS) is possibly the most important and potentially treatable cause for hypertension. The common causes for RAS are atherosclerotic disease of aorta, fibromuscular dysplasia (involving the renal artery) and Takayasu's arteritis.

Atherosclerotic RAS is typically seen in patients over 60 years of age who may be having underlying long-standing hypertension and/or diabetes. It is suspected when hypertension suddenly becomes uncontrolled or if sharp elevation of serum creatinine occurs soon after initiation of therapy with ACE inhibitors or angiotensin receptor blockers. Other situations where atherosclerotic RAS is suspected are patients with diabetes and macrovascular complications, CV disease, smoking, dyslipidemia, presence of abdominal bruit and disparity in renal sizes on ultrasound scan. Angiography shows involvement of aorta and major branches. The stenosis is typically seen at ostium and proximal part of renal artery.

Fibromuscular dysplasia (FMD) lesions produce distortions of the luminal diameter of large- and medium-sized arteries due to non-atherosclerotic arteriopathies. Clinically apparent FMDs are most common among young females between the ages of 15 and 50 years. On angiography, FMD causes small stenotic lesions along a vessel with intervening areas of dilatation (small aneurysms), creating a "string of beads" appearance. The lesions usually involve the mid to distal vessel beyond the first 1 to 2 cm from the aorta.

Takayasu arteritis is a rare, systemic, inflammatory large-vessel vasculitis of unknown etiology that most commonly affects women of childbearing age. It is defined as "granulomatous inflammation" of the aorta and its major branches including the renal arteries. It causes discrete stenosis of the aorta and its main branches, including the common carotid, subclavian and the renal arteries. Renal artery involvement is not uncommon in Asian and African patients and is a major cause of renovascular hypertension in these countries.

Pathophysiology

Narrowing of the renal artery may be present without causing significant hemodynamic changes in the renal circulation. Only when more than 70% of the vascular lumen is narrowed it is considered critical because, with such lesion the renal perfusion gets affected. The resultant renal ischemia initiates multiple mechanisms in an attempt to restore renal perfusion and maintain GFR, and stimulates release of renin from juxtaglomerular apparatus.

Harry Goldblatt demonstrated in experimental models, the role played by the kidney in hypertension. A metal clip was applied to one renal artery sufficient enough to cause ischemia of the kidney and opposite kidney was removed (1 clip, 1 kidney model) or retained (1 clip, 2-kidney model). The ischemic kidney releases renin. Renin promotes the conversion of angiotensinogen to a decapeptide, angiotensin I. In a rate-limiting step, angiotensin-converting enzyme (ACE) converts angiotensin I to an octapeptide, angiotensin II, which is a potent vasoconstrictor and also stimulates aldosterone secretion, sodium and water retention and hypertension. If the opposite kidney is normal (1 clip, 2-kidney model), pressure natriuresis in normal kidney results in excretion of sodium and water, decrease in intravascular volume, further decrease in the perfusion to the ischemic kidney, further activation of RAAS and renin dependent sustained hypertension. In the 1 clip, 2-kidney model, if the clip is removed early, renin activity returns to normal and hypertension is reversed. However, if the clip is removed after a long period of hypertension, despite restoration of blood flow to the kidney, the hypertension persists due to irreversible changes in the opposite kidney, systemic circulation, sympathetic activity and increase in peripheral vascular resistance. This is analogous to unilateral renal artery stenosis in humans (Fig. 35.2). The exact onset of critical stenosis and extent of permanent damage is uncertain and renin levels alone does not predict the outcome of revascularization procedures.

In the 1 clip, 1 kidney model, since the opposite kidney is absent, there is no pressure natriuresis. The increased intravascular volume suppresses further release of renin but hypertension is maintained by expanded volume and other microvascular events. In clinical practice, this 1 clip, 1 kidney model resembles bilateral renal artery stenosis (Fig. 35.3) or stenosis of solitary native kidney or transplant renal artery stenosis. These patients develop volume dependent hypertension, impairment of renal functions, left ventricular hypertrophy, increase in left atrial and pulmonary venous pressure, left ventricular failure and episodes of 'flash pulmonary edema' or other hypertensive urgencies.

Clinical Features

These patients have higher nocturnal blood pressure. The lower levels of blood pressure observed during sleep in ambulatory blood pressure monitoring as seen in normal individuals are not seen in patients with RVH

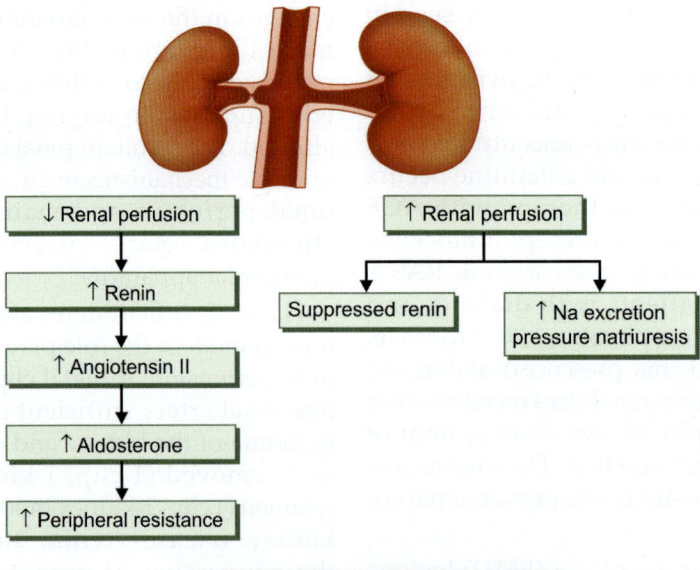

Fig. 35.2: Stenosis (narrowing) in one renal artery causes increased renin, angiotensin II, aldosterone and increase peripheral resistance and blood pressure. On the other side, increased perfusion suppresses renin and increases sodium loss (so, there is no edema). As a result there is disparity in the renal vein renin level between stenosed and contralateral kidney

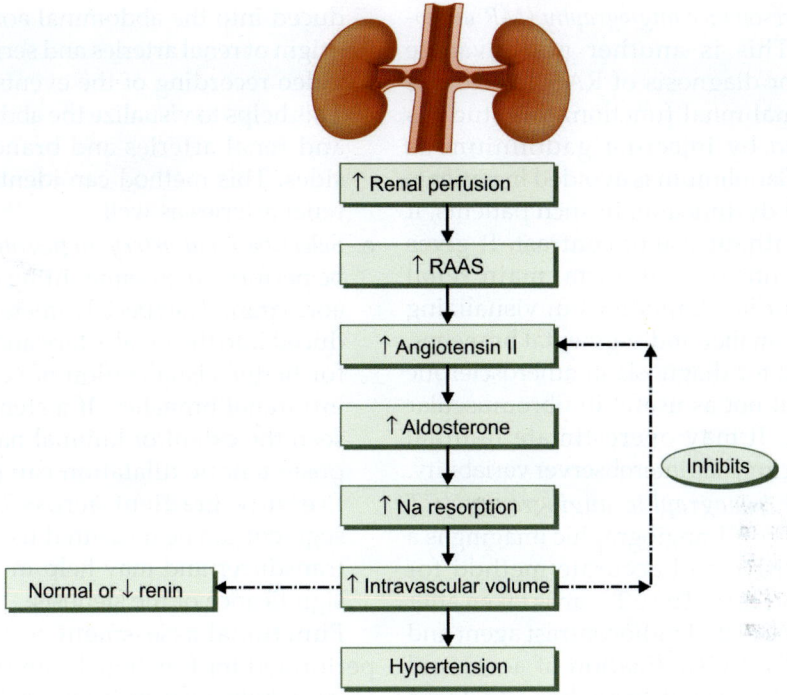

Fig. 35.3: Narrowing of both renal arteries increase renin, angiotensin, aldosterone, sodium retention and intravascular volume but hypervolemia suppresses RAAS and renin level comes down. Hypertension is mainly volume mediated

('nondippers'). They often have 'resistant hypertension' requiring 3 or more drugs for control especially if the renal functions are also impaired. Sometimes they present with hypertensive urgency with neuroretinopathy and evidence of target organ involvement. Patients with bilateral disease who have tendency for volume expansion can present with 'flash pulmonary edema'. They may develop deterioration of renal functions following treatment with ACE inhibitor or angiotensin receptor blocker (ARB). On physical examination disparity in blood pressure between upper and lower limbs would suggest a possibility of aortoarteritis. Presence of a systole-diastolic bruit in epigastrium on either side of midline is highly suggestive of renal artery stenosis but is observed in only half of the cases, hence, its absence does not rule out renovascular disease.

Diagnostic Tests

Renal artery stenosis can be diagnosed in retrospect, when the blood pressure returns to normal after revascularization procedure. In clinical practice, tests to detect anatomical narrowing of the renal arteries and functional tests to establish significant narrowing and its effect on blood pressure are done. Some of the available tests are:

a. *Color Doppler ultrasonography:* This is a simple non-invasive test with sensitivity and specificity of >85% if performed by experienced hands. It can identify lesions in major renal arteries. In very sick/non-cooperative patients, obese individuals, those with multiple renal arteries or if lesions involve accessory/smaller branches, Doppler study may not give the required information. The method has the advantage of being able to detect both unilateral and bilateral renal artery disease.

b. *Magnetic resonance angiography (MR angiography):* This is another non-invasive method for diagnosis of RAS. In patients with normal renal function, this study is performed by injecting gadolinium as contrast. Gadolinium is avoided in patients with renal dysfunction. In such patients, it is done without use of contrast. It gives excellent imaging of aorta, main renal arteries but has limitations in visualizing lesions in smaller and segmental branches. It is useful for diagnosis in atherosclerotic disease but not as useful in fibromuscular dysplasia. It may overestimate luminal narrowing and has interobserver variability.

c. *Computed tomographic angiography (CT angiography):* CT angiographic imaging is a very sensitive and accurate method for diagnosis of RAS. The CT scan is taken after injecting iodinated radiocontrast agent and it gives good visualization of aorta and even smaller renal branches. As large volume of contrast is used it has limitations in patients with impaired renal functions.

d. *Abdominal aortogram:* Flush abdominal aortogram via percutaneous femoral, brachial or radial artery puncture is the 'gold standard' for diagnosis of renal artery stenosis (Fig. 35.4). Here, the dye is introduced into the abdominal aorta above the origin of renal arteries and serial pictures or video recording of the events is recorded. This helps to visualize the abdominal aorta, and renal arteries and branches on both sides. This method can identify accessory renal arteries as well.

e. *Selective renal artery angiography:* This can be performed on same sitting as abdominal aortogram. The special catheter can be introduced into the renal artery and dye injected for better visualization of segmental and intrarenal branches. If a stenotic lesion is seen the extent of luminal narrowing and post-stenotic dilatation can also be seen. Pressure gradient across the stenosed segment can be measured using a pressure transducer and may help in assessing the significance of the stenosis.

Functional assessment certain tests are performed for functional significance and to assess whether corrective procedure would be beneficial.

i. *Radionuclear imaging with ACE inhibition:* It provides important functional data and helps in diagnosis and management of patients with suspected renal artery stenosis. Technetium 99m labeled diethylenetriamine penta-acetic acid (99mTcDTPA)

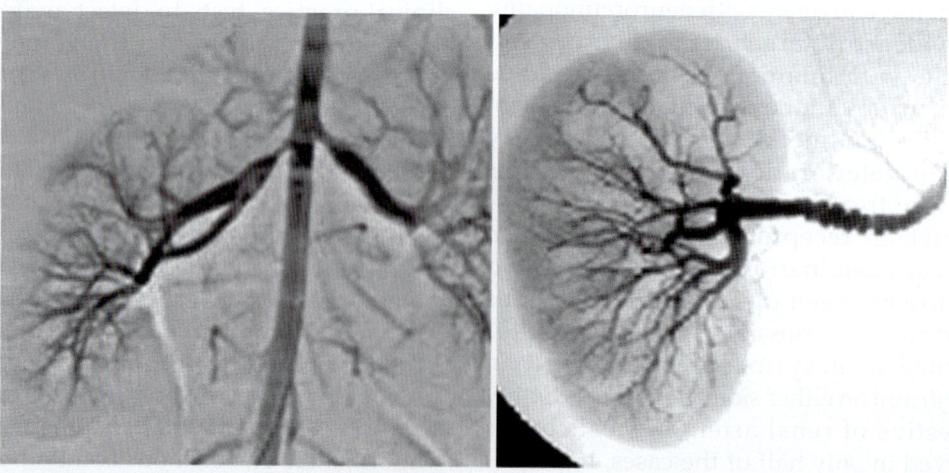

Fig. 35.4: Bilateral atherosclerotic narrowing of early part of renal artery (left). Beaded appearance of renal artery due to fibromuscular dysplasia (right)

is filtered freely in the glomerulus and is excreted in urine. It is often used to measure GFR. Renal scan using DTPA after administering captopril tablet is a reliable imaging technique for identification of functionally significant RAS. Captopril, 25–50 mg, is administered 1 hour prior to the renal scan. In patients with a functionally significant renal artery stenosis, the renogram shows decrease in renal uptake of DTPA on the affected side as compared to the baseline scan.

ii. *Plasma renin activity and renal vein renin:* Hemodynamically significant RAS causes ischemia and stimulates renin release from the kidney and suppresses renin from the other kidney. So, all patients of RAS will not have elevated plasma renal activity (PRA). Moreover, some patients with essential hypertension also have elevated PRA. Therefore, PRA has low predictive value to identify which patient should be evaluated in detail for RVH. Estimation of PRA after single dose of ACE inhibitor (in patients who are not on medications) helps in improving the predictive value. Estimation of renin from renal vein was used for diagnosis and to identify patients for revascularization procedures. If the renal vein renin is high on the side to arterial stenosis and that from the opposite side is suppressed, it gives a clue that hypertension may still be renin dependent and improvement can be expected after revascularization. However, since this is an invasive test, it is seldom used in clinical practice.

Management

If the stenosis of renal artery is found to be responsible for hypertension, efforts to restore the renal circulation are undertaken. The options available are:

a. Medical therapy with ACE inhibitors/ ARBs along with other antihypertensive drugs are used to control blood pressure.

(*see* Chapter 36). In most patients, target blood pressures are achieved. In the event of 'resistant hypertension' or when there is risk of progression of the disease, revascularization procedures may help to control blood pressure and preserve renal functions.

b. Percutaneous transluminal renal angioplasty (PTRA) followed by placement of a stent across the stenosed segment an accepted procedure for management of RAS (Fig. 35.5).

c. Surgical revascularization: Aortorenal bypass by using a synthetic polytetrafluoroethylene (PTFE) or polyester (Dacron) graft from aorta to the renal artery bypassing the stenosed segment helps to restore blood flow to the ischemic areas of the kidney. In suitable cases, hepatorenal anastomosis (on right side) and splenorenal anastomosis (left side) can be done to by-pass the obstruction and avoiding synthetic grafts.

Endocrine Disorders

Disorders of endocrine glands are another important cause for secondary hypertension (Table 35.2).

Pheochromocytoma

This is a catecholamine secreting tumor arising from chromaffin cells of adrenal medulla. Sometimes it may arise from extra adrenal sites like sympathetic ganglia (paraganglioma). Pheochromocytoma is commonly seen in fourth and fifth decades of life. Patients may be asymptomatic and adrenal mass may be detected during abdominal scan for other indications. The classical triad of paroxysmal hypertension, headache and palpitations/ sweating is seen in only 25% of the cases and can also be observed in cases of essential hypertension. Hence, these symptoms are not a reliable indicator for presence of pheochromocytoma. Some of the other non-specific symptoms are orthostatic hypotension (low plasma volume), wide fluctuations in blood pressure, hypertension with tachycardia,

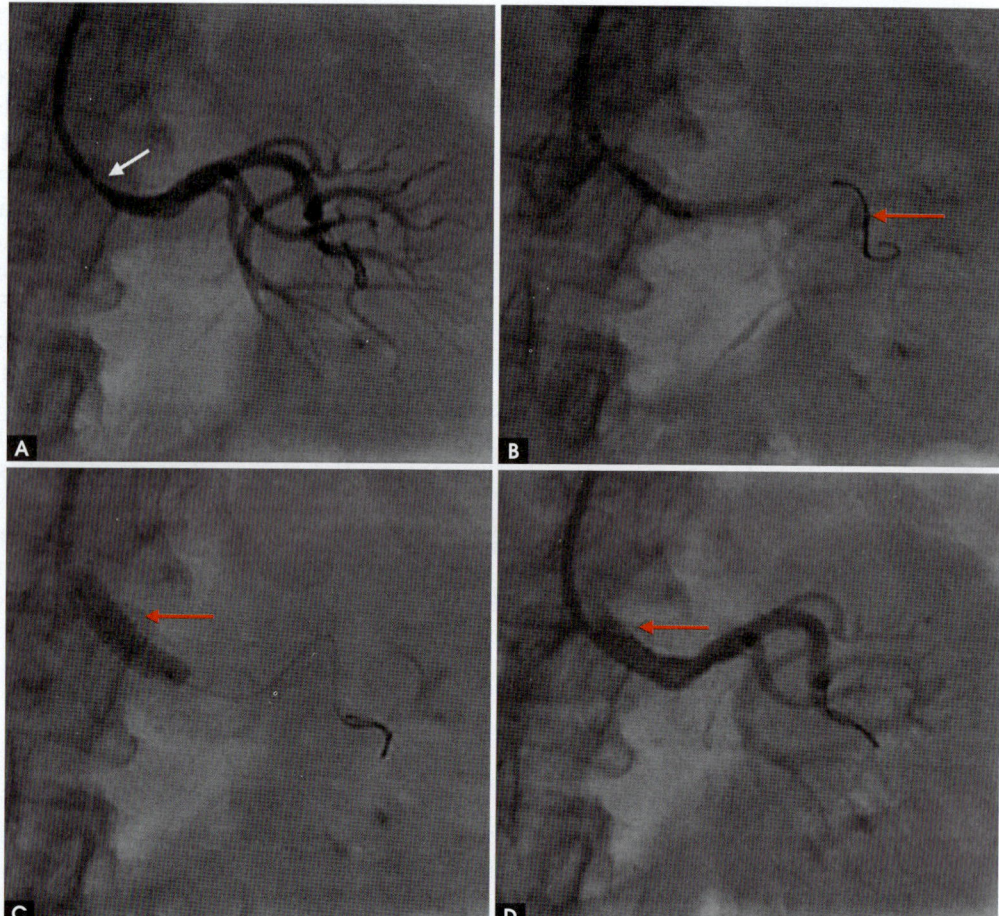

Fig. 35.5A to D: (A) In a 70-year-old lady with recent onset uncontrolled hypertension, angiogram reveals stenosis of proximal segment of left renal artery (white arrow). (B) Guidewire is negotiated across the stenosed segment (red arrow). (C) Stent placed and inflated (red arrow). (D) Follow-up angiogram shows patent stent with restored flow (red arrow)

visual blurring, papilledema, weight loss, polyuria and polydipsia. Abnormalities in carbohydrate metabolism with insulin resistance, impaired fasting glucose, and 'apparent' type 2 diabetes mellitus may occur due to excessive secretion of catecholamines.

Diagnosis in pheochromocytoma, the metabolism of catecholamine and formation of metanephrine and normetanephrine occurs within the tumor. The method of reliably identifying catecholamine secreting tumors is by measuring fractionated catecholamines (dopamine, norepinephrine, and epinephrine) from serum and fractionated metanephrines and normetanephrine in a 24-hour urine by high performance liquid chromatography. With this, the chances of false positive results due to use of drugs like α-methyldopa and labetalol and false-negative results caused by imaging contrast agents can be avoided. Once the diagnosis is established the tumor should be localized, in adrenal or extra-adrenal sites using ultrasound, radiological or imaging procedures. Multiple tumors are also common.

About 25% of pheochromocytoma tumor may be malignant. Isotope study using iodine-131 metaiodobenzylguanidine (MIBG) is highly reliable and have high sensitivity for localizing the tumor.

Management: During surgical procedure some patients are at risk of developing hypertensive emergencies. These patients require good control of blood pressure with combined α-adrenergic and β-adrenergic blockade, calcium channel blockers for 10–14 days preoperatively to normalize blood pressure and saline infusions to expand the contracted blood volume. Treatment options for hypertensive crises include intravenous sodium nitroprusside, phentolamine or nicardipine. Following surgery there is prompt reduction in BP. Persistence of BP suggests a residual tumor, multiple tumors or coexistent essential hypertension.

Primary Hyperaldosteronism (Conn's Syndrome)

In a patient presenting with hypertension, hypokalemia and metabolic alkalosis, hyperaldosteronism should be suspected. It may also be detected incidentally as enlarged adrenal gland on abdominal scan and is relatively less common cause for secondary hypertension. Angiotensin II and serum potassium are two important stimulants for secretion of aldosterone from adrenal glands. Classical primary aldosteronism (Conn's syndrome) is characterized by excessive aldosterone secretion which promotes renal tubular sodium reabsorption, renal K^+ loss, extracellular volume expansion, hypertension and suppressed renin levels. Most common subtypes of primary aldosteronism are bilateral adrenal hyperplasia (idiopathic hyperaldosteronism) and unilateral aldosterone-producing adenoma.

Diagnosis: As discussed earlier, expanded volume in hyperaldosteronism suppresses plasma renin concentration (PRC) and plasma renin activity (PRA). For diagnosis of primary hyperaldosteronism, plasma aldosterone levels has no diagnostic value in isolation. Ratio of plasma aldosterone concentration and plasma renin activity (PAC/PRA ratio) would be a sensitive screening test for diagnosis. The mean value in normal subjects or patients with essential hypertension is 4 to 10, whereas, it is more than 30–50 in most patients with primary aldosteronism. In hypokalemic subjects raising serum potassium levels into the mid-normal range with potassium supplementation will increase PAC and optimize the PAC/PRA ratio. It is unaffected by posture and antihypertensive drugs and the mineralocorticoid receptor antagonists. Drugs like spironolactone and eprenalone must be discontinued for at least 6 weeks prior to testing. More cases are being identified by this screening method.

Other clinically important causes for hypertension, hypokalemia and alkalosis are:

i. Renovascular disease (in which hyper-secretion of renin leads to increased angiotensin II and aldosterone secretion), the ratio between plasma aldosterone concentration and PRA is <10.

ii. When both PRA and plasma aldosterone concentration are high, diuretic use should be considered which could be surreptitious and characterized by low intravascular volume, metabolic alkalosis and hypokalemia.

iii. Renin secreting tumor (rare)

iv. Rarely mineralocorticoid receptor stimulation (e.g. hypercortisolism, licorice root ingestion) when both the PRA and plasma aldosterone concentration are suppressed.

Although hyperaldosteronism is observed in both RAS and primary aldosteronism, in RAS the initiating event is high renin and low intravascular volume, whereas primary aldosteronism it is expanded volume and suppressed renin level (Fig. 35.6).

Obstructive sleep apnea: This disorder is usually seen in obese individuals who present with excessive somnolence during daytime. Recurrent episodes of airway obstructions result in hypoxia and hypercapnia increasing sympathetic neural tone, which in turn causes vasoconstriction and hypertension. Treatment of primary problem, weight reduction and non-invasive ventilator ('CPAP') therapy at night helps in control of BP. Some of these patients may have resistant hypertension which is due to excessive aldosterone levels. The ratio of serum aldosterone to plasma renin activity is most often used to diagnose the condition. Treatment with aldosterone antagonists, spironolactone is helpful in controlling blood pressure.

Apparent mineralocorticoid excess: Certain unusual diseases present with features of hypokalemia, hypertension and cushingoid features. In contrast to other types of hyperaldosteronism, these patients have suppressed plasma aldosterone levels. The most common type, classical congenital adrenal hyperplasia, is due to one of several autosomal recessive genetic deficiencies in enzymes involved in adrenal steroidogenesis, resulting in mineralocorticoid and androgen excess. Although common in infants and children, in some patient the diagnosis is established only by adolescent age. Hypertension is due to deficiency of either 11β-hydroxylase or 17α-hydroxylase which results in high circulating levels of deoxycortico-sterone and 11-deoxycortisol, with increased production of adrenal androgens. After diagnosis is established these patients are treated with glucocorticoids. This suppresses corticotropin secretion and reduction in signs and symptoms of mineralocorticoid excess.

Miscellaneous: It is important to take a proper history during evaluation of a patient for hypertension since use of drugs is a common cause of secondary hypertension. Oral contraceptive pills, use of NSAIDs, sympathomimetic drugs, calcineurin inhibi-

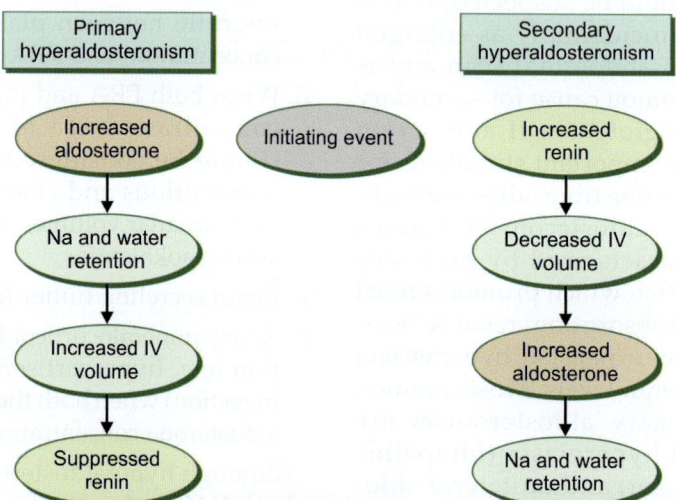

Fig. 35.6: Hypertension with hypokalemia could be due to hyperaldosteronism. In adrenal hyerplasia or adenoma the primary event is excessive aldosterone production, expanded IV volume and suppressed renin, whereas in renal artery stenosis the renin levels are high, intravascular volume is low and resultant secondary hyperaldosteronism

tors (cyclosporine) are some commonly used drugs that cause hypertension. The mechanisms include salt and water retention, increase in sympathetic activity, release of vasoconstrictors, endothelins and inhibitory effect on vasodilatory prostacyclines. Identification of the offending agent and its withdrawal if possible would ameliorate hypertension in many of these cases.

Summary

A variety of conditions are identifiable as underlying cause for secondary hypertension. A proper history, detailed clinical examination, necessary laboratory tests and imaging tests help in proper diagnosis. In high risk individuals, more detailed and even invasive investigations are undertaken to make the correct diagnosis and plan the treatment. Newer non-invasive radiological and nuclear medicine investigations along with availability of accurate laboratory methods for estimation of various hormones and chemicals have further widened our scope for diagnosis of some of these potentially curable causes for hypertension.

Management of Hypertension

• KC Gurudev

Hypertension is an important independent risk factor for coronary artery disease, stroke, heart failure and chronic kidney disease. The extent of blood pressure control determines the reduction in morbidity and mortality. In younger and older patients with hypertension, the degree of blood pressure reduction is more important compared to the choice of anti-hypertensive drug. With the same level of blood pressure control, most antihypertensive drugs provide the same degree of protection against target organ damage. Majority of the patients with confirmed hypertension require lifelong medications often with more than one drug. Most organizations and professional bodies recommend that normal blood pressure should be less than 120 mm Hg systolic and less than 80 mm Hg diastolic. In individuals with blood pressure above 140/80 mm Hg drug therapy is required.

Lowering the systolic blood pressure by 10–12 mm Hg and diastolic blood pressure by 5–6 mm Hg reduces relative risk for stroke by 35–40% and coronary heart disease by 12–16% in the first five years of starting treatment. The risk of heart failure is also reduced by 50%. Control of hypertension is the single most effective intervention to slow down the rate of progression of hypertension-related kidney disease.

Before starting drug therapy, a thorough evaluation should be performed to determine the extent of target organ damage and an assessment of secondary causes of hypertension. Initial evaluation should include careful history, clinical examination, urine analysis (including testing for microalbuminuria), complete blood count, fasting blood sugar, renal function tests, lipid profile, thyroid profile, ECG, chest X-ray, ophthalmoscopic evaluation and ultrasonography of abdomen.

Those who have a systolic blood pressure of 120–129 mm Hg and diastolic less than 80 mm Hg require counseling on non-pharmacological therapy and reassessment every 3–6 months. According to the new American College of Cardiology/American Heart Association (ACC/AHA) hypertension guidelines 2017, persons who have systolic blood pressure of 130–139 mm Hg and diastolic of 80–89 mm Hg are in stage 1 hypertension. If they have no clinical cardiovascular disease, non-pharmacological therapy and periodic reassessment is advised. In those with clinical features of atherosclerotic cardiovascular disease, additional blood pressure lowering medication is required. In type 2 diabetes with or without chronic kidney disease and stage 1 hypertension, drug therapy is required in addition to non-pharmacological intervention from the beginning. Persons with a systolic blood pressure of more than 140 mm Hg or diastolic more than 90 mm Hg are considered to be in stage 2 hypertension. They need to be treated with drugs and non-pharmacological measures.

In persons under the age of 50 years, extent of diastolic blood pressure elevation is a better predictor of higher cardiovascular risk and mortality, whereas in those above 50 years, systolic blood pressure is a better predictor. In diabetic patients the target goal for blood pressure control is less than 125/80 mm Hg. Angiotensin converting enzyme inhibitors (ACEIs) or angiotensin receptor blockers (ARBs) are the first choice and can be used as monotherapy. ACEIs/ARBs are the ideal drugs which also help in reducing the proteinuria and retard the progression of the disease. A rise of creatinine up to 25% above the baseline is acceptable while using ACEI/ARB. However, these drugs may cause sudden decrease in GFR and hyperkalemia. If necessary, calcium channel blocker drugs are added to achieve the target. In patients with CKD, the target goal is less than 130/80 mm Hg. Theoretically, too high or too low blood pressures may overwhelm the autoregulatory capacity of cerebral, coronary and renal blood flow, thereby increasing overall morbidity and mortality. The concept of 'J' curve suggests that the risk of a cardiovascular event is high when the blood pressure is too high or too low.

Non-pharmacological Measures in the Management of Hypertension

Adoption of a healthy lifestyle is most important for both prevention and management of high blood pressure. Lifestyle interventions, not only lower the blood pressure but also enhance the efficacy of the antihypertensive medications. The critical lifestyle changes that reduce overall cardiovascular risk are:

1. Smoking cessation
2. Weight reduction
3. Avoiding/moderation of alcohol intake
4. Reduction of salt intake
5. Physical exercise
6. Increase in consumption of fruits and vegetables
7. Reduce intake of saturated and total fat
8. Patient education
9. Periodic follow-up.

The benefits of non-pharmacologic measures in terms of the benefits are summarized in Table 36.1.

Pharmacological Methods (Drug Treatment) in Hypertension

Primarily, 4 types of antihypertensive drugs are commonly used. The choice of drugs depends on the proven or presumed cause of hypertension and should be individualized.

1. *Diuretics:* Diuretics are the first choice in patients who have volume overload hypertension. Generally, older individuals, those who have water retention due to CKD should be given diuretics. Thiazide like diuretics (chlorthalidone and indapamide/hydrochlorothiazide cause more sodium loss and hyponatremia is a common complication. Loop diuretics (frusemide, torsemide, bumetinide) predominantly excrete water but may cause hypokalemia. The use of diuretics should be monitored and individualized.

2. *Long-acting calcium channel blockers:* They are primarily vasodilator drugs which reduce peripheral resistance and thereby the blood pressure (amlodipine, nifedipine).

3. *Angiotensin-converting enzyme blockers:* They block the enzyme which causes conversion of angiotensin I to angiotensin II which is a powerful vasoconstrictor. All drugs ending with 'PRIL' belong to ACE inhibitor group (e.g. enalapril, ramipril, lisinopril, captopril, perindopril).

4. *Angiotensin II receptor blockers:* This group of drugs block the receptors through which angiotensin II exerts its action. All drugs in this group end as 'sartan' (e.g. losartan, telmisartan, irbesartan, candesartan).

Table 36.1: Recommended modifications and potential benefits

Modification	Recommendation	Average range Systolic BP reduction
Smoking	Absolute stoppage of smoking	Overall benefit
Weight reduction	Maintain normal body weight and BMI (BMI = 18.5–24.9 kg/m^2)	5–20 mm Hg/10 kg weight loss
DASH* eating plan	Diet rich in fruits, vegetables, and low-fat dairy products with reduced the content of saturated and total fat	8–14 mm Hg
Dietary sodium restriction	Reduce dietary sodium intake to 100 mmol/day (2.4 g sodium or 6 g sodium chloride)	2–8 mm Hg
Aerobic physical activity	Regular aerobic physical activity (e.g. brisk walking) at least 30 m in/day, most days of the week	4–9 mm Hg
Moderation of alcohol consumption	Men: Limit to 2 drinks per day; women and lighter-weight persons: Limit to 1 drink per day	2–4 mm Hg

*DASH → Dietary approaches to stop hypertension

Important drugs used in treatment of hypertension, their indications, dosage, adverse effects and contraindications are summarized in Table 36.2.

The choice of the drug is influenced by its other favorable actions in addition to anti-hypertensive effect. β blockers are preferred for controlling heart rate in atrial fibrillation or in ischemic heart disease. ACE inhibitors and ARBs are first-line therapy in all patients who have heart failure, myocardial infraction, systolic dysfunction, and in patients with proteinuric chronic kidney disease. Diuretics have an added benefit of volume control in patients with heart failure or chronic kidney disease. Non-DHP calcium channel blockers can be given for rate control in patients with atrial fibrillation or for control of angina in patients with coronary disease and normal left ventricular systolic function. Calcium channel blockers also may be preferred in patients with obstructive airway disease. α blockers are preferred in older men with symptoms of prostatism and if they are not at high cardiovascular risk.

Monotherapy

Three main classes of drugs, namely thiazide-like and type diuretics, long-acting calcium channel blockers and ACEI/ARB group of drugs are the first line drugs used for initial monotherapy. If prescribed for the right indication, each of these categories of drugs is equally effective in attaining the target blood pressure.

Younger patients are more likely to have renin mediated hypertension and are more likely to respond best to ACEI/ARB. Older patients above the age of 60 respond better to diuretics or long-acting calcium channel blockers. However, older patients with history of heart failure, myocardial infarction or proteinuric chronic kidney disease are treated with ACEI/ARB. Patients are reassessed 4–6 weeks after initiation of monotherapy. If the response is inadequate and the patient has not achieved the goal blood pressure, the dose is increased step-wise. If the maximum dose is administered directly as the second step, the side effects of medicines may occur and override the advantage of control of blood pressure.

Table 36.2: Class of drug, indications, dosage, adverse effects and contraindications of common antihypertensive drugs

Class	Hemodynamic effect	Advantages	Side effects	Contraindications
Diuretics Hydrochloro- thiazide (12.5–50 mg/day) Furosemide (40– 200 mg/day)	Initial volume shrinkage	Effective in elderly Enhances efficiency of other agents May be used in renal insufficiency Useful in patients with fluid retention	Weakness Palpitation Hypokalemia Metabolic alkalosis Hypomagnesemia Hyperlipidemia Glucose intolerance Hypercalcemia Hyperuricemia	Pre-existing volume contraction
β blockers Propranolol (40–320 mg/ day) Metoprolol (50–200 mg/day) Atenolol 25–100 mg/day) Labetalol (200– 1800 mg/day)	Reduce cardiac output	Secondary prevention of MI Low cost Good patient acceptability Reduce mani- festation of anxiety Hepatic metabolized Co-existing angina, migraine, glaucoma	Bronchospasm Fatigue Hypoglycemia Glucose intolerance Hypertriglyceridemia Decrease HDL cholesterol Sleep disturbance Nightmares Impotence GI distress	Asthma Heart block Careful use in PVD Insulin-requiring diabetes Allergy Coronary spasm Withdrawal angina
ACEI Enalapril (2.5–40 mg/day) Ramipril (2.5–20 mg/day)	Peripheral vasodila- tation	No CNS side effects Unload congestion Congestive heart failure No coronary vasoconstriction Possible renal protection	Dry cough Taste disturbance Rash Leukopenia	Pregnancy Cautious use in renal failure and bilateral renovascular disease
ARB Losartan (25–100 mg/day) Telmisartan (20–160 mg/day) Azilsartan (20–80 mg/day)		Same as ACEI	Angioedema Hyperkalemia	Same as ACEI
Vasodilators Hydralazine (50–300 mg/day)	Vasodilatation Lupus-like syndrome Hirsutism Pericardial effusion		Fluid retention Reflex cardiac stimulation Headache	Uncontrolled angina pectoris

Contd.

Table 36.2: Class of drug, indications, dosage, adverse effects and contraindications of common antihypertensive drugs *(Contd.)*

Class	Hemodynamic effect	Advantages	Side effects	Contraindications
Minoxidil (2.5–80 mg/day)			Orthostatic hypotension Impotence	
α receptor blocker	Peripheral vasodilatation	Effective in elderly No decrease in cardiac output No sedation No alteration in blood lipids	Postural dizziness Fatigue Malaise GI upset Cost	Orthostatic hypotension
Prazosin (1–20 mg/day)				
Central acting agents α methyldopa (250–2000 mg/day) Clonidine (0.1mg– 0.6 mg/day)	Reduce cardiac output	No alteration in blood lipids No fluid retention	Sedation Dry mouth Withdrawal syndrome Autoimmune syndrome	Orthostatic hypotension Liver disease Heart failure
Calcium channel blocker Verapamil (120–240 mg/day) Diltiazem (90–270 mg/day) Nifedipine (30–180 mg/day)	Peripheral vasodilatation	Effective in elderly No CNS side effects Coronary vasodilatation	Flushing Local edema Constipation Blunt AV node conduction	

In patients with a normal renal function, the maximum therapeutic dose of ACE/ARB, can be administered as a monotherapy.

In the elderly, thiazide diuretic as monotherapy may have an advantage as they have beneficial effects on bone mineral density. However, the disadvantage of development of hyponatremia should also be borne in mind. β blockers are not useful for initial use as monotherapy. If the patient remains in the range of 20/10 mm Hg above the targeted goal, a strategy of sequential monotherapy may be tried in which different classes of drugs are tried as monotherapy if the present drug does not achieve control. If monotherapy fails, it will be necessary to switch to combination therapy.

Combination Therapy

In combination therapy, an additional drug is needed. Monotherapy may be suitable only when the blood pressure at the time of diagnosis is only 20/10 mm Hg above goal. If the initial blood pressure is >20/10 mm Hg, starting combination therapy initially it increases the chances of attaining target blood pressure early. The recommended drugs for combination therapy are long-acting DHP calcium channel blocker plus a long-acting ACEI/ARB. In obese patients, a combination of thiazide diuretic and a long-acting ACEI/ARB is ideal. In non-obese patients, if the combination therapy is required ACEI/ARB and a long-acting calcium channel blocker is recommended.

Timing of Dose: Bedtime Vs Morning Doses

Ordinarily, nocturnal blood pressures are 15% lower than daytime values. Failure of the blood pressure to fall by 10% during sleep is called "non-dipping" and is a predictor of adverse cardiovascular outcome. The lack of nocturnal dip has a greater prognostic significance compared to daytime mean blood pressures. Bedtime/evening dosing in monotherapy and timing of one of medication from morning to evening in a combination therapy may restore nocturnal blood pressure dip. This strategy reduces overall 24 hours mean pressure and decreases the incidence of cardiovascular disease.

Hypertensive Emergency

Patients with a systolic blood pressure more than 180 mm Hg and diastolic blood pressure more than 120 mm Hg, with end-organ damage, is considered to be having hypertensive emergency. This condition requires immediate attention with parenteral antihypertensive medications since failure to control the blood pressure can lead to life-threatening complications. The common backgrounds under which hypertensive emergencies occur and the management strategies are outlined in Table 36.3.

Hypertensive Urgency

Patients with blood pressure more than 180/120 mm Hg who are asymptomatic and have no end organ damage are in 'hypertensive urgency'. Although there is no proven benefit in rapidly lowering their blood pressure with parenteral antihypertensive medications, it is necessary to reduce the blood pressure gently since they may develop hypertensive emergency at any time (Table 36.4).

Resistant Hypertension

Resistant hypertension is defined by the 2017 American College of Cardiology/American Heart Association (ACC/AHA) hypertension guideline and by the 2013 European Societies of Hypertension and Cardiology (ESH/ESC) statement as blood pressure that remains above goal (office SBP/DBP = 130/80 mm Hg)

Table 36.3: Treatment of hypertensive emergencies

Causes and parenteral drugs used for hypertensive emergencies	
Hypertensive encephalopathy	Nitroprusside, nicardipine, labetalol
Malignant hypertension (when IV therapy is indicated)	Enalaprilat, labetalol, nicardipine, nitroprusside
Stroke	Nicardipine, labetalol, nitroprusside
Myocardial infarction/unstable angina	Nitroglycerine, esmolol, nicardipine, labetalol
Acute left ventricular failure	Nitroglycerine, enalaprilat, loop diuretics
Aortic dissection	Nitroprusside, esmolol, labetalol
Adrenergic crisis	Phentolamine, nitroprusside
Postoperative hypertension	Nitroglycerine, nitroprusside, labetalol, nicardipine
Pre-eclampsia/eclampsia of pregnancy	Hydralazine, labetalol, nicardipine

Table 36.4: Parenteral antihypertensive drugs

Parenteral antihypertensive drug doses in emergencies

Nitroprusside	Initial 0.3 (µg/kg)/min; usual 2–4 (µg/kg g)/min; maximum 10 (µg/kg)/min for 10 min
Nicardipine	Initial 5 mg/h; titrate by 2.5 mg/h at 5–1 5 min intervals; max 1 5 mg/h
Nitroglycerine	Initial 5 µg/min, then titrate by 5 µg/min at 3–5 min intervals; if no response is seen at 20 µg/min, incremental increases of 10–20 µg/min may be used
Labetalol	2 mg/min up to 300 mg or 20 mg over 2 min, then 40–80 mg at 10 min intervals up to 300 mg total
Enalaprilat	Usual 0.625–1.25 mg over 5 min every 6–8 h; maximum 5 mg/dose
Esmolol	Initial 80–500 µg/kg over 1 min, then 50–300 (µg/kg)/min
Phentolamine	5–15 mg bolus
Hydralazine	10–50 mg at 30 min intervals

in spite of concurrent use of three antihypertensive agents of different classes at optimal doses and one should be a diuretic. Patients also have resistant hypertension if they require at least four medications to achieve adequate blood pressure control. Nearly 15% of patients considered as resistant hypertension have pseudoresistance rather than actual resistance.

The reasons for pseudoresistance are as follows:

1. Inaccurate blood pressure measurement (use of inappropriate sized cuff)
2. Poor adherence to blood pressure medications
3. Poor adherence to lifestyle modifications
4. Sub-optimal antihypertensive therapy
5. White coat resistance (while well-controlled blood pressure on ambulatory monitoring)

The reasons for truly resistant hypertension are:

1. Extracellular volume expansion
2. Increased sympathetic activity
3. Simultaneous use of NSAIDs and stimulants
4. Undetected secondary hypertension
5. Substance abuse

When to Discontinue Antihypertensive Therapy

In few patients with stage I hypertension, well controlled with monotherapy, there is a possibility of gradually lowering of medication. After the withdrawal of medicines 5–55% of these patients may remain normotensive for a couple of years, but it is ideal to keep them on a small dose of medication rather than completely withdrawing. Well controlled patients on multiple drugs do well with the decrease in number and dosage of pills that they are taking. One should be cautious in tapering the drug dose and withdrawing. It should be done gradually since the abrupt cessation of therapy especially short-acting β blockers (propanol), short-acting α_2-agonists (clonidine) can lead to rebound hypertension and even hypertensive emergency.

Management of Renal Parenchymal and Renovascular Hypertension

Renal parenchymal hypertension often presents with edema, impaired kidney functions, and active urinary sediments in all age groups. Renovascular hypertension has a bimodal distribution, being common in younger and elderly patients (fibromuscular dysplasia and atherosclerotic renal artery stenosis respectively) and may present with impaired kidney functions when it is bilateral.

The mainstay of management of renal parenchymal hypertension is lifestyle modifications, especially salt and water restriction in the diet, ACEI, and ARB. The usefulness of ACEIs and ARB is that they slow down the rate of progression of renal disease and reduce proteinuria. ACEIs and ARB may cause sudden deterioration in GFR and life-threatening hyperkalemia. One should start with lowest possible dose and increase the dosage with frequent monitoring of creatinine and potassium. An increase of serum creatinine up to 25% from baseline is accepted, and in case the rise is beyond this, the dose is reduced or withdrawn.

Unilateral renal artery stenosis leading to hypertension is primarily treated medically with ACE and ARB along with statins, anti-oxidants, and anti-platelet drugs. Thiazide diuretics and long-acting calcium channel blockers, mineralocorticoid receptor antagonist or a β-blocker should be added if necessary for control of hypertension. There are specific situations when a patient requires intervention in the form of percutaneous transluminal renal angioplasty (PTRA). They are:

1. Patient with a short duration of blood pressure elevation, before diagnosis.
2. Failure or intolerance to optimal medical therapy for control of blood pressure.
3. Recurrent 'flash' pulmonary edema and refractory heart failure.

Patients with bilateral renal artery stenosis often have impaired renal function at presentation and rapidly worsening of kidney function. Even in these patients, the primary aim is to control the blood pressure with medical treatment unless there is a compelling indication for surgical intervention as with unilateral renal artery stenosis. One should be cautious as ACE and ARB can cause a sudden decline in GFR and lead to increase in serum creatinine and potassium.

Management of Endocrine Causes of Hypertension

Endocrine pathology is suspected in individuals with resistant hypertension or those with additional features. Treatment is aimed at the cause and is rewarding. Primary hyperaldosteronism is a common endocrine cause of secondary hypertension. It is classified as lateralizing (unilateral) or non-lateralizing (bilateral) hyperaldosteronism. Investigations include CT, MRI, adrenocortical scintigraphy, and adrenal venous sampling. Spironolactone and eplerenone are the main drugs for control of hypokalemia. Calcium channel blockers are used for control of blood pressure. Curative treatment involves surgery.

Both hypothyroidism and hyperthyroidism can present with hypertension. After treatment of the primary thyroid disorder, the blood pressure usually gets controlled. Thyroxine is used for the treatment of hypothyroidism while either surgery or pharmacotherapy involving methimazole or carbimazole coupled with a nonspecific β-blocker (propranolol) for hyperthyroidism.

Cushing's syndrome with hypertension needs correction of hypercortisolism. For ectopic and bilateral or unilateral Cushing's syndrome, the treatment is surgical excision. Cushing's disease requires trans-sphenoidal resection of the ACTH secreting pituitary tumor.

Pheochromocytoma is a rare cause of hypertension and presents with sweating, headache, and flushing. Patients have a significant postural drop in blood pressure. It is often amenable to surgical treatment. However, care must be taken to achieve adequate adrenal blockade and plasma volume expansion before the surgery by starting α-blockade with phenoxybenzamine 10–14 days before surgery, and two days after beginning α-blockers with β-blockade. β-blockade before α-blockade may precipitate hypertensive crisis. During preoperative preparation, a patient must be well hydrated with fluid and salt to achieve plasma volume expansion.

Pregnancy and Kidneys

IX

Pregnancy and Kidneys

Maternal Changes in Pregnancy

• Jasmine Sethi • Manish Rathi

During pregnancy, the pregnant mother undergoes significant anatomical and physiological changes in order to nurture and accommodate the developing fetus. These changes begin after conception and affect every organ system in the body (Table 37.1).

On an average, pregnant woman gains 12 kg of weight which is equally distributed between enlarging conceptus and maternal organs. About 50–60% of weight gain is contributed by retention of water which is distributed in the fetus, placenta, amniotic

Table 37.1: Physiological changes in organ systems during pregnancy in mother	
Cardiovascular	Cardiac output increases
	Resting heart rate rises, physiological/dilutional anemia
	Fall in blood pressure
	Hypercoagulable state
Respiratory	Increased resting minute ventilation and tidal volume
	Compensated respiratory alkalosis
	Decreased functional residual capacity
Gastrointestinal	Gastrointestinal reflux increases
	Increased gall stones, hemorrhoids, fecal incontinence
Renal	Increased renal perfusion and GFR
	Hyponatremia, hypouricemia, respiratory alkalosis
	Polyuria and diabetes insipidus
	Hydronephrosis and hydroureter
Hematological	Physiological anemia
	Increased procoagulable factors—hypercoagulable state
	Increased iron and folate requirements
Musculoskeletal	Increased joint laxity
	Widening and increased mobility of sacroiliac joints
	Vaginal lengthening, exaggerated lumbar lordosis
Endocrine	Increased total T3 and T4, increased thyroxin binding globulin
	Increased ACTH, cortisol
	Insulin resistance

fluid, maternal blood, uterus and breasts. Water retention is clinically evident as edema of the ankles and legs. Almost all pregnant women develop increased skin pigmentation, most disturbing of which is melasma. Stria gravidarum develop due to connective tissue changes mostly on the abdomen, breasts and thighs. This chapter highlights the maternal changes in pregnancy that occur in every organ system with a special emphasis on changes in kidney and urinary tract. This will help the clinician to differentiate normal physiological changes from adaptations that are abnormal.

Cardiovascular and Hemodynamic Changes

Total plasma volume increases by 40–45% above nonpregnant values and the peak increase is seen at 28–34 weeks of gestation. Resting heart rate begins to increase in first trimester and returns to baseline quickly postpartum. Cardiac output increases 30–50% above the pre-pregnant state. This increase in cardiac output is accounted by increased stroke volume in early half of pregnancy and increased heart rate in later half. Systolic and diastolic blood pressures fall early in gestation due to reduction in systemic vascular resistance. The fall reaches a nadir by the end of second trimester and gradually reach pre-pregnant levels by term.

Pregnancy is associated with changes in several coagulation factors that result in physiological hypercoagulable state predisposing to venous thrombosis during pregnancy.

Respiratory Changes

Resting minute ventilation rises in pregnancy by about 50% mainly due to increase in tidal volume. Respiratory rate remains essentially unchanged. This increased minute ventilation is attributed to the direct stimulation of the central respiratory centers by progesterone. This maternal hyperventilation causes a fall arterial pCO_2 which is associated with

compensatory fall in serum bicarbonate to 18–22 mmol/L. Thus, persistent mild compensated respiratory alkalosis is present in normal pregnancy.

Gastrointestinal Changes

Gastroesophageal reflux is seen in 40–80% of women during pregnancy. This is because of decreased lower esophageal sphincter tone. Pregnancy also decreases gall bladder motility and predisposes to gallstones. Prolonged intestinal transit times and decreased gut motility predisposes to abdominal bloating and constipation.

Renal and Urinary Tract

There are profound changes in renal physiology during normal pregnancy that leads to marked alterations from non-pregnant physiological norms. These changes are summarized in Table 37.2.

Structural Changes

Increased Renal Size

Both the kidneys increase by 1–1.5 cm during pregnancy. This growth is mainly due to increased kidney vascular and interstitial volume. The nephron number remains unchanged. Overall the volume of the kidneys increases up to 30%.

Hydroureter and Hydronephrosis

The renal pelvis and calyceal system dilate due to the effect of progesterone and mechanical compression of ureters at pelvic brim. The dilated collecting system leads to urinary stasis which may lead to increased risk of pyelonephritis in pregnancy. Dilatation of ureters and renal pelvis (hydroureter and hydronephrosis) is more common on right side due to dextrorotation of the uterus and seen in up to 80% of women by the second trimester of pregnancy. In clinical practice, 24-hour urine collections may be affected by incomplete emptying of ureters, and women should be instructed to lie on their left side for

Table 37.2: Renal changes in pregnancy

Anatomical changes	Increased renal size
	Hydroureter and hydronephrosis
	Bladder wall relaxation and decreased capacity
	Ureteric smooth muscle relaxation—urinary stasis
Renal hemodynamics	Increased renal perfusion and GFR
	Decreased systolic blood pressure
	Increased renin and aldosterone
	Sodium retention
	Volume expanded state
	Increased proteinuria
Other changes	Chronic respiratory alkalosis
	Mild hyponatremia
	Hypouricemia
	Decreased serum anion gap
	Decreased serum osmolality
	Impaired tubular function (glucosuria, aminoaciduria)

an hour before emptying the bladder at the start of the collection and an hour before passing the last urine at the end of a collection period.

Bladder

The enlarging uterus displaces the bladder superiorly and anteriorly, thus decreasing bladder capacity. This may be responsible for increased urinary frequency during pregnancy.

Renal Hemodynamics

Increased Glomerular Filtration Rate

Decreased peripheral vascular resistance and increased arterial compliance lead to increased renal perfusion and glomerular filtration rate (GFR) during pregnancy. The increase in GFR is seen within one month of conception and peaks at approximately 40–50% above baseline levels by the early second trimester and then declines towards normal by term. The physiologic increase in GFR during pregnancy normally results in a decrease in concentration of serum creatinine, which falls by an average of 0.4 mg/dl to normal range of 0.4–0.8 mg/dl in normal pregnancy. Hence, a serum creatinine of 1.0 mg/dl, although normal in a non-pregnant

female, reflects renal impairment in a pregnant woman. GFR estimation based on modification of diet in renal disease (MDRD) and chronic kidney disease epidemiology collaboration (CKD-EPI) equations underestimates true GFR during pregnancy and should not be used in pregnant women. Endogenous creatinine clearance, measured by 24-hour urine collection remains the standard of care for GFR estimation in pregnancy.

Decreased Plasma Osmolality

There is altered osmoregulation in pregnancy. There is a decrease in plasma osmolality by 10 mOsm/kg below the non-pregnant state due to decrease in the plasma sodium and associated anions. In pregnancy, plasma sodium concentration decreases up to 4–5 mEq/L below the non-pregnancy levels. This has been attributed to pregnancy related vasodilatation and arterial underfilling stimulating anti-diuretic hormone (ADH) release and thirst. In non-pregnant state, fall in plasma osmolality of this magnitude will completely suppress the release of ADH. In pregnancy, osmotic thresholds for ADH release and thirst are lowered to recognize the reduced plasma osmolality as normal. This can also cause transient diabetes insipidus during pregnancy.

Renal Tubular Function in Pregnancy

Increased Urine Protein Excretion

In pregnancy, there is an increase in total urinary protein and albumin excretion, notable after 20 weeks of gestation. The protein content in urine is mostly Tamm-Horsfall, with a small amount of albumin and other circulating proteins. Abnormal proteinuria in pregnant women is defined as protein levels of 300 mg/24 hours or more, which is twice the normal limit of that in non-pregnant women.

Hypouricemia

During pregnancy, there are alterations in tubular handling of wastes and nutrients. Uric acid excretion increases due to the increases in GFR, decreases in proximal tubular reabsorption, or a combination of both. Serum uric acid levels fall in early pregnancy, reaching a nadir of 2–3 mg/dl by 22 to 24 weeks, followed by gradual rise to normal by term. The late gestational rise in serum uric acid level is attributed to increased renal tubular reabsorption of urate.

Increased Urinary Excretion

Glucosuria that occurs in pregnancy is attributed to the increased GFR and filtered glucose load that exceeds the capacity of the proximal tubule to reabsorb. There is also reduction in fractional reabsorption of amino acids. Vitamins like nicotinic acid, ascorbic acid, and folic acid are all excreted in increased amounts during pregnancy and this emphasizes the need for adequate vitamin supplementation. Calcium excretion increases 2–3 times during normal pregnancy such that supersaturation of urine occurs. However, the combined effects of increased acid glycoprotein excretion, including Tamm-Horsfall protein and nephrocalcin inhibits stone formation.

Electrolyte Balance and Anion Gap

Retention of sodium and water in the mother throughout pregnancy result in an increase of 6 to 9 L in total body water, 900 mEq of sodium. This excess water and sodium are eliminated in the process of diuresis and natriuresis which occurs postpartum. Potassium excretion decreases, and there is net potassium retention in pregnancy that is distributed equally between maternal tissues and developing fetus. For reasons that are not well understood, a small reduction in serum anion gap occurs in pregnancy.

To summarise, a proper understanding of the physiological alterations in the mother during normal pregnancy is essential to recognize understand both normal and abnormal situations and diseases in pregnancy.

Blood Pressure Changes and Hypertensive Disorders in Pregnancy

• Manisha Sahai

BLOOD PRESSURE CHANGES IN PREGNANCY

Systolic and diastolic blood pressure (BP) typically fall early in gestation and are about 5–10 mm Hg below baseline in the second trimester, declining to a mean of about 105/60 mm Hg. In the third trimester, blood pressure gradually increases and may normalize to nonpregnant values by term. The fall in BP is induced by a reduction in systemic vascular resistance (SVR). This is seen despite the increase in cardiac output in 2nd and 3rd trimesters and increase in blood volume during pregnancy. This occurs due to the decreased response to the angiotensin hormone which is seen despite an increase in renin. This insensitivity to angiotensin II is due to the effects of progesterone and vascular endothelial growth factor (VEGF) mediated prostacyclin production, as well as modifica-

tions in the angiotensin I receptors during pregnancy. VEGF is produced from placenta. Relaxin produced from corpus luteum also reduces BP.

HYPERTENSIVE DISORDERS IN PREGNANCY: CLASSIFICATION

Hypertension complicates up to 10% of pregnancies. Hypertensive disorders in pregnancy are classified differently by various guidelines (Table 38.1). The 4 important disorders are:

1. Gestational hypertension is seen in 5% and is defined as BP of 140/90 mm Hg or greater with no hypertension before pregnancy. BP returns to normal levels within 12 weeks postpartum. Patients are asymptomatic or have symptoms like pre-eclampsia. It usually affects nulliparous females after 20 weeks. Proteinuria does not occur and

Table 38.1: Classification of hypertensive disorders in pregnancy

National high BP education program (NHBPEP, 2000)	Society of Obstetricians and Gynecologists of Canada (SOGC), 2014	International society for the study of hypertension in pregnancy (ISSHP) guidelines, 2014
Gestational hypertension	Gestational hypertension	Gestational hypertension
Chronic hypertension	Pre-existing hypertension	Pre-existing hypertension
Pre-eclampsia	Pre-eclampsia	Pre-eclampsia
Pre-eclampsia superimposed on chronic hypertension	Other hypertensive disorders	Other hypertensive disorders
		White coat hypertension

serum uric acid is normal. It may progress to PE in 25% and also predicts development of hypertension later in life.

2. Chronic hypertension, seen in 2%, is defined as BP of 140/90 mm Hg or greater before pregnancy or before 20 weeks' gestation, or by persistent hypertension long after delivery. Causes include essential hypertension or hypertension secondary to renal disease, renovascular hypertension, endocrine disorders or drugs, i.e. oral contraceptive pills, steroids, NSAIDs, etc. Complications include superimposed pre-eclampsia in 25%, abruptio placentae, growth restriction and fetal death.

3. *Pre-eclampsia (PE):* Occurs in 7% of all pregnancies. Incidence is 1.5–2 times higher in first pregnancies. It was earlier defined as triad of hypertension, proteinuria and edema occurring after 20th week of gestation with few cases developing postpartum within hours. In 2013, ACOG removed proteinuria as an essential criterion for diagnosis and included end organ damage (Table 38.2). International Society for the Study of Hypertension in Pregnancy (ISSHP) defines pre-eclampsia as hypertension and proteinuria, organ dysfunction, or fetal growth restriction consistent with placental insufficiency. Risk factors for PE are described in Table 38.3. Most common symptom is swelling of feet. Abdominal pain, visual disturbances, nausea, vomiting, headache, increased reflexes, worsening edema or hypertension may indicate impending eclampsia in a pre-eclamptic female.

4. Pre-eclampsia superimposed on chronic hypertension is defined as new-onset proteinuria (i.e. >300 mg/d) after 20 weeks' gestation in a hypertensive patient or as a sudden increase in proteinuria or BP in a patient with hypertension and proteinuria before 20 weeks' gestation.

Complications of HT Disorders of Pregnancy

Hemolytic Anemia, Low Platelets and Elevated Liver Enzymes (HELLP)

Pre-eclampsia may be associated with HELLP. Occurs antepartum, peripartum or post-

---

Table 38.2: Definition of pre-eclampsia

American College of Obstetricians and Gynecologists, 2013

- Hypertension
  - Rise in systolic BP >30 mm Hg
  - Diastolic BP >15 mm Hg
  - Blood pressure of greater than or equal to 140 mm Hg (systolic) or 90 mm Hg (diastolic) on at least two measurements, ideally separated by a period of rest
- Proteinuria
  - Greater than or equal to 300 mg per 24-hour urine collection (or this amount extrapolated from a timed collection) or
  - Protein/creatinine ratio greater than or equal to 0.3 : 1
  - Dipstick reading of 1+ (used only if other quantitative methods not available)
- If no proteinuria any other evidence of end organ damage
  - Thrombocytopenia (platelet count less than 100,000/μl)
  - Liver dysfunction (elevated blood levels of liver transaminases 2 times normal)
  - Pulmonary edema
  - Renal insufficiency (elevated serum creatinine >1.1 mg/dl or a doubling of serum creatinine in absence of other renal disease)
  - New-onset cerebral disturbances
  - Visual disturbances

Pre-eclampsia is associated with intrauterine growth retardation and small for gestational age (SGA) babies

Table 38.3: Risk factors for pre-eclampsia
• Multiple pregnancies
• Chronic hypertension
• Renal disease
• Diabetes
• Autoimmune diseases
• Nulliparity
• Previous history of PE

partum in 5% of pre-eclampsia or 10–20% of severe pre-eclampsia, and maybe associated with disseminated intravascular coagulopathy (DIC), placental abruption, liver failure, subcapsular liver hematoma, retinal detachment, ARDS, ascites, pleural effusion and acute kidney injury (AKI). Perinatal mortality is seen in 6–17%.

Eclampsia

It is characterized by seizures/CNS complications after 20 weeks and is the most dangerous complication. Occurs in 0.2–0.6% of pregnancies, and in 10–20% of pre-eclampsia in developing countries (1–2% in developed countries). Cerebral damage is caused by failure of autoregulation related to endothelial damage, exacerbated by acute changes in BP. Posterior reversible leukoencephalopathy syndrome (PRES) may be seen in eclampsia due to vasogenic edema in posterior cerebral circulation. Coexistent endothelial damage in PE predisposes to CNS complication even at lower BP.

Acute Kidney Injury (AKI)

AKI is seen if there is HELLP, significant bleeding or hemodynamic instability or DIC. AKI in pregnancy is discussed in detail in Chapter 39.

Disseminated Intravascular Coagulation (DIC)

Severe preeclampsia may be associated with DIC with prolongation of PT, APTT, low clotting factors, elevated FDP and D-dimer. There is activation of coagulation cascade.

Fibrin forms crosslinked networks in small blood vessels (MAHA). The abnormalities may resolve within 2 weeks postpartum.

Pre-eclampsia maybe associated with intrauterine growth retardation, small for gestational age (SGA) babies and fetal demise.

Long-term Complications

These women are at increased risk of cardiovascular disease throughout life, and their children are likely to suffer from metabolic syndrome, cardiovascular disease, and hypertension at earlier ages.

Pathophysiology

Uteroplacental ischemia: In normal pregnancy vascular endothelial growth factor (VEGF) and placental-induced growth factor (PIGF) are synthesized by placenta. VEGF and PIGF induce synthesis of nitric oxide and prostacyclin in endothelial cells decreasing vascular tone and BP. In pre-eclampsia genetic and environmental factors result in inadequate invasion of uterine spiral arteries by placental trophoblasts. Uterine vessels do not transform from low-caliber resistive channels to a high-caliber capacitance system resulting in uteroplacental ischemia. The uteroplacental ischemia results in oxidative stress and release of soluble cytokine, sFlt-1 (soluble fms-like tyrosine kinase-1). sFlt-1 is potent antagonist of VEGF and PIGF. In PET, sFlt-1 rises in 2nd trimester with decrease in VEGF and PIGF. Increased concentration of circulating preeclamptic factors—angiotensin I and agonistic antibodies to angiotensin I receptor and soluble endoglin are seen in PE.

Diagnosis

Any pregnant woman presenting with hypertension before 20 weeks is likely to have chronic hypertension. Those presenting after 20 weeks may have gestational hypertension or PE. Presence of proteinuria and other evidence of end organ damage differentiates preeclampsia from gestational HT. Proteinuria is tested by urine dipstick or PCR, but 24-hour urine is the gold standard. Complete blood count (CBC) in pre-eclampsia shows anemia, thrombocytopenia, schistocytes, indicating microangiopathic hemolytic anemia; and abnormal renal and liver function tests and elevated uric acid (Table 38.4).

Management of Pregnancy-related Hypertension

HT in pregnancy is associated with several complications and management includes not only control of blood pressure but avoidance of complications.

Screening and Prevention for PE

All pregnant women must undergo screening for pre-eclampsia.

- *First trimester screening:* Medical history and history of previous PE is recorded. BP and urine protein are checked. Newer tests like urinary PlGF and sFlt-1 are used for early diagnosis. PIGF rises at 12 weeks while sFlt rises 5 weeks before onset of PE. The ratio of PIGF/sFlt is useful. Combining first trimester uterine artery Doppler findings with maternal characteristics (obesity, maternal history, age, number of fetuses) and serum markers may help in early diagnosis of PE. Those with early onset PET should be tested for anti-phospholipid antibody syndrome.

- *Second trimester screening:* Uterine artery Doppler at 20–22 weeks should be done in those with new-onset hypertension after 20 weeks or for those identified as high risk in first trimester. Abnormal Doppler is strongly associated with risk of pre-eclampsia and IUGR. Aspirin reduces risk of PE by 50–60% and should be initiated at 12 weeks in following situations: (i) as soon as diagnosis of PE is made or (ii) if chronic hypertension or (iii) PIH in earlier pregnancy. Controversial prevention strategies include calcium supplementation, fish oils, sodium restriction, and antioxidants.

Management of Pre-eclampsia

Patients should be evaluated for signs of severe PE (Table 38.4). If these are absent then OP management can be allowed. Women with stable BP on treatment, normal labs, normal fetus and able to understand their condition are candidates for outpatient management while those with severe pre-eclampsia are admitted.

Table 38.4: Severe pre-eclampsia (any of these findings)

- Systolic blood pressure of 160 mm Hg or higher, or diastolic blood pressure of 110 mm Hg or higher on two occasions at least 4 hours apart while the patient is on bed rest (unless antihypertensive therapy is initiated before this time)
- Thrombocytopenia (platelet count less than 100,000/microliter)
- Impaired liver function as indicated by abnormally elevated blood concentrations of liver enzymes (to twice normal concentration), severe persistent right upper quadrant or epigastric pain unresponsive to medication and not accounted for by alternative diagnoses, or both
- Progressive renal insufficiency (serum creatinine concentration greater than 1.1 mg/dl or a doubling of the serum creatinine concentration in the absence of other renal disease)
- Pulmonary edema
- New-onset cerebral or visual disturbances
- Photopsia, scotomata, cortical blindness, retinal vasospasm
- Severe headache (headache that persists and progresses despite analgesic therapy
- Altered mental status

In contrast to older criteria, the 2013 criteria do not include proteinuria >5 g/24 hours and fetal growth restriction as features of severe disease

Outpatient Management

- Patient education—all symptoms and signs of impending eclampsia (headache, abdominal pain, visual disturbances, vaginal bleeding) should be explained with instructions to report immediately to hospital in emergency.
- BP monitoring should include regular BP measurement twice a week in OP.
- Lab monitoring: Once pre-eclampsia is diagnosed based on the tests mentioned above regular lab monitoring is needed (Table 38.5).
- *Management of hypertension:* American College of Obstetricians and Gynecologists Committee (ACOG) guidelines recommend treatment above (160–170/100–110 mm Hg). The target of treatment should be to maintain BP <150/100 mmHg. BP should not be lowered <110/80. Nifedipine, methyldopa and hydralazine are used in OP patients (Table 38.6).
- *Diet and exercise:* Women with preeclampsia should be offered advice on a healthy diet and light exercise. Strict bedrest is not advisable and may be harmful.

Table 38.5: Laboratory tests if pre-eclampsia

Urine protein-dipstick, urine protein creatinine ratio 24-hour urine protein (at diagnosis)

Biochemical weekly (more frequently if needed)
- Serum creatinine, blood urea, serum electrolytes
- Serum uric acid
- Serum bilirubin
- SGOT/PT

Hematological parameters weekly
- Hemoglobin
- Peripheral smear
- Platelet count
- LDH

Fetal growth—USG assessment of fetal growth, liquor volume fortnightly if abnormal weekly

Fetal well being—nonstress test, biophysical profile (twice a week)

Umbilical artery Doppler if fetal growth restriction (weekly, more frequent if abnormal)

Kick count daily

Table 38.6: Management of hypertension

Oral (acute, severe before IV line placement)
Nifedipine
Labetalol
Methyldopa

Intravenous (acute, severe, i.e. >180/110 mm Hg)
Labetalol 200 mg can be repeated at 30 min
Hydralazine
Sodium nitroprusside if emergency

Admission

- If severe PE is suspected most guidelines recommend admission for evaluation. (ACOG, ISSHP and WHO).
- *Glucocorticoids* should be given for fetal lung maturity at the diagnosis of severe early onset preeclampsia especially if <34 weeks gestational age.
- *Thromboprophylaxis:* Patients on bedrest or with nephrotic proteinuria should receive low molecular weight heparin unless contraindicated.
- *Magnesium sulfate:* Women with severe PE or those with impending eclampsia (severe headache, clonus, neurological impairment) should be given magnesium sulfate for eclampsia prophylaxis. Mg sulphate is also given as treatment for seizures in eclampsia (Table 38.7).
- *Hypertension:* Oral nifedipine retard or a 200 mg dose of labetalol can be administered orally as first-line therapy. The latter can be repeated in 30 minutes if needed. Intravenous (IV) labetalol and hydralazine are used for management of acute-onset, severe hypertension (BP >180/110) or in eclampsia. Magnesium sulfate is not recommended as antihypertensive agent. Sodium nitroprusside should be reserved for extreme emergencies.
- *Eclampsia:* Mother should be stabilized. Seizures should be controlled with magnesium sulfate. IV labetalol is used for management of hypertension. Once stabilized, early delivery is planned either vaginally or cesarean.

Table 38.7: Indications of magnesium sulfate

- Women with severe PE
- Those with impending eclampsia (severe headache, clonus, neurological impairment) for eclampsia prophylaxis
  - 4 g loading dose with a maintenance infusion of 1 g/h with close monitoring, observation of urine output, respiratory rate, and deep tendon reflexes
- Those with eclampsia/seizures should be controlled with magnesium sulfate
  - If already given another bolus is given with increase of infusion rate to 2 g/hour

Indications for Delivery

- At any gestation, delivery is indicated for life-threatening maternal disease, severe refractory hypertension, eclampsia, placental abruption or rapidly deteriorating HELLP syndrome, DIC, pulmonary edema or renal dysfunction. Otherwise expectant treatment with close monitoring is done.
- 34–36 weeks after the age of viability, delivery may be indicated for serious fetal compromise (abnormal biophysical profile, non-reactive non-stress test and oligohydramnios, reversed diastolic flow).
- After 37 weeks, in any woman with gestational hypertension or mild to moderate disease, delivery is preferred.

Management during Delivery

All women with hypertensive disorders in pregnancy should have continuous fetal monitoring in labor. BP should be measured hourly in labor, and antihypertensive medication continued. In women with severe preeclampsia, more frequent BP measurement is required even invasive monitoring is recommended, particularly if intravenous antihypertensive therapy is required. A maintenance infusion of a balanced salt or isotonic saline solution at about 80 ml/hour is often adequate for a patient who is nil by mouth and has no ongoing abnormal fluid losses, such as bleeding. Platelet transfusion should not be used to normalize the platelet count in non-bleeding patients, as long as the platelet count is above 10,000 to 20,000/μl. However, platelets should not be withheld from a patient with potentially life-threatening bleeding.

Post-delivery and long-term management: BP settles by 1st week, sometimes may take as long as 6 weeks. Beyond that other causes of BP should be considered. Some patients may have postpartum PE which is diagnosed if HT develops post-delivery and this should be managed like antepartum PE. Women should be monitored for CKD and cardiovascular morbidity in later life.

Conclusion

Hypertensive disorders are common problems in pregnancy. Most common disorder after 20 weeks gestation is preeclampsia. Early identification and management helps in reducing short-term and long-term fetal and maternal morbidity and mortality.

Renal Disease and Pregnancy

• Manisha Sahay

INTRODUCTION

Pregnancy may be associated with acute kidney injury (PRAKI) or may worsen underlying renal disease.

ACUTE KIDNEY INJURY IN PREGNANCY

In developed countries only 1 in 20,000 pregnant women develop severe AKI. However, in India, the incidence of PRAKI is reported to be 10–20%.

Causes of PRAKI are listed in Table 39.1.

Etiology—PRAKI

Septic abortion: Common with illegal abortions performed by quacks. Commonest causative organism is Clostridium. It manifests few hours to 1–2 days after abortion with fever, vomiting, occasionally jaundice, pain abdomen and ashen grey skin. Progression to shock and death is rapid. Anemia, leukocytosis, thrombocytopenia and DIC may be seen. Septic abortions have decreased after legalization of abortions.

Hyperemesis gravidarum is characterized by severe vomitings, volume loss and rarely acute kidney injury.

Pre-eclampsia (PE)

Pre-eclampsia is discussed in the chapter on hypertension. In most women with pre-

Table 39.1: Causes of PRAKI

Causes in early pregnancy
a. Sepsis
b. Hyperemesis gravidarum

Causes in late pregnancy
a. PE and complications
b. HELLP syndrome
c. Disseminated intravascular coagulation (DIC)
d. Abruptio placentae
e. Eclampsia
f. Amniotic fluid embolism
g. Thrombotic microangiopathy (TMA)
h. Hemolytic uremic syndrome

Other causes (same as in pregnant females)
a. Thrombotic thrombocytopenic purpura (TTP)
b. Acute fatty liver of pregnancy (AFLP)
c. Volume loss
d. Antepartum hemorrhage (APH)
e. Postpartum hemorrhage (PPH)
f. Puerperal sepsis.

Other causes (same as in nonpregnant females)
a. Nephrotoxic drug intake
b. Stones and obstruction
c. Volume depletion due to diarrhea
d. Infections
e. Acute pyelonephritis
f. Bacterial, viral, fungal or parasitic
g. Malaria, dengue, leptospirosis
h. Spider, snake and scorpion bites

eclampsia, the glomerular filtration rate (GFR) decreases by 30–40%, which results in only minor increases in serum creatinine. AKI requiring renal replacement therapy (RRT) is uncommon except in patients with severe preeclampsia or its complications or when there is accompanying hemorrhage and ischemic ATN. The incidence of AKI in preeclampsia with hemolysis, elevated liver enzymes and low platelets (HELLP) is 15%, and AKI in abruption, disseminated intravascular coagulation (DIC) and ecclampsia may be 30%. AKI begins to resolve spontaneously within two to three days postpartum, and complete recovery occurs within 8 weeks. Some cases may be fatal. Renal histology shows glomerular endotheliosis. Moderately increased albuminuria (30–300 mg/day) may persist. Women who develop preeclampsia may be at increased risk of developing end-stage renal disease (ESRD) later in life, but absolute risk is small.

Thrombotic Microangiopathy (TMA)

TMA is an important cause of PRAKI. TMA is characterized by microangiopathy, i.e. abnormality of microcirculation with resultant hemolysis due to passage of RBC through constricted blood vessels leading to hemolytic anemia (MAHA) and thrombocytopenia. Hemolysis is identified by presence of schistocytes on peripheral smear and increased serum LDH >600 units/L, increased reticulocyte count, low haptoglobin and high unconjugated bilirubin. Liver enzymes are normal. TMA differs from disseminated intravascular coagulation (DIC) as coagulation parameters are normal in TMA. TMA includes hemolytic uremic syndrome (HUS) and thrombotic thrombocytopenic purpura (TTP).

HUS occurs commonly in primipara and is characterized by AKI, MAHA and severe HT. Symptoms can begin before delivery, but onset is usually delayed for 48 hours or more after delivery (mean four weeks). HUS may follow a normal pregnancy or be preceded by

findings indistinguishable from pre-eclampsia. The cause is obscure and viral illness, retained placental fragments, drugs, e.g. oxytocics, ergot and oral contraceptives have been implicated. Recently it has been determined that HUS maybe due to inherited defects in regulation of complement system. Complement proteins play an important role in defense against infections and inflammation and are regulated by proteins like factor H, factor I, monocyte chemoattractant protein (MCP), factor B, etc. Defects in complement regulatory proteins lead to overactivity of complement and formation of membrane attack complexes which damage endothelium. This microvascular damage is responsible for microangiopathy and hemolytic anemia. Renal biopsy shows mesangiolysis, glomerular simplification and thrombi in glomeruli and vascular changes. There may be hypocomplementemia, deficiency in prostaglandin (PG) or antithrombin levels. Outcome is poor with high maternal mortality (18–44%) and fetal loss (80%). 45% progress to CKD. Recurrence in subsequent pregnancies is low. HUS needs to be differentiated from preeclampsia. History of preceding proteinuria and hypertension favor pre-eclampsia); absence of DIC, onset more than two days after delivery, and/or persistent disease for >1 week favor HUS. Treatment includes plasmapheresis, and plasma infusion.

TTP was earlier described as pentad of MAHA, thrombocytopenia, AKI, fever, and neurologic abnormalities. Currently it is defined as TMA associated with ADAMTS-13 deficiency. This protease enzyme cleaves von Willebrand factor (vWF) which prevents formation of platelet thrombi. Deficiency leads to platelet thrombi and thrombocytopenia. AKI is often mild. TTP almost always occurs antepartum, many cases begin before 24 weeks but the disease also occurs in third trimester. Diagnosis is by demonstrating the reduced levels or activity of ADAMTS-13 enzyme. However, the test is not freely available. TTP is an uncommon cause of renal failure in pregnancy.

Acute Fatty Liver of Pregnancy

AFLP is a rare complication of pregnancy that is associated with AKI in 60%. It is due to mutation in enzyme for long chain 3-hydroxy-acyl-CoA dehydrogenase. It is characterized by jaundice, mild AKI in last trimester, DIC, pancreatitis and encephalopathy. The diagnosis should be suspected in a woman with preeclampsia who has hypoglycemia, hypofibrinogenemia, and a prolonged PTT (in the absence of abruptio placentae), high bilirubin, normal/high transaminases, microvesicular steatosis and rarely liver necrosis. Renal biopsy shows acute tubular necrosis (ATN). Treatment includes IV fluids, treatment of DIC, i.e. cryoprecipitate, fresh frozen plasma, and correction of hypoglycemia. AFLP reverses with delivery. C section is preferred. Liver transplant is the treatment of choice in patients with liver necrosis. 20–25% maternal and fetal mortality is seen, 25% recur.

Antepartum and Postpartum Hemorrhage

APH/PPH leads to volume loss and decrease in blood supply to kidneys leading to AKI. If the insult is mild and transient, kidneys recover completely. However, prolonged and significant hypotension may lead to ATN and cortical necrosis. The latter is irreversible and contributes to permanent kidney failure.

Puerperal Sepsis (PS)

PS is any bacterial infection of female reproductive tract following abortion or delivery. Signs and symptoms include fever > 38.0°C, chills, lower abdominal pain, and foul-smelling vaginal discharge. It usually occurs after first 24 hours to first ten days following delivery. Risk factors include cesarean section, presence of bacteria such as group B streptococcus in vagina, premature rupture of membranes, multiple vaginal exams, manual removal of placenta, and prolonged labor. Origin of sepsis is generally from female genital tract. Mastitis and urinary tract infections also may serve as source for sepsis. Severe sepsis is characterized by hypotension and DIC and multiorgan failure. High vaginal swabs, urine and blood cultures should be sent. Patient needs treatment with appropriate antibiotics. IV fluids, dobutamine, norepinephrine and vasopressin may be needed for maintaining blood pressure. Any septic focus including retained products of conception need to be evacuated. Puerperal sepsis has a poor prognosis.

Amniotic Fluid Embolism

AFE is a life-threatening obstetric emergency. AFE occurs in 2–8/100,000 deliveries and causes 10% maternal mortality. In AFE, amniotic fluid, fetal cells, hair, or other debris enters mother's bloodstream via placental bed of uterus and triggers an allergic-like reaction. This results in cardiorespiratory collapse, DIC and AKI. Use of drugs to induce labor, such as misoprostol, doubles the risk of AFE. Maternal age >35 years, cesarean or instrumental vaginal delivery, polyhydramnios, cervical laceration or uterine rupture, placenta previa or abruption, eclampsia, and fetal distress are also associated with increased risk. There is no specific treatment, and initial emergency management consists of cardiovascular and respiratory resuscitation and correction of the coagulopathy.

Acute Pyelonephritis

Urinary tract infections (UTIs) are common and range from asymptomatic bacteriuria to pyelonephritis. UTIs are associated with small for gestational age (SGA) babies, premature labor, intrauterine fetal death (IUD) and anemia and hypertension in mother. Pregnant females are at risk for development of UTIs (2–10%), because of anatomic and physiologic changes that occur in normal pregnancy. Asymptomatic bacteriuria (AB) (>100,000 organisms/ml in urine culture) is common in pregnancy. 30% develop pyelonephritis especially in 2nd trimester if asymptomatic bacteriuria is left untreated. Onset is abrupt with fever, chills, flank pain, anorexia, nausea, vomiting and costovertebral tenderness. Etiologic organisms include *Escherichia coli*, Klebsiella, Enterobacter, Proteus and gram-positive organisms. 15% patients have concurrent bacteremia. Other complications include hemolysis, sepsis, adult respiratory distress syndrome, hepatic dysfunction and death. Some pregnant women develop AKI. Renal biopsy may reveal focal microabscesses and recovery after antimicrobial therapy may be incomplete due to irreversible injury.

Universal screening for AB is recommended. Dipstick has a sensitivity of <50% and routine microscopy and culture are needed. Treatment with a 10-day course of oral antibiotics (nitro-furantoin, ampicillin, amoxicillin, sulfonamides, cephalexin or co-amoxiclav) reduces incidence of pyelonephritis. Urinalysis with culture should be performed on a monthly basis after resolution. Recurrence occurs in 35%. If bacteriuria is persistent, suppressive therapy (nitrofurantoin 100 mg, cephalexin or amoxicillin) is indicated till term.

Pyelonephritis requires hospitalization and fluids. Effective IV antibiotics include ampicillin plus gentamicin or a third-generation cephalosporin followed by oral administration (14 days).

Urinary Tract Obstruction

Functional hydronephrosis rarely cause renal failure. Renal functions are normal in the lateral recumbent position and oliguria occurs when patient is supine. In some cases, either insertion of a ureteral catheter or delivery of fetus is required. Rarely, acute urinary tract obstruction in pregnancy may result from renal calculus and may need stenting.

Lab Diagnosis of AKI

Tests are enumerated in Table 39.2. Renal biopsy is done if there is no recovery of

Table 39.2: Laboratory evaluation in PRAKI

a. Urine examination
b. Urine culture
c. Complete blood picture (anemia, schistocytes, thrombocytopenia)
d. Serum creatinine, blood urea, electrolytes
e. ABG
f. Blood cultures
g. LFT
h. Uric acid
i. Ultrasound of kidneys
j. Renal biopsy

Table 39.3: Renal histology in PRAKI

Renal biopsy
a. Acute tubular necrosis (ATN)
b. Cortical necrosis—diffuse or patchy
c. Thrombotic microangiopathy
d. Interstitial nephritis
e. Glomerular endotheliosis in PE

renal function in 1–2 weeks or if cause of renal failure is unknown. Renal histology may be varied (Table 39.3).

Renal cortical necrosis (RCN): It is a pathological abnormality seen in severe cases of PRAKI. Causes include abruptio, septic abortion, placenta previa, prolonged IUD or amniotic fluid embolism which may cause significant endothelial damage with formation of fibrin thrombi and impaired NO release which causes impaired circulation. It may be patchy or total. Patients develop abrupt onset of oligoanuria, gross hematuria, flank pain and hypotension. The triad of oliguria/anuria, gross hematuria, and flank pain in pregnancy is characteristic. Renal calcifications on plain film abdomen (6 weeks) or hypoechoic areas in renal cortex or cortical tram track calcification on CT films (3 weeks) may be seen. Angiography shows abrupt cut off of vascularity. No specific therapy is effective. Many patients develop chronic kidney disease.

Management of AKI in Pregnancy

The cause of AKI should be treated. Septic abortion should be treated with antibiotics, volume resuscitation, hyperbaric oxygen, antitoxin and exchange transfusion. Hysterectomy is rarely indicated as a lifesaving procedure.

Hyperemesis gravidarum is treated by volume replacement and antiemetics.

Pre-eclampsia requires BP control (*refer* to Chapter 38).

HUS or TTP may need plasmapheresis or plasma infusions. Platelet transfusions should be avoided. Heparin and fibrinolytic agents and antithrombin III concentrates may be used. Dilatation and curettage should be considered when TMA occurs close to delivery. Newer drugs such as eculizumab have been recommended for treatment in complement regulator deficiencies.

APH and PPH need volume and blood replacement apart from therapy to stop bleeding.

Therapy of AKI includes four "D" therapy: **D**ialysis, **d**iet, **d**yselectrolytemia correction and **d**elivery.

If the fetus is viable and period of gestation is >34 weeks pregnancy can be terminated. If the fetal lung maturity is uncertain the pregnancy can be continued and dialysis can be done for renal failure if there is no threat to maternal well-being. Antenatal steroids may be used to hasten fetal lung maturity.

Pregnancy in Patients with Underlying Renal Disease

Obstetricians may get to see ladies with high creatinine (chronic kidney disease) or proteinuria in their practice. All such patients including those who plan to conceive should be referred for nephrology opinion.

Pregnancy in Nephrotic Syndrome (NS)

Nephrotic syndrome worsens in pregnancy in about 50% with increasing proteinuria and edema. NS is associated with thrombo-embolism, IUGR, preterm labor and poor long-term maternal and renal prognosis. Some patients with nephrotic syndrome with massive proteinuria may need biopsy and this can be done safely till 32 weeks otherwise biopsy is deferred till delivery. These patients may need low molecular weight heparin prophylaxis till 6 weeks postpartum. Diuretics are avoided as these can cause intravascular volume depletion. Steroids may be used in severe cases.

Pregnancy and Systemic Lupus Erythematosus (SLE)

Lupus nephritis may affect fetal and maternal outcomes. Fetal loss occurs in 50%. Fetal complications include abortion, intrauterine growth retardation, low birth weight, small for gestational age and preterm delivery. Anemia, thrombocytopenia, infections and flares and deterioration of renal function are more common in mother. Pregnancy should be planned in lupus only when dsDNA has remained negative for 6 months. If the patient is on renin-angiotensin system blocker, it should be withdrawn before conception. The treatment for LN during pregnancy should be modified. Steroids and hydroxychloroquine (HCQ) should be continued during pregnancy in all patients with SLE. MMF should be substituted by azathioprine about 6 weeks prior to conception. If treatment regimen consists of tacrolimus or cyclosporine, it may be continued. Cyclophosphamide is avoided because it is teratogenic. Rituximab should also be avoided. When flares occur, the dose of prednisone is increased. Therapeutic abortion is recommended if a lupus flare is associated with worsening renal function or worsening hypertension prior to 34 weeks' gestation. Induction of labor is recommended after 34 weeks' gestation if fetal maturity is satisfactory. Fetal survival rates are good (95%).

APLA, i.e. lupus anticoagulant (LA), IgG/IgM-anticardiolipin (aCL) antibodies, IgG/

IgM-anti-β_2-glycoprotein (GP) I antibodies, Ro/La antibodies should be tested pre-pregnancy and repeated periodically during pregnancy. APLA leads to thrombosis and pregnancy losses. Ro and La are associated with congenital heart block in baby. If APLA is positive, anticoagulation with heparin (LMW or conventional) and aspirin should be given throughout pregnancy. HCQ reduces APLA titres. Serial assessment with fetal Doppler echocardiography from 16 to 28 weeks of gestation is recommended. If fetal bradycardia is noted, β-agonists are administered to the mother. Fetal pacing can be considered if facilities exist.

Pregnancy in Chronic Kidney Disease (CKD)

Current consensus suggests degree of renal insufficiency, proteinuria and hypertension rather than underlying renal diagnosis are the primary determinants of outcome (Table 39.4). Pre-eclampsia (PE) in CKD is characterized by worsening of hypertension and proteinuria. Although it generally occurs in third trimester, women with underlying renal disease are at greater risk for second trimester PE. In fact, second trimester PE is considered a pointer to pre-existing renal disease.

Pregnancy in Patients on Chronic Dialysis

Those patients who have CKD stage 5 (GFR <15 ml/min) often need lifelong dialysis for survival. Pregnancy occurs only in 1% per year in such patients and even if conception occurs, it may end up in abortions, small for gestational age (SGA), intrauterine growth retardation, PE, preterm labor, fetal death and maternal complications. More frequent and prolonged dialysis to keep BUN levels less than 50 mg/dl may decreases morbidity and mortality. Dialysis prescription should be for a minimum 20 hours per week instead of standard 12 hours. Peritoneal dialysis can be done till 2nd trimester, hemodialysis is safe even in 3rd trimester.

Pregnancy in Patients after Transplantation

Fertility rates increase 6 months after successful transplantation. An elevated pre-pregnancy creatinine (>1.4 mg/dl), proteinuria and uncontrolled hypertension are associated with a higher risk of decline of maternal renal function and decreased fetal survival. Patients should wait at least 1 year after living related donor transplant and 2 years after a cadaveric transplant before planning pregnancy. The renal function should be stable (serum

Table 39.4: Treatment strategies and outcomes in pregnancies complicated by CKD		
Stage of CKD	*Outcomes*	*Decision*
Mild CKD Creatinine <1.5 mg/dl No proteinuria Normal BP	Normal maternal and fetal outcome	Pregnancy continued
Moderate CKD Cr 1.5–2.5 mg/dl Proteinuria Hypertension	Live births—90% 50% IUGR Preterm labor Decline in renal function PE 50% progress to ESRD	Counselled against pregnancy Contraception may include barrier methods or progesterone-only pills IUDs are associated with higher infection rate
Severe CKD Serum creatinine >2.5 mg/dl Nephrotic proteinuria	High maternal and fetal mortality	Strictly counseled to avoid pregnancy

creatinine <2.0 mg/dl) and they should be on minimal stable immunosuppression, i.e. prednisone 10 mg/d, azathioprine 2 mg/kg/d, cyclosporine 5 mg/kg/d or tacrolimus 0.08 mg/kg/day. If the condition of the recipient is stable, without any episode of rejection, well maintained renal function and blood pressure, pregnancy may be considered. About 12% of such women conceive. 20% pregnancies may end in spontaneous abortions whereas, if the pregnancy crosses the 1st trimester, the successful outcome may be 90%. Pregnancy does not increase risk for rejection. Mycophenolate mofetil has potentially teratogenic effects and should be changed to azathioprine. Although azathioprine crosses the placenta, the immature fetal liver cannot convert it to its active form, 6-mercaptopurine hence fetal toxicity does not occur. Acute rejection may occur and high-dose steroids and antithymocyte globulin (ATG) may be used for treatment. Patients should receive antibiotic prophylaxis before all surgical procedures. UTI in pregnancy warrants long-term prophylaxis. Obstruction of transplant ureter by pregnant uterus is rare. Neonatal outcome is good except a higher rate of preterm birth (50%), SGA (30%), and neonatal mortality (3%) *vs* general population (12.3, 5, 0.68%, respectively). Long-term outcome of surviving infants is good.

Monitoring of pregnant patients in CKD and transplant is given in Table 39.5.

Table 39.5: Monitoring during pregnancy in CKD and transplant

Prenatal visits every 2 weeks until 28 weeks' gestation and then weekly

BP daily

Lab work
- Urine protein by dipstick (24-hr protein if dipstick abnormal)
- Monthly CBC
- Monthly RFT (electrolytes, BUN, creatinine)
- Monthly ultrasounds
- Monthly urine cultures
- Screening for CMV—IgM, IgM for HSV in transplant
- Biweekly fetal surveillance with a biophysical profile in 3rd trimester

Obstetric management: The most common cause of morbidity and mortality in patients with any renal disease is preterm labor. Elective early delivery can be performed at 34–36 weeks in CKD or dialysis, when fetal lung maturity is achieved. In stable transplant recipients, delaying delivery until the onset of labor is prudent. Vaginal delivery is preferred. Steroids dose is increased peripartum.

Conclusion

Pregnancy may be associated with risk of AKI. Prompt diagnosis and management results in good outcomes. Patients with underlying kidney disease may become pregnant. Adequate monitoring, control of hypertension and timely delivery results in a successful maternal and fetal outcome.

Approach to
Common Renal Problems

Approach to an Edematous Patient

• Satish Balan

INTRODUCTION

Edema can be due to a number of causes but a careful analysis will lead us to the diagnosis in almost all cases. One of the most common manifestations of renal diseases is edema. It is defined as swelling due to accumulation of fluid in any part of the body. Edema can be localized or systemic. In the former, the edema is due to local causes such as cellulitis, lymphangitis, lymphedema or other causes which are beyond the scope of this discussion. Thus, we shall discuss the various causes of generalized edema due to systemic causes. Fluid in the body exists in two compartments, the intracellular and extracellular fluid compartments. Edema always implies an increase in the extracellular fluid compartment.

Why Does Edema Occur?

Edema occurs due to excessive fluid exudation from the capillaries in the peripheries wherever there is loose interstitium. Thus, there should be an imbalance in the Starling forces in the peripheral tissues which cause the edema to form. As we are aware, the Starling forces which keep the fluid from exuding are a combination of the hydrostatic and oncotic pressures in the vascular tree against the same forces in the extravascular tissue. The following values summarize the Starling forces in the capillaries (Table 40.1).

From the above table we can see that at the arterial end of the capillary, the net driving force is to move the fluid from intravascular to interstitial space and at the venous end of the capillary, the reverse happens. Thus, under normal circumstances, no edema can form. In order for edema to occur either the capillary hydrostatic pressure (Pc) must be high (as occurs in cardiac failure) or the capillary oncotic pressure (πc) must be low (as occurs in hypoproteinemic states such as nephrotic syndrome). The other factor driving edema when there is a failure of the Starling forces as

Table 40.1: Starling forces in the capillaries		
In mm Hg	*Arteriolar end of capillary*	*Venous end of capillary*
Capillary hydrostatic pressure **(Pc)**	25	15
Capillary oncotic pressure **(πc)**	25	25
Interstitial hydrostatic pressure **(Pi)**	−6	−6
Interstitial oncotic pressure **(πi)**	5	5

The equation for the net driving pressure across the capillary is (Pc − πc) − (Pi − πi)

Table 40.2: Causes of edema

Allergic reactions and angioedema	Due to increased capillary permeability
Cardiac diseases	Increased systemic venous pressure and fluid overload (increased Pc)
Chronic liver disease	Decreased oncotic pressure and increased systemic venous pressure (decreased πc)
Malabsorption—protein calorie malnutrition	Decreased oncotic pressure due to reduced protein synthesis and protein losses (decreased πc)
Renal disease	Fluid overload or decreased plasma oncotic pressure due to protein losses (both mechanisms may be seen in different diseases)
Obstructive sleep apnea	Pulmonary hypertension leading to cardiac failure (increase Pc)
Hypothyroidism	Non-pitting edema is characteristic
Pregnancy	Increased plasma volume and increased venous pressure due to the gravid uterus pressing on the great veins
Idiopathic edema	Occurs in middle-aged women and the cause is not known
Drug-induced—calcium channel blockers	Due to venodilatation and reduced Pc on the venous side
Drug-induced edema—NSAIDs	Due to increased fluid retention by the kidneys (increased Pc)

occurs when the capillaries become inflamed, permeable and leaky leading to fluid losses. From the above equation it is easy to understand the various causes of edema as summarized in Table 40.2.

CLINICAL FEATURES OF EDEMA

History

A careful history will be the first point of evaluation in the edematous patient. A history of jaundice and prominent ascites suggests hepatic edema. Edema presenting periorbitally is more suggestive of nephrotic syndrome but may also be a feature of chronic liver disease. Edema associated with breathlessness and inability to lie flat is suggestive of cardiac edema or fluid overload and edema or renal failure. A history of thyroid disease and of obstructive sleep apnea symptoms is also important. Drug intake especially of calcium channel blockers and of NSAIDs strongly suggests drug-induced edema.

Clinical Examination

The clinical examination should firstly involve a careful search for edema. Edema fluid gravitates to the dependent parts of the body.

Commonly dependent edema occurs in the legs or feet. In recumbent patients it can be present only in the sacral area. In these days of very successful intensive care treatment, edema can be seen at the elbow region in the ICU patient who is nursed in the semi-recumbent position. Periorbital puffiness particularly on rising from sleep which subsides after a few hours is characteristic of edema of nephrotic syndrome. Evaluation of the jugular venous pressure, auscultation of the chest for basal crepitations is essential in all patients. A grossly edematous patient is said to have anasarca which includes ascites and pleural effusions.

Pitting is a characteristic sign in edema when mild finger pressure over the edematous area leaves an indentation that remains for some time. Pitting should be examined against a bony surface, e.g. over the tibia, medial malleolus, the dorsum of foot or the sacrum. Raised skin temperature or tenderness suggests infection or cellulitis or deep vein thrombosis.

In long-standing edema, the skin may become hardened and sclerotic leading to a thickened, woody feel. Lymphedema is due to progressive accumulation of lymph and though the edema may be pitting in the early stages, later on the skin becomes fibrotic and thickened and the edema is non-pitting. In chronic lymphedema the skin may have a 'verrucous' appearance which was commonly referred to picturesquely as elephantiasis. peau d' orange or orange peel appearance is also seen in chronic lymphedema.

Presence of asterixis, clubbing, jaundice and spider nevi suggest liver disease. Goitre may suggest thyroid disease, though often, thyroid disease may present with edema without goitre.

Diagnosis of Edema

A careful history and clinical examination can help us reach a diagnosis in a large number of cases. However, some investigations are mandatory in all patients. The investigations which can help use reach the diagnosis are noted below:

1. Urinalysis—for significant proteinuria
2. Evaluation of serum urea and creatinine— for abnormal renal function leading to edema.
3. Liver function tests and prothrombin time—for hepatic diseases.
4. ECG, chest X-ray and echocardiogram—for evaluating cardiovascular system.
5. Brain natriuretic peptide estimation—a more specific test and is raised in cardiac failure. (The test is expensive and usually is used only when there is a need to differentiate pulmonary edema from infection.) Good clinical examination in most cases will make such investigations unnecessary.
6. Thyroid function tests in all cases to evaluate for hypothyroidism.
7. Sleep study in an obese patient with daytime somnolence.
8. Ultrasound of the abdomen can be useful to identify chronic liver disease or kidney disease.

Treatment

The objectives of treatment are to reduce the edema as well as to treat the underlying disease which is causing the edema. Since edema implies an increase in total ECF volume, the primary aims should be to limit salt and water intake so that the patient is able to achieve a negative balance as far as fluids are considered. In most cases of edema, restriction of salt and water alone may not be sufficient to control edema. In such circumstances, diuretics are used. All diuretics act by increasing salt and water excretion by the kidneys.

Diuretics

Diuretics belong to five different groups (Table 40.3):

1. *Osmotic diuretics and proximal tubular diuretics:* These act on the proximal tubule and decrease total reabsorption of solutes as a result of their osmotic activity (e.g. mannitol). Another example of a diuretic acting on the proximal tubule is acetazolamide which acts by blocking bicarbonate reabsorption and leading to salt and water loss. However, both these diuretics are weak and cannot be used for their diuretic properties in patients with edema.
2. *Loop diuretics:* These diuretics act on the loop of Henle specifically inhibiting sodium transport in this segment of the nephron. The loop of Henle is responsible for generating an osmotic gradient in the medulla. The resulting high medullary osmolarity leads to passive reabsorption of water if water channels are active in the medullary collecting duct. Thus, blocking the transporter in the loop of Henle will lead to excretion of salt and water. Because of the relatively high water loss with these drugs, hyponatremia seldom occurs. These are some of the most powerful diuretics in use today. These drugs are effective even if the GFR is low and thus can be used even when the renal function is poor.

Table 40.3: Some properties of the 5 common groups of diuretics

Class and name	Maximal dose	Length of action
1. Osmotic diuretics, e.g. mannitol	Not used for edema	NA
2. Proximal tubular diuretics Acetazolamide	Not used for edema	NA
3. Loop diuretics		
Furosemide	80–240 mg orally max depending on condition Up to 500 mg IV per day	Lasts 6 hours; slightly more orally since absorption can be delayed
Bumetanide	2–10 mg depending on the condition	4–6 hours
Torsemide	10–100 mg depending on condition	6–8 hours
4. Distal tubular diuretics		
Hydrochlorothiazide	Max 100 mg per day in 2 divided doses	6–12 hours
Metolazone	Up to 20 mg per day	>24 hours
Chlorthalidone	Max 200 mg per day	24–48 hours
5. Potassium sparing diuretics		
Spironolactone (aldosterone antagonist)	Max 200 mg per day	2–3 days
Eplerenone (aldosterone antagonist)	Max 100 mg in 2 divided doses	6 horus
Amiloride (sodium channel blocker)	30 mg twice daily max	24 hours
Triamterene (sodium channel blocker)	300 mg daily max	7–9 hours

3. *Thiazide and thiazide-like diuretics:* These act on the distal convoluted tubule. The thiazide sensitive channels in the DCT are responsible for reabsorbing around 5% of sodium that escapes the loop of Henle. This is still a large quantity of sodium in absolute terms, so these drugs can cause significant diuresis. They are not effective when the renal function is low and so cannot be used in renal failure. The thiazide group of diuretics result in more sodium loss compared to water loss and are called 'saliuretics'. Both loop diuretics and thiazide group of diuretics lead to electrolyte abnormalities, predominantly hypokalemia. Hyponatremia can also occur, though more common with thiazides than with loop diuretics.

4. Potassium sparing diuretics act on the sodium channel in the collecting duct segments of the nephron. By blocking the sodium channel, sodium is not reabsorbed in these segments and so gets excreted. As sodium channels are required for potassium secretion here, potassium is not lost in the urine. Thus, these are known as potassium sparing diuretics, and therefore the important side effect is hyperkalemia.

Clinical use of Diuretics

Use of diuretic must be tailored to the requirements of the condition and the extent of edema. Typically lower doses are used in the edema of cirrhosis of liver and nephrotic syndrome. Higher doses are needed with worsening severity of cardiac failure but the highest doses are needed in patients with stage 4 or 5 of chronic kidney disease. When diuretics are used, one should have a treatment goal in mind, which is usually a target weight to be achieved. This is especially important in the case of loop diuretics since one can easily cause excess diuresis resulting in volume depletion and hypotension. A close follow-up is needed at least initially to assess the response and to titrate the dosing.

The type of diuretic chosen depends on the condition. The most important use of the aldosterone antagonist spironolactone or eplerenone is in heart failure but here it is usually combined with other diuretics for better efficacy. These drugs are also useful in cirrhosis and nephrotic syndrome as they are effective. The main drawback is that these drugs take several days for their action to begin so in the initial period, some other diuretics are needed to control the edema. Thiazide and thiazide-like agents are used usually in the management of hypertension. However, in the management of edema, they are used mainly in addition to loop diuretics for management of edema in renal and cardiac disease.

A combination of thiazide and sodium channel blocker like amiloride or triamterene can be used in milder edema since the effect on potassium would be neutral. The loop diuretics are usually the drugs of choice in the management of edema. The dosage can be titrated to effectively control edema up to maximum doses as stated in Table 40.3.

In all cases where diuretics are used, the treatment of the clinical condition should also proceed simultaneously since control of the primary lesion will lead to resolution of edema in the long-term and reduce the need for diuretics.

Other Measures to Control Edema

In addition to diuretics and salt and fluid excretion, edema can be controlled in some situations in nephrotic syndrome and in cirrhosis by administration of salt-poor albumin along with a loop diuretic. However, the use of albumin should be done only in consultation with an expert. Lastly, refractory edema can respond to dialysis or ultrafiltration.

Conclusion

Edema is a symptom which prompts us to think of diseases of the heart, kidney, liver or endocrine system. The importance of edema is that it can be life-threatening but there are some general unifying principles in management as stressed above. Management of edema should go hand in hand with diagnosis of the cause and treatment of the primary ailment which alone can lead to long-term resolution of the edema.

Approach to Proteinuria

• Umesh Sharma

In health, the normal urinary protein excretion is <150 mg/24 hours. About 50–60% of the normally excreted urinary proteins are low molecular weight tubular mucoproteins called Tamm-Horsfall protein. The other proteins excreted in urine include some blood group-related proteins, immunoglobulins (usually IgA), 2 microglobulin, apoproteins, urokinase, and very small amounts of enzymes and peptide hormones. The daily urinary excretion of albumin will be less than 30 mg. Proteinuria more than 150 mg/day can occur in various forms and varying severity. It can be classified as tubular, glomerular and overflow proteinuria depending on the source of excreted proteins. It may be transient or persistent. Dipstick test is used for the evaluation of proteinuria. Dipstick is used for detection in semiquantitative terms the presence of proteins or albumin. Urinary proteins include predominantly albumin and a small amount of globulins. Dipsticks are sensitive to albumin but fail to pick up globulins and smaller amounts of other proteins mentioned above. The reading is reported as nil, trace, 1+ (30 mg/L), 2+ (100 mg/L), 3+ (300 mg/L) and 4+ (2000 mg/L). False-positive results are obtained if the urine is very concentrated or contaminated with blood, or if the pH of urine is >7.0 and false-negative tests if the urine is very dilute. Urine examination by dipstix cannot detect Bence Jones protein in urine, whereas conventional heat coagulation acetic acid test can detect the same.

Quantitation of proteinuria can be done on a spot urine sample by measurement of albumin to creatinine ratio (ACR) expressed as mg (albumin)/gm of creatinine. This helps assess 24-hour urinary albumin excretion rate (AER). A more precise AER can be measured by a timed collection of a 24-hour urinary sample, and is expressed as mg/24 hours.

Definitions

Glomerular proteinuria: When the glomerulus is the source of proteins excreted in the urine, the condition is called glomerular proteinuria. It is usually associated with pathological damage to the glomerulus. When the damage is milder, predominantly loss of albumin occurs. If the damage is more severe, other proteins also are excreted in the urine. Glomerular proteinuria is classified as per the albumin excretion rate (AER) and is termed "significant" if AER is >500 mg, 'non-nephrotic' when AER is <3.5 gm/24 hours and 'nephrotic' if AER of >3.5 gm/1.73 m^2 body surface area (BSA)/24 hours. In a spot urinary sample, if the albumin/creatinine excretion ratio is 3.5:1 (or 3.5 g albumin/g of creatinine), it denotes significant glomerular disease.

Tubular proteinuria: This occurs as a result of diseases predominantly affecting the tubulo-interstitial component of the kidney. It usually comprises low molecular weight proteins such as 2 microglobulins. The amount excreted is usually <2 g/day and the dipstick test may be negative.

Overflow proteinuria: This is also called overproduction proteinuria and is commonly due to increased production of abnormal low molecular weight proteins. The glomerular filtration of these abnormal proteins over-whelms the reabsorptive capacity of the renal tubules and the proteins are excreted in the urine. Such types of proteinuria may result in acute tubular injury. Excessive levels of immunoglobulin light chains as in multiple myeloma, myoglobulin in rhabdomyolysis or hemoglobin in intravascular hemolysis are the common clinical conditions associated with overflow proteinuria.

Transient proteinuria. Glomerular proteinuria may occur transiently without any glomerular pathology as seen following high fever or severe physical exertion. It is usually self-limiting and does not cause any long-term damage to the glomerulus.

Orthostatic proteinuria: In tall and thin adolescents and young adults <30 years of age, there is mild proteinuria (usually <2 g in a day), more towards the evening, though there is no proteinuria in the first morning urine sample after overnight rest in bed. These individuals often show an exaggerated lumbar lordosis. The proteinuria has no deleterious effect on the renal glomeruli. Such patients need follow-up only.

Significant proteinuria: If the proteinuria of more than 500 mg in 24 hours is present, it is called 'significant' and needs further evaluation.

Microalbuminuria: In this condition, the urinary excretion of albumin is between 30 mg and 300 mg in 24 hours or 20 µg and 200 µg per minute. This amount is too small to be detected by routine tests and can be detected only by radioimmunoassay (RIA) for albumin or by special dipsticks called microalbumin ('micral') test strips. Microalbuminuria is an early feature of diabetic nephropathy and hypertensive nephrosclerosis. Microalbuminuria has also been shown to be associated with poor long-term prognosis in cardiovascular disease.

Physiology and Pathophysiology

Proteins in plasma circulate through the glomerular capillaries. The glomerular capillary filtration barrier consists of the capillary endothelium, basement membrane and the epithelial foot processes which offer a 'size-selective' and 'charge-selective' barrier to filtration albumin, globulins and other high molecular weight plasma proteins. The foot processes of podocytes or the visceral epithelial cells rest on the glomerular basement membrane. They are arranged in such a way that they produce a series of narrow channels called 'slit diaphragm' that allow passage of solutes and water but not large molecular weight proteins. This is the 'size selective' barrier. The molecular weight of albumin is 66,500 daltons and the oblong shape of the molecule may permit its passage through the filter. Since the filtration barrier is negatively charged, it repels negatively charged protein molecules like albumin thus acting as a 'charge selective' barrier.

In glomerular diseases, when the podocytes are affected, the function of the slit diaphragm is compromised and fusion of foot processes and subsequent damage to capillary endo-thelial fenestrae occurs. The endothelial damage occurs due to reduction in vascular endothelial growth factor (VEGF). This allows significant quantities of albumin to escape into the urinary space and lost in urine. In other

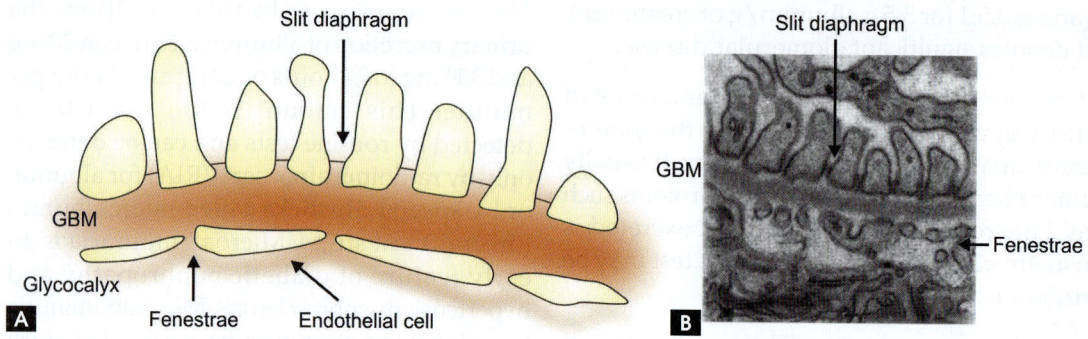

Fig. 41.1A and B: (A) Schematic diagram; (B) Electron microphotograph showing normal glomerular basement membrane with endothelial cell and its fenestrae on one side, and foot processes of podocytes with slit diaphragms on the other side

glomerular diseases associated with more severe damage, disruption of the glomerular basement membrane occurs resulting in formation of large pores through which other plasma proteins may also escape into the urine (Figs 41.1 and 41.2)

The proteinuria results in exposure of mesangial and tubular cells to the filtered proteins. Mesangial cells have an important role in maintenance of normal glomerular hemodynamics and clearance of immune complexes. The exposure leads to mesangial cell proliferation and release of cytokines which initiate an inflammatory response further causing endothelial cell damage, glomerulosclerosis and tubulointerstitial fibrosis.

Etiology

Proteinuria can be due to either abnormal amount or type of protein excreted.

- Defective glomerular barrier that allows abnormal amounts of proteins to enter Bowman space with resultant damage to the kidneys (glomerular proteinuria).
- Systemic diseases that compromise the ability to reabsorb proteins normally in the renal tubules (tubular proteinuria).
- Excessive plasma proteins that are filtered across the glomerular capillary and overwhelm the capacity of reabsorption by renal tubules (overflow proteinuria).

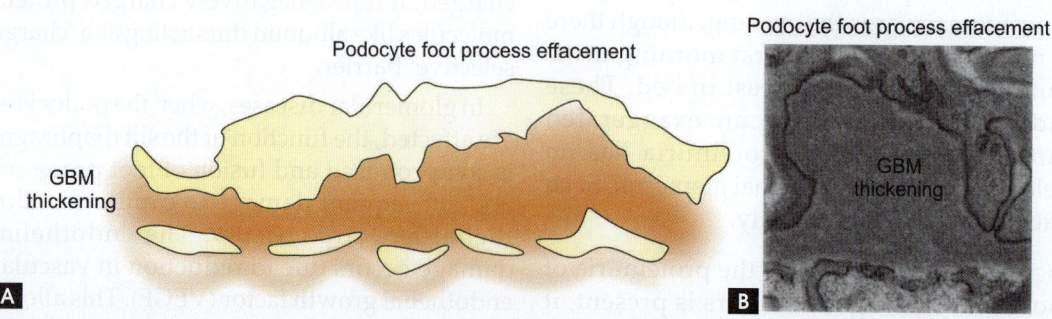

Fig. 41.2A and B: (A) Schematic diagram; (B) Electron microphotograph showing foot process effacement and thickened glomerular basement membrane in a patient with nephrotic syndrome

Glomerular Disease

The causes of glomerular disease may be classified as primary (when there is no evidence of any systemic disease) or secondary (when the kidney is involved secondary to a systemic disease). Primary glomerular disease may be either a proliferative glomerulonephritis (with a nephritic or active urinary sediment) or non-proliferative glomerulonephritis, with a bland urinary sediment (Table 41.1).

Evaluation

Occurrence of significant proteinuria merits detailed evaluation for the cause. This can often be carried out on outpatient basis unless there is an obvious renal disease which merits hospitalization. It is important to ascertain that proteinuria is persistent, through repeated dipstick tests. A detailed history is recorded. Mild to moderate proteinuria may be entirely asymptomatic. There may be urinary symptoms such as frothy, smoky or red urine, especially in relation to an upper respiratory tract infection. History of facial puffiness and/or pedal edema is relevant. History of a systemic disease such as diabetes, hypertension, chronic inflammatory disease such as lupus, joint pains, skin rash, eye symptoms, sleep apnea, chronic congestive heart failure and chronic renal disease should be obtained.

Detailed physical examination should include search for pedal edema, facial puffiness, anasarca, anemia and hypertension. Skin rashes, joint swelling, petechiae, purpura,

Table 41.1: Proteinuria due to glomerular diseases and correlation with urinary sediment

Non-proliferative GN with bland urinary segment	Proliferative GN (active urinary sediments)	Secondary glomerular diseases with active urinary sediment	Secondary glomerular diseases with bland urinary sediment
Minimal change disease	IgA nephropathy, anti-GBM disease, diabetic nephropathy		
Membranous glomerulo-nephritis (MGN)	Mesangioproliferative GN (MesPGN)	Renal vasculitis [including diseases associated with anti-neutrophil cytoplasmic antibodies (ANCA)]	Hypertensive nephrosclerosis
Primary focal and segmental glomerulo-sclerosis (FSGS)	Membranoproliferative (syn. Mesangiocapillary GN) (MPGN) • Immune complex mediated GN • Complement mediated GN	Lupus nephritis	Amyloidosis
Fibrillary glomerulonephritis	–	Cryoglobulinemic glomerulonephritis	Secondary FSGS
Immunotactoid glomerulonephritis	–	Bacterial endocarditis-associated GN	Light chain deposition disease
–	–	Henoch-Schönlein purpura	–
–	–	Post-infectious glomerulonephritis (PIGN)	–

alopecia, jaundice, heart murmurs, organ enlargement and eye changes should also be carefully looked for.

Laboratory Examination

Laboratory investigations should include the following:

- Urinalysis including microscopic examination on at least three separate occasions, preferably on first morning sample of urine.
- Urine ACR on a random urine sample.
- In suspected orthostatic proteinuria, split urine collection from 7 am to 7 pm and from 11 pm to 7 am should be done for quantitation of proteinuria.
- 24 hour/timed urinary collection for quantitation of albumin excretion.
- Complete hemogram including erythrocyte sedimentation rate (ESR).
- Biochemistry including serum creatinine, blood urea, serum proteins and albumin: Globulin ratio, serum lipids, and blood glucose.

Special tests are undertaken after the preliminary tests as indicated.

- Serological tests including anti-streptolysin O (ASO) titres
- Antinuclear antibodies (ANA)/anti-double-stranded DNA antibodies (anti-dsDNA)
- C-reactive proteins (CRP)/procalcitonin
- Complement levels (C3/C4)/cryoglobulins.
- Viral markers [hepatitis B surface antigen (HBsAg), anti-hepatitis C antibodies (anti-HCV) and anti-human immunodeficiency virus antibodies (anti-HIV)].
- Serum protein electrophoresis and urine electrophoresis
- Anti-glomerular basement membrane antibodies (anti-GBM Ab) and anti-neutrophil cytoplasmic antibodies (ANCA).
- Imaging studies like ultrasonography of the kidneys, chest X-ray, and CT scan.

Renal biopsy: If proteinuria is documented in an adult and is suspected to be of glomerular origin, as evidenced by 'active' sediment or nephrotic range proteinuria, renal biopsy should be performed to determine the exact diagnosis, guide the choice of therapy and assess the prognosis.

In children, most cases of nephrotic syndrome are due to minimal change disease (MCD), and usually respond to steroids. Biopsy is usually reserved for steroid-unresponsive patients. It is best to refer such patients to a nephrologist to arrive at a decision on renal biopsy.

An algorithm for investigation of a dipstick-positive proteinuria is shown in Fig. 41.3.

Treatment

Treatment can be broadly classified as general and specific. The general measures are instituted to reduce proteinuria and manage complications of nephrotic syndrome. In view of the loss of immunoglobulins and complement components in urine, patients are particularly prone to contracting bacterial infections. Spontaneous bacterial peritonitis, skin and pulmonary are common in children with nephrotic syndrome due to reduced humoral as well as cell-mediated immunity. Immunization with pneumococcal vaccine is strongly recommended. Though there is no role for prophylactic antibiotics, any infection should be promptly treated with appropriate antibiotics.

Diet: Salt restriction in diet is an effective measure to reduce edema/anasarca and hypertension. Fluid management is of utmost importance. Often, edematous proteinuric patients are wrongly advised to consume excessive fluids to 'increase' the urine volume. The high fluid intake actually results in more fluid retention and worsening of edema. Strict fluid control and salt restriction are necessary till the edema subsides. In nephrotic subjects with heavy proteinuria and normal renal function, protein supplementation with high

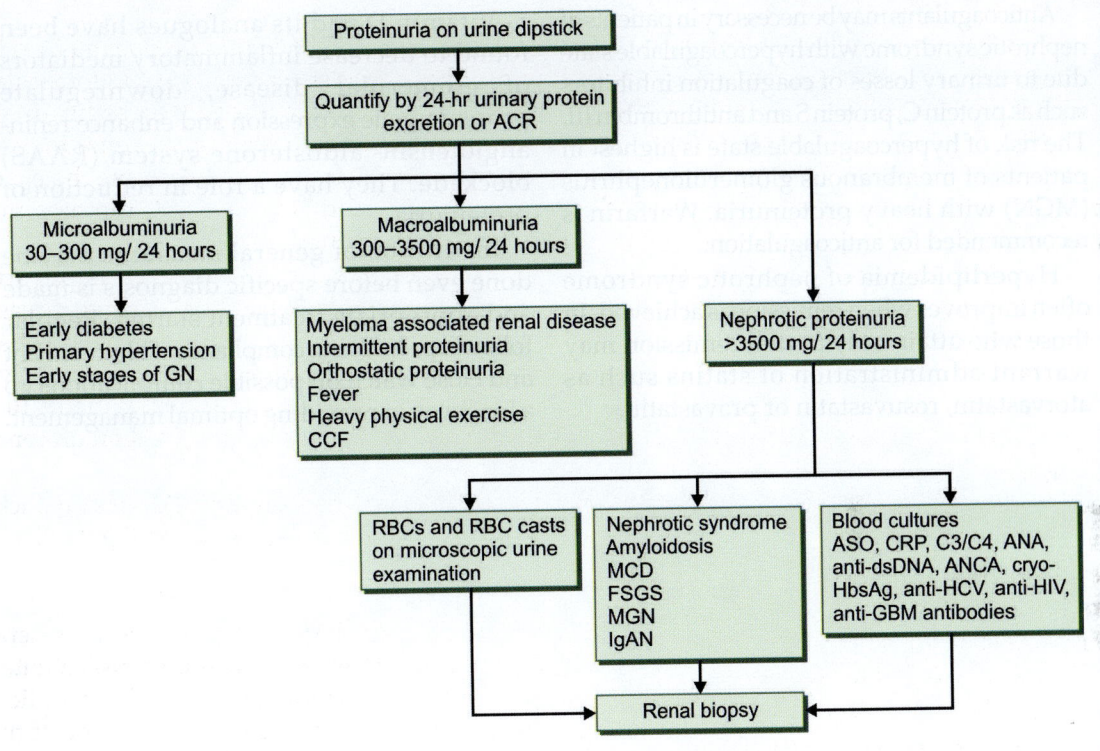

Fig. 41.3: An algorithm for evaluation of proteinuria

biological value proteins may be required to prevent protein malnutrition. Since most of the patients are on a protein restricted diet, a blanket prescription of 'low protein' diet is inappropriate since a minimum protein intake of 0.6 gm/kg body weight is necessary to prevent breakdown of body's own protein. In patients with elevated serum creatinine, who are taking more than 1 gm protein/kg body weight, a diet restricting protein to 0.6–0.8 gm/kg first class protein should be recommended. This level of protein intake not only prevents negative nitrogen balance but also delays progression of renal failure.

Drug treatment with either angiotensin-converting enzyme (ACE) inhibitors or angiotensin receptor blockers (ARB) in best tolerated dose may help reduce proteinuria and rate of progression of renal disease. They act by inhibiting angiotensin-mediated efferent arteriolar vasoconstriction thereby reducing intraglomerular capillary pressure. They also help control blood pressure in patients of glomerular disease with hypertension. Other effects include restoration of size- and charge-selectivity of glomerular capillary filtration barrier, reduction in breakdown of bradykinin and reduction in production of cytokines that promote glomerulosclerosis and fibrosis.

Diuretics may be required for management of edema/anasarca and fluid overload. If a single loop diuretic such as frusemide or torsemide fails to reduce fluid overload, a combination of a loop diuretic and metolazone may be used. The fluid balance chart should be maintained and fluid intake closely monitored to prevent occurrence of intravascular volume contraction. In severely hypoalbuminemic subjects, intravenous infusion of human albumin may help to eliminate more fluid from the body.

Anticoagulants may be necessary in patients of nephrotic syndrome with hypercoagulable state due to urinary losses of coagulation inhibitors such as protein C, protein S and antithrombin III. The risk of hypercoagulable state is highest in patients of membranous glomerulonephritis (MGN) with heavy proteinuria. Warfarin is recommended for anticoagulation.

Hyperlipidemia of nephrotic syndrome often improves when remission is achieved. In those who attain only partial remission may warrant administration of statins such as atorvastatin, rosuvastatin or pravastatin.

Vitamin D and its analogues have been found to decrease inflammatory mediators of glomerular disease, downregulate prorenin gene expression and enhance renin-angiotensin- aldosterone system (RAAS) blockade. They have a role in reduction of proteinuria.

Institution of general measures may be done even before specific diagnosis is made and appropriate treatment started. Regular follow-up, ensuring compliance with treatment and close watch on possible complications go a long way in providing optimal management.

Approach to Hematuria

• Sanjay D'Cruz

Hematuria can be sign of disease anywhere in the genitourinary tract or can rarely be factitious. In young adults particularly, hematuria may be transient and of no consequence. On the other hand, there is an appreciable risk of malignancy in older patients even if transient. Gross hematuria is often alarming; and it prompts the patient to seek early medical attention. Unexplained hematuria associated with no obvious underlying condition (e.g. cystitis, ureteral stone) is also common. All cases of hematuria should be investigated by appropriate investigations to identify the cause.

Hematuria may be visible to the naked eye (called gross hematuria) or detectable only on examination of the urine sediment by microscopy (called microscopic hematuria). Gross hematuria can result from as little as 1 ml of blood in a liter of urine. Dipstick tests that use orthotoluidine can detect as low as 2–3 RBCs per high power field with a sensitivity of 91–100% and specificity of 65–99%, but they also may be positive in the presence of free hemoglobin or myoglobin. Therefore, a positive dipstick test merits microscopic examination for confirmation. Approximately 1 million RBCs pass into the urine daily; this corresponds to 1 to 3 RBCs/high power field in centrifuged urine sediment examined microscopically. Microscopic hematuria is defined as 3 or more RBCs/high power field on microscopic examination of the centrifuged urine specimen, in two of three freshly voided, clean catch, midstream urine samples.

Microscopic hematuria following catheter-related urothelial trauma is indeed rare. Likewise, anticoagulants do not increase the risk of hematuria. Hence, it seems prudent not to outright neglect microhematuria in catheterized patients or those on anticoagulants. Reddish urine need not necessarily indicate hematuria. Intermittent excretion of red to brown urine can be seen in a variety of clinical situations other than bleeding into the urinary tract. Numerous substances and drugs that can discolor the urine red are given in Table 42.1.

The prevalence of asymptomatic hematuria varies from 0.19 to 16.1%. This wide variation is due to difference in age, sex, amount of follow up and number of screening studies performed. In older population with higher risk of urologic diseases, the prevalence rates are as high as 21%. Risk factors for significant disease in patients with microscopic hematuria are shown in Table 42.2.

Hematuria can be further classified as glomerular and extraglomerular; separating nephrologic and urologic diseases. Disruption

Table 42.1: Substances causing reddish urine

Endogenous	Food products	Drugs	
Bilirubin	Rhubarb	Adriamycin	
Hemoglobin	Blackberries	Phenothiazine	
Myoglobin	Blueberries	Chloroquine	Phenytoin
Porphyrins	Paprika	Desferrioxamine	Prochlorperazine
	Beetroot	Levodopa	Quinine
	Fava beans	Methyldopa	Riboflavin
	Artificial food color	Metronidazole	Rifampicin
		Nitrofurantoin	Sulphonamides
		Phenazopyridine	Warfarin
		Phenolphthalein	

Table 42.2: Risk factors for significant disease in microscopic hematuria

a. Male gender
b. Age (>35 years)
c. Past or current smokers
d. History of irritative voiding symptoms
e. History of pelvic irradiation
f. Occupational or exposure to chemicals or dyes (benzenes or aromatic amines)
g. Analgesic abuse
h. History of gross hematuria
i. History of urologic disorder/disease
j. History of chronic urinary tract infection
k. Exposure to known carcinogenic/chemotherapeutic (alkylating) agents
l. History of chronic indwelling foreign body

of the glomerular filtration barrier leads to glomerular hematuria. Presence of dysmorphic RBCs, significant proteinuria (more specifically, albuminuria) exceeding 1 g/day and red cell casts in the urine signifies glomerular disease. Urinary albumin/protein ratio >0.59:1 points towards glomerular disease. Dysmorphic RBCs are distorted, variable in shape and less hemoglobinized. This change of shape occurs due to passage of RBCs through slit membranes of glomerulus and through urine of different osmolality within the tubule. Some of these RBCs can be ring-shaped with vesicle-shaped protrusions on their surface called acanthocytes. Acanthocytes appear to be most predictive of glomerular disease. Hematuria without proteinuria or casts is termed isolated hematuria. Isolated hematuria is more consistent with extraglomerular bleeding. Anything that disrupts the urothelium such as irritation (stone), inflammation (infection/drugs) or invasion (malignancy) can result in RBCs in the urine. Trauma, infarction, arteriovenous malformations or bleeding diathesis are some other causes of extraglomerular hematuria. Presence of bright red color blood clots in urine suggests urothelial trauma/tumor.

Rarely, hematuria is factitious, when blood is added to an 'un-witnessed' urine collection (e.g. from a fingerstick or spitting to the sample after injuring the gum). Factitious hematuria can be documented by the absence of hematuria in a urine specimen obtained under direct observation and supervision. Patients who malinger hematuria are capable of 'dodging' and baffling the observer and successfully produce a bloodstained sample. The causes of hematuria (Table 42.3) vary with age, with the most common being inflammation or infection of the prostate or bladder, stones and, in older patients, kidney or urinary tract malignancy or benign prostatic hyperplasia.

Detailed history and physical examination provide important clues to the nature of the underlying disease, narrow the differential diagnosis and separate glomerular from extraglomerular bleeding. Transient microscopic hematuria can be caused by vigorous exercise,

Table 42.3: Common causes of hematuria

Drugs	*Renal causes of hematuria*
Analgesics	Vasculitides
Anticoagulants	Henoch-Schönlein purpura, microscopic polyangiitis,
Amitriptyline	granulomatosis with polyangiitis (GPA)
Busulfan	
Cyclophosphamide	*Glomerular disease*
Oral contraceptives	Infection-related glomerulonephritides
Penicillins (extended spectrum)	Immunoglobulin A nephropathy
Quinine	Lupus nephritis
Vincristine	Mesangial proliferative glomerulonephritis
	Alport syndrome
Systemic causes of hematuria	Thin basement membrane disease
Bleeding diathesis	Nail-patella syndrome
Sickle cell disease	Fabry disease
	Goodpasture's syndrome
	Other types of GN (MPGN, mesangioproliferative GN)
Infections	*Tubulointerstitial disease*
Tuberculosis of GU tract	Polycystic kidney disease
Schistosomiasis	Hereditary nephritis
Metabolic causes of hematuria	Medullary cystic disease
Hypercalciuria	Interstitial nephritis
Hyperuricosuria	Analgesic nephropathy
Factitious hematuria	Renal papillary necrosis
Trauma, exercise	Reflux nephropathy
Menstruation	Loin pain—hematuria syndrome
Endometriosis	Tumors (primary renal cell, leukemic
	infiltrate, metastatic)
	Infections (syphilis, toxoplasmosis, cytomegalovirus, Epstein-Barr virus)
	Renal masses (vascular, neoplastic, congenital)
Renal vascular causes of	Urinary tract diseases
hematuria	Infection or cancer of the ureter, bladder,
Arteriovenous malformation	prostate and urethra
Renal artery disease: Thrombosis,	Nephrolithiasis
embolus, dissecting aneurysm,	
malignant hypertension	
Renal vein thrombosis	

sexual intercourse, trauma, digital rectal prostate examination or menstrual contamination. If transient microscopic hematuria is suspected, follow-up urine studies should demonstrate resolution 48 hours after the discontinuation of these activities. The initial step in the evaluation of patients with red urine is centrifugation of the specimen to see if the red or brown color is in the urine sediment or the supernatant. Hematuria is responsible if the red to brown color is seen only in the urine sediment, with the supernatant being clear.

Clinical Clues

By proper history and thorough clinical examination, a number of clues to identify the site and cause of bleeding can be obtained. The important clues are:

a. Hematuria occurring throughout urination suggests upper urinary tract or upper bladder disease suggesting that the urine in the bladder is already well mixed with blood. Hematuria occurring at the end of urination suggests a problem in the trigone, bladder neck or the prostatic urethra whereas, if it occurs at the start and clears midway, it suggests a problem in the urethra distal to the urogenital diaphragm. Although the 'three-glass test' is a crude method, it is still a useful means by which the clinician gets to see the initial, middle and last part of urinary stream.

b. History of last menstrual period and history of vaginal bleeding is important in women to rule out contamination with blood from vagina.

c. Cyclic hematuria in women during and shortly after menstruation, suggests endometriosis of the urinary tract.

d. Lower urinary tract symptoms suggest presence of UTI or urothelial malignancy.

e. In cases of sterile pyuria the patient should be evaluated for stone/tumor/genitourinary TB) and nephrological causes like acute interstitial nephritis.

f. A recent infective episode raises the possibility of infection related glomerulonephritis, IgA nephropathy, or hereditary nephritis.

g. Colicky flank pain suggests a stone disease.

h. Passage of blood clots, indicates a urological problem, e.g. bladder stone, tumor, or trauma.

i. A brief travel and occupation history may reveal risk factors for pathogen or chemical exposure associated with hematuria.

j. Painless hematuria in the absence of signs and symptoms of renal disease or UTI should prompt an investigation for genitourinary malignancy or tuberculosis.

k. Weight loss, extrarenal manifestations such as rash, arthritis, arthralgia, or pulmonary symptoms suggests a variety of systemic illnesses, including vasculitic syndromes, malignancy and tuberculosis.

l. A thorough drug history should be taken, since many drugs can cause either hematuria or reddish discoloration of the urine.

m. A family history of hematuria would suggest certain heridofamilial diseases like hereditary nephritis, polycystic kidney disease, or sickle cell disease.

Physical Examination

In the general physical examination, the prostate, external genitalia including urethral meatus should be examined. Phimosis and balanitis in diabetic men are a common cause of persistent microscopic hematuria which is often overlooked. New-onset hypertension may be a sign of renal disease. Petechiae, arthritis, mononeuritis multiplex, and rash suggest immunologic disease, vasculitis or coagulopathy. Ocular examination and hearing should be evaluated if Alport syndrome is suspected. An abdominal lump could point to an enlarged kidney and should be further evaluated with imaging tools.

Laboratory Examination

Urinalysis is the first and most important investigation. It is necessary to distinguish hematuria from pigmenturia (discoloration of the urine). This can be done by inspecting the urine and subjecting it to a dipstick test. Dipstick positive urine for heme should be subjected to microscopy to look for RBCs and crystals. The urine sediment (or direct counting of RBC per ml of uncentrifuged urine) is the gold standard for the detection of microscopic hematuria. Once hematuria is confirmed the next step is to look for protein in urine. If the urine protein is greater than trace it should be followed up with either a random albumin/creatinine ratio or a 24-hour quantitative proteinuria. Increased urinary protein excretion can be an extremely important diagnostic discriminator. The next step is to perform a microscopic examination of the sediment of a recently obtained and centrifuged urine sample under both low and high power. Presence of RBC casts and dysmorphic RBCs (best detected with phase-contrast microscopy/scanning electron microscope) strongly suggests a glomerular origin of the bleeding. Casts are best looked for at the periphery of the coverslip. Pyuria with hematuria necessitates testing for UTI.

If there are pointers to nephronal hematuria, further tests to delineate the cause would depend on the history and examination. Various tests depending on the differential diagnosis include, ASO, CRP, throat swab, C3/C4 levels, ANA and ANCA. A renal biopsy may be indicated in such cases. In painless isolated hematuria with an otherwise unremarkable laboratory evaluation, especially in those at risk for urothelial malignancies, patients should undergo imaging of the kidney and genitourinary tract, urine cytology for malignant cells as well as cystoscopy.

Diagnostic Imaging Tools

A variety of imaging tools are available, the choice depends on the cost, availability of equipment and expertise and more importantly the diagnostic possibility based on history and physical examination.

Intravenous Pyelography/ Intravenous Urography (IVU)

This is the traditional modality to evaluate the anatomy of the urinary tract and provides details of the collecting system. It is cheap and readily available; however, it is not sensitive to identify lesions smaller than 3 cm. IVU is superior to CT in detecting transitional cell carcinoma involving the kidney or ureter but has limited application in the evaluation of tumors of the bladder and urethra.

Ultrasonography

Ultrasonography has the advantage of being readily available, being cheap and can be used in pregnant ladies and patients with renal insufficiency, as it does not require intravenous contrast. It is a good modality for confirming and characterizing a cyst, calculi and hydronephrosis. However, its accuracy is lower for detecting solid lesions smaller than 3 cm in diameter and for evaluating the urothelium.

CT Scan

Microscopic hematuria associated with renal colic is best evaluated with CT. Non-contrast CT has the advantage of higher accuracy, decreased radiation dose, faster examination time, and improved sizing and localization of stones. Contrast CT is the best imaging test for small renal parenchymal masses, and renal and perinephric abscesses. CECT also enables detection of aneurysms in vessels. It is approximately as good as MRI at detecting small parenchymal masses, and it is less expensive. The major limitations of contrast CT is that it cannot be used in patients with renal insufficiency and it lacks sensitivity in detecting uroepithelial malignancies.

CT Urography (CTU)

Multidetector CTU provides global imaging of the genitourinary tract as it combines the benefits of conventional CT scanning (with and without contrast) with the ability of an IVP to accurately visualize ureteral and pelvicalyceal surfaces. CTU is the preferred imaging study in patients with otherwise unexplained hematuria. The drawbacks are the high dose of ionic radiation and that it cannot be used in patients with renal failure.

Magnetic Resonance Imaging (MRI)

MRI can be used to assess the upper urinary tract in whom intravenous contrast is contra-indicated. Its high cost and lack of availability in many locations are major drawbacks.

Angiography

If the above tests are negative, then an arteriovenous malformation or any other vascular causes could be the culprit and an angiography may be considered.

Renal Biopsy

If urine shows dysmorphic RBCs, RBC casts, significant proteinuria and if there is recent onset hypertension and declining renal function a glomerular pathology is likely.

Flowchart 42.1: Algorithm for evaluation of asymptomatic microscopic hematuria

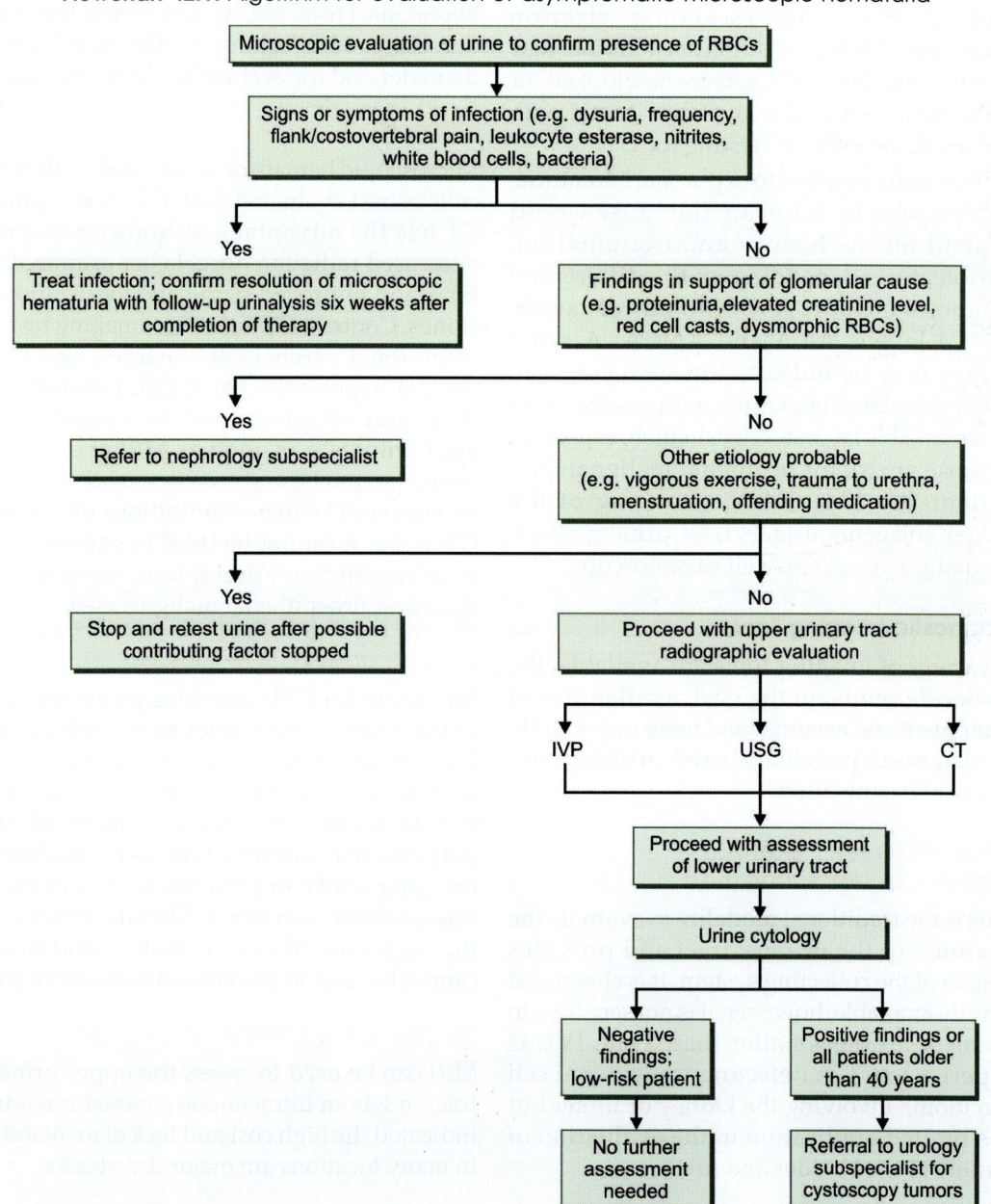

Renal biopsy is indicated in such patients. Renal biopsy is not usually performed for isolated glomerular hematuria since there is no specific therapy for these conditions and since the renal prognosis is excellent in such patients.

Urine Cytology

High risk patients with isolated hematuria, following radiographic assessment of the upper urinary tract, should undergo urine cytology studies. The sensitivity can be increased by sending first voided urine sample on three consecutive days. Advantage of urine cytology over cystoscopy is cheap, non-invasive and causes less discomfort to the patient. The sensitivity of urine cytology is highest for detection of high-grade lesions in the bladder and carcinoma *in situ*. It is of limited value in detecting low-grade lesions in the bladder as well as renal cell cancer.

Cystoscopy

As none of the above tests can completely evaluate the bladder mucosa, in patients of isolated hematuria over 40 years of age and younger patients having underlying risk factors for genitourinary malignancy cystoscopy is indicated. Cystoscopy is the only reliable method of detecting transitional cell carcinoma of the bladder and the urethra.

The algorithm for evaluation of asymptomatic microscopic hematuria is given in Flowchart 42.1.

Follow-up

In patients with non-glomerular hematuria with no evidence of primary renal disease, if high risk factors are present, complete urologic evaluation including upper tract imaging, cystoscopy and cytology should be done. Even if all tests are negative, the patient should be followed up at 6 monthly intervals for 3 years. Evaluation should include urinalysis, blood pressure, renal function tests, cytology and cystoscopy if indicated.

Summary

Microscopic hematuria is a common urinary abnormality across all age groups. Etiology varies with age and sex but infections, stone disease, prostate related diseases and urothelial malignancies are dominant causes. Patients with dysmorphic RBCs, RBC casts, proteinuria, freshly diagnosed hypertension or deranged renal functions generally have an identifiable cause and need renal biopsy. Every patient with persistent isolated hematuria needs thorough evaluation. Despite thorough evaluation a large proportion of patients still remain undiagnosed and need periodic follow-up.

Approach to Oliguria and Polyuria

• Sreejith Parameswaran

Changes in urine volume often alerts the patient to approach for medical help. A systematic analysis is necessary for arriving at the correct cause and plan appropriate management. Simple remedies like modification of fluid intake alone may be necessary in a few cases. Therefore, a clear understanding of the causes, consequences and management of oliguria and polyuria are important.

Oliguria defined as the reduction in the urine output in a previously healthy individual. The criteria for diagnosis of oliguria are:

a. In infants—<1 ml/kg/hour.

b. In children—<0.5 ml/kg/hour for 6–12 hours (KDIGO, *see* chapter on AKI) or <0.5 ml/kg/hour for 8 hours (RIFLE criteria, chapter on AKI) or <300 ml/24 hours

c. In adults—0.5 ml/kg/hour for 6–12 hours (KDIGO).

The objective of hourly monitoring is to detect oliguria as early as possible so that pre-renal failure can be diagnosed and corrected promptly. This helps to prevent development of tubular necrosis and established AKI. Anuria is defined as urine output <100 ml/ 24 hours in adults or <0.1 ml/kg/24 hours in children. Oliguria often occurs secondary to reduction in GFR resulting from acute kidney injury: Historically, the etiology of AKI was divided into three categories: Pre-renal, renal

and post-renal. Conditions associated with effective hypoperfusion in which there is no parenchymal damage to the kidney are grouped as 'pre-renal' causes (Table 43.1).

If the pre-renal causes persist, the renal tubules may undergo acute tubular necrosis (ATN) and the AKI is established. Other renal parenchymal diseases can also cause AKI. This is called intrinsic renal failure and can be caused by diseases of small renal arterioles, glomeruli, tubules or interstitium (Table 43.2).

The next group of diseases causing AKI are 'post-renal causes which imply obstruction to various levels in the urinary tract due to various causes (Table 43.3).

History and physical examination findings are important for categorizing oliguria: Proper history and physical examination are important for categorizing oliguria. Important points in the history are history of fluid loss from the body (vomiting, diarrhea, diuretics, hemorrhage, burns), reduced fluid intake, hypotension, cardiac disease, liver disease and use of nephrotoxic medications including over-the-counter drugs, illicit or herbal preparations. History of trauma, myalgia and recent exposure to radiographic contrast agents should be ascertained. Symptoms suggesting systemic diseases like skin rash, arthritis, uveitis, weight loss, fatigue or

Table 43.1: Conditions causing pre-renal AKI	
1. Intravascular volume depletion → hypovolemia and hypotension	c. Congestive heart failure
a. Hemorrhage (external /internal:	d. Valvular diseases
i. Trauma	e. Pulmonary diseases
ii. Surgery	i. Pulmonary hypertension
iii. Post-partum	ii. Pulmonary embolism
iv. Gastrointestinal	f. Sepsis
b. Other gastrointestinal losses:	3. *Systemic vasodilation* (diminished relative circulating volume):
i. Diarrhea	a. Sepsis
ii. Vomiting	b. Cirrhosis
iii. Nasogastric tube loss	c. Anaphylaxis
c. Renal losses:	d. Drugs
i. Diuretics	4. Renal vasoconstriction
ii. Osmotic load (diabetes mellitus) with diuresis	a. Early sepsis
iii. Diabetes insipidus	b. Hepatorenal syndrome
d. Skin and mucous membrane losses:	c. Acute hypercalcemia
i. Burns	d. Drugs:
ii. Hyperthermia	i. Norepinephrine
e. Nephrotic syndrome	ii. Vasopressin
f. Cirrhosis of liver	iii. Nonsteroidal anti-inflammatory drugs (NASIDs)
g. Capillary leak syndrome	iv. Angiotensin converting enzyme inhibitors (ACEI)
2. Reduced cardiac output (hypotension due to pump failure)	v. Calcineurin inhibitors (CNIs)
a. Cardiogenic shock	vi. Iodinated contrast media
b. Pericardial diseases	5. Increased intra-abdominal pressure (intra-abdominal pressure >15 mm Hg)
i. Restrictive cardiomyopathy	Abdominal compartment syndrome
ii. Constrictive pericarditis	
iii. Pericardial tamponade	

evidence of infections like HIV, hepatitis B or C should be looked for. Presence of hematuria, foamy urine, cough, sinusitis, hemoptysis, edema, nephrotic syndrome, trauma, flank pain, anticoagulation use recent surgery should be ascertained.

In the physical examination, weight loss, orthostatic hypotension and tachycardia, dry mucosal surfaces, poor skin turgor elevated JVP, third heart sound, pulmonary rales, peripheral edema, ascites, caput medusae, spider angiomas, muscle tenderness, compartment syndrome, assessment of volume status periorbital, sacral, and lower-extremity edema; rash; oral/nasal ulcer, fever, arthralgia, drug-related rash and funduscopic examination

will be useful. The following algorithm summarizes the clinical approach to an oliguric patient (Fig. 43.1).

Certain urinary indices calculated from physical and chemical constituents or the urine helps to differentiate between the stage of pre-renal to the stage of established acute tubular necosis (Table 43.4). Clinical features, urinary findings, and confirmatory tests in the differential diagnosis of AKI are summarized in Table 43.5.

APPROACH TO POLYURIA

Polyuria may be defined as the excretion of excessive amount of urine above 3 liters per day and 2 liters per m^2 in children. Nocturia is

Table 43.2: Causes of intrinsic AKI

Diseases involving the renal parenchyma
1. Acute tubular injury → acute tubular necrosis (ATN)
    a. Ischemia due to hypoperfusion (pre-renal conditions causing hypovolemia / hypoperfusion /
    b. Endogenous toxins:
        i. Myoglobin
        ii. Hemoglobin
        iii. Paraproteins
        iv. Uric acid
    c. Exogenous toxins:
        i. Antibiotics
        ii. Chemotherapeutic agents
        iii. Radiocontrast media
        iv. Phosphate preparations
2. Tubulointerstitial Injury
    a. Acute allergic interstitial nephritis:
    b. NSAIDs
    c. Antibiotics
    d. Infections: Viral/bacterial/fungal
    e. Infiltration: Lymphoma/leukemia/sarcoidosis
    f. Allograft rejection
3. Glomerular Injury:
    a. Immune mediated inflammation:
        i. Anti-GBM disease
        ii. ANCA associated vasculitis
        iii. Cryoglobulinemia
        iv. Membranoproliferative glomerulonephritis (MPGN)
        v. IgA nephropathy
        vi. Systemic lupus erythematosus (SLE)
        vii. Henoch-Schönlein purpura
        viii. Polyarteritis nodosa
    b. Hematologic disorders:
        i. Hemolytic uremic syndrome (HUS)
        ii. Thrombotic thrombocytopenic purpura (TTP)
4. Renal microvasculature:
    a. Malignant hypertension
    b. Pre-eclampsia/eclampsia
    c. Hypercalcemia
    d. Radiocontrast media
    e. Scleroderma
    f. Drugs
5. Damage to large vessels
    a. Renal arteries and arterioles:
        i. Thrombosis
        ii. Vasculitis
        iii. Dissection
        iv. Thromboembolism
        v. Atheroembolism
        vi. Trauma
    b. Renal venules and veins:
        i. Thrombosis
        ii. Compression
        iii. Trauma

nocturnal polyuria. The day/night ratio of urine output is 2:1 for young healthy adults, but this ratio falls with increasing age, so that by age 60, the ratio is closer to 1:1. Nocturia is defined as passage of large amounts of urine at night changing the day/night ratio of urine output to 1:1 in young adults and below 0.6 : 1 in the elderly.

Polyuria can be due to either water diuresis, solute diuresis or mixed water-solute diuresis. For a healthy adult, the 24-hour urine volume averages about 1.6 liters and is associated with the excretion of approximately 800 mOsm of total solute. Polyuria is defined based on the age of the individual (Table 43.6).

There are three basic mechanisms for polyuria:

1. Polydipsia (refers to increased intake of fluids and is defined by a fluid intake of more than 100 ml/kg/day or 6 L per day).
    a. Psychogenic polydipsia (compulsive water drinking)
    b. Stress and anxiety
2. Increased urinary loss of solutes
    a. Diabetes mellitus
    b. Hyperthyroidism
    c. Hyperparathyroidism
    d. Drugs
        i. Diuretics
        ii. Mannitol
        iii. Glycerol
        iv. Radiocontrast agents

Table 43.3: Causes of post-renal acute kidney injury	

1. Intratubular obstruction (obstruction occurring in renal tubules)
  a. Crystalluria
2. Extrinsic causes in upper urinary tract:
  a. Retroperitoneal compression (lymph nodes/ tumors)
  b. Retroperitoneal fibrosis (radiation/drugs/ inflammation)
  c. Pelvic or intra-abdominal tumors (carcinoma cervix, uterus, ovary, prostate)
  d. Ureteral ligation or surgical trauma
  e. Granulomatous diseases
3. Intrinsic causes in upper urinary tract:
  a. Nephrolithiasis and stones
  b. Strictures
  c. Edema
  d. Tissue debris
  e. Blood clots
  f. Sloughed papillae
  g. Fungal ball
  h. Malignancy
4. Causes in the lower urinary tract:
  a. Urethral causes:
	i. Posterior urethral valves
	    ii. Urethral strictures
	    iii. Trauma
	    iv. Infections
	    v. Tuberculosis
	    vi. Tumors
	  b. Lesions in prostate:
	    i. Benign prostatic hypertrophy
	    ii. Carcinoma
	    iii. Infection
	  c. Bladder involvement:
	    i. Bladder neck obstruction
	    ii. Bladder calculi
	    iii. Carcinoma
	    iv. Schistosomal infection (Africa)
	  d. Functional:
	    i. Neurogenic bladder (spinal cord injury)
	    ii. Diabetes (autonomic neuropathy)
	    iii. Multiple sclerosis
	    iv. Stroke
	    v. 'Pharmacologic' (side effects of drugs— anticholinergics/antidepressants)

e. Inability of the kidney to reabsorb water/ salt

f. Diabetes insipidus (central/nephrogenic DI)

g. Drugs (diuretics/mannitol/glycerol/ radiocontrast agents)

h. Early renal failure in CKD

i. Recovering stage of acute tubular necrosis/post-obstructive diuresis

j. Adrenal insufficiency

k. Cerebral salt wasting (CSW)

l. Renal salt wasting (aldosterone resistance/ salt diuresis/renal tubular acidosis)

When a patient presents with polyuria, it is necessary to confirm the same by measuring 24-hour urine volume. Next step is to determine whether polyuria is due to water diuresis or solute diuresis. This is possible by looking into urinary osmolality (Uosm). If the Uosm is >250 mOsm/kg, it indicates a solute diuresis and if <150 mOsm/kg (dilute urine) indicates a water diuresis. The ratio of urine/plasma osmolality (Uosm/Posm) also helps to differentiate between water diuresis (Uosm/ Posm <0.9) or solute diuresis (Uosm/Posm >0.9). It will be possible to identify the solute responsible for solute diuresis by analyzing the urine for electrolytes, glycosuria, urea and other solutes.

The differential diagnoses of water diuresis are: (1) Primary polydipsia, (2) central diabetes insipidus, (3) nephrogenic diabetes insipidus. Central DI can be congenital or acquired. Important acquired causes are 'post-neuro-trauma', cerebral hemorrhage or infarction, brain death, brain metastatasis (breast), craniopharyngioma, pinealoma, histiocytosis, drug or toxin-induced (ethanol, diphenyl-hydantoin, snake venom, demeclocycline, cisplatin, lithium), electrolyte abnormalities (hypercalcemia/hypokalemia), polycystic kidney disease/bilateral partial ureteric obstruction and genetic disorders.

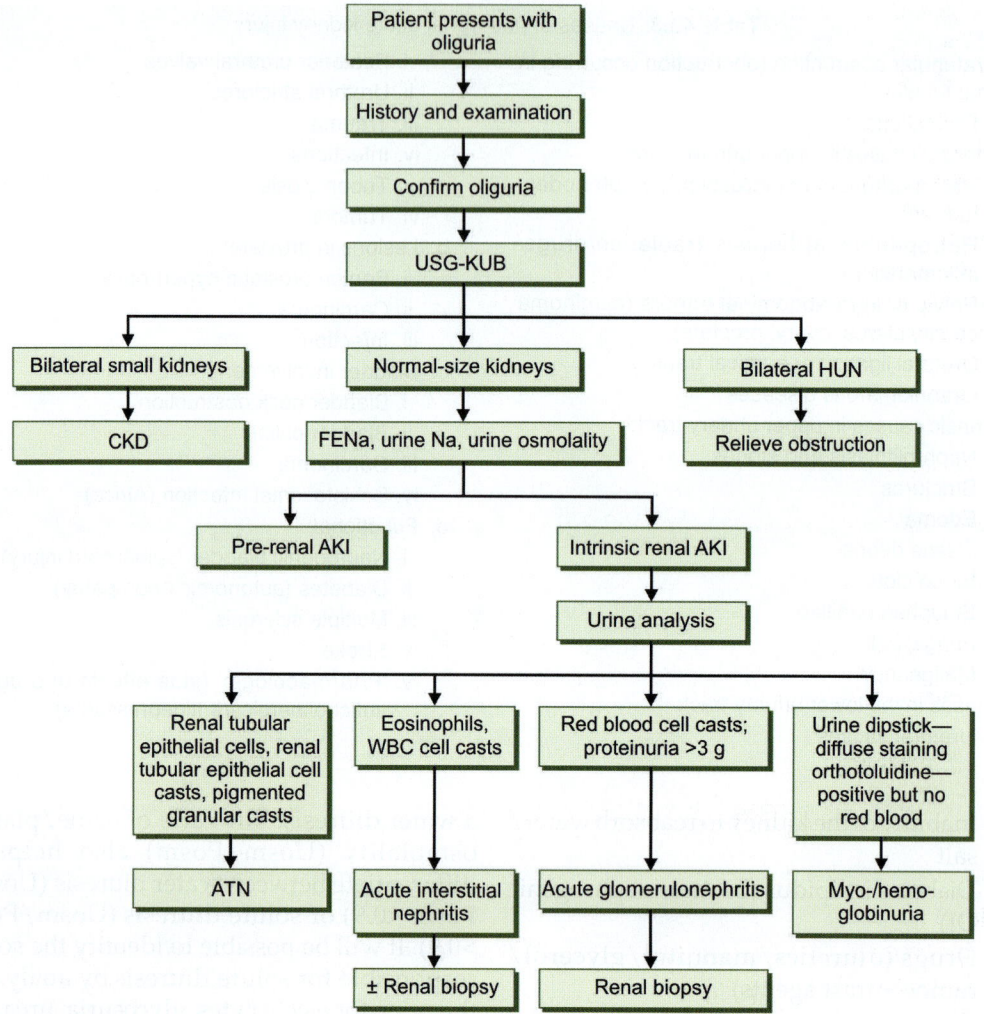

Fig. 43.1: Algorithmic approach for oliguria. The first step in diagnosis is to rule out obstruction

Clinical Features

Certain clinical features, identified from a careful case history or meticulous physical examination may provide clue towards the etiology of polyuria. Clinical clues from history and physical examination are shown in Table 43.7.

Investigations

1. *Urine examination*
   a. 24-hour urine volume. To confirm polyuria. Confirming presence of polyuria by

measurement of urine volume is essential and should be the first step, before further evaluations are undertaken, because a significant number of patients may be having only increased frequency of urine and not necessarily increased volume of urine.
   b. Urine osmolality <300 mOsm/kg of water and/or urine specific gravity <1.010 suggests dilute urine.
   c. Urine sugar, and other routine tests including microscopy.

Table 43.4: Urine indices used in the differential diagnosis of pre-renal acute kidney injury and acute tubular necrosis

Diagnostic index	Pre-renal AKI	Intrinsic ATN
Urinary Na (mmol/L)	<20	>20
Fractional excretion of Na (%)	<1*	>2*
Fractional excretion of urea (%)	<35	>50
Renal failure index	<1	>1
Serum BUN/serum creatinine	>20	≤10
Urine Cr/plasma Cr	>40	<20
Urine urea nitrogen/plasma urea nitrogen	>8	<3
Urine osmolality	>500	~350
Urine specific gravity	>1.018	~1.010
Urine sediments	Hyaline casts	Muddy-brown granular casts

*Fractional excretion of sodium $FENa = \dfrac{Urine\ Na/plasma\ Na}{Urine\ Cr/plasma\ Cr}$

Pre-renal AKI with FENa <1%	1. Adrenal insufficiency
	2. Bicarbonaturia in metabolic alkalosis
	3. CKD
	4. Diuretics
Intrinsic-renal AKI with FENa >1%	1. Contrast-induced nephropathy
	2. Pigment nephropathy
	3. Sepsis (early stages)
	4. Acute vasculitis
	5. Acute interstitial nephritis

$$Renal\ failure\ index = \dfrac{Urine\ Na}{Urine\ Cr/plasma\ Cr}$$

2. Blood tests
   d. Blood counts
   e. Random blood sugar (rule out hyperglycemia)
   f. HbA1C
   g. Blood urea
   h. Serum creatinine (rule out kidney disease)
   i. Serum electrolytes including corrected calcium
   j. Thyroid functions
3. Ultrasonogram of kidneys and urinary tract (rule out obstructive uropathy).

   The algorithm for initial work up of a case of polyuria is provided in Fig. 43.2.
4. *Water deprivation test:* Once presence of polyuria is confirmed and urine is found to be hypo-osmolar (dilute), water deprivation test is undertaken to differentiate the causes of polyuria with water diuresis. The technique includes complete fluid deprivation for a specific duration while monitoring urine volume, urine osmolality, serum osmolarity and vitals. Interpretation of findings from water deprivation test is described.

Water deprivation test must be performed and interpreted in a systematic manner so that correct conclusions can be made. Overall findings in water deprivation test are summarized in Table 43.8.

Plasma osmolality of more than 295 mOsm/kg suggests central DI, and less than 270 mOsm/kg suggests compulsive water drinking. Lithium is the most common cause of nephrogenic DI, occurring in up to 50% of patients receiving long-term lithium therapy.

Table 43.5: Useful clinical features, urinary findings, and confirmatory tests in the differential diagnosis of AKI

Cause of AKI	Clinical features	Typical urinalysis results	Confirmatory tests
Pre-renal azotemia	Pre-renal azotemia: E/o true volume depletion (thirst, postural or absolute hypotension and tachycardia, low JVP, dry mucous membranes and axillae, weight loss, fluid output greater than input) or decreased effective circulatory volume (e.g. heart failure, liver failure), treatment with NSAID, diuretic, or ACEI/ARB	Hyaline casts FENa <1% UNa <10 mmol/L SG >1.018	Occasionally requires invasive hemodynamic monitoring; rapid resolution of AKI with restoration of renal perfusion
Diseases of small renal vessels and glomeruli			
Glomerulonephritis or vasculitis	Glomerulonephritis or vasculitis compatible clinical history (e.g. recent infection), sinusitis, lung hemorrhage, rash or skin ulcers, arthralgias, hypertension, edema	RBC or granular casts, RBCs, white blood cells, proteinuria	Low complement levels; positive ANCA, anti-GBM antibodies, ASLO antibodies, anti-DNAse, cryoglobulins; renal biopsy
HUS/TTP	Compatible clinical history (e.g. recent gastrointestinal infection, cyclosporine, anovulants), pallor, ecchymoses, neurologic findings	May be normal, RBCs, mild proteinuria, rarely RBC or granular casts	Anemia, thrombocytopenia, schistocytes on peripheral blood smear, low haptoglobin level, increased LDH, renal biopsy
Malignant hypertension	Severe hypertension with headaches, cardiac failure, retinopathy, neurologic dysfunction, papilledema	May be normal, RBCs, mild proteinuria, rarely RBC casts	LVH by echocardiography or ECG, resolution of AKI with BP control
Ischemic or nephrotoxic acute tubular necrosis			
Ischemia	Recent hemorrhage, hypotension, surgery often in combination with	Muddy-brown granular or tubular epithelial cell casts FENa >1%,	Clinical assessment and urinalysis usually inform diagnosis

Contd.

Table 43.5: Useful clinical features, urinary findings, and confirmatory tests in the differential diagnosis of AKI (*Contd.*)

Cause of AKI	Clinical features	Typical urinalysis results	Confirmatory tests
	vasoactive medication (e.g. ACE inhibitor, NSAID)	UNa >20 mmol/L SG ~1.010	
Exogenous toxin	Recent contrast medium-enhanced procedure; nephrotoxic medications; often with coexistent volume depletion, sepsis, or CKD	Muddy-brown granular or tubular epithelial cell casts FENa >1%, UNa >20 mmol/L SG ~1.010	Clinical assessment and urinalysis usually inform diagnosis
Endogenous toxin	History suggestive of rhabdomyolysis (coma, seizures, drug abuse, trauma)	Urine supernatant tests positive for heme in absence of RBCs	Hyperkalemia, hyperphosphatemia, hypocalcemia, increased CK, myoglobin
	History suggestive of hemolysis (recent blood transfusion)	Urine supernatant pink and tests positive for heme in absence of RBCs	Hyperkalemia, hyperphosphatemia, hypocalcemia, hyperuricemia, and free circulating Hb
	History suggestive of tumor lysis (recent chemotherapy), myeloma (bone pain), or ethylene glycol ingestion	Urate crystals, dipstick—negative proteinuria, oxalate crystals, respectively	Hyperuricemia, hyperkalemia, hyperphosphatemia (for tumor lysis); circulating or urinary monoclonal protein (for myeloma); toxicology screen, acidosis, osmolal gap (for ethylene glycol)
Diseases of the tubulointerstitium			
Allergic interstitial nephritis	Recent ingestion of drug and fever, rash, loin pain, or arthralgias	WBC casts, white blood cells (frequently eosinophiluria), RBCs, rarely RBC casts, proteinuria (occasionally nephritic)	Systemic eosinophilia, renal biopsy
Acute bilateral pyelonephritis	Fever, flank pain and tenderness, toxic state	Leukocytes, occasionally WBC casts, RBCs, bacteria	Urine and blood cultures
Post-renal AKI	Abdominal and flank pain, palpable bladder	Frequently normal, hematuria if stones, prostatic hypertrophy	Plain abdominal radiography, USG-KUB post-void residual bladder volume, CT, urography, retrograde or antegrade pyelography

5. *Other investigations:* Magnetic resonance scan of brain/pituitary is performed rarely to confirm central diabetes insipidus. Absence of 'bright spot' in the posterior pituitary give a clue to the diagnosis of central DI.

Table 43.6: Urine volumes in polyuria in different age groups

Age	Urine volume
At birth	150 ml/kg /24 hr
Till the age of 2 years	100–110 ml/kg/24 hr
Older child	40–50 ml/kg/24 hr
	2000 ml/m²/24 hr
Adults (>18 years)	3–3.5 L/24 hr
	>4–5 ml/kg/hr
	> 6000 ml/day

Treatment

Since central DI is due to deficiency of vasopressin, the treatment is by supplementation with 1-desamino-8-D-arginine vasopressin. Several formulations of DDAVP are available. These include intranasal spray 10 µg/spray, parenteral preparation of 4 µg/ml for IV/IM injections and oral 100/200 µg tablets (roughly 1 µg IV = 10 µg intranasal = 100 µg oral tablet). DDAVP administration is used to differentiate between central DI and nephrogenic DI in a patient with polyuria whose initial workup is suggestive of DI. A lack of response to DDAVP indicates a diagnosis of nephrogenic DI. Management of nephrogenic DI is less rewarding. Treatment with chlorpropamide, chlorothiazide, are tried.

Learning Points

- In patients with increased urination, a thorough clinical history can determine whether it is urinary frequency or polyuria; correct 24-hour urine volume measurement may help to make the distinction.
- Psychogenic polydipsia/compulsive water drinking should be ruled out.
- Exclude use of drugs like caffeine, alcohol, diuretics and lithium.
- Metabolic causes like diabetes mellitus, uremia, hypokalemia, hypercalcemia in all patients with polyuria.

Table 43.7: Clinical clues from history and physical examination in a case of polyuria

History	Physical examination findings
Age of onset—congenital/acquired	Ambiguous genitalia, polyuria, shock in newborn period—congenital adrenal hyperplasia
Polyhydramnios in antenatal period	Failure to thrive—diabetes mellitus, nephrogenic diabetes insipidus, renal tubular defects, congenital adrenal hyperplasia
Abrupt onset, preferential for cold drinks, nocturia—cranial diabetes Insipidus	Diabetes mellitus, optic atrophy, deafness—Wolfram syndrome
Family history—diabetes mellitus or diabetes insipidus	Rash, seborrhea, ear discharge—histiocytosis
Weight loss/hyperphagia or loss of appetite—diabetes mellitus	Wasting or cachexia—malignancy, diabetes mellitus
Neurosurgery, meningitis or deceleration injury—central diabetes insipidus	Hemiparesis/brainstem stroke—ICH
Polydipsia and psychiatric illness—nocturnal, abnormal behavior	Bitemporal hemianopia—craniopharyngioma
Constipation and paresthesia—hypercalcemia	Muscle weakness, floppiness—hypokalemia, RTA, Bartter
Salt craving—adrenal insufficiency	Hyperpigmentation, vitiligo—adrenal insufficiency
Drugs—diuretics, lithium, vitamin D supplements, nephrotoxic drugs, mannitol, ethanol	Lymphadenopathy—infiltrative disorders and malignancy
Urinary tract obstruction, polycystic kidney disease	Anemia, half and half nails—CKD
Weight loss, increased sweating, diarrhea—hyperthyroidism	Tremor, tachycardia: Signs of thyrotoxicosis

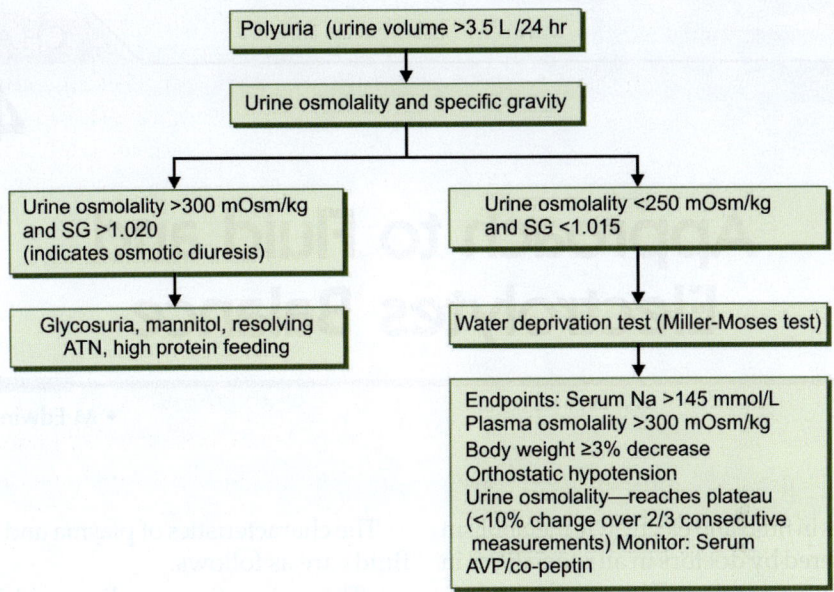

Fig. 43.2: Initial workup for polyuria

Condition	Urinary osmolality with water deprivation (mOsm/kg H₂O)	Plasma vasopressin after dehydration (pg/ml)	Increase in urinary osmolality with exogenous vasopressin

Table 43.8: Interpretation of water deprivation test

Condition	Urinary osmolality with water deprivation $(mOsm/kg\ H_2O)$	Plasma vasopressin after dehydration (pg/ml)	Increase in urinary osmolality with exogenous vasopressin
Normal	>800 mOsm/kg	>2	Less or no increase
Complete central diabetes insipidus	<300	Undetectable	>50% increase
Partial central diabetes insipidus	300–800	1.5	>10% increase in urinary osmolality
Complete nephrogenic diabetes insipidus	<300	>5	<10% increase in urine osmolality
Partial nephrogenic diabetes insipidus	300–800	>2	<10% increase in urine osmolality
Primary polydipsia	>500	<5	A little or no increase

- Urine dipstick testing is useful, and specific gravity can direct further investigations/referral.
- Plasma/urine osmolality may help to distinguish between different diagnoses.

Approach to Fluid and Electrolytes Balance

• M Edwin Fernando

Disturbances in fluid and electrolyte metabolism are encountered by doctors in all specialities in their routine practice. Thorough understanding of the mechanism of the disturbances and the potential dangers of therapy will enable timely recognition and proper management.

1. MAJOR FLUID COMPARTMENTS IN THE BODY

Water makes up 60% (50–70%) of the total body weight in humans. The amount of body fat, which varies with age, sex and nutritional status affect the water content in the body. Water is distributed in several compartments. The main compartments are as follows:

i. Intracellular fluid (ICF) compartment bounded by cell membranes (inside the cells) is equal to 40% of body weight.

ii. Extracellular fluid (ECF) compartment is separated from the external medium by epithelia and from ECF by cell membranes. This forms 20% of body weight. The ECF is subdivided into intravascular (plasma— 4%) and extravascular compartments (interstitial 16%—lymph and transcellular 1–3%).

2. IONIC COMPOSITION OF BODY FLUIDS

The average normal electrolyte concentration in ECF and ICF are given in Table 44.1.

The characteristics of plasma and interstitial fluids are as follows:

i. The main cation is sodium which accounts for most of the osmolality of both fluids.

ii. The concentrations of potassium, calcium and magnesium are small although extremely important for physiological function.

iii. Chloride and bicarbonate are the principal anions. Bicarbonate is the main ECF buffer.

iv. The important difference between plasma and interstitial fluid is the high protein content in plasma.

The prominent features of the ICF are:

i. Potassium is the principal cation

ii. Magnesium is far more concentrated than in ECF

iii. The main intracellular anions are protein and organic phosphates are very low.

3. OSMOLALITY OF BODY FLUIDS

The osmotic effect of a substance in a solution is dependent on the number of particles dissolved and is independent of their weight, charge and chemical formula. The common unit is milliosmole (mOsm). When 1 g molecular weight of the substance is dissolved in 1 g water, the osmolality is 1 or 1000 mOsm. The plasma osmolality is 285 ± 15 mOsm/kg

Table 44.1: Normal electrolyte concentrations in body fluid compartments

	ECF		ICF
Cations (mEq/L)	Plasma	Interstitial	-
Sodium	142	145	10
Potassium	4	4	155
Calcium	5	3	-*
Magnesium	2		26
Anions (mEq/L)			
Chloride	103	114	3
Bicarbonate	26	31	10
Phosphate	1		95
Sulphate	1		20
Proteins	16		55
Organic acids	6		

*Calcium concentration in mitochondria is very high.

water. This can be calculated from the formula:

Plasma osmolality = 2 (Na + K) + urea in mg/6+ glucose in mg/18

The osmolality can be measured more accurately using an osmometer which measures the freezing point of a solution. A solution with osmolality of 1 (1000 mOsm) freezes at negative 1.860 C. So, by noting the freezing point of the test solution, the osmolality can arrived at.

4. BALANCE OF WATER AND ELECTROLYTES

1. *Concept of balance:* Normally, the volume and composition of body fluids remains essentially constant, that is the gains and losses of ions and water are equal, hence the net balance is zero. Persistent deviation from zero balance is abnormal and physiological feedback mechanisms always tend to bring back the two parameters to steady state.
2. *Pathways of gains and losses:* There are 2 normal sources of water gain:
   a. Water intake—as fluids or as constituent of solid food.
   b. Metabolic water production—from catabolism of carbohydrate, protein and fat.

Water losses can be classified as insensible that occurs due to evaporation through respiratory tract and skin and measurable losses in urine and feces. Rough estimates of losses and gains are given in Table 44.2.

Table 44.2: Gain and loss of fluids from the body

	Intake (ml/day)
Water as fluid	+ 1200
Water in food	+1000
Water of oxidation	+300
Fluid balance	
Total fluid gain	+2500
	Output (ml/day)
Urine	−1500
Insensible loss	−900
Respiratory loss	−400
Loss through skin	−500
Water in stool	−100
Fluid balance	−2500
Total fluid loss	

The distribution of water and electrolytes in a day for an average adult is shown in Table 44.3.

5. REGULATION OF SALT AND WATER BALANCE

1. Control of Salt Balance

Sodium salts are the principal osmotic component of ECF fluid. The amount of

Table 44.3: Approximate average gain and loss of water and elements in a normal person

Substance	Intake Oral	Metabolic	Output Urinary	Fecal	Insensible
Water as fluid (ml)	1200	300	1500	100	900
Water in food (ml)	1000	–	–		
Sodium (mEq/L)	155	–	150	2.5	2.5
Potassium (mEq/L)	75	–	70	5	
Chloride (mEq/L)	155	–	150	2.5	2.5
Nitrogen (g)	10	–	9	1	–
Acid (mEq/L)	–	–	–	–	–
Nonvolatile	–	50	50	–	–
Volatile	–	14,000	–	–	14,000

sodium determines the ECF volume and also the total body water. As the cell membrane is permeable to water, changes in plasma sodium lead to water movement between extracellular and intracellular compartments. Sodium balance is achieved by regulation of intake, excretion or both. Sodium excretion is regulated by 3 factors: Glomerular filtration rate, aldosterone and 'third' factor—natriuretic hormones, hydrostatic and colloid osmotic pressure difference across the tubular lumen.

2. Control of Water Balance

ECF osmolality is controlled by water balance. Unlike sodium, water balance is controlled by the changes in intake and excretion. Control of intake is by the sensation of thirst. Excretion is controlled by antidiuretic hormone (ADH). The stimulus for both is increased plasma osmolality. Fluid and electrolyte disturbance must be viewed, not as isolated entities, but in the context of specific settings in which they occur. They often occur in various combinations. As example, a patient with acute gastroenteritis can have volume depletion, hyponatremia, hypokalemia and metabolic acidosis. The clinician should be aware of these facts and apply them in the management of his patients.

Fluid and electrolyte disturbances can be classified as disorders of:

1. Volume regulation (volume depletion, volume excess)

2. Sodium balance (hyponatremia, hypernatremia)
3. Potassium balance (hypokalemia, hyperkalemia)
4. Acid–base balance.

VOLUME DEPLETION

The most common disturbance of fluid and electrolyte equilibrium is body fluid volume depletion. This can be classified as:

A. Simple dehydration—loss of water without electrolytes.

B. Hypovolemia—combined loss of water and electrolytes.

A. Simple Dehydration (Loss of Water Without Electrolytes)

The fluid requirement of body is determined by the insensible losses through skin and lungs and by the amount of water required to excrete the daily solute. Thirst ordinarily maintains water intake well above the basic level. If access the fluid intake is sharply decreased, either due to illness otherwise, dehydration will develop.

The causes of dehydration are:

1. Inadequate water intake: Impaired conscious state—post-surgical, comatose.

2. Increased free water loss: Insensible losses— increased sweating, elevated ambient temperature, fever, respiratory tract losses— hyperventilation.

3. Renal losses
   a. Vasopressin deficiency—central diabetes insipidus
   b. Renal defect—nephrogenic diabetes insipidus.

Clinical Features

Pure water depletion produces hypernatremia (plasma Na 150 mEq/L) and hypertonicity of the plasma. With pure water depletion, vascular collapse and shock are rare. This is due to fact that hypernatremia extracts fluid from intracellular fluid (ICF) compartment to extracellular fluid (ECF) compartment. Pure water-loss should be suspected whenever hypernatremia is found without any evidence of volume depletion or shock. Hypernatremia produces cerebral dehydration and clinical features of restlessness, irritability, lethargy, seizures and coma.

Treatment

The principle is to calculate free water deficit and correct with plain water.

Example: A 60 kg man is found unconscious with high fever and his serum Na is 165 mEq/L.

Free water deficit

$$= 0.6 \times \text{Body weight (kg)} \times (\text{serum Na}/140 - 1)$$
$$= 0.6 \times 60/100 \times (165/140) - 1. = 36 \times (1.17 - 1)$$
$$= 36 \times 0.17$$
$$= 6.12 \text{ L}$$

This is usually corrected by giving water as a 5% dextrose infusion (dextrose is metabolized leaving pure water in the body). Blood sugar must be monitored and appropriate doses of insulin given as needed. This correction is usually done over a period of 48–72 hours.

B. Hypovolemia (Combined Depletion of Water and Sodium)

The causes of volume depletion are:
1. *Gastrointestinal losses*
   a. Vomiting
   b. Diarrhea
   c. Gastric or small bowel drainage
   d. Bowel fistula (colostomy, ileostomy)
2. *Skin losses*
   a. Sweating
   b. Burns
3. Renal losses
   a. Osmotic diuresis (diabetes mellitus)
   b. Diuretics
   c. Post-obstructive diuresis
   d. Chronic kidney disease
   e. Addison's disease

1. Gastrointestinal (GI) Losses

This is a very common cause of volume depletion. The composition of fluid lost from the GI tract varies according to the segment from which the fluid lost (Table 44.4).

Most GI secretions are approximately isotonic as plasma. Therefore, usually no change in ECF osmolality occurs, unless fluid replacement is incorrect. Excessive GI losses tend to cause potassium depletion. Gastric

Table 44.4: Volume and electrolyte concentration of gastrointestinal secretions

	Mean volume (ml/day)	Na	K	Cl	HCO₃	H
Saliva	1300	56	16	16	53	–
Gastric	–	–	–	–	–	–
Secretions	1200	40–65	10	100–140	6	90
Bile	700	135–155	5	80–110	35–50	–
Pancreatic secretions	800	135–155	5	55–75	70–90	–
Jejunal secretions	2500	130–150	7	110–130	25–35	–
Ileal secretions	1500	120–130	10	50–60	50–70	–
Diarrheal fluids		116	30	100	40	–

fluid has a high hydrogen ion concentration therefore loss by vomiting causes metabolic alkalosis. Intestinal and pancreatic juice as well as bile have a high bicarbonate concentration and therefore losses from these segments will produce metabolic acidosis. Fluid losses can be isotonic or hypotonic. In isotonic losses there is no change in plasma sodium and plasma osmolality while in hypotonic losses hypernatremia and increased plasma osmolality occur.

2. Cutaneous Losses

The important causes of cutaneous sodium loss are sweating, heat stroke and burns. Sweat is hypotonic, water loss is greater than Na loss. Burns cause a loss of plasma protein in addition to salt and water.

3. Renal Losses

a. *Osmotic diuresis:* Severe diabetes mellitus (hyperosmolar non-ketotic diabetic coma), high osmotic loads of urea (from high-protein infant formula and in adults from high-protein tube-feeding), mannitol and glycerol (during therapeutic use) can produce osmotic diuresis where water content is more than salt, producing hypotonic volume depletion.

b. *Diuretics:* Abuse of diuretics results in ECF volume depletion especially if another mechanism of loss develops (vomiting or diarrhea).

c. *Renal diseases:* Renal losses of sodium and water intake place during the diuretic phase of acute kidney injury, relief of obstruction and in chronic tubulointerstitial nephritis.

Clinical Features

The most frequent symptoms and physical signs are given below:

   i. Thirst, weakness, cold.
  ii. Dryness of mucous membranes
 iii. Decreased skin turgor
  iv. Decreased sweating
   v. Sunken eyes and cheeks
  vi. Orthostatic hypotension
 vii. Tachycardia
viii. Hypothermia
  ix. Weight loss
   x. Shock

Volume depletion can be classified as mild if associated with loss of <5% of body weight or severe if >10% of body weight is lost. In mild volume depletion there is no circulatory disturbance. As the severity worsens, postural tachycardia, postural hypotension, persistent hypotension followed by hypotension and shock in severe cases.

Laboratory Diagnosis

There are no pathognomonic laboratory signs of sodium depletion. Since plasma sodium concentration depends not only on the amount of sodium in the ECF, but also on the amount of water, it can increase or decrease or remain within the normal (hypertonic, hypotonic or isotonic depletion). Reduction in plasma volume results in hemoconcentration and the hematocrit rises. The changes in potassium, bicarbonate and pH depend on the actual causes of volume depletion.

Management

The treatment of volume depletion includes prophylaxis, prompt restoration of ECF volume and correction of the cause of sodium loss. The type of replacement therapy necessary to prevent volume depletion can be estimated from the type of loss and severity of volume depletion. When faced with a patient who had developed signs and symptoms of severe volume depletion, rapid restoration of ECF volume is needed. After stabilization of vital signs, other appropriate fluids can be given. Composition of various intravenous fluids is given in Table 44.5.

Fluid therapy in various disorders is discussed below:

1. *Acute gastroenteritis:* This is one of the most common causes of volume depletion.

Table 44.5: Composition of various commonly used intravenous fluids

Solutions	Glucose	Na	Cl	K	Ca	Lactate	HPO₄	Acetate	NH₄
5% GDW	50	–	–	–	–	–	–	–	–
5% GDW/0.9% NaCl	50	154	154	–	–	–	–	–	–
5% GDW/0.45% NaCl	50	77	77	–	–	–	–	–	–
0.45% NaCl	–	77	77	–	–	–	–	–	–
0.9% NaCl	–	154	154	–	–	–	–	–	–
3% NaCl	–	513	513	–	–	–	–	–	–
Ringer lactate	–	130	109	4	3	28	–	–	–
Isolyte M	50	40	40	35	–	–	15	20	–
Isolyte E	50	140	103	10	–	–	–	47	–
Isolyte G	50	63	150	17	–	–	–	–	70

GDW: Glucose in distilled water, Na: Sodium, Cl: Chloride, K: Potassium, Ca: Calcium, HPO₄: Phosphate, NH₄: Ammonium

Intravenous rehydration is required only for initial rehydration of the severely ill-patient who is in shock or is unable to drink. The recommended solutions are isotonic saline, isotonic sodium bicarbonate solution (isotonic sodium bicarbonate solution is prepared by adding 150 ml of 7.5% sodium bicarbonate solution to 1 liter of 5% GDW) or Ringer lactate solution. Since 0.9% saline is freely available, it is given initially. It is not an ideal solution because it will not correct acidosis and potassium losses. Although Ringer lactate contains some lactate and potassium, it may not be sufficient to correct the deficit. Bicarbonate and potassium containing solutions will be needed in some cases. The recommended dose of IV fluids is dependent on the severity of volume depletion. In severe losses, 100 ml/kg body weight is the amount required (10% volume depletion). The initial rehydration should be fast (1000 ml in 15 min) until the pulse is felt. After infusion of 1 to 2 litres, rehydration can be carried out at a slower rate (1000 ml in 30 to 45 min) till BP returns to normal. Patients with severe volume depletion may need 4 to 5 liters of fluids. In patients who can take fluids orally, a change from IV to oral route is made. 5% dextrose solution should never be used for volume depletion as the sole replacement fluid. Oral rehydration therapy is based on the observation that in glucose and salt given orally enhances the initial absorption of salt and water, corrects electrolyte and water deficiency.

Composition of oral rehydration fluid

Ingredient	Quantity
Sodium chloride	3.5 g
Sodium bicarbonate	2.5 g
Potassium chloride	1.5 g
Glucose	20 g
Potable water	1 liter

During the initial stages of oral therapy, an adult can consume up to 750 ml per hour (100 ml/kg within 4 hours). In addition to deficit replacement, maintenance fluid (2 liters per day) should be given and concurrent losses replaced.

Vomiting/nasogastric losses

1. Patients with hypotension should be treated with isotonic saline till shock is corrected.
2. Later, 0.45% saline (half normal saline) is preferred as the sodium content of gastric fluid is low.
3. Potassium replacement has to be given depending on plasma levels.
4. In severe metabolic alkalosis, acidifying agents have to be given (isolyte G).

2. *Fluid therapy in diabetic ketoacidosis:* Patients are severely dehydrated, have high blood glucose and ketone bodies in blood.

1. If patient is in shock, isotonic saline should be used (2 to 3 liters).
2. After shock is corrected; hypotonic (0.45%) saline should be used.
3. Insulin therapy is usually enough to correct the acidosis.
4. Bicarbonate should be given only if acidosis is severe.
5. Potassium supplements should be given monitoring plasma levels once the acidosis is corrected.

3. *Fluid replacement for renal losses*

1. If patient has severe volume depletion, isotonic saline should be used.
2. Later, replacement should be either with 0.45% saline or 50% as isotonic saline and 50% as 5% dextrose for the amount lost.
3. For patient who can take orally, salt can be given, depending on the severity, which can range from 4 to 10 g (1 g = 17 mEq).

HYPONATREMIA

Hyponatremia is defined as a plasma sodium concentration less than 135 mEq/L and is a frequent occurrence in the hospitalized patients. It always means excess water in relation to sodium.

The following must ascertained to evaluate hyponatremia:

1. Is it true or 'pseudohyponatremia'? The most common causes of pseudohyponatremia are hyperlipidemia or when plasma protein concentration is more than 10 g. Such high levels of serum proteins occur in plasma cell dyscrasias. Under normal circumstances, sodium is distributed only in the aqueous phase of serum. In both above conditions, the non-aqueous phase of the serum containing the lipids/abnormal proteins will show reduced serum levels of sodium when examined by 'flame photometry'. If the test is done by 'ion selective' method, accurate sodium levels are obtained.
2. Does the hyponatremia reflect hypotonicity or is it associated with normal or high tonicity? Normally, hyponatremia is associated with hypotonicity. In conditions like hyperglycemia, glucose in the extracellular will draw water out from intracellular space until both the compartments have the same osmolar concentration. The Na^+ concentration drops by 1.6 mEq/L for every 100 mg/dl increase in glucose. This can also occur with mannitol infusion. This is called 'translocational hyponatremia' and the sodium corrects itself when the blood sugar is controlled. Sodium chloride supplementation is needed only if hyponatremia persists in spite of correction of glucose.
3. Having ruled out 'pseudohyponatremia' and 'translocational hyponatremaia', it is confirmed that the hyponatremia is associated with hypotonicity or 'true hyponatremia'.

Hyponatremia is classified depending on the time over which it developed, severity of symptoms and ECF volume status.

1. Acute (<48 hours) vs chronic (>48 hours)
2. Mild (130–134 mEq/L), moderate (120–129 mEq/L), severe (<120 mEq/L)
3. Hypovolemic/euvolemic/hypervolemic

An understanding of brain volume regulation is important to understand the classification based on duration and symptomatology of hyponatremia.

The time lapse required for the brain to expel osmotic moieties discriminates between acute (<48 hr) and chronic (>48 hr) hyponatremia.

Acute Hyponatremia

Acute hyponatremia is usually more symptomatic than chronic hyponatremia.

Acute hyponatremia is characterized by 'hyponatremic encephalopathy' a known consequence of brain swelling due to decrease in extracellular osmolality that favors movement of water into brain cells through aquaporin 1 and aquaporin 4 in astrocytic foot process. It results from insufficient time for brain cells to adapt to the hypotonic environment. Symptoms usually include nausea and vomiting in the earlier stages of cerebral edema followed by seizures and coma from herniation. It is associated with an overall mortality of 38%.

Patients at risk for hyponatremic encephalopathy are those in postoperative period due to inadvertent postoperative administration of hypotonic fluids, menstruating women due to estrogen that downregulates $Na^+/K^+/$ ATPase activity in brain cells—thereby impeding brain adaptive response to hyponatremia and prepubertal children resulting from the discrepancy between skull and brain size that predisposes them to cerebral injury from hyponatremia.

Chronic Hyponatremia

In chronic hyponatremia the adaptive mechanisms are in place and brain edema is curtailed as a result of which patients are usually asymptomatic or paucisymptomatic. Patients with chronic hyponatremia (present >48 hours), exhibit subtle neurocognitive or neuromotor symptoms, including gait disturbances, falls, and concentration deficit. Chronic hyponatremia is also associated with osteoporosis and fractures as a substantial amount of sodium is bound to proteoglycans, which make up the ground substance of bone, connective tissue, and cartilage.

Classification-based on ECF Volume Status

a. *Hyponatremia and decreased ECF volume (hypovolemia):* Volume depletion causes loss of both sodium and water. Signs of hypovolemia include reduced skin turgor (in elderly patients reduced skin turgor in inner aspect of thigh and skin overlying the sternum), dry skin, axilla, tongue and oral mucosa, postural hypotension with dizziness, flat neck veins, elevated BUN creatinine ratio.

b. *Hyponatremia with normal ECF volume (normovolemia):* In this category of hyponatremia, the major clinical manifestations

are due to hypotonicity *per se*. The severity of the clinical picture depends on the rapidity of development of hyponatremia rather than on the level of plasma sodium.

c. *Hyponatremia with increased ECF volume (hypervolemia):* These patients have excess of body fluids often related to cardiac failure, cirrhosis of liver, nephrotic syndrome or renal failure. Its presence is an independent predictor of mortality.

SIADH

SIADH, despite being a common cause euvolemic hyponatremia, is a diagnosis of exclusion. Arginine vasopressin (ADH) is a peptide hormone released from posterior pituitary. The main stimulus for its release is increased plasm osmolality with other non-osmotic stimuli being nausea, postoperative pain and pregnancy. In SIADH, ADH secretion is considered inappropriate as neither hypertonicity nor hypovolemia stimulates its release. This syndrome is now known as syndrome of inappropriate antidiuresis (SIAD).

Etiology of SIADH

a. Carcinoma—lung, duodenum, pancreas
b. Pulmonary disorders—pneumonia, lung abscess, tuberculosis, aspergillosis.
c. CNS disorders—encephalitis, meningitis, stroke, acute psychosis, brain tumor, brain abscess, head trauma, subdural hematoma, Guillain-Barre syndrome.
d. Drugs—SSRI, cyclophosphamide, vincristine, carbamazepine.

Essential Diagnostic Criteria for SIADH

1. Hypotonic hyponatremia (plasma osmolality <270 mOsm/kg of water)
2. Inappropriate antidiuresis, i.e. urine osmolality higher that would be anticipated for the degree of hyponatremia (>100 mOsm/kg of water).
3. Normal adrenal, thyroid, renal and pituitary function.

4. Absence of clinical symptoms of hypo-volemia or generalized edema.
5. Urine sodium >40 mmol/L with normal dietary sodium intake.

The increased ADH secretion in SIADH initially increases total body water by water retention. The increased TBW transiently expands the ECF volume which triggers urinary sodium loss thereby restoring ECF volume to normal and causing further hyponatremia. This explains the euvolemia and absence of edema in SIADH.

Differential Diagnosis

A close differential for hyponatremia in central nervous system disorders is cerebral salt wasting. In this condition the primary defect is salt wasting secondary to release of brain natriuretic peptide that leads to volume depletion and secondary ADH release. It mimics SIADH in all aspects except for signs for volume depletion. The distinction between the two entities are important from a therapeutic point of view.

Treatment of Hyponatremia

Key principles of management
1. Determine the duration of hyponatremia
2. Assess severity of clinical symptoms and decide need for hospitalization.
3. Determine goal rate of correction and avoid overcorrection.
4. Diligent search for underlying etiology.

A. Acute Symptomatic Hyponatremia

If plasma Na is below 130 mEq/L and the patient has CNS symptoms, the best approach is to increase ECF osmolality by administra-tion of hypertonic (3%) saline. The goal of therapy is to rapidly increase the serum sodium by 4 to 6 mEq/ L over a period of a few hours. Hypertonic saline may be administered at the rate of 1 to 5 ml/kg/hour depending on the severity of neurological symptoms for acute hyponatremia. Coadministration of furosemide enhances free water clearance.

B. Chronic Hyponatremia

The maximum rate of correction should be restricted to 8 mEq/L in any 24-hour period. Therapeutic strategies include:
• Hypertonic saline in the event of seizures/isotonic saline for less severe symptoms.
• Coadministration of furosemide
• Water restriction
• Treatment of reversible etiologies
• Demeclocycline, vaptans.

Be wary of osmotic demyelination syndrome (ODS): During correction of chronic hyponatremia, brain cells try to reverse the adaptive process by increasing the production of organic osmolytes and increase the intracellular inorganic ion content but requires time. Risk factors for ODS include serum sodium <105 mEq/L, chronic alcoholism, hypokalemia, malnourished patients. Central pontine myelinosis which is the common type of ODS presents with quadriparesis, pseudobulbar palsy, locked in state.

Treatment: Re-inducing a mild level of hyponatremia within 12–24 hours with desmopressin and hypotonic fluids with 5% dextrose reduces neurological manifestations and decreases mortality in ODS.

C. Hypovolemic Hyponatremia

Treatment involves administration of isotonic sodium solution until volume deficit is corrected. There is usually no need to use hypertonic salt solutions because isotonic saline reverses the pathophysiological factors leading to impaired water excretion.

D. Euvolemic Hyponatremia

SIADH

a. *Restriction of water intake:* Adequate fluid restriction is restriction to an amount less than the urine output and estimated insensible losses, e.g. if a hyponatremic patient has a daily urine output of 500 ml and daily insensible losses of 500 ml daily, restriction to 1000 ml of water daily would prevent further lowering of plasma sodium, while more severe fluid restriction is needed (less than 1000 ml/day) to increase plasma sodium.

b. Isotonic saline should not be used in treatment of SIADH, as it is a source of free water. Hypertonic saline with or without loop diuretic is advocated.

c. *Vaptans:* They are drugs which act on the V2 receptors by directly blocking binding of AVP to its renal receptors. They have the unique ability to induce an aquaresis—the excretion of electrolyte-free water without accompanying solutes.

Conivaptan is a nonselective V1a/V2 receptor antagonist approved for the treatment of euvolemic and hypervolemic hyponatremia. Tolvaptan is the first oral vaptan. They are superior to conventional diuretics in view of less electrolyte abnormalities. Common side effects include thirst, increased daytime urination, dry mouth and hepatotoxicity.

E. Hypervolemic Hyponatremia

a. Water restriction
b. Treatment of underlying cause
c. Diuretics/vaptans

HYPERNATREMIA

Hypernatremia is defined as plasma sodium concentration greater than 150 mEq/L.

Signs and Symptoms

The signs and symptoms of hypernatremia depend upon the degree and rapidity with which it develops. The initial symptoms include lethargy, irritability, tremor, hyperreflexia, ataxia, seizures and may progress to coma. As with hyponatremia, a diagnostic approach is based on a classification on the basis of ECF volume.

A. Hypovolemic Hypernatremia

This may be due to renal or extrarenal water loss. Renal loss occurs when associated with osmotic diuresis as in diabetes mellitus. Hypotonic losses may occur in urine which leads to hypernatremia. Extrarenal losses occur due to excessive sweating and diarrhea in children. The primary therapeutic goal is to administer isotonic saline (0.9%) until restoration of ECF volume is achieved and then hypotonic (0.45%) sodium chloride or 5% dextrose can be used to correct plasma osmolality and sodium.

B. Euvolemic Hypernatremia

These patients suffer primarily from water losses without electrolyte losses. The causes are insensible water loss occurring in hospitalized ill patients who do not receive adequate replacement for insensible losses. Any patient also has primary water loss without electrolyte loss and prolonged sweating and may become hypernatremic. Other causes are diabetes insipidus (DI), both central and nephrogenic. Central DI may be idiopathic (50%), or following trauma, neoplasms or surgical procedures in the region of pituitary.

The common causes of nephrogenic DI are:
1. Chronic renal disease
   a. Chronic interstitial disease
   b. Polycystic kidney disease
   c. Obstructive nephropathy
   d. Medullary cystic disease
2. Drugs
   a. Lithium
   b. Amphotericin
3. Electrolyte disorders
   a. Hypokalemia
   b. Hypercalcemia

Central DI and nephrogenic DI can be differentiated by administering exogenous vasopressin. Since central DI is due to vasopressin deficiency, it will respond to ADH whereas, since the defect is at the level of renal tubule, there will be no response to vasopressin.

These patients must be treated primarily with water replacement either orally or parenterally with 5% dextrose. Free water deficit (in litres) is calculated by the formula:

Free water deficit = 0.6 × body weight (kg) ×
(serum Na/140 − 1)

$$[150 − 140/(140 − 1)] = 10/139 = 0.07$$
$$= 0.6 × 60 × 0.07$$
$$= 2.5 \text{ liters}$$

This deficit should be corrected over 48 hours with a view to reduce serum sodium level no more than 2 mEq/L/hour initially (in emergencies) and not more than 8 mEq/L/day.

C. Hypervolemic Hypernatremia

This is a rare cause of hypernatremia. Those patients who have received excessive amounts of hypertonic saline or sodium bicarbonate infusions as in resuscitation from cardiac arrest are prone to develop hypernatremia with excess ECF volume. Treatment is usually by using diuretics, restricting salt and water and in rare cases, hemofiltration/dialysis.

Disorders of potassium (K⁺): Total body potassium is about 50 mEq/L of body weight or 3000 mEq in a 60 kg person. This is the most abundant intracellular cation and approximately 98% is located within the cells. The normal intracellular concentration of potassium is 150–160 mEq/L, while the extracellular K⁺ is 3.5–5 mEq/L.

HYPOKALEMIA

Hypokalemia is defined as a plasma potassium concentration below 3.5 mEq/L.

The important causes of potassium deficiency are:

a. *Diuretics:* Drugs, osmotic diuresis (diabetes mellitus).
b. *GI losses:* Diarrhea, vomiting, laxatives, surgical drainage.
c. *Renal disease:* Interstitial nephritis, Fanconi syndrome, Bartter's syndrome.
d. *Excess adrenal corticosteroids:* Hyperaldosteronism, excess of glucocorticoids.
e. Metabolic alkalosis
f. *Metabolic acidosis:* Renal tubular acidosis, diuretics and GI losses are the most common cause of hypokalemia.

Clinical Features

Neuromuscular: Gastrointestinal tract dysfunction with hypokalemia can manifest as ileus or constipation. Skeletal muscle abnormality can vary from mild weakness to overt paralysis, with life-threatening respiratory paralysis. Potassium depletion can also predispose to rhabdomyolysis, myoglobinuria and acute kidney injury.

Cardiac: Hypokalemia alters the ECG with flattening of T waves and development of prominent U waves, which may give the impression of a prolonged QT interval. It predisposes to atrial and ventricular ectopic beats. Hypokalemia increases the sensitivity to digitalis and predisposes towards life-threatening arrhythmias.

Renal: The most commonly recognized defect of hypokalemia is an inability to concentrate the urine maximally, resulting in polydipsia and polyuria. Chronic potassium depletion can lead to hypokalemic nephropathy.

Renal ammonia production is stimulated by hypokalemia. This may provoke hepatic encephalopathy in patients with cirrhosis.

Management

Prevention: Patients treated with diuretics should be advised to take adequate dietary potassium (e.g. fruits and vegetables). The serum potassium should be measured regularly and if therapy is prolonged potassium supplements should be prescribed.

Treatment: Hypokalemia is not usually an emergency. Therapy always runs the risk of hyperkalemia.

Oral therapy: The drug of choice is 10% potassium chloride syrup (15 ml = 20 mEq). It is best administered in liquid form and should be diluted in juice and given immediately after meals to minimize gastric irritation.

But if metabolic acidosis occurs in combination with hypokalemia, potassium with bicarbonate or metabolic precursors (gluconate, acetate or citrate) is preferable.

Alternatively, the aldosterone antagonist, spironolactone, can be used to correct hypokalemia. As a general rule the comcomitant administration of potassium supplements and potassium-sparing diuretics should be avoided to prevent hyperkalemia.

Intravenous therapy: If the patient cannot take potassium orally or if hypokalemia is severe parenteral therapy is necessary. The serum potassium level must be known and adequate urine output established before therapy. IV potassium should be rarely given to oliguric patients.

Dosage: Oral potassium, or if necessary, IV administration in dosages of 80–120 mEq/day is usually sufficient.

When IV therapy is employed in a non-urgent situation (K >2.5 mEq/L) the potassium concentration should not exceed 40 mEq/L and the rate of administration should not exceed 10 mEq/hr.

If urgent therapy is required (K <2.0 mEq) potassium can be administered more rapidly but should not exceed 40 mEq/hr. The ECG should be monitored continuously and serum potassium should be checked frequently. For IV use potassium chloride is available as 15% solution (1 cc = 2 mEq) which should be administered in saline (unless contraindicated) rather than dextrose in water, since infusion of glucose-containing fluids may cause serum potassium level to fall further.

Complications
1. Hyperkalemia
2. Ulcers in the small bowel (oral)
3. Phlebitis (IV)

HYPERKALEMIA

Hyperkalemia is defined as a plasma potassium concentration above 5 mEq/L. This is a medical emergency.

Causes

1. *Renal failure:* Hyperkalemia is an important complication of acute kidney injury and later stages of chronic kidney disease.

2. *Mineralocorticoid deficiency:* Addison's disease.
3. *Drugs:* Spironolactone, triamterene, angiotensin converting enzyme inhibitors/angiotensin receptor blocking drugs, nonsteroidal anti-inflammatory drugs.
4. Metabolic acidosis.

While interpreting the result of serum K^+, 'pseudohyperkalemia' should be ruled out. The most common cause is the tourniquet method for drawing blood. Collection errors like a tight tourniquet, repeated fist clenching or exercise and hemolysis of the blood sample may cause elevation of plasma K^+ by as much as 2.7 mEq/L or more. Leukocytosis and thrombocytosis can also elevate K^+. ECG changes may be helpful in differentiating true hyperkalemia from pseudohyperkalemia.

Clinical Features

The most important clinical manifestation of hyperkalemia is its effect on cardiac function. With plasma K^+ concentration less than 6.5 mEq/L the early ECG abnormally is peaking or tenting of the T wave. With the potassium concentration more than 6.5 mEq/L, flattering of the P wave, prolongation of PR interval and widening of QRS complex with development of deep S wave are seen. With severe hyperkalemia (K >8.0 mEq/L), a sine wave pattern develops with imminent ventricular fibrillation or cardiac arrest.

Therapy

If the ECG findings reflect any change attributable to hyperkalemia or if serum K^+ exceeds 6.5 mEq/L, aggressive and prompt therapy should be instituted:

i. *IV calcium gluconate:* 10–30 ml of 10% solution. This acts immediately by antagonizing membrane effect of K^+, but the action lasts only about 30 minutes.

ii. *IV sodium bicarbonate:* 50–150 ml of 7.5% solution.

iii. IV glucose 50 g + regular insulin 10 units. These act within 15–30 minutes, and are effective for several hours. These act by redistributing K^+ from extracellular space to intracellular space.

iv. *Cation exchange resin:* Sodium polystyrene sulfonate (kayexalate). This can be given orally or as an enema.

v. *Calcium polystyrene sulphonate:* 15 g three times a day orally.

vi. *Newer potassium binders:* Patiromer and sodium zirconium cyclosilicate.

Patiromer is a nonabsorbable polymer that binds potassium in exchange for calcium in the distal colon. It is safe and efficacious in CKD patients. Zirconium cyclosilicate is an inorganic sodium/potassium cation exchanger which acts throughout the intestine.

vii. Hemodialysis effectively removes nearly 25–30 mEq of K^+ per hour. If K^+ free dialysate is used, removal can be faster. However, close monitoring is necessary because, fatal hypokalemia may develop while using K^+ free dialysate. Peritoneal dialysis also can remove 10–15 mEq of K^+ per hour.

Approach to Arterial Blood Gas (ABG) Analysis

• A Vimala

Blood gas analysis is a valuable tool to assess ventilation and tissue perfusion. This is only an aid and not a substitute for clinical analysis. Though there are many values in the printout, blood gas analyzer measures only pH, pCO_2 and PO_2. All the other values are calculated and generated using the software in computer. Blood sample should be collected meticulously since any error in collection, storage or transport to the laboratory can alter the blood gas values. The basic procedure is a simple arterial puncture.

Radial artery is the most common site of puncture because of ease of access but should be performed only by experienced personnel. Before puncturing radial artery Allen's test is performed to ensure that collateral blood supply is adequate from ulnar artery. Needle is inserted at point of maximum pulsation just proximal to the proximal transverse skin crease at the wrist.

The other arteries used for puncture are brachial artery and femoral artery. In the case of brachial artery puncture, the needle is inserted medial to the biceps tendon over the point of maximum pulsation. For femoral artery puncture, the needle is introduced at the point of maximum pulsation in mid-inguinal region 2 cm below the inguinal ligament. In neonates, umbilical artery is chosen for puncture.

Samples collected from central vein can be used for finding out mixed venous O_2 saturation in conditions like sepsis syndrome. While drawing blood from peripheral vein for analysis, tourniquet should not be applied and artery should not be compressed.

Certain precautions are necessary for collecting blood sample:

a. Heparin is acidic in pH and it will lower pH of the sample. Therefore, only low strength (1000 U/ml) heparin is used. Ideally, syringe and needle are heparinized by drawing 0.5 ml of heparin into the syringe and is expelled so as to coat the lumen of the syringe and needle. This is to prevent dilution of blood sample with heparin.

b. Glass syringe should be used instead of plastic syringe as plastic syringe is permeable to air.

c. Syringe should get filled spontaneously and not by suction.

d. Presence of air bubbles in the sample, might interfere with PaO_2 values. Hence, care should be taken to avoid air bubbles.

e. Direct contact of blood with atmospheric air is avoided by putting a rubber cap over the needle and bending the needle.

The sample should be transported and processed immediately (<30 minutes). Since blood is a living medium with continuous metabolism, the cells will consume oxygen and produce CO_2. So, any delay in processing may lead to low PaO_2 and high pCO_2. To prevent this, the sample should be stored in ice slush at 4°C. Sample should be shaken well before feeding into the equipment. The values of pH and pCO_2 change with changes in temperature. Normal blood gas values at sea level are shown in Table 45.1 (the values vary slightly in higher altitudes).

If venous sample is used for blood gas analysis, the pH may be the same but PO_2, is lower and pCO_2 and HCO_3 are higher in venous compared to arterial samples.

Explanation of Parameters in the ABG Printout

1. pH

pH is the negative logarithm to the base 10 of H^+ ion concentration. It is expressed in gram ions/L. When the concentration of hydrogen ions increase, the solution becomes more acidic and the pH falls. When the concentration of hydrogen ions decrease, the solution becomes more alkaline and the pH increases. Therefore, pH is inversely proportional to H^+ ions. In a normal person, pH is closely controlled between 7.35 and 7.45. pH is the measured value. To convert pH into H^+ ions, 2 formulae are used. (a) 0.1 pH change rule and (b) 'rule of thumb'.

a. 0.1 change pH rule

pH 7 H^+ ions = 100 nanomoles/L.

For every 0.1 increase in pH, H^+ ions, multiply by 0.8.

pH 7.1 = 100 × 0.8 = 80.

pH 7.2 = 100 × 0.8 × 0.8 = 64

For every 0.1 decrease in pH below 7, multiply 100 by 1.25.

pH 6.9 = 100 × 1.25 = 125

pH 6.8 = 100 × 1.25 × 1.15 = 156

b. Rule of thumb

To convert pH to H^+ ions in the range 7.25–7.55, drop the number seven and subtract from 80. Thus, the approximate nanomole concentration for H^+ ions can be found by subtracting the number in the decimal from 80. This rough rule is applicable within the physiologic range of body pH.

Example, pH 7.34 = (80 – 34 = 46 nanomoles)

7.25 = (80 – 25 = 55 nanomoles)

7.50 = (80 – 50 = 30 nanomoles)

When acids or alkali are added to the body, they are immediately buffered by chemical buffers inside the cells and extracellular compartments. They serve to blunt the changes in pH. The important 'first-line' buffer systems are hemoglobin, proteins, organophosphates and bone apatite. ECF buffers are plasma proteins and HCO_3. The intracellular buffers are proteins, phosphate and hemoglobin. HCO_3 acts as H^+ ion acceptor and H_2CO_3 acts as H^+ ion donor for the buffering actions. The 'second-line' of defense against drastic pH change occur as a result of elimination of CO_2 by the respiratory system. The lungs can eliminate up to 15000 mmols of CO_2 per day. The excretion of acid ions as

Table 45.1: Normal blood gas values at sea level		
	Adults	Neonates
1. Arterial pH	7 .35–7.45	7.4 ± 0.05
2. $PaCO_2$	35–45 mm Hg	35–45 mm Hg
3. HCO_3	22–26 mEq/L	20–28 mEq/L
4. PaO_2	80–100 mm Hg	50–70 mm Hg
5. Base excess	−2 to +2	+ 4 to −4
6. Anion gap	7–14	7–14

titratable acid and ammonium occurs in the kidney. The kidneys are capable of reabsorbing all the filtered bicarbonate and regenerate new bicarbonate but it takes between 48 and 72 hours when an acid–base imbalance occurs. For every H^+ ion eliminated by the body, it gains one HCO_3. Thus, the kidneys regulate concentration of pH through buffering and excretion of acids. In later stages, bone is used up as a buffer. In renal failure there is failure to excrete H^+ ions and continuous accumulation overwhelms the buffering systems resulting in acidosis. The lungs regulate CO_2 by retaining or washing out of CO_2 by hypo- or hyper-ventilation. Hypoventilation and or decreased CO_2 exchange leads to accumulation of pCO_2 and cause respiratory acidosis. Hyper-ventilation leads to wash out of CO_2 and cause respiratory alkalosis.

2. Bicarbonate (HCO_3)

Bicarbonate is produced by the kidneys and acts as an important buffer to maintain normal pH. The normal range for bicarbonate is 22–26 mmol/L. HCO_3 is used to buffer the excess H^+ ions and HCO_3 level will fall. If there is chronic respiratory acidosis, additional bicarbonate is produced by the kidneys to keep the pH within normal range. This is the mechanism for raised bicarbonate level in chronic (type 2) respiratory failure where the pH remains normal despite a raised CO_2.

Actual bicarbonate: In the ABG machine, actual bicarbonate ($aHCO_3$) is calculated using Henderson's equation using the measured pH, pCO_2. This value is dependent on pCO_2 and will be high if pCO_2 is high and vice versa. So, it is necessary to look at the standard bicarbonate.

Standard bicarbonate ($sHCO_3$) is the concentration of bicarbonate in the plasma which is equilibrated with normal $PaCO_2$ of 40 mm Hg, normal PO_2 of 100 mm Hg at normal body temperature of 37 degrees. The $sHCO_3$ thus eliminates the respiratory changes and reflects the metabolic change.

Base excess (BE): Base excess (BE) is the amount of base that needs to be removed to bring the pH to normal when pCO_2 is corrected to 40 mm Hg. It is calculated from $sHCO_3$. The BE is between −2 to +2 under normal circumstances. In acidosis, there is deficiency of base and BE will be ≥2. If the base deficit is −13, it means that the $sHCO_3$ is 11 mmol/L. If BE is reported as +7, it would suggest that the $sHCO_3$ is 31 mmol/L.

3. Partial Pressure of CO_2 (pCO_2)

pCO_2 is the partial pressure of carbon dioxide in blood. It is in the range of 40 +/− 4 mm Hg. pCO_2 is always higher in venous blood. In arterial blood, it increases when there is hypoventilation resulting in CO_2 accumulation and decreases when hyperventilation and carbon dioxide wash out occurs. In acute respiratory disorders, which affect pCO_2 concentration, the renal compensatory mechanism is to change the HCO_3 concentration correspondingly. Since the renal compensation takes time, the change in pH may be considerable in the acute stage and by 48–72 hours, the renal compensation is complete and the change in pH is minimized.

4. Partial Pressure of Oxygen (PaO_2)

PaO_2 is the partial pressure of oxygen in arterial blood.

[PAO_2 (Capital letter 'A' is used for partial pressure of alveolar oxygen) is the term used for denoting the oxygen tension in the alveoli].

FiO_2 is the fraction of O_2 in inspired air and is 21% in normal atmospheric air at sea level. [It increases in those administered oxygen.] SO_2 is the percentage of Hb saturated with O_2.

SpO_2 is the oxygen saturation of hemoglobin measured in the peripheral capillary blood using 'pulse oximeter'. This has many fallacies as this is dependent on the peripheral blood flow and is not part of ABG measurement.

In health, the partial pressure of oxygen in arterial blood (PaO_2) is close to the partial pressure of oxygen in the pulmonary alveoli

(PAO$_2$). (Note: Alveolar oxygen → capital 'A' and arterial oxygen → small 'a'). Normal [A-a] O$_2$ difference in patients on room air is 15 mm Hg. In disease processes affecting the respiratory system, [A-a] O$_2$ gradient varies. In a hypoxic patient, Alveolar to arterial oxygen gradient ([A-a] O$_2$ gradient/difference) is used to differentiate between primary abnormalities in ventilation from diffusion defects. The [A-a] O$_2$ gradient will be normal in primary defects in ventilation.

Respiratory failures are of 2 types

Type 1, the oxygen delivered to the alveoli is not adequately transferred to the blood. There is hypoxia (low PaO$_2$) and nearly normal pCO$_2$ (only in very severe cases of type 1 respiratory failure, the pCO$_2$ may increase) and A-a O$_2$ gradient increased, e.g. pneumonia, pulmonary embolism or ARDS. There is ventilation/perfusion mismatch and the volume of air moving in and out of the alveoli is not matched with the flow of blood in the lung.

Example: If PAO$_2$ is 98 mm Hg and PaO$_2$ is 65 mm Hg [A-a], O$_2$ difference is 98–65 = 33. This suggests that although oxygen is delivered to the alveoli, it does not oxygenate the blood and indicates a defect in diffusion. If PaO$_2$ is less than 50 mmHg, and [A-a] O$_2$ gradient increased, diffusion defect is likely.

Type 2 respiratory failure is caused by inadequate alveolar ventilation and is characterized by hypoxia (low PaO$_2$) and hypercarbia (high pCO$_2$). Because of this, the alveolar oxygen and arterial oxygen are low, and carbon dioxide is also not removed resulting in retention of CO$_2$. There is no diffusion defect since whatever oxygen is present in the alveoli is being taken up and the A-a oxygen difference is normal (<15). This can occur in chronic obstructive pulmonary disease, suffocation, respiratory paralysis/exhaustion, brainstem lesions/motor neuron disease/Guillian-Barré syndrome, opioid poisoning, severe chest wall deformities or even extreme obesity.

Example: If PAO$_2$ is 70 mm Hg, and PaO$_2$ is 65 mm Hg, the gradient is within normal limits (70–65 = 5 mm Hg). The cause is defective ventilation.

---

5. Lactate

Lactate is produced as a by-product of anaerobic respiration. A raised lactate can be caused by any process which causes tissue to use anaerobic respiration and is a good indicator of poor tissue perfusion.

6. Base Excess (BE)

This is the amount of strong base which would need to be added or subtracted from a substance in order to return the pH to normal (7.40). A value outside of the normal range (–2 to +2 mEq/L) suggests a metabolic cause for the acidosis or alkalosis. 25% of buffer base is constituted by Hb, 50% by HCO$_3$ and 25% by proteins, phosphate, sulfate. In terms of interpretation, base excess more than +2 mEq/L indicates metabolic alkalosis and base excess less than –2 mEq/L indicates metabolic acidosis.

7. Anion Gap (AG)

Total anions and cations in the body are equal and thus the electrical neutrality is maintained. Cations (positively charged) in ECF are mainly sodium. Other cations are potassium, calcium, magnesium and lithium (in patients taking treatment). Anions (negative charge) in ECF include mainly chloride and bicarbonate. Many unmeasured anions like lactate, ketone, phosphate, sulphate and organic anions are also present in blood (Fig. 45.1). For calculation of anion gap (AG), only sodium as a measured cation and chloride and bicarbonate as measured anions are considered in the calculation. Thus, there appears to be a 'gap' between the two, which is the difference between unmeasured anions and unmeasured

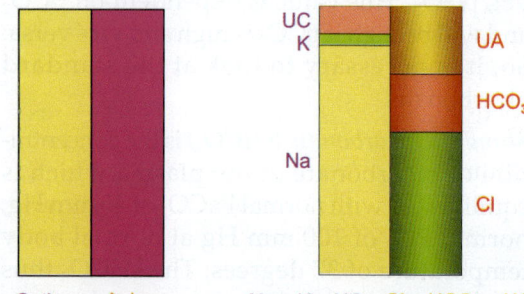

Cations = Anions   Na + K + UC = Cl + HCO$_3$ + UA

Fig. 45.1: Anions and cations in blood

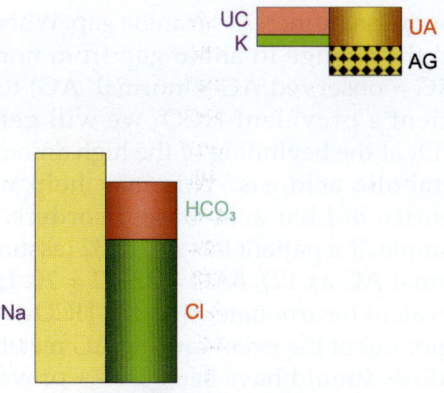

Fig. 45.2: Showing anions gap

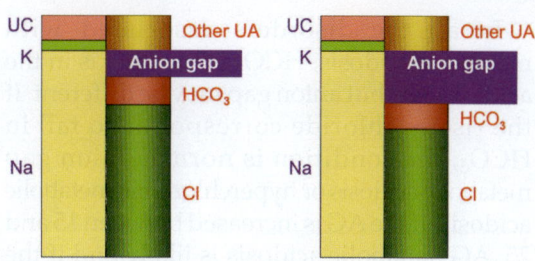

Fig. 45.3: Showing normal anion gap (Left) and high anion gap metabolic acidosis (right). *Note:* In normal anion gap metabolic acidosis, the HCO₃ level is reduced and this is compensated by increase in chloride. In high anion gap metabolic acidosis, the HCO₃ is reduced, anion gap high, and chloride is normal

cations. This is computed as AG and equals the difference between $Na - (Cl + HCO_3)$ (Fig. 45.2). Since there are more unmeasured anions than cations AG in blood is always a positive (12 ± 3 mmol/L).

Anion Gap: Normal Value(s) and Interpretation

The normal value for anion gap with the equation $(AG) = Na - (Cl + HCO_3)$ is 12 ± 3. Generally, Na and Cl are measured by ion specific electrodes and HCO_3 obtained from arterial blood gas analysis. If the HCO_3 is estimated from venous blood, the value of total CO_2 content (tCO_2) is about 1–3 mmol/L higher than estimated HCO_3. Therefore when tCO_2 is used in the equation instead of HCO_3 the normal anion gap for that patient is 9 ± 3 mmol/L. Since albumin is negatively charged ion, AG depends on albumin concentration as well. Thus, for every drop of albumin of 1.0 g/dl below the normal 4.5 g/dl will reduce AG by 2.5 mmol/L. Thus, if the serum albumin is 3.0 g/dl, normal anion gap is assumed to be $12 - (1.5 \times 2.5) = (12 - 3.75) = 8.25$. If serum albumin is 2.5 g% and observed AG = 20, the corrected AG = $20 + (2 \times 2.5) = 25$. In other words, in a patient with serum albumin of 2.5 g%, normal anion gap is assumed to be $12 - [2 \text{ mmol/L} \times (4.5 \text{ g} - 2.5 \text{ g})] = 12 - (2.5 \times 2) = 9$.

The concept of anion gap helps us in probing the mechanism of generation of metabolic acidosis (Fig. 45.3). Whenever an endogenous acid like keto acid, lactic acid, uremic organic acids or exogenous acid like methanol (which gets converted in humans to formic acid) is added to plasma, the H⁺ ions in the acid titrates the bicarbonate down and the corresponding anion remains in plasma as an unmeasured anion. The bicarbonate is used up and cause 'high anion gap' metabolic acidosis. The chloride levels remain unchanged. Thus, high anion gap metabolic acidosis implies existence of an acid with an anion other than chloride.

(UA = unmeasured anion, UC = unmeasured cation, AG = anion gap)

On the other hand, in situations like HCO₃ depletion as in gut HCO₃ wasting (diarrhea) or renal HCO₃ wasting (proximal RTA), the bicarbonate compartment shrinks and the chloride compartment increases proportionately. When large amounts of ammonium chloride is ingested, it produces systemic acidosis and the H⁺ titrates HCO₃ down and chloride is added to plasma. In both the above situations, one chloride is gained for every HCO₃ lost. Thus, the AG remains intact. There is a proportionate increase of chloride for the drop in HCO₃. The normal AG metabolic acidosis is 'hyperchloremic'.

In all the disorders associated with metabolic acidosis, HCO_3 is low, pH is in the acidic range, but anion gap may be different. If the rise in chloride corresponds to fall in HCO_3, the condition is normal anion gap metabolic acidosis or hyperchloremic metabolic acidosis. If the AG is increased between 15 and 25, AG metabolic acidosis is likely and if the AG is over 25, high AG metabolic acidosis is surely present.

If increased anion gap is present, the relationship between the increase in the anion gap and the decrease in $[HCO_3^-]$ is assessed. For each millimole of acid added, one millimole of HCO_3 is used up in buffering. However, *in vivo*, about 50% of buffering occurs intracellularly and the change in AG is not exactly equal to the change in HCO_3. Difference in the AG is represented as 'delta' AG (δAG) and the difference in bicarbonate represented is represented as delta HCO_3 (δHCO_3).

δAG = Observed AG – normal AG.

δHCO_3 = Normal HCO_3 – observed HCO_3.

The ratio of delta anion gap (δAG) to the delta bicarbonate (δHCO_3) helps to differentiate between uncomplicated high AG metabolic acidosis from non-AG metabolic acidosis and associated metabolic alkalosis. Examples:

i. δAG/$\delta HCO_3 \rightarrow 1.0$ to 2.0 = Uncomplicated AG metabolic acidosis.

ii. δAG/$\delta HCO_3 \rightarrow <1$ = Non-AG metabolic acidosis.

iii. δAG/$\delta HCO_3 \rightarrow >2$ = Coexisting metabolic alkalosis.

Assuming normal AG of 12, AG of 17–25 mmol/L is suggestive of high anion gap metabolic acidosis and values over 25 are confirmatory. If the anion gap is more than 25, irrespective of pH and HCO_3, one can be certain that high anion gap metabolic acidosis exists. The increase in anion gap is due to unmeasured excess acid anions in serum. The H^+ of the corresponding anion would have titrated the HCO_3 down. This would mean that in a case of high anion gap metabolic acidosis, for every drop in HCO_3 there is a proportionate increase in anion gap. When we add the change in anion gap from normal (δAG = observed AG – 'normal' AG) to the patient's prevalent HCO_3 we will get the HCO_3 at the beginning of the high anion gap metabolic acidosis. This may help us to identify hidden acid–base disorders. For example, if a patient has AG of 32 (assuming normal AG as 12), δAG = 32–12 = 20. If the prevalent bicarbonate is 10, the HCO_3 at the beginning of the event causing AG metabolic acidosis should have been δAG + prevalent HCO_3 (20 + 10 = 30) which would suggest metabolic alkalosis.

Conditions causing high AG are more common (Table 45.2) compared to those causing low serum AG (Table 45.3).

In a patient with high AG, if obvious causes like diabetic ketoacidosis, lactic acidosis or renal failure are not present, toxic ingestion should be suspected. In such situations, calculation of osmolal gap helps to differentiate between the two. Osmolality is measured by an instrument called 'osmometer' which finds the actual osmolality of liquids from the freezing point. The calculated osmolality depends on the blood/urine levels of certain electrolytes.

Osmolal gap = measured osmolality – calculated osmolality [2 (Na^+) + glucose/18 + BUN/2.8].

Normally, the osmolal gap should be <10. For example, if the measured osmolality is 310 and calculated osmolality is 280, osmolal gap is 30 and presence of toxins like methyl alcohol should be suspected.

Table 45.2: Disorders associated with high serum anion gap

Mnemonic: **KUSMALE**

K—Ketoacidosis (diabetic/starvation)
U—Uremia
S—Salicylates
M—Methanol
A—Alcohol
L—Lactic acidosis
E—Ethylene glycol

Table 45.3: Disorders associated with low serum anion gap

Cause	Comments
Laboratory error	Most frequent cause
Hypoalbuminemia	common cause of low serum anion gap (apply corrections)
Multiple myeloma	Correlates with severity of hyperglobulinemia (positively charged paraprotein)
Halide intoxication	Depends on serum halide concentration (bromide, lithium, iodide). Low anion gap with lithium ≥4 mEq/L (patients on lithium treatment)
Hypercalcemia	Common in hypercalcemia associated with hyperparathyroidism
Polymyxin B	Depends on serum level
Underestimation of serum sodium	Most frequent with hypernatremia or hypertriglyceridemia
Overestimation of serum chloride	Rare with ion selective electrodes

Classification of ABG Abnormalities

Based on abnormalities of pH, ABG abnormalities are classified into acidosis and alkalosis. If the primary event is metabolic or respiratory, it can be labeled respectively as metabolic and respiratory. Thus, there can be four primary acid–base disorders. If the primary abnormality is in pCO_2, and it can due to respiratory causes either be respiratory acidosis or respiratory alkalosis. If the change is mainly HCO_3, a metabolic abnormality either metabolic acidosis or metabolic alkalosis is the primary cause. In special situations, two or three independent acid–base disorders may coexist. Metabolic acidosis with respiratory alkalosis is the most common mixed acid–base abnormality seen in ICU setting. Metabolic acidosis with increased anion gap can coexist with non-anion gap acidosis ('hybrid' metabolic acidosis). Metabolic acidosis can be combined with metabolic alkalosis as in diabetic ketoacidosis or uremic acidosis associated with vomiting.

ASSESSMENT OF ACID–BASE DISORDER AND INTERPRETATION OF ABG

It is necessary to identify the primary acid–base disorder in order to understand the severity of the underlying pathophysiologic mechanisms and guide the treatment. Although the body can tolerate variations in pH to some extent, extreme levels may be fatal (Table 45.4).

Interpretation of ABG

While interpreting the ABG, a systematic approach is needed. It can be approached in numerous ways. It is advisable that one familiarizes oneself with one method and follow the same systematically. In this chapter, the approach is simplified into essentially 7 steps.

Step 1: Clinical assessment.

Step 2: Understand working formula for anlaysis.

Step 3: Is the pH normal δ or is academia or alkalemia present δ?

Step 4: Identify the primary acid–base disorder.

Table 45.4: Significance of pH changes

pH range	Disorder	Significance	Remarks
7.35 to 7.45	Normal	May also indicate mixed disorder	
7.34 to 7.1	Acidemia	Treat primary condition	Bicarbonate correction not always required
7 to 7.1	Severe acidemia	Correct pH to 7.1	Correction with bicarbonate in metabolic acidosis
<7.0	Severe acidemia	Urgent correction	Can be fatal
7.46–7.69	Alkalemia	Clinically important	
>7.7	Severe alkalemia		Can be fatal

Step 5: What is the appropriate response to the primary event?

Step 6: Is the secondary response is as expected, more or less?

Step 7: Identify mixed acid–base disorders.

Step 1: Clinical assessment is of paramount importance and ABG should be interpreted only with the clinical background. A proper clinical assessment will include detailed history, physical examination and preliminary investigations. Most of the interpretations on ABG are made based on the clinical background.

Step 2: Working formula for ABG analysis: pH, HCO_3/pCO_2.

The working formula is a simplification of the basic Henderson-Hasselbach equation as follows:

$$pH = pK + \log(\text{base}/\text{acid}) \text{ where}$$
$$HCO_3 \text{ is the base and}$$
$$H_2CO_3 \text{ (carbonic acid)}.$$
$$H_2CO_3 \rightarrow H_2O + CO_2$$
$$CO_2 \text{ is measurable as } pCO_2$$
$$\text{Therefore, } H_2CO_3 = 0.03 \times pCO_2$$
$$pH = pK + \log HCO_3/(0.03 \times pCO_2)$$

By removing the constants (pK, log sign and 0.03) and substituting equal to (=) sign by proportional to (α) sign, we can derive the following formula:

$$pH \propto CO_3/pCO_2$$

Step 3: Is the "pH" normal? Is there alkalemia or acidemia? [Acidemia means 'acid content' and alkalemia means 'alkali content' in blood beyond normal range.]

Normal pH ranges from 7.35 to 7.45. If the pH is <7.35, it suggests acidemia and if it is >7.45 alkalemia. Normal pH may indicate either 'normal acid–base status' or a 'mixed' acid–base disorder. The term acidosis or alkalosis represents the disease condition/situation causing acidemia or alkalemia. Combination of acid–base abnormalities may be present even if the pH is in the normal range of 7.35–7.45.

However, pH alone should not be considered while interpreting the ABG.

Example 1. pH = 7.4, HCO_3 = 12 mmol/L, pCO_2 = 60 mm Hg.

Interpretation of pH alone shows that the pH is normal. If we analyze the pCO_2 (60 mm Hg—very high) and HCO_3 (12 mmol/L—very low), both are grossly abnormal both suggesting acid–base disorder (mixed).

Step 4: Identify the primary acid–base disorder.

Three parameters pH, HCO_3 and pCO_2 are considered initially for interpreting an acid base disorder.

When the pH increases (alkalemia), if the HCO_3 (numerator) also increases, the disorder is primarily metabolic (because of increase in HCO_3) and alkalosis (because pH increases). In other words, when there is a primary increase in HCO_3, the pH will increase and primary decrease in HCO_3 decreases the pH. If the pH increase is accompanied by a fall in pCO_2 (denominator) the disorder is primarily respiratory (because pCO_2 falls) and alkalosis (because pH increases). Similarly, when the pCO_2 increases (accumulation of CO_2), the pH will fall suggesting respiratory acidosis.

Thus, the ratio of bicarbonate to pCO_2 determines the acid–base status. There are 4 primary acid–base disorders. Diagnosis of simple acid–base disorder based on pH is given in Table 45.5.

Step 5: What is the response of the body to a primary acid–base disorder?

When the offending disorder has exhausted the capacity of the buffer systems, the second line of defense comes into play to prevent excessive deviation of pH from normal. This 'secondary' response aims to counterbalance the primary change and causes the opposite effect on pH.

In any fraction, if the numerator and denominator change correspondingly (in the same direction), the change in value of the fraction will be only minimal. In the case of the equation pH HCO_3/pCO_2, if the numerator

Table 45.5: The initial change in parameters in primary acid–base disorders

Disorder	pH	pCO2	HCO3
Respiratory acidosis	Decreased	Increased	
Respiratory alkalosis	Increased	Decreased	
Metabolic acidosis	Decreased		Decreased
Metabolic alkalosis	Increased		Increased

(HCO3) and denominator (pCO2) move in the same direction, the change in pH is minimized. For example, if the HCO3 has decreased and pCO2 has also decreased, the impact on pH may be lesser. This is the basis for the secondary response. The body elicits a secondary response to a primary acid–base event by altering the numerator or denominator of the formula correspondingly (Table 45.6).

It is important to understand 'magnitude of secondary response' to a given primary acid–base disorder. For any change in the parameter of primary change, there is a proportionate and predictable change in its counterpart. Magnitude of this change varies between 'metabolic' vs 'respiratory' acid–base disorders, as well as between 'acute' vs 'chronic' disorders. Hence, the next step is to assess whether the 'secondary' response is appropriate and

adequate. There is a limit to which the secondary response could occur.

Step 6: Is the secondary response is as expected, more or less?

For every primary response, there is a secondary change within a certain range. Table 45.7 summarises the range of expected change to a primary acid–base response.

In metabolic acidosis, the primary event is drop in bicarbonate and secondary response is drop in pCO2 of about 1–1.5 times the drop in HCO3.

Example 2: pH: 7.27, HCO3: 12 mmol/L and pCO2: 27 mm Hg.

The pH is in the acidic range (7.27), and low HCO3 (12) explains the change in pH. This is metabolic acidosis. Note that pCO2 is low in this report. If low pCO2 were the primary event we would have expected a rise in pH.

Table 45.6: Secondary response to a primary acid–base event

Primary disorder	Primary event response	'Secondary' and change	Secondary event and change
a. Metabolic acidosis	HCO3↓	Respiratory alkalosis	pCO2↓
b. Metabolic alkalosis	HCO3↑	Respiratory acidosis	pCO2↑
c. Respiratory acidosis	pCO2↑	Metabolic alkalosis	HCO3↑
d. Respiratory alkalosis	pCO2↓	Metabolic acidosis	HCO3↓

Table 45.7: Expected change to a primary acid–base disorder

Disorder	pH	HCO3	pCO2	Expected change (δ = 'Delta' = deviation from normal)
Metabolic acidosis	↓	↓ (primary)	↓ (secondary)	$\delta pCO_2 = \delta HCO_3 \times 1{-}1.5$
Respiratory acidosis	↓	↑ (secondary)	↑ (primary)	$\delta HCO_3 = \delta pCO_2 \times 0.1$ (acute)
				$\delta HCO_3 = \delta pCO_2 \times 0.4$ (chronic)
Metabolic alkalosis	↑	↑ (primary)	↑ (secondary)	$\delta pCO_2 = \delta HCO_3 \times 0.25{-}1.0$
Respiratory alkalosis	↑	↓ (secondary)	↓ (primary)	$\delta HCO_3 = \delta pCO_2 \times 0.1$ (acute)
				$\delta HCO_3 = \delta pCO_2 \times 0.4$ (chronic)

Therefore low pCO_2 does not explain the pH change and is a secondary response. Therefore, the disorder is primarily metabolic acidosis with attempt to compensation by respiratory alkalosis.

Is the compensation adequate/more or less?

To find this, we use the formula $\delta pCO_2 = \delta HCO_3 \times 1\text{-}1.5$ which says, the change in pCO_2 should be 1 to 1.5 times the change in HCO_3. Here, the change is HCO_3 is $24 - 12 = 12$. So, the change in pCO_2 should be between 12 and 18 or between 40–12 and 40–18 or between 22 and 28 mm Hg. Here, it is 28. Therefore, the compensation is adequate.

There is another method to calculate the expected pCO_2 in a patient with metabolic acidosis. If 15 is added to the prevailing HCO_3, we get the expected pCO_2. Therefore, the expected pCO_2 in this case will be $12 + 15 = 27$.

Example 3: pH: 7.30, HCO_3: 30 mmol/L and pCO_2: 60 mm Hg.

The fall in pH (7.3) to acidotic range is explained by the rise in pCO_2 to 60 mm Hg. If high bicarbonate (30) was the primary event, it should have increased the pH. So, the primary event is high pCO_2 caused by respiratory acidosis. The high bicarbonate is due to secondary metabolic alkalosis by renal alkali retention in an attempt to offset major change in the pH.

Is the secondary response/compensation appropriate?

In respiratory acidosis, the expected change is $\delta HCO_3 = \delta pCO_2 \times 0.1$ (acute) and $\delta HCO_3 = \delta pCO_2 \times 0.4$ (chronic). Therefore, in the acute setting, for every 10 mm Hg rise in pCO_2 rise in HCO_3 is just 1 mmol/L. Since the kidney takes about 3–5 days to reach its maximal secondary response, in chronic respiratory acidosis, there is up to 4 mmol/L rise of HCO_3 for every 10 mm Hg rise of pCO_2.

Here, the $\delta pCO_2 = 60 - 40 = 20$ and the expected δHCO_3 should be in the range of 8 (HCO_3 $24 + 8 = 32$). The value is close to the expected range considering chronic respiratory acidosis. However, it is more than the expected compensation for acute respiratory acidosis and may suggest a combined respiratory acidosis and metabolic alkalosis.

This example also explains the importance and need for history regarding onset of illness before interpreting the results. The combination of respiratory acidosis and metabolic alkalosis could occur in patients with chronic obstructive pulmonary disease when they develop superadded metabolic events like vomiting or diuretic use.

Example 4: pH: 7.49, HCO_3: 34 mmol/L and pCO_2: 45 mm Hg.

The pH in alkaline range (7.49) is well explained by the high HCO_3 (34 mmol/L), but not by the high pCO_2 and so, metabolic alkalosis is the primary event. The secondary response is rise in pCO_2 by hypoventilation.

Is the secondary response/compensation appropriate?

In metabolic alkalosis for every 1 mmol/L rise of HCO_3 there will be 0.25–1.0 mm Hg rise in pCO_2 or $\delta pCO_2 = \delta HCO_3 \times 0.25\text{-}1.0$. Here, the δHCO_3 is $34 - 24 = 10$. The expected δpCO_2 should be between 2.5 and 10 or pCO_2 should be in the range of 42.5 to 50. Here, the value is 45 mm Hg and is within normal range. Therefore, the secondary response is adequate and appropriate.

Example 5: pH: 7.49, HCO_3: 22 mmol/L and pCO_2: 30 mm Hg.

The pH in the alkaline range (7.49) is well explained by the low pCO_2 but not by the low HCO_3. Therefore, this is respiratory alkalosis and low HCO_3 is the 'secondary' response.

Is the secondary response/compensation appropriate?

In respiratory alkalosis, the expected change is $\delta HCO_3 = \delta pCO_2 \times 0.2$ (acute) and $\delta HCO_3 = \delta pCO_2 \times 0.4$ (chronic). Therefore, in the acute setting, for every 10 mm Hg fall in pCO_2, the HCO_3 falls by 2 mmol/L and in chronic, there is up to 4 mmol/L fall. Here, the δpCO_2 is 10 and the fall in HCO_3 should be between 2 and 4 mmol/L, i.e. HCO_3 should be between 20 and 22. Therefore, the response is adequate and appropriate.

These figures are only approximate, and may vary in a given case. It is evident from Table 45.7 that, in 'metabolic' acidosis or alkalosis, the secondary response is very energetic, whereas in 'respiratory' acidosis or alkalosis secondary response lags behind. This is because the lung has enormous functional reserve and smartly 'overworks'. Note that in the examples 2–5 above, the numerator [HCO_3] and denominator [pCO_2] have moved in the same direction.

Step 7: Identify mixed acid–base disorders: Combinations of two or three acid–base disorders, in the same patient constitute 'mixed' acid–base disorders. Double disorders are common, triple disorders are not as frequent. Respiratory acidosis and alkalosis cannot co-exist in the same patient at the same time. However, disorders with high anion gap metabolic acidosis with non-anion gap metabolic acidosis may occur in combination with other types. Double disorders may be of various types. Combinations of acidosis both metabolic and respiratory as well as combinations of alkalosis both metabolic and respiratory are dangerous, because this combination causes profound shift of pH.

One of the easiest ways to identify mixed acid–base disorders is to see whether the numerator and denominator in the equation have moved in opposite directions. If it has occurred, invariably there will be more than one disorder.

Example 6: pH: 7.18, HCO_3: 16 mmol/L and pCO_2: 50 mm Hg.

Here, the pH is acidic (7.18) and both low HCO_3 (16 mmol/L) and high pCO_2 (50 mm Hg) could explain the pH change. Note that the numerator and denominator have moved in different directions [numerator (HCO_3) downwards and denominator (pCO_2) upwards]. Therefore, this represents a combination of metabolic and respiratory acidosis. Such a combination occurs in patients with sepsis, diabetic ketoacidosis or uremic acidosis with respiratory failure.

Example 7: pH: 7.60, HCO_3: 30 mmol/L and pCO_2: 31 mm Hg.

The pH in alkaline range (7.6) is explained by both high HCO_3 (30 mmol/L) and low pCO_2 (31 mm Hg). Here also, the numerator and denominator have moved in opposite directions, numerator upwards and denominator downwards. So, it is a combination of metabolic alkalosis and respiratory alkalosis.

In some cases, HCO_3 and pCO_2 will be abnormal with pH being normal. In such cases, in order to identify the primary acid–base disorder it is essential to critically assess the quantity of change of both HCO_3 and pCO_2 from normal and figure out whether the primary disorder is 'metabolic' or 'respiratory' by ascertaining in which argument is the magnitude of secondary response fitting appropriately.

Example 8: pH: 7.38, HCO_3: 28 mmol/L, pCO_2: 50 mm Hg.

In this example, the pH is within normal range (7.38). But the HCO_3 is high (28 mmol/L) and pCO_2 is also high (48 mm Hg). This could be respiratory acidosis compensated by metabolic alkalosis, or metabolic alkalosis well compensated by respiratory acidosis or combination of independent disorders.

Firstly, assuming that the primary event is metabolic alkalosis with increase of HCO_3 by 4, the expected secondary response is a rise in pCO_2 by 4 to 6 mm Hg. So, the pCO_2 should have been 44–46 mm Hg. The observed pCO_2 is 50, above the anticipated value. Now, if we assume that the primary event to be respiratory acidosis, the pCO_2 has gone up by 8 mm Hg. The expected rise in HCO_3 is 4 and HCO_3 is 28. Thus, the interpretation as primary respiratory acidosis with 'compensatory' metabolic alkalosis is more appropriate. The clinical presentation will provide the guide correct diagnosis.

Example 9: pH: 7.42, HCO_3: 18 mmol/L and pCO_2: 25 mm Hg.

In this example, the pH is normal and both HCO_3 and pCO_2 are low. This could be either metabolic acidosis or respiratory alkalosis or a combination. Now, if we consider that this is predominantly a metabolic acidosis, in which HCO_3 has come down by around 6 mmol/L (from a normal of 24 mmol/L) and you would expect pCO_2 to have come down by around 6–9 mm Hg to around 31 to 34 mm Hg (from a normal of 40 mm Hg). However, the observed pCO_2 is 25 and is below the anticipated value. If we consider the primary event as respiratory alkalosis, pCO_2 has come down by around 15 mm Hg (40–25 mm Hg)/ The expected fall in HCO_3 will be around 5 mmol/L (15 × 4/10 = 6) to 18 mmol/L. Thus, primary respiratory alkalosis with compensation by metabolic acidosis or primary respiratory alkalosis with associated trivial primary metabolic acidosis appears appropriate. This combination can occur in salicylate overdose, where salicylate causes metabolic acidosis and stimulation of respiratory center will cause respiratory alkalosis. A similar situation can occur in pneumonia and sepsis. The clinical scenario will help to settle the issue.

Triple or complex acid–base disorders are combinations of metabolic acidosis, metabolic alkalosis with either respiratory acidosis or alkalosis. Common clues to the presence of a hidden third acid–base disorder in such a setting include presence of a very high anion gap or elevated HCO_3 or a more than anticipated secondary response.

Example 10: pH: 7.32, HCO_3: 16 mmol/L, pCO_2: 36 mm Hg, anion gap: 24.

In this example, pH in acidic range is explained by low bicarbonate but not low pCO_2. So, we will assume the primary disorder as metabolic acidosis and minimal attempt to compensation by respiratory alkalosis. The AG is 24 and is high. The δAG is 12 and δHCO_3 is 8 and the 'δ ratio' is 1.5 (*see* page 401 on anion gap earlier in this chapter). So, the above result suggests uncomplicated AG metabolic acidosis. There is feeble compensation by respiratory alkalosis.

Example 11: pH: 7.30, HCO_3: 16 mm Hg, pCO_2: 32 mm Hg, Na: 140 mmol/L, chloride: 110 mEq/L, anion gap: 14 (serum albumin 4.5 g%).

In this example, metabolic acidosis with respiratory compensation can be inferred easily. The anion gap is 14 (normal). The δAG is 2 and δHCO_3 is 8 and the 'δ ratio' is 0.25. Since the ratio is <1, the condition is non-AG metabolic acidosis. (Note that the AG will be more when serum albumin levels decrease. For every gram reduction in albumin from 4.5 g%, the AG increases by 2.5.)

Example 12: pH: 7.20, HCO_3: 8 mmol/L, pCO_2: 26 mm Hg, anion gap: 20.

In this example also, the presence of metabolic acidosis (pH: 7.23 and HCO_3: 8 mmol/L) with respiratory compensation (pCO_2: 26 mm Hg) can be inferred easily. The AG is 20 and δAG is 8. If it was purely AG metabolic acidosis, the prevalent HCO_3 should have been less by only 8 mmol/L and should have been in the range of 16 mmol/L. Since it is only 8 mmol/L, additional non-AG metabolic acidosis may be coexisting.

Example 13: pH = 7.44, pCO_2 = 12, HCO_3 = 8, AG = 38.

The pH is in towards alkaline side of normal range and both HCO_3 and pCO_2 are grossly abnormal. So, there is a mixed acid base disorder. Since AG is 38, metabolic acidosis is present. δAG is 38–12 = 26 and prevailing HCO_3 is 8 mmol/L. Therefore, the HCO_3 at the time of the event causing metabolic acidosis should have been 26 + 8 = 34 mmol/L suggesting metabolic alkalosis. Moreover, δAG is 26 and δHCO_3 is 34–24 = 10 and the 'δ ratio' is 26:10 (>2) suggesting coexisting metabolic alkalosis. The expected pCO_2 when the prevalent HCO_3 is 8 [normal (24 mmol/L), prevalent HCO_3 (8 mmol/L) = 16 × 1 to 1.5] or between 20 and 24. Here, it is 12 mm Hg suggesting additional respiratory alkalosis.

Thus, there are 3 acid–base disorders in this example, pre-existing metabolic alkalosis, AG metabolic acidosis and respiratory alkalosis. The clinical scenario would be a patient:

a. On nasogastric suction, developing metabolic alkalosis (due to acid loss) [pH: 7.49, HCO_3^- 32, pCO_2: 45, AG: 12].

b. Developing septic shock and AG metabolic acidosis (lactic acidosis) [pH: 7.2, HCO_3: 10, pCO_2: 24, AG: 36].

c. Developing endotoxemia and respiratory alkalosis [pH: 7.44, HCO_3: 8, pCO_2: 12, AG: 38].

Potassium abnormalities are common in acid–base disorders. K shifts from ICF to ECF during acidosis and may cause hyperkalemia. A normal K with severe acidosis suggests K depletion and needs to be followed up closely because shift of K back to ICF can lead to life-threatening hypokalemia during correction of acidosis. This is important during correction of diabetic ketoacidosis. Metabolic alkalosis is often associated with hypokalemia. Interestingly, in metabolic alkalosis, the configuration of albumin molecule is altered. This increases its negative charges so that there is an increase in 'normal' anion gap up to 5 mEq/L. Therefore, a high AG is of no consequence in metabolic alkalosis unless patient has associated metabolic acidosis.

Some typical clinical scenarios of combinations of mixed acid–base disorders are given in Table 45.8.

Metabolic acidosis: Some important causes of metabolic acidosis are given in Table 45.9.

Metabolic alkalosis: Loss of hydrochloric acid from stomach (vomiting/nasogastric suction) or loss of chloride through kidney (diuretic use/mineralocorticoid excess) results in metabolic alkalosis. If the kidneys are normal, they respond by excreting bicarbonate and conserving chloride. If urinary chloride is <10 mmol/L in a patient with metabolic alkalosis, it suggests extrarenal loss of chloride loss or remote diuretic use. Patients are volume depleted, and alkalosis responds to sodium chloride infusion. It is called chloride responsive metabolic alkalosis. In some conditions, metabolic alkalosis results from renal chloride wasting. These conditions are often associated with volume expansion and alkalosis is not easily corrected with chloride replacement. These patients are categorized as chloride resistant metabolic alkalosis. Patients with Bartter's syndrome have ongoing renal chloride leak, are often volume depleted, but replacing chloride does not improve alkalosis. Some common causes of metabolic alkalosis are shown in Table 45.10.

Treatment of acid–base disorders: Very often, acid–base disorders do not require any specific treatment other than treatment of the underlying condition. Presence of an acid–base disorder as part of systemic disease generally indicates its severity and special

Table 45.8: Some scenarios of mixed acid–base disorders	
Mixed metabolic disturbance	*Examples of combination of clinical diosrders*
Metabolic acidosis + respiratory acidosis	Septic shock* + chronic obstructive pulmonary disease (COPD)
	Diabetic ketoacidosis (DKA) + COPD
Metabolic alkalosis + respiratory alkalosis	Severe vomiting + high fever#, hyperemesis gravidarum
Metabolic acidosis + respiratory alkalosis	Pneumonia with septic shock*, salicylate overdosage
Metabolic alkalosis + respiratory acidosis	Diuretic use + COPD, vomiting + COPD
Metabolic acidosis + metab.alkalosis	Uremic acidosis + vomiting, DKA + vomiting
Metabolic alkalosis + metabolic acidosis	Endotoxemia# + NG suction + septic shock*
+ Respiratory alkalosis	Salicylate overdosage with vomiting

*Due to associated lactic acidosis; #Fever and endotoxemia produce hyperventilation.

Table 45.9: Common causes of metabolic acidosis

High anion gap metabolic acidosis	Conditions
Endogenous acids	Ketoacidosis:
	Diabetic
	Alcoholic
	Starvation
	Lactic acidosis:
	Type A
	(tissue hypoxia, shock)
	Type B
	(liver disease, drugs)
	D-lactic acidosis
	Uremic acidosis
Exogenous acids	Methanol intoxication*
	Ethylene glycol intoxication*
	Formic acid*
	Salicylate poisoning
Normal anion gap metabolic acidosis	
GI loss of bicarbonate	Diarrhea
	Enterocutaneous fistulas
	Ureterosigmoidostomy
Renal loss of bicarbonate	Proximal RTA
Renal acid secretory defect	Distal RTA
	Hyperkalemic (type IV) RTA
	Aldosterone deficiency
Miscellaneous	NH_4Cl ingestion
	Massive isotonic dilution

Causes marked* are associated with a high osmolar gap.

Table 45.10: Common conditions causing metabolic alkalosis

Chloride responsive (volume depleted)	Chloride resistant (volume repleted)
Vomiting	Mineralocorticoid excess
Nasogastric suction	Hyperaldosteronism
Chloriuretic drugs (diuretics)	Bartter's syndrome
Overcorrection following hypercapnia	Cushing's syndrome
	Liddle's syndrome
	Severe potassium depletion

attention should be paid to volume status, electrolyte imbalance especially disturbances of potassium, magnesium, calcium and phosphate. Potassium disturbances are common and important and the risk of development of profound hypokalemia during treatment of acidosis needs monitoring. Respiratory exhaustion may occur in a patient with severe metabolic acidosis. A patient with severe metabolic acidosis who is compensated reasonably well with very low HCO_3 and CO_2 might develop life-threatening acidosis, when respiratory muscle fatigue occurs. This leads to CO_2 retention and development of respiratory acidosis with sharp fall in pH. Such a catastrophe should be anticipated and prevented.

Actual treatment of acidosis with alkali is required only when pH is less than 7.1–7.2 and if the primary condition cannot be brought under control quickly with measures like use of insulin in diabetic ketoacidosis, normalization of tissue oxygenation in lactic acidosis or by dialysis in uremic acidosis. If such control might take a longer time or when respiratory exhaustion is anticipated, treatment with alkali is indicated. Objective of treatment is to improve hemodynamics and prevent respiratory exhaustion. At a cellular level, bicarbonate therapy may be disadvantageous. It is to be noted that HCO_3 is not diffusible across the cell, but CO_2 generated from HCO_3 being a gas, diffuses easily into the cell. This leads to intracellular paradoxical acidification which might be harmful. When alkali therapy is indeed indicated, it can be given as a bolus or infusion. 50 ml of 7.5% sodium bicarbonate contains 44.5 mmol of HCO_3. The amount of bicarbonate to be administered is estimated by multiplying the HCO_3 space (volume of distribution of HCO_3) with the number of mmol/L change desired. HCO_3 space in healthy person is about 50% of body weight, but increases with acidosis and drop in HCO_3

level and can be up to 80% of body weight. Bicarbonate injections are hypertonic and should be given as infusion unless patient is volume overloaded or oliguric. Response to therapy should be periodically monitored. Once desired pH is attained, bicarbonate therapy can be stopped and attention should be paid to treatment of the primary condition. In conditions like lactic acidosis and keto-acidosis, once the primary disorder is checked, risk of overshoot alkalosis should be monitored for.

Volume depleted alkalotic patient is treated with large amounts of chloride, either as sodium or potassium salt depending on requirements. Treatment of volume repleted (chloride resistant) patients focuses on amelio-rating hyperaldosterone state, by surgery in adenoma, spironolactone in mineralocorticoid excess not due to adenoma, amiloride in Liddle's syndrome, ACE inhibitors, prosta-glandin inhibitors, etc. in Bartter's syndrome, etc. Non-sodium, non-potassium combinations of chloride like ammonium chloride and hydrochloric acid are used in exceptional situations to treat metabolic alkalosis.

Careful analysis of ABG report combined with correlation with the clinical scenario and associated electrolyte disorders helps in the precise diagnosis and appropriate management of the primary cause.

Chronic Kidney Disease– Mineral Bone Disease (CKD–MBD) and Renal Osteodystrophy

• Dilip K Pahari • N Roychaudhuri

Chronic kidney disease (CKD) is an important cause of morbidity and mortality. Prevalence of CKD 8–16%. It is defined as an irreversible, progressive reduction in renal function at least for a period of three months and is staged as stages 1 to 5 as shown in Table 46.1.

As kidney function declines, there is a progressive deterioration in mineral homeostasis, with a disruption of normal serum and tissue concentration of phosphorus and calcium, and changes in circulating levels of hormones. These include parathyroid hormone (PTH), 25-hydroxyvitamin D (25(OH) D), 1,25-dihydroxyvitamin D metabolites, fibroblast

growth factor-23 (FGF-23), and growth hormone.

1. Chronic kidney disease–mineral and bone disorder (CKD–MBD) is a common complication of chronic kidney disease and is a part of broad-spectrum disorders of mineral metabolism that occur in this clinical setting. It involves biochemical abnormalities of serum phosphorus, PTH, vitamin D levels, and alkaline phosphatase which are closely related to bone metabolism. The disorders of the bone have to be considered not only with regard to the bone itself but also with regard to the

Table 46.1: Staging of CKD (NKF KDOQI—National Kidney Foundation's Kidney Disease Outcomes Quality Initiative)

Stage	Description	GFR (ml/min/1.73 m²)	Plan
1	Kidney disease with normal or elevated GFR	>90	Diagnosis and treatment of underlying condition and comorbidities, cardiovascular risk reduction
2	Kidney damage with mildly decreased GFR	60–89	Estimating progression
3a	Kidney damage with mildly decreased GFR	30–44	Evaluating and treating complications
3b	Moderate to severely decreased GFR	45–30	Moderately to severely decreased GFR
4	Moderately decreased GFR	15–29	Preparation for renal replacement therapy
5	Kidney failure (ESRD)	<15	Renal replacement therapy

Table 46.2: KDIGO classification

1. CKD–MBD (systemic disorder of mineral and bone metabolism due to CKD) (Fig. 46.1).
   a. Abnormalities of calcium, phosphorus, PTH, or vitamin D metabolism
   b. Abnormalities in bone turnover, mineralization, volume, linear growth, or strength
   c. Vascular or other soft-tissue calcification
2. Renal osteodystrophy (alteration of bone morphology in patients with CKD)

consequences of disturbed mineral metabolism of extraskeletal sites, including the vasculature. Kidney disease improving global outcome (KDIGO) has classified mineral bone disorder in CKD and renal osteodystrophy (Table 46.2). Renal osteodystrophy is one measure of the skeletal component of the systemic disorder of CKD–MBD that is quantifiable by histomorphometry of bone biopsy.

Pathogenesis of metabolic bone disease in CKD: Renal bone disease is a common complication of chronic kidney disease. It results in both skeletal complications (e.g. abnormalities of bone turnover, mineralization, and linear growth) and extraskeletal complication (e.g. vascular or soft tissue calcification).

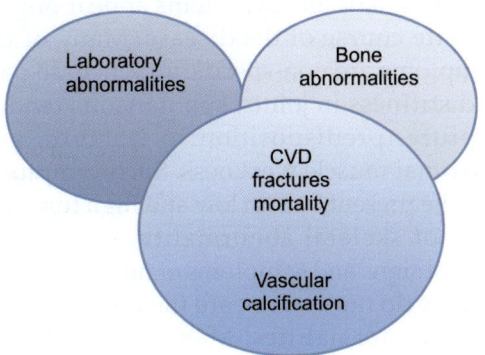

Fig. 46.1: Chronic kidney disease–mineral and bone disorder. Showing the spectrum and overlapping clinical, biochemical and bone changes in CKD–MBD

Several types of bone diseases are known to occur in CKD patients

a. Excessive secretion of parathyroid hormone (PTH) due to secondary hyperparathyroidism (SHPT) causes high turnover bone disease, called otitis fibrosa.
b. Low turnover bone disease (LTBD), like osteomalacia is characterized by calcification defect (defective mineralization) and is often complicated with vit D deficiency and/or aluminum accumulation.
c. Adynamic bone disease caused by PTH suppression, another type of LTBD, is encountered more and it may be related to use of calcium salts as phosphate binder with or without vit D treatment.
d. Mixed disease
e. β_2-microglobulin associated bone disease.

High turnover bone disease is the result of secondary hyperparathyroidism. Factors involved in the pathogenesis of secondary hyperparathyroidism are:

a. *Retention of phosphorus:* Phosphate retention begins in early chronic kidney disease; when the GFR falls. As functional mass declines, the fractional excretion of phosphate drops, leading to an increase in the serum phosphate level.
b. *Hypocalcemia:* Development of hyperphosphatemia is accompanied by a reciprocal decrease in serum calcium concentration. Hypocalcemia is a stimulus for parathyroid hormone (PTH) release. PTH has a phosphaturic effect and thus, results in the return of phosphate and calcium to normal levels. As GFR continues to decline, this cycle maintains serum calcium and phosphate concentrations within the normal ranges, at the expense of rising PTH levels (this phenomenon was called 'Bricker's trade-off hypothesis'). When further renal mass is lost and GFR drops below 30 ml/min/1.73 m² (chronic kidney disease stage 4–5) despite all the compensatory mechanisms, hyperphosphatemia and hypocalcemia becomes sustained.

c. *Decreased renal synthesis of 1,25-dihydroxy-cholecalciferol (1,25-dihydroxyvitamin D_3, or calcitriol):* As nephron mass decreases, the β-hydroxylation in the kidney of inactive 25-hydroxyvitamin D_3 [25-(OH) vitamin D_3] declines, leading to lower serum levels of calcitriol [active vit D_3] otherwise called 1,25-dihydroxyvitamin D_3 [1,25-(OH) D_3]. Hyperphosphatemia also suppresses the renal hydroxylation of inactive 25-hydroxyvitamin D3 to calcitriol. So, serum calcitriol levels are low when the GFR is less than 30 ml/min/1.73 m^2. Under normal conditions, calcitriol enhancs calcium absorption in the gut and PTH-mediated calcium release from bone. The lack of 1,25-(OH)$_2$ vitamin D_3 contributes to the development of hypocalcemia. The combination of these factors results in secondary hyperparathyroidism and renal osteodystrophy. Calcitriol levels decline slowly and progressively throughout the course of CKD.

d. *Role of intrinsic alterations in the parathyroid gland:* Hypocalcemia is a powerful stimulus for PTH secretion and for parathyroid growth. Decreased levels of calcitriol also may contribute to the parathyroid abnormalities. Calcitriol is a major regular regulator of PTH secretion, and vitamin D receptor is expressed in the parathyroid glands. Decreases in vit D receptor and calcium sensing receptor in the parathyroid glands render them more resistant to the action of vit D and calcium, and accelerate parathyroid cell growth.

e. *Skeletal resistance to the actions of PTH:* Many factors are involved in skeletal resistance, including phosphorus retention, possibly decreased levels of calcitriol, downregulation of the PTH receptor and the potential actions of PTHB fragments that have shown to blunt the calcemic effect of PTH.

The factors involved in the pathogenesis of secondary hyperparathyroidism are summarized in Fig. 46.2.

Low turnover bone disease (LTBD) is commonly observed in patients with kidney disease, especially in patients who are on dialysis, and is characterized by an extremely slow rate of bone formation and turnover. LTBD has two subgroups, osteomalacia and adynamic bone disease. Bone lesions are characterized by a decrease in bone turnover or remodelling, with a reduced number of osteoclasts and osteoblasts, and decreased osteoblastic activity.

In osteomalacia there is an accumulation of mineralized bone matrix or increased osteoid volume, which may be caused by vitamin D deficiency or excess aluminum.

Adynamic bone disease is characterized by reduced bone volume and mineralization and may be due to excess aluminum or over-suppression of PTH production with calcitriol.

Therefore, both forms facilitate the availabilty of Ca and P, which ends up being deposited in soft tissues such as arteries. Dialysis-related amyloidosis from β$_2$ microglobulin accumulation in patients who have required chronic dialysis for at least 8–10 years is another form of bone disease. It manifests with cysts at the ends of long bones.

Clinical signs and symptoms of metabolic bone disease in CKD: Patients are often asymptomatic and symptoms appear only in the late course of the disease. Many of the symptoms are non-specific and include pain and stiffness in joints, spontaneous tendon rupture, predisposition to fracture, and proximal muscle weakness. Such symptoms may be present both in low and high turnover type of skeletal abnormality. Absence of critical signs and symptoms of metabolic bone disease do not underscore the importance of these abnormalities. Many of the factors contributing to metabolic bone disease also have consequences at extraskeletal sites as well. Therefore, the control of these factors helps to decrease the morbidity and mortality.

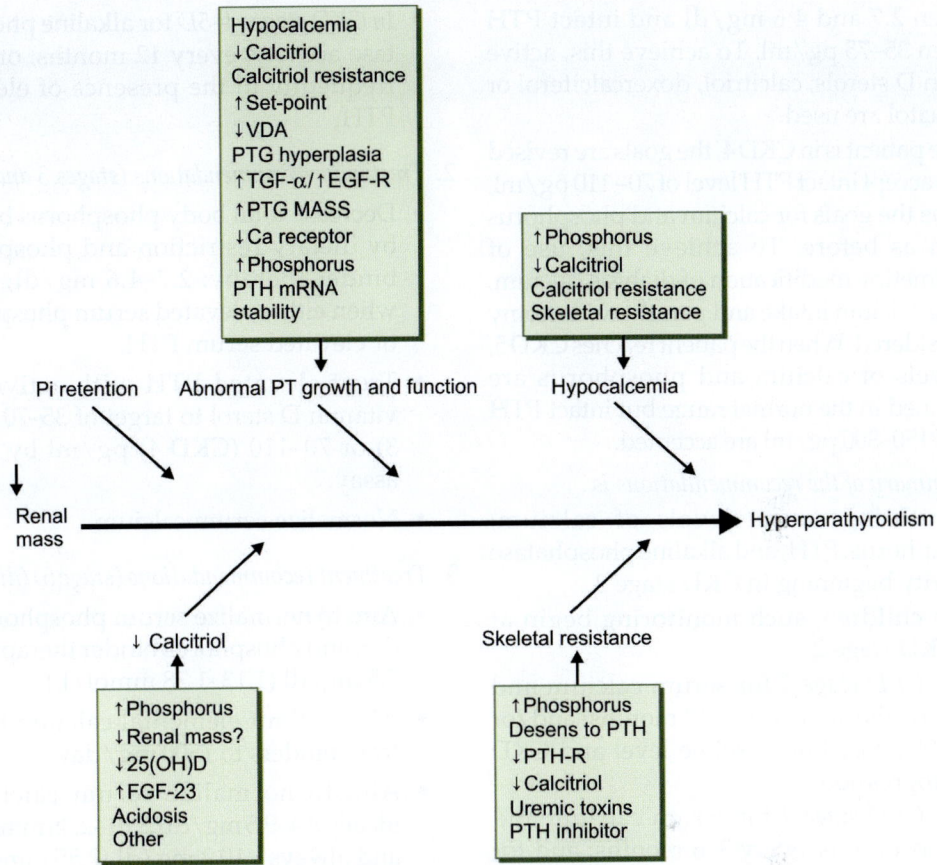

Fig. 46.2: Factors in the pathogenesis of secondary hyperparathyroidism

Diagnosis of CKD–MBD: Diagnosis of CKD–MBD relies on biochemical measurements of calcium, phosphorus, PTH and vit D concentrations. A number of biologic markers of bone formation and bone resorption might be used in conjunction with measurement of the mineral ions and PTH to gauge cell activity. Of these, alkaline phosphatase and bone-specific alkaline phosphatase are most useful. Although histologic examination of un-decalcified sections of bone remains the gold standard for the precise diagnosis of renal bone disease, bone biopsy is not widely used in clinical practice because of the invasive nature of the technique.

Prevention and management of metabolic bone disease in CKD: A "stepped-care" approach to the prevention and treatment of secondary hyperparathyroidism in CKD. The important steps are:

a. Monitor PTH levels
b. Check vitamin D status and correct if deficient
c. Correct acidosis
d. Dietary phosphate restriction
e. Add calcium based phosphate binders if hypocalcemia. Otherwise use non-calcium based phosphate binders.

The goal is to maintain calcium level between 8.4 and 10.2 mg/dl, phosphorus between 2.7 and 4.6 mg/dl and intact PTH between 35–75 pg/ml. To achieve this, active vitamin D sterols, calcitriol, doxercalciferol or paricalcitol are used.

If the patient is in CKD 4, the goals are revised so as to accept intact PTH level of 70–110 pg/ml, whereas the goals for calcium and phosphorus remain as before. To achieve this, use of calcimimetics, modification of dialysis calcium, limiting calcium intake and parathyroidectomy are considered. When the patient reaches CKD 5, the levels of calcium and phosphorus are maintained in the normal range but intact PTH level of 150–300 pg/ml are accepted.

The summary of the recommendations is

1. Monitoring serum levels of calcium, phosphorus, PTH, and alkaline phosphatase activity beginning in CKD stage 3.
   - In children, such monitoring begin at CKD stage 2.
   - *In CKD stage 3* for serum calcium and phosphorus, every 6–12 months; and for PTH, based on baseline level and CKD progression.
   - *In CKD stage 4* for serum calcium and phosphorus, every 3–6 months; and for PTH, every 6–12 months.
   - *In CKD stage 5, including 5D* for serum calcium and phosphorus, every 1–3 month; and for PTH, every 3–6 months.

   - *In CKD stages 4–5D* for alkaline phosphatase activity, every 12 months, or more frequently in the presence of elevated PTH.

2. *Treatment recommendations (stages 3 and 4)*
   - Decrease total body phosphorus burden by dietary restriction and phosphorus binder therapy: 2.7–4.6 mg/dl; begin when either elevated serum phosphorus or elevated serum PTH.
   - Treat elevated PTH with active oral vitamin D sterol to target of 35–70 (CKD 3) or 70–110 (CKD 4) pg/ml by intact assay.
   - Normalize serum calcium.

3. *Treatment recommendations (stage 5) (dialysis)*
   - Aim to normalize serum phosphorus by diet and phosphorus binder therapy 3.5–5.5 mg/dl (1.13–1.78 mmol/L).
   - Aim to limit elemental calcium intake from binders to 1500 mg/day.
   - Aim to normalize serum calcium—ideally 8.4–9.5 mg/dl (2.10–2.38 mmol/L), and always <10.2 mg/dl (2.55 mmol/L); Ca × P <55 mg^2/dl^2. Treatment advised for elevated PTH with active vitamin D sterol to target of 150–300 pg/ml (16–32 pmol/L) by intact assay.

Inherited Renal Diseases

• Alan Fernandes Almeida • Richard Savio Fernandes Almeida

INTRODUCTION

Advances in molecular genetics have contributed greatly to our understanding of many kidney diseases. Many renal diseases have been identified to be the result of single gene defect. Genetic causality is strongest with monogenic disorders and weakest with polygenic diseases. Mutations may determine the age of onset and treatment response. In the future, greater number of rare single gene defects may be identified, permitting preventive diagnostics.

Inherited kidney diseases may be divided into:

1. Glomerular disorders presenting with proteinuria consequent to a single gene defect that affects the glomerulus.
2. Renal cystic, interstitial disorders or renal tumors.
3. Tubular and metabolic diseases (transport diseases related to enzymatic disorders or deficiencies).
4. Renal stone disease.
5. Congenital abnormalities of the kidney and urinary tract (CAKUT).

Inherited renal disorders described in this chapter are given as follows.

Inherited Kidney Diseases

- *Glomerular:* Structural abnormalities of proteins normally present in the glomerular basement membrane or accumulation of non-glomerular basement membrane extracellular components:
  - Nephrotic syndrome (NS)
    - o Congenital NS
    - o Infantile NS
  - Alport syndrome
  - Thin basement membrane disease
  - Fabry disease
  - Nail patella syndrome
- *Tubular disorders:* Altered tubular function:
  - Fanconi syndrome
  - Cystinuria
  - Dent disease
  - Cystinosis
  - Hereditary hypophosphatemic rickets
  - Primary hyperoxaluria
  - Renal tubular acidosis
  - Bartter syndrome
  - Liddle syndrome
  - Gordon syndrome
  - Gitelman syndrome
  - Nephrogenic diabetes insipidus

- *Cystic disorders of the kidney*
  - Autosomal recessive polycystic kidney disease (ARPKD)
  - Autosomal dominant polycystic kidney disease (ADPKD)
  - Juvenile nephronophthisis—medullary cystic disease
  - Tuberous sclerosis
  - von Hippel-Lindau disease

[CAKUT (congenital abnormalities of the kidney and urinary tract) (*see* Chapter 9)]

Congenital nephrotic syndrome (CNS): Children with CNS present in the first three months of life with nephrotic syndrome. This syndrome having autosomal recessive inheritance pattern was first described in a Finnish population. The defect is in the (nephrin precursor *Homo sapiens* 1 (NPHS1) gene that codes for the protein nephrin that is found in the podocyte which forms part of the glomerular capillary filter. Massive proteinuria begins *in utero* and the child is born with or develops a difficult to manage nephrotic edema shortly after birth. The eventual management would be nephrectomy and transplantation.

There are other genetic defects, e.g. podocin (NPHS2), an autosomal recessive form of familial focal segmental glomerulosclerosis, which could result in nephrotic syndrome and rapid progression to end-stage renal disease. These are not steroid responsive, though a few may respond to cyclosporine.

Infantile nephrotic syndrome: Denys-Drash syndrome (Wilms' tumor 1 (WT1) gene mutation) presents with infantile nephrotic syndrome, gonadal dysgenesis and a renal biopsy showing a diffuse mesangial glomerulosclerosis. Wilms' tumor may develop in a few. Progression to renal failure ensues by the age of 3 years.

Genetic mutations may also result in adolescent and adulthood nephrotic states, which are usually autosomal dominant in inheritance with the histopathological pattern of focal segmental glomerulosclerosis (FSGS).

Alport syndrome: This is a generalized inherited disorder affecting all the basement membranes in the body. Type IV collagen, a major component of the basement membrane, has a collagenous (C) and a non-collagenous (NC) domain. Mutation of the –3, 4 or 5 chain in the NC domain produces the defect in Alport syndrome. The inheritance is variable—either X-linked (80%), autosomal recessive (15%) and autosomal dominant (5%). Males are more affected, females are either mildly affected or are carriers. Episodic hematuria precipitated by upper respiratory infections, proteinuria and hypertension increasing with age (occasionally nephrotic syndrome in adolescents or young adults) are the clinical presentations. The glomerular basement membrane abnormality results in hematuria, glomerulonephritis and progressive renal failure. Sensorineural hearing deficit, lenticonus and keratoconus are due to abnormalities in cochlear, lenticular and corneal basement membranes respectively. The anterior lenticonus appears as "oil droplet in water" by direct oblique illumination of the eyeball with torchlight. Persistent microscopic or gross hematuria, if accompanied by visual or auditory defects and positive family history of any of the above, should point towards a diagnosis of Alport syndrome. Whereas the renal biopsy may appear 'normal' on light microscopy and immunofluorescence, pathognomonic findings of areas of thickening, thinning and lamellation of the GBM ("Basket weave" appearance) are seen on electron microscopy. There is no effective treatment for the primary condition. Renal transplantation may be necessary when renal failure ensues in the 2nd or 3rd decade of life. Because the kidney allograft contains the normal –3 and 4 the recipient may identify this protein as foreign and produce antibodies against the glomerular basement membrane. These anti-GBM antibodies in the recipient may result in anti-GBM disease in the post-transplant period.

Thin basement membrane disease: This autosomal dominant (AD) –3 or –4 chain defect, also known as benign familial hematuria, presents in early childhood with isolated microscopic hematuria and rarely as significant proteinuria. No hypertension, progressive renal failure or extrarenal manifestations are associated. Electron microscopic examination reveals thinning of the glomerular basement membrane (usually <250 nm compared to mean normal (female adults: 320 ± 50 nm; male adults: 370 ± 50 nm). These patients need regular monitoring for hypertension, proteinuria or renal insufficiency, though development of renal failure is rare.

Fabry disease: Fabry disease is the second most prevalent lysosomal storage disorder—an X-linked inborn error of the glycosphingolipid metabolic pathway that results in accumulation of globotriaosylceramide within lysosomes of vascular endothelial cells, smooth muscle cells and epithelial cells throughout the body. Affection of the kidneys, heart, nervous system (peripheral and central) is consequent to deficiency of enzyme galactosidase A. Angiokeratomas, acroparesthesiae, hypohidrosis, corneal and lenticular changes are the early clinical manifestations. In the 3rd decade of life, hypertension, proteinuria and microscopic hematuria precede the development of progressive renal failure. Renal biopsy reveals enlarged glomerular and tubular epithelial cells with clear vacuoles (accumulated glycosphingolipid), accompanied by segmental and global glomerulosclerosis. Electron microscopically, lysosomal inclusions, 'myelin figures' are seen in the visceral epithelial cells. Enzyme replacement therapy, using recombinant human α galactosidase A, may safely reverse the major clinical manifestations and stabilize renal function in these patients.

Nail patella syndrome: This rare autosomal dominant inherited disorder, related to the LIM homeobox transcription factor 1β (LMX1B) gene defect, is usually manifest at birth or in early childhood. Hypoplastic or rudimentary patellae, dysplastic nails and elbows (head of radius abnormally small and underdeveloped), ocular changes (abnormally dark and cloverleaf shaped irides), iliac 'horns', proteinuria (nephrotic syndrome in adolescence or young adulthood), microhematuria, hypertension, progressive renal failure in a minority, characterizes this syndrome. Here again, characteristic histologic changes (multiple irregular lucencies in the GBM-'moth-eaten') confirms the diagnosis. No specific treatment is available.

Inherited tubular disorders: Fanconi syndrome: This is a disorder of proximal renal tubular function related to either a genetic defect or acquired. Mainly toxin-induced damage to the proximal tubular function is responsible for the acquired forms. Multiple transport abnormalities including increased urinary loss of several organic substances (aminoacids, glucose, bicarbonate and organic acids like uric acid) or loss of inorganic ions essential for mineral homeostasis, viz. calcium, magnesium, sodium, potassium and phosphorus, occur. Clinically, Fanconi syndrome is characterized by renal rickets (hypophosphatemic), hyperchloremic metabolic acidosis (bicarbonaturia), dehydration (electrolyte, fluid and mineral losses), electrolyte imbalance, osteomalacia and growth failure. Some of the inherited metabolic disorders that could present with Fanconi syndrome include (cystinosis (described below), hereditary fructose intolerance (deficiency of aldolase B), tyrosinemia (fumaryl acetoacetate hydrolase enzyme deficiency disrupts metabolic breakdown of tyrosine), Wilson disease (disorder of copper transport leading to toxic accumulation of copper) and Lowe syndrome (genetic disorder affecting the eyes, brain and kidneys). Management of these disorders include correction of metabolic abnormalities/ deficiencies and supplementation of fluids, phosphates and alkali. Bone disease would require adequate doses of active vitamin D. Specific therapy should be directed to the underlying etiology.

Cystinuria: Abnormal dibasic aminoacid (COAL) transport in the intestines and renal tubule characterizes this autosomal recessive disorder. Increased excretion of poorly soluble cystine crystals (flat hexagonal) in the urine form yellow-brown radiopaque cystine stones. Reduction in urinary cystine concentration (<300 mg/dl) by increasing fluid intake, a high urine output (2–4 liters/day), alkalinizing the urine with sodium potassium citrate and occasional use of penicillamine (250 mg up to 2 gm/day in patients with recurrent stone disease), helps.

Dent's disease: A rare X-linked recessive disorder is characterized by defective or absent proximal tubule renal chloride channel (CIC-5). Proximal tubule chloride entry determines protein reabsorption and the functions of various receptors, resulting in low molecular weight proteinuria, glucosuria, aminoaciduria, hypercalciuria, phosphaturia, kaliuresis, hyperuricosuria, impaired urinary acidification with resultant nephrocalcinosis, nephrolithiasis and rickets.

Cystinosis: This autosomal recessive metabolic genetic disorder results in an accumulation of cystine crystals in the kidneys, eyes, liver, muscles, pancreas, brain and white blood cells. Multiorgan involvement may be mild to severe. Dehydration, vomiting, polyuria, polydipsia, accompany metabolic acidosis. Hypophosphatemic rickets may ensue. Hypothyroidism is an associated disorder. Constipation, poor/loss of appetite and failure to thrive are evident. Fanconi's syndrome, with subsequent renal failure constitutes the renal manifestations. Treatment is symptomatic. High fluid intake, alkali administration,

carnitine, phosphates and vitamins are required. Cysteamine, a cysteine-depleting agent that lowers cysteine levels within the cells, has been proven to be effective in delaying or preventing renal failure.

Hereditary hypophosphatemic rickets: This is a rare inherited disorder (X-linked dominant, autosomal dominant and recessive) characterized by impaired transport of phosphate ($NaPO_4$ transporter) and often altered vitamin D metabolism in the kidneys. Hereditary hypophosphatemic rickets with hypercalciuria is a rare bone disorder manifesting with muscle weakness, short stature, skeletal deformities and bone pain. Treatment of hypophosphatemia includes phosphate supplementation and activated forms of vitamin D (calcitriol).

Primary hyperoxaluria: Enzyme deficiency in this autosomal recessively inherited disorder results in excessive oxalate production in the body. There are 3 main types—type 1: Defect in the alanine glyoxyalate aminotransferase; type 2: Failure of conversion of glyoxyalate to glycolate; and type 3: Due to a mutation in the HOGA1 gene. Oxalate accumulation may also be seen in bone, skin, retina, myocardium, blood vessels, joints, nervous system and elsewhere, explaining the cardiomyopathy, nephrocalcinosis (not identified in type 3), recurrent nephrolithiasis, renal failure, arthritis, skin lesions, etc. Good hydration, alkalinization of urine, supplementation of potassium citrate, magnesium and pyridoxine, constitute part of the conservative management. Liver transplantation replaces the missing hepatic enzymes and corrects the biochemical abnormalities. In advanced renal failure, combined liver and renal transplantation needs consideration.

RENAL TUBULAR ACIDOSIS

A normally functioning renal tubule helps maintain acid–base balance. Dysfunctional tubules could produce metabolic acidosis.

Renal tubular acidosis—types 1, 2 and 4 have been described.

Type 1 RTA

Type 1 or distal RTA (dRTA) results from secretory or permeability defects in the tubule. Defective secretion of protons (in the collecting duct) or permeability defects reduce the capacity to maintain a high intratubular H$^+$ ion concentration. Hyperchloremic metabolic acidosis occurs (normal anion gap). Urine pH cannot be lowered below 5.5. Decreased renal production of citrate, hypocitraturia and hypercalciuria predisposes to nephrocalcinosis and nephrolithiasis. Osteomalacia and rickets could occur. The autosomal recessive varieties of dRTA present in infancy with severe symptoms of acidosis, dehydration, failure to thrive and stone-related renal dysfunction. The autosomal dominant variants present in adulthood and are detected during the investigation of renal calculus disease. Bicarbonate supplementation in the doses of 1–4 mEq/kg body weight is warranted.

Type 2 RTA

The proximal tubule defect (inability to reclaim bicarbonate) accompanies type 2 RTA (proximal RTA). This acidification defect may occur either in isolation or may be associated with other generalized proximal tubule dysfunction, namely Fanconi syndrome. Fanconi syndrome is characterized by glycosuria, aminoaciduria, enzymuria, hypercitraturia (in dRTA, there is hypocitraturia), phosphaturia and losses of various electrolytes like sodium, potassium and calcium. Hypercitraturia prevents renal stone formation. In proximal RTA, the excretion of bicarbonate exceeds 15% when the serum bicarbonate exceeds 17 mmol/L. Once the HCO$_3^-$ falls below 15 mmol/L, with the establishment of a new transport maximum, all bicarbonate absorption is ensured. Therefore, the urine acidification to pH <5.5 becomes possible. Thiazide diuretics, by creating a volume contraction, stimulate bicarbonate reabsorption.

Type 4 RTA

Hyperchloremic metabolic acidosis, hyperkalemia, salt wasting with co-existent renal dysfunction, is a feature. The inherited forms of this disorder could be related to resistance of the intracellular mineralocorticoid receptor (milder dominant form) or a defect in the epithelial Na channel (ENaC). Therapy is based on severity of hyperkalemia.

Bartter Syndrome

Bartter's syndrome is an autosomal recessive disorder due to mutations affecting the sodium-potassium-2 chloride channel (NKCC$_2$), amongst other channels, in the thick ascending limb of the loop of Henle. In fact, Bartter's can be variably classified as a tubulopathy, a salt wasting disorder and a channelopathy. Impaired kidney ability to reabsorb salt, consequent fluid, electrolyte (hypokalemia) and acid–base (hypochloremic metabolic alkalosis) issues are noted. Volume contraction (normal or low BP) activates RAAS (hyperreninemia, hyperaldosteronism). PGE$_2$ levels rise in the chronically volume contracted and hypokalemic state. The anticipated blood pressure rise is not evident, despite high plasma renin activity due to the effects of PGE$_2$, kallikrein and volume contraction. Nephrocalcinosis accompanies the hypercalciuric state. The onset of symptoms (polyuria, polydipsia, vomiting, dehydration, failure to thrive) start in infancy or early childhood. Correction of dehydration, potassium and sodium supplementation and use of prostaglandin synthase inhibitors, like indomethacin or ibuprofen, constitute the mainstay of treatment.

Liddle Syndrome

Also known as pseudohyperaldosteronism, this autosomal dominant disorder is associated with an overactive amiloride-sensitive epithelial sodium channel (ENaC) in the cortical collecting duct. Hypokalemic metabolic alkalosis, volume expansion (excessive sodium reabsorption), hypertension and suppression of renin/aldosterone (due to volume expansion) result. It manifests most often in adolescents or in young adults with early-onset hypertension, hypokalemia, metabolic alkalosis in the setting of low plasma renin and aldosterone. Sodium restriction and potassium supplementation helps. Hypertension responds well to triamterene and amiloride, but spironolactone is ineffective since the increased activity of ENaC is not aldosterone-mediated.

Gordon Syndrome

This autosomal recessive disorder, also known as pseudohypoaldosteronism type 2 or chloride shunt syndrome, is characterized by hyperchloremia, hyperkalemia (decreased distal sodium delivery to cortical collecting duct), metabolic acidosis, severe hypertension (low plasma renin) with short stature, intellectual impairment, muscle weakness, hypercalciuria and renal stones. Treatment is with a low salt diet or thiazide diuretics (hydrochlorothiazide) aimed at decreasing chloride intake and blocking NaCl co-transporter activity.

Gitelman Syndrome

This autosomal recessive disorder results from a mutation of the thiazide-sensitive sodium chloride co-transporter (NCCT) in the distal convoluted tubule. This defect impairs the kidney's ability to retain electrolytes such as potassium, calcium, magnesium, sodium and chloride. Common symptoms include episodes of varying severity such as salt craving, fatigue, muscle weakness, cramps, tetany, abdominal pain, nocturia, nausea and vomiting. The later age of presentation and magnesium wasting differentiates it from Bartter's syndrome. Liberal salt intake, oral magnesium and potassium chloride supplementation are the mainstay of treatment and long-term prognosis is excellent. Amiloride, spironolactone, and eplerenone are helpful.

Nephrogenic Diabetes Insipidus

Mutations in the AVPR2 gene or AQP2 gene result in the kidney's inability to absorb water. Polydipsia and polyuria are the two main symptoms. Excessive urination at night (nocturia) occurs. Some infants may present with vomiting, retching, unexplained fevers, lethargy and irritability. Poor feeding, constipation and diarrhea may also occur. Dehydration develops. While managing infants with this disorder, treatment should be aimed at minimising the polyuria and avoiding hypernatremia and volume depletion.

INHERITED CYSTIC DISORDERS OF THE KIDNEY

Autosomal Recessive Polycystic Kidney Disease (ARPKD)

ARPKD results from mutations of a single gene (PKHD1). Defective remodeling of ductal plates occurs with tubular (fusiform and/or saccular dilation of collecting ducts) and biliary duct abnormal development. The spectrum of clinical phenotypes depends on the age at presentation. Enlarged echogenic kidneys, oligohydramnios (poor fetal urine output) help in prenatal or at birth identification of the affected fetuses. The 'Potter' phenotype with characteristic facies, pulmonary hypoplasia with spinal and limb deformities, is noted. Children presenting in the neonatal period, have a more rapid decline to end stage renal disease, whereas in children presenting later in childhood or in adolescence, portal hypertension predominates. Large echogenic kidneys in the fetus and neonate, with hyper-echogenic medulla are characteristic. The liver is normal sized or somewhat enlarged. Portal fibrosis progresses. Hepatosplenomegaly with patchy increase in hepatic echogenicity is noted. For children who survive the perinatal period, aggressive blood pressure control is necessary. With failing kidney function, management plans as for children with CKD are followed. Close monitoring of portal hypertension is warranted.

Renal transplantation, with or without a combined liver transplant, is the treatment of choice for ESRD in ARPKD patients.

Autosomal Dominant Polycystic Kidney Disease (ADPKD)

Mutations are noted in 2 genes; PKD1 and PKD2, with variable expression. The resultant multisystem disorder is characterized by multiple bilateral renal cysts which may be associated with cysts in other organs like, liver, spleen, pancreas and arachnoid membranes. The genes code for ADPKD proteins (polycystin-1, polycystin-2). Cysts of variable sizes are distributed throughout the cortex and medulla. Parenchymal distortion results. Age at detection and course of the disease vary. The mean age at presentation is 55 years in PKD1 and 71 years in PKD2. Incidental detection on ultrasound of the abdomen can occur in one-third of adults. Pain and hematuria (60%) and hypertension (80%) are the common features with hypertension often preceding detection of ADPKD with renal dysfunction. Renal calculus disease may be associated. Urinary tract infections within the cysts or in the intervening parenchyma may be noted. Appropriate antibiotic therapy of sufficient duration is required to successfully treat the cyst infections. Extrarenal manifestations such as cysts in the liver, seminal vesicles, prostate, pancreas and arachnoid are noted. Herniae (abdominal, inguinal and hiatus) and colonic diverticuli could also exist. Intracranial hemorrhage from a ruptured arterial aneurysm and mitral valve prolapse are other notable occurrences. Ultrasound imaging, coupled with a family history corroborates the diagnosis. CECT imaging is a sensitive tool and aids in identifying calcification in the cyst walls, renal calculi and hemorrhage in the cyst.

Hypertension control: Use of ACEI or ARB drugs is preferred. Renal transplantation would be the option of choice when renal failure occurs. Pretransplant nephrectomy, hemorrhage or infected cysts may require exercising of a surgical option earlier in the course. Medical management of cysts (sirolimus) and vasopressin receptor 2 (V2R) antagonist (tolvaptan) have been tried to retard cyst growth.

JUVENILE NEPHRONOPHTHISIS—MEDULLARY CYSTIC DISEASE COMPLEX

Autosomal Recessive Juvenile Nephronophthisis

Three distinct forms of NPHP exist (based on age at onset)—infantile, juvenile, adolescent. The infantile form occurs before the age of 5, the more common juvenile form occurs at a mean age of 13 years. Decreased urinary concentrating capacity, salt wasting occurs. Polyuria and polydipsia are common. Anemia and retinal dystrophy have been described.

Autosomal Dominant Medullary Cystic Kidney Disease

This condition is less common than the autosomal recessive NPHP. The diagnosis is usually made based on the family history, the clinical associations of hyperuricemia and gout and the ultrasound finding of medullary cysts.

Tuberous sclerosis complex: An autosomal dominant disorder with a high rate of spontaneous mutations, presents in childhood or adulthood with a clinical triad of mental retardation, seizure disorder and facial angiofibromas. CNS hamartomas, cardiac rhabdomyomas, renal angiomyolipomas, ash-leaf spots (hypomelanotic) and subependymal giant cell astrocytomas may be noted.

von Hippel-Lindau syndrome: This autosomal dominant inherited disorder presents in adulthood. Tumors of the cerebellum, spinal cord, renal and pancreatic cysts, tumors of the eyes, pheochromocytoma, renal carcinoma, retinal hemangioblastomas and angiomas may occur.

Approach to Urinary Tract Obstruction

• V Ramasubramanian

Urinary tract obstruction is a common problem encountered in clinical practice. Obstruction can be at any point from the kidney to the urethral meatus. Functionally the urinary tract obstruction can be divided into upper and lower as the etiologies. Symptoms and treatments differ depending on the site of obstruction. The 'upper' urinary tract is from the kidney to the vesicoureteric junction (VUJ) which include the pelviureteric junction (PUJ) and the ureter. The 'lower' urinary tract consists of the bladder, bladder neck, the urethra, the urethral meatus and in males the prostatic urethra. As long-term obstruction can lead to irreversible renal damage, early detection and relief of obstruction are essential to preserve renal function.

The incidence of undetected obstruction is high since autopsy studies have shown incidence of hydronephrosis to be 3.8% in adults and 2% in children. In many of these instances, no clinical manifestations were present prior to death. Most of the hydronephrosis in children occur below 1 year of age. There are many causes for congenital urinary tract obstructions (Table 48.1). Until the age of 20 years, no substantial sex difference is observed. In women between 20

Table 48.1: Common causes of congenital urinary tract obstruction

a. PUJ obstruction
b. Ureteral valves/folds
c. Ureteric strictures and obstructed megaureter
d. Fibroepithelial polyps
e. Retrocaval ureter (compression by IVC)
f. VUJ obstruction
g. VUR
h. Ureterocele
i. Bladder diverticula
j. Spina bifida (neurogenic bladder)
k. PUV
l. Urethral atresia/phimosis
m. Labial fusion (female)

and 60 years of age, it is more frequent secondary to pregnancy and gynecologic malignancies. In men, the frequency is high above 60 years due to benign prostatic hyperplasia or prostatic malignances.

Etiology

Upper Urinary Tract Obstruction

Anatomic narrowing of certain points in the drainage system from the kidney to the VUJ predispose to obstruction to urine flow in these sites. They are the pelviureteric junction, the pelvic brim and the vesicoureteric junction. At the pelvic brim, the ureter crosses over to run anterior to the common iliac vessels before entering the pelvis. The narrowest site is the UVJ. In women, an additional area of narrowing can occur as the ureter crosses posterior to the pelvic vessels and broad ligament. Hence, these are the usual sites susceptible for obstruction to urine follow. The obstruction may be intraluminal (intrinsic) or less commonly extraluminal (extrinsic). The common intraluminal causes are due to crystal deposition (uric acid, sulfonamides, acyclovir, indinavir and ciprofloxacin). Acute intraluminal obstruction is commonly caused by calculi, blood clots, tumors or a sloughed papilla which is the common cause in diabetics. Nephrolithiasis represents the most common cause in younger men. Calcium oxalate stones occur most commonly. Chronic obstruction can be caused by ureteral stricture due to stones, cancer or iatrogenic injury from ureteroscopy. In women, ureteric compression by advanced gynecological malignancies, uterine prolapse can lead to urinary tract obstruction. In children, the obstruction may be due to PUJ or VUJ obstruction, a ureterocele, ectopic ureter or an obstructed megaureter. PUJ obstruction is the most common with a frequency of 5 cases per 100,000 population per year. Intrinsic intramural processes that cause obstruction include failure of micturition or more rarely of ureteral peristalsis.

Extrinsic causes of obstruction include a lower pole vessel arising from aorta, abdominal aortic or common iliac vessel aneurysms, vascular graft placement, retrocaval ureter and retroperitoneal fibrosis. Endometriosis though rarely results in ureteral obstruction it should be included in the differential diagnosis in premenopausal women. Inadvertent ligation of the ureter may occur rarely following pelvic procedures. Dilatation of the right upper ureter up to the pelvic brim may be seen in some women during the second and third trimesters of pregnancy. This is due to the combined effect of progesterone action and the gravid uterus mainly on the right ureter. This resolves by 6–8 weeks postpartum.

Lower Urinary Tract Obstruction

Posterior urethral valve is the commonest cause of lower tract obstruction in male children. In older men, benign prostatic hypertrophy (BPH) is the most common cause. Urethral stricture, bladder cancer, prostate cancer, uterine prolapse, meatal stenosis are other causes. Neurologic dysfunction occurring in diabetes mellitus, multiple sclerosis, spinal cord injury, cerebrovascular disease and parkinsonism produce a variety of functional bladder disturbances. Genitourinary tuberculosis leads to irreversible ureteral or bladder fibrosis and obstruction. Chronic schistosomiasis is a cause of chronic lower tract obstruction and hematuria in the African continent. Some gastrointestinal diseases like Crohn's disease, appendicitis, diverticulitis, chronic pancreatitis with pseudocyst and faecaloma may rarely cause symptoms and signs suggestive of obstructive uropathy.

Pathogenesis

The experiment to study the glomerular hemodynamics following acute unilateral and bilateral ureteric ligation and response to removing obstruction after 24 hours helps us to understand the pathogenesis of the two types of acute ureteric obstruction. Within one to 2 hours of acute unilateral ureteric obstruction, the afferent arteriolar resistance decreases, glomerular capillary hydraulic pressure increases and the proximal tubular pressure increases. By 24 hours, afferent arteriolar resistance increases, glomerular capillary hydrostatic pressure decreases and the proximal tubular pressure is normalized. 24 hours after release of obstruction, the afferent arteriolar resistance increases, glomerular capillary hydrostatic pressure decreases and the proximal tubular pressure also decreases.

In the case of bilateral obstruction, the afferent arteriolar resistance remains normal, glomerular capillary hydrostatic pressure normalizes, and the proximal tubular pressure remains elevated. 24 hours after removal of obstruction, the afferent arteriolar resistance is high, glomerular capillary hydrostatic pressure is low and proximal tubular pressure remains normal. In all these situations, the GFR decreases within 24 hours of obstruction and recovers only later. This combined with the tubular dysfunction causes the postobstructive diuresis.

Clinical Features

The clinical presentation varies according to the site, duration and the degree of obstruction. Obstruction in the kidney and ureter can manifest as flank pain, ipsilateral back pain or ipsilateral groin pain. Pain may be absent in chronic obstruction. Pain due to stone in the ureter may be waxing and waning. During the episode of colicky pain, the patient may not be comfortable in any position and will often be 'rolling in the bed'. This is in contrast to pain in acute appendicitis or peritonitis where, any movement exacerbates the pain and the patient prefers to remain still. With PUJ obstruction the pain worsens with ingestion of large quantity of fluids or administration of diuretics. Often PUJ is detected in the antenatal ultrasonography these days. Flank pain with an abdominal mass may be the presentation of PUJ in neonates. Hematuria may or may not be present. Fever, chills may be present if infection accompanies obstruction. Presence of costovertebral angle tenderness may indicate acute pyelonephritis. Bilateral obstruction or obstruction in a solitary kidney can lead to anuria and uremic symptoms. In conditions associated with severe hydronephrosis, the kidney will be palpable.

The symptoms of lower urinary tract obstruction include urgency, frequency, nocturia, incontinence, decreased force of urinary stream, split urinary stream in stricture urethra, hesitancy, post-void dribbling and a sense of incomplete emptying. Suprapubic pain and palpable bladder may be present in acute urinary retention. Infection can lead to dysuria, mild hematuria. Gross hematuria may be due to tumor, stone, infection or due to a bleeding vessel in the urinary tract. Digital rectal examination reveals prostate enlargement or prostatitis. Urethral meatal stenosis or urethral diverticulum will be apparent on clinical examination. A pelvic examination in women will reveal uterine or bladder prolapse.

Investigations

Urine Analysis

WBCs in urine may be present in infection, ureteral stent placement, stones in the urinary tract, malignancy or recent urinary tract instrumentation. Leukocyte esterase and nitrate positive urine samples should be sent for culture and sensitivity. Hematuria may be due to various causes already mentioned which need further investigations.

Blood Chemistry

Blood urea or BUN, creatinine and electrolyte estimation help to assess the degree of renal insufficiency and electrolyte abnormalities.

Imaging

Ultrasound is a noninvasive and relatively inexpensive modality useful for detecting hydronephrosis. It can be performed in patients with renal insufficieny, children, pregnant women, and in those who are allergic to radiocontrast media. It is sensitive for the detection of renal masses, hydro-ureteronephrosis and distended bladder. However, interobserver variability may compromise the quality and accuracy. The combination of USG with radiography of KUB can make initial evaluation complete. Increased renal cortical echogenicity, parenchymal rims greater than 5 mm, contralateral hypertrophy, resistive index (RI) ratio of 1.1 or higher are features to differentiate obstructing and non-obstructing hydronephrosis. Renal ultrasound elastography measures kidney elasticity by shear wave technique and provides information about renal stiffness related to fibrosis. Routine antenatal ultrasonography has facilitated early diagnosis of fetal hydronephrosis. Approximately one-third of fetal hydronephrosis is due to congenital *abnormalities of the kidney and urinary tract (CAKUT)*. Congeintal abnormalities of kidney and urinary system (CAKUT) (*see* Chapter 9 for detailed description. Various causes include PUJ obstruction (44%), VUJ obstruction (21%), dysplasias (12%), posterior urethral valves (9%) and VUR (12%). The anteroposterior diameter of the fetal renal pelvis helps to predict the chances of persistence of postnatal abnormalities. If the anteroposterior diameter is more than 6 mm at less than 20 weeks, more than 8 mm at 20 to 30 weeks and more than 10 mm at 30 weeks, significant hydroureteronephrosis is likely to persist postnatally. Between 5% and 25% of infants and children with antenatal hydronephrosis will need surgical intervention.

Intravenous pyelography (IVU) involves injection of contrast material and a series of abdominal X-rays taken over 15 to 30 minutes. It gives anatomic and functional information of the upper urinary tract. Delayed calyceal filling, contrast excretion or pronged nephrogram and dilatation of the proximal tract above the obstruction are findings in an obstruction.

Computerized tomography (CT) scan is often considered as a first-line radiographic test. It gives information about the urinary tract and also about retroperitoneal and pelvic conditions that compress the urinary tract. A noncontrast CT scan helps to detect renal stones, whereas a contrast CT scan is very useful in neoplasms, strictures and sloughed papilla. CT can identify even radiolucent stones because even uric acid stone (density 100 Hounsfield units) has higher than soft

tissue density compared to the soft tissue density of 10 to 70 Hounsfield units. An exception to using a noncontrast CT is nephrolithiasis secondary to HIV protease inhibitors primarily indinavir as the stones are non-radiopaque and signs of obstruction may be minimal. Intra-abdominal causes for urinary tract obstruction like abdominal aneurysms, small and large bowel masses can also be detected with a CT scan.

Magnetic resonance imaging (MRI) is not a first-line investigation. It is not sensitive for renal stones. It is useful in delineating specific tissue planes for surgical planning and also to evaluate the presence and extent of renal vein and inferior vena caval thrombus. MR contrast gadolinium produces irreversible nephrogenic systemic fibrosis (NSF) in patients with renal impairment exposed to gadolinium.

Radionucleotide studies using mercaptoacetyltriglycine also called MAG-3 is useful to determine the differential function of the kidneys as well as the concentrating ability, excretion and drainage of the urinary tract. Administration of furosemide can help to verify delayed excretion in PUJ obstruction. Renal excretion of the tracer with t½ of more than 20 minutes is diagnostic of obstruction.

Retrograde urethrogram is done by injecting dye through a catheter with tip placed into the urethral meatus. It is useful mainly in the setting of trauma when urethral disruption and clot obstruction is suspected. It is also useful to define the extent of urethral stricture before surgery.

Retrograde pyelogram is done by injecting dye into the catheter placed in the ureteric orifice by cystoscopy. Images will show the anatomic outline of the ureters and renal pelvis up to the level of obstruction and show filling defects in the presence of a mass, stone or clot. As there is insignificant contrast absorption, it may be useful in patients with renal failure and allergy to contrast.

Nephrostogram is done by injecting dye into the nephrostomy tube and is useful in evaluating kidneys and ureters when retrograde access is difficult and also for planning interventions.

Treatment

The mainstay of management of urinary tract obstruction is to tackle any life-threatening situation, stabilize the patient, relieve obstruction, and preserve as much renal function as possible. Once the cause is identified, it is treated appropriately.

Medical

Septicemia with pyelonephritis is a complication of severe or complete obstruction which presents with fever, elevated WBC count, hypotension and severe flank pain. Relief of obstruction along with administration of broad-spectrum antibiotics on an emergent basis is needed. Once, results of culture are available, antibiotics can be tailored. Patients with renal insufficiency need immediate attention. Dialysis may be required in patients with hyperkalemia, acidosis, convulsions, coma or pericarditis. Partial obstruction without infection or renal failure can be managed on an outpatient basis with analgesics of opioid group and antibiotic prophylaxis to cover commom uropathogens.

Surgical

Lower Urinary Tract

Temporary form of relief can be provided by using with urethral Foley's catheter or suprapubic catheter to relieve the obstruction. Definitive treatment includes:

a. Dilatation of meatal stenosis with urethral sounds.
b. Dilatation of urethral strictures with filiform bougies.
c. Endoscopic incision of urethral strictures.
d. Transurethral resection of prostate (TURP) for prostate.
e. Bladder neck incision for bladder neck obstruction.

Upper Urinary Tract

Obstruction to the ureter is managed temporarily by inserting a ureteric stent across the stenotic segment using a cystoscope. The groove in the stent will facilitate passage of urine through the stenotic segment. A percutaneous nephrostomy tube can be placed through the flank directly into the renal pelvis. Ureteric stent can also be inserted through the nephrostomy tube. Definitive treatment includes:

a. Removal of distal ureteric stones using lithotripsy through ureteroscope.
b. Proximal and midureteric stones using laser lithotripsy.
c. Extracorporeal shockwave lithotripsy (ESWL).
d. Renal calculi removal through flexible ureteroscopy.
e. Percutaneous removal through a nephrostomy tract.
f. Open surgery is reserved for renal or ureteric stones above 2 cm size.

PUJ obstructions are commonly treated with a pyeloplasty which can be performed by open or laparoscopic methods. Small ureteral strictures are dilated endoscopically with balloon dilator, whereas larger strictures require resection and reanastomosis. Distal ureteral strictures can be treated with ureteral reimplantation either directly or using a psoas hitch or a 'Boari' flap. Neoplasms can be managed by segmental resection or by nephroureterectomy.

Pathophysiology

Volume of an unobstructed collecting system is 5–10 ml. Following obstruction, the collecting system gets dilated and intraluminal pressure increases proximal to the obstruction. This pressure and dilatation eventually will affect the medulla, and the increasing pressure in the tubules of the cortex cause cortical thinning and atrophy. Renal failure occurs due to:

a. Pressure atrophy

b. Intrarenal reflux of urine (which causes damage to both the cortex and medulla)

c. Ischemia due to lack of renal blood flow.

d. Hypertension due to extracellular fluid volume expansion.

e. Increased renin secretion.

f. Decreased prostaglandin synthesis.

Dynamics

Propulsion of urine from the kidneys to the bladder is the result of three forces.

a. Hydrostatic pressure

b. Ureteral and pelvic peristalsis

c. Rate of urine flow.

Action potentials originating in the smooth muscles of the minor calyx in the renal pelvis are conducted along the renal pelvis and down the ureter. Though the ureteral pressure rises to 20–25 cm during coaptation during peristalsis, retrograde transmission does not occur and the renal pelvic pressure seldom rises above 4–5 cm. After acute obstruction smooth muscle fibers increase in tension and contract with greater force. With persistent obstruction the tension may decrease and contraction becomes weaker and is associated with less force. Finally dilatation may occur with loss of force. The glomerular filtration rate (GFR) is initially increased due to increased glomerular capillary pressure and later decreases due to increased intratubular pressure. An increase in the intratubular pressure without an increase in the glomerular capillary pressure will result in a decrease in GFR.

Immediately after unilateral or bilateral ureteral obstruction, renal blood flow increases up to 25%, accompanied by an increase in the tubular pressure. This is due to decrease in the renal vascular resistance mediated by vasodilator prostaglandins. With persistent obstruction the renal blood flow decreases by 40–50% of the normal and GFR to 20–30%. The drop in GFR is more marked. In unilateral obstruction, afferent arteriolar resistance increases resulting in drop in GFR. Proximal intratubular pressure becomes normal. In bilateral obstruction the persistent increase in the proximal intratubular pressure leads to drop in GFR with renal blood flow and glomerular capillary pressure remaining normal. The predominant site of vascular resistance appears to be the efferent arteriole.

Post-obstructive Diuresis

After relief of complete bilateral obstruction or obstruction in a solitary kidney, there is a prolonged diuresis due to massive loss of water, sodium and other solutes due to a dramatic decrease in the reabsorptive ability of the nephron. It may be physiologically appropriate due to the retained urea within the bloodstream and nephrons that act as an osmotic diuretic. It could be iatrogenic also due to intravenous fluid administration which maintains high ECF volume and stimulates atrial natriuretic peptide (ANP) which stimulates diuresis. Recovery of GFR depends on the duration of obstruction and determines the duration of post-obstructive diuresis. Replacement of appropriate fluids is essential during the phase of post-obstructive diuresis because the patient may go into a state of volume contraction, hypotension and irreversible shock.

Approach to Renal Stone Disease

• Pinaki Mukhopadhyay

INTRODUCTION

Nephrolithiasis is a common and complex disorder. Kidney stones, or renal calculi, are solid masses made of crystals that usually originate in kidneys, but can develop anywhere along the urinary tract. Depending on their location, they are classified as nephrolithiasis (in the kidney), ureterolithiasis (in the ureter) or cystolithiasis (in the bladder). They are also classified by their chemical composition as calcium oxalate, uric acid, struvite or cysteine stone. The prevalence of stone disease increases with age, and the lifetime risk of stone formation. In men, the incidence begins to rise after age 20, peaks between 40 and 60 years.In women, the incidence is higher in their late twenties.

Epidemiology

Stones are more common in men than in women, and the type of stones differ somewhat between the sexes. In children, reported frequency of stone disease and type of stones is not clear but is different compared to adults. In adults, the prevalence of stones has been increasing over the past 30 years in both sexes. The prevalence of stone disease in adults differs depending on the race, genetic factors, water consumed, atmospheric temperature and other geographic factors. The reasons for the increasing prevalence are not clear, but one factor may be increased rates of obesity, as risk of stones increases along with body mass index and waist circumference, especially in women.

Calcium oxalate (CaOx) is the predominant component of most stones either as the monohydrate (whewellite) or dihydrate (weddelite), often admixed with some calcium phosphate (CaP) which may form the initial nidus of the stone. Stones composed predominantly of CaP (as apatite or brushite) are less common, and are seen more frequently in women. Rarely, insoluble drugs such as indinavir, triamterene or ephedrine, may form stones. Stone disease through unknown mechanisms is associated with an increased risk of hypertension, especially in women. In some forms of nephrolithiasis associated with systemic disease progressive loss of renal function may occur.

Risk Factors

Numerous risk factors are associated with stone formation and are generally divided into nondietary, dietary, and urinary.

1. Non-dietary Factors

 i. *Family history:* The risk of stone formation is twofold higher in individuals with a family history of stone disease. The increased risk is likely due to both genetic predispositions, similar dietary and environmental exposure.

ii. *Race/ethnicity:* There is wide variation in the pattern of the disease in different parts of the world, thus projecting the significance of the 'stone belt' areas. Stone disease of the urinary tract is more common in Northern India, Pakistan, Afghanistan and 'Gulf' countries and is due to various etiopathological factors prevailing there.

iii. *Systemic disorders:* There is substantial evidence that nephrolithiasis is a systemic disorder. Well-known conditions associated with calcium containing stones include primary hyperparathyroidism, renal tubular acidosis, and Crohn's disease. Several other common conditions, including obesity, gout, and diabetes mellitus (DM), have recently been convincingly linked to nephrolithiasis.

iv. *Environmental factors:* Occupations or settings with higher insensible fluid losses, such as working in hot environment increases the risk of stone formation. The risk will also be higher when individuals have restricted access to water or toilet facilities, leading to lower fluid intake and lower urine volume.

2. Dietary Factors

Since the type of diet influences urine composition, the risk of nephrolithiasis is related to diet. High dietary intake of animal protein, sodium, refined sugars, fructose and high fructose corn syrup, oxalate, grapefruit juice, and apple juice may increase the risk of kidney stone formation.

i. *Calcium:* Although it was considered earlier that high calcium in diet causes stone disease, studies have shown that individuals with a higher intake of dietary calcium actually had a lower risk of nephrolithiasis, independent of other risk factors.

ii. *Oxalate:* Urine oxalate is clearly an important risk factor for calcium oxalate stone formation. Use of high oxalate containing edible fruits/vegetables may cause AKI due to precipitation of oxalate in the renal tubules with intratubular obstruction. The role of dietary oxalate in the pathogenesis of calcium oxalate nephrolithiasis is less clear.

iii. *Other nutrients:* A variety of other nutrients has been implicated in stone formation. For example, higher animal protein intake may increase urinary calcium and decrease urinary citrate, thereby increasing the risk of stone formation.

iv. *Fluid intake and beverages:* Fluid intake is the main determinant of urine volume. Stone formation occurs more frequently if the urine is concentrated and dilute urine does not favor crystal growth. Therefore reduced fluid intake and formation of concentrated urine is an important risk factor for stone formation. The risk of stone formation is markedly higher when the urine output is less than 1 L/day. Carbonated drinks, other drinks with hoigh fructose content, hard liquour are avoided. Dehydration from low fluid intake is a major factor in stone formation.

3. Urinary Factors

i. Hypercalciuria is commonly defined as urine calcium excretion 300 mg/day (7.5 mmol/day) in men and 250 mg/day (6.25 mmol/day) in women while on a diet containing 1,000 mg/day calcium. Using these traditional definitions, approximately 20–40% of patients with calcium stone disease will have hypercalciuria.

ii. Hyperoxaluria is defined as urinary oxalate excretion >45 mg/day (0.5 mmol/day). Elevated urinary oxalate excretion is an important independent risk factor for stone formation and is three to four times more common among men than in women. This may explain the higher incidence of stone disease in men.

Pathogenesis

Pathophysiological Mechanism(s) of Calcium Stones

The pathogenetic mechanisms of kidney stone formation are complex and diverse. Factors like low urine volume, concentrated urine, hypercalciuria, hyperuricosuria, hypocitraturia, hyperoxaluria, and abnormalities in urine pH, metabolic and environmental risk factors play an important role. The stones may form in any part of the urinary system from kidneys, ureters, bladders and prostate. Approximately 80% of calcium kidney stones are calcium oxalate (CaOx) with a small percentage (15%) of calcium phosphate (CaP).

Depending on the relative concentration of solids and liquids, a solution can be unsaturated, saturated or supersaturated. In the case of urine, the free ion activity of the stone components is critical. In an unsaturated state, crystallization does not occur. In a saturated state, depending on the other factors in the urine and the presence of a 'nidus' or site for attachment of crystal, it may get attached to the nidus and grow. In supersaturated state, the spontaneous crystal formation is called nucleation. If the nucleation involves the same ions, it is called homogeneous nucleation. If different ions or substances are involved, it is called heterogenous nucleation. Continued exposure of the crystal to saturated or supersaturated urine results in the growth of the crystal to form stone.

Hypercalciuria

In the case of calcium kidney stone formers, hypercalciuria is the most common abnormality and is detected in 30–60% of adults with nephrolithiasis. The pathophysiological mechanisms for "idiopathic hypercalciuria" are numerous and hypercalciuria is a heterogeneous disorder.

   i. Increased intestinal calcium absorption ("absorptive" hypercalciuria)
  ii. Enhanced calcium mobilization from bone ("resorptive" hypercalciuria)
 iii. Decreased renal calcium reabsorption.

Increased intestinal calcium absorption is the most common abnormality and the term "absorptive hypercalciuria" is used to denote this condition. Increased intestinal calcium absorption may be dependent or independent of 1,25-dihydroxyvitamin D [1,25(OH)2D]. Hypercalciuria is classified into two different groups.

a. The most severe variant is characterized by normocalcemia, hypercalciuria, intestinal hyperabsorption of calcium, and normal or suppressed serum PTH and/or urinary cAMP.

b. A less severe form also shares many of the above biochemical characteristics, but hypercalciuria normalizes after a restricted calcium diet (<400 mg/d).

Resorptive Hypercalciuria

The most common prototype of resorptive hypercalciuria is primary hyperparathyroidism. Since the diagnosis of primary hyperparathyroidism is made earlier because of greater awareness and diagnostic facilities, the prevalence of nephrolithiasis in this condition is low. The exact relationship between hypercalciuria and the risk of nephrolithiasis with primary hyperparathyroidism is not fully understood. Hypercalciuria could occur due to increased calcium mobilization from bone or by increased intestinal calcium absorption. It is noted that kidney stones are more prevalent in younger populations with primary hyperparathyroidism and may be due to enhanced synthesis of $1,25(OH)2D3$ with normal kidney function and consequent increased intestinal calcium absorption. Bone disease may occur in older subjects due to lower serum $1,25(OH)2 D_3$ levels resulting in diminished intestinal calcium absorption.

Renal Leak Hypercalciuria

Renal leak hypercalciuria is a second, less common variety of hypercalciuria in which defective renal tubular calcium reabsorption is accompanied by enhanced PTH, calcitriol, and net intestinal calcium absorption.

Hyperuricosuria

Hyperuricosuria as an isolated abnormality is detected in 10% of calcium stone formers. However, in combination with other metabolic abnormalities it may be present in 40% of such persons. The pathophysiological mechanism underlying hyperuricosuria is attributed to a high purine diet the end-product of purines being uric acid. However, in approximately one-third of patients, endogenous uric acid (UA) overproduction results in hyperuricosuria and dietary restriction does not significantly alter urinary UA excretion. The physicochemical basis involved in this process has not been well established. Any relationship between urinary UA and CaOx stone formation has not been established as yet.

Hypocitraturia

Citrate is an endogenous inhibitor of calcium stone formation, and low urine citrate excretion (hypocitraturia) is encountered in 20–60% of calcium nephrolithiasis. The major determinant of urinary citrate excretion is acid–base balance. Hypocitraturia commonly occurs with metabolic acidosis or following diet-rich in acid content. This is possibly related to increased (upregulation of) proximal renal tubular reabsorption of citrate. The main conditions associated with hypocitraturia are distal renal tubular acidosis (dRTA), use of carbonic anhydrase inhibitors and normal bicarbonatemic states including incomplete dRTA, thiazide treatment with hypokalemia, primary aldosteronism, high protein consumption, excessive salt intake, and converting enzyme inhibitors.

Hyperoxaluria

Urinary oxalate and calcium are equally important in raising urinary CaOx supersaturation. Hyperoxaluria is detected in 10–50% of calcium stone formers. The underlying mechanisms of hyperoxaluria can be divided into:

   i. Oxalate overproduction as a result of an inborn error in metabolism:

     a. Type I hyperoxaluria resulting from a deficiency or mistargeting of hepatic alanine glyoxylate transferase enzyme.

     b. Type II primary hyperoxaluria due to a deficiency in glyoxylate reductase/hydroxypyruvate reductase enzyme.

     c. Type III hyperoxaluria (rare) as a result of the gain of function of hepatic or renal mitochondrial 4-hydroxy-2-oxoglutarate aldolase.

In addition to hyperoxaluria, these disorders are associated with multiple other kidney stone risk factors including low urine volume, hypocitraturia, hypomagnesuria, and highly acidic urine.

   ii. Increased dietary intake and bioavailability.

   iii. Increased intestinal oxalate absorption.

Disturbances in Urinary pH

Both highly acidic urine (pH ≤5.5) and highly alkaline urine (pH ≥6.7) predispose patients to calcium kidney stone formation. With unduly acidic pH, urine becomes supersaturated with undissociated UA that participates in CaOx crystallization. Significantly alkaline urine increases the abundance of monohydrogen phosphate which, in combination with calcium transforms finally to hydroxyapatite. In clinical practice, conditions associated with CaP stone formation include dRTA, primary hyperparathyroidism, and use of carbonic anhydrase inhibitors.

The composition and characteristics of common types of stones are summarized in Table 49.1.

Histopathological Mechanisms of Calcium Kidney Stone Formation

Increased urinary supersaturation of a stone-forming salt, leads to homogeneous nucleation in the lumen of the nephron, followed by

Table 49.1: Composition and characteristics of common type of stones

Kidney stone type	Population	Circumstances	Color	Sensitivity	Details
Calcium oxalate	80%	When urine is acidic (decreased pH)	Black/dark brown	Radio-paque	Some of the oxalate in urine is produced by the body. Calcium and oxalate in the diet play a part but are not the only factors that affect the formation of calcium oxalate stones. Dietary oxalate is found in many vegetables, fruits, and nuts. Calcium from bone may also play a role in kidney stone formation.
Calcium phosphate	5–10%	When urine is alkaline (high pH)	Dirty white	Radio-paque	Tends to grow in alkaline urine especially when proteus bacteria are present.
Uric acid	5–10%	When urine is persistently acidic	Yellow/reddish brown	Radiolucent	Diets rich in animal proteins and purines: substances found naturally in all food but especially in organ meats, fish, and shellfish.
Struvite	10–15%	Infections in the kidney	Dirty white	Radio-paque	Prevention of struvite stones depends on staying infection-free. Diet has not been shown to affect struvite stone formation.
Cystine	1–2%	Rare genetic disorder	Pink/yellow	Radio-paque	Cystine, an amino acid (one of the building blocks of protein), leaks through the kidneys and into the urine to form crystals
Xanthine		Extremely rare	Brick red	Radiolucent	

crystal growth and consequent obstruction in the distal nephron. Patients with higher urinary calcium excretion develop an interstitial apatite plaque called Randall's plaque that covers the renal papillary surface. CaOx stones use these plaques as a nidus, anchor and grow there. The extent of plaques is more in persons who have hypercalciuria and lower in those with dilute (unsaturated) urine. In the case of CaP stone formers, apatite crystal deposition occurs in the inner medullary collecting duct, producing plugs associated with interstitial scarring. Thus, the pathogenesis and histology of CaOx and CaP stone formation are different.

Genetic Basis of Calcium Stone Formation

Higher incidence of kidney stones has been reported if first-degree relatives and family members have kidney stones. This genetic link is supported by the observation that there is greater concordance with renal stone incidence in monozygotic than dizygotic twins. Although the functional significance of gene polymorphisms have not been established, association between the calcium sensor receptor (CaSR) gene polymorphism and recurrent nephrolithiasis has been identified.

Pathophysiological Mechanism(s) of Non-calcium Stones

UA Stone Formation (Fig. 49.1)

The etiological causes of UA stone formation are genetic, acquired, or a combination of both. Over the past decade, the metabolic syndrome has been characterized as the most prevalent cause of UA stone formation. The underlying pathophysiological mechanisms responsible for UA nephrolithiasis are: (1) Low urine volume; (2) hyperuricosuria; and (3) unduly acidic urine. Acidic urine with pH ≤5.5 is an invariable feature in UA nephrolithiasis. The two principal causes for acidic urine are: (1) Impaired ammonium (NH_4^+) excretion; and (2) increased endogenous acid production.

Cystinuria (Fig. 49.2)

Cystine stone forms only a small fraction of kidney stones in adults but is prevalent among children and adolescents. Cystinuria may be inherited as either autosomal recessive, usually associated with normal urinary cystine excretion or autosomal dominant with incomplete penetrance with increased urinary cystine excretion. It is characterized by an inherited defect in renal cystine reabsorption. This genetic defect is due to defective renal tubular reabsorption dibasic amino acids including cystine, ornithine, lysine, and arginine. Out of this, only cysteine has low solubility in urine. Therefore, the main complication is development of cystine stones.

Infection Related Stones (Fig. 49.3)

The most important factors for the formation of infection related stones are highly alkaline urine pH (>7.2), presence of urease-producing organisms and supersaturated urinary environment with respect to magnesium, ammonium, and phosphate ions. Rare forms of kidney stones such as dihydroxyadenine, ammonium urate, and stones resulting from protease inhibitor drugs may also occur.

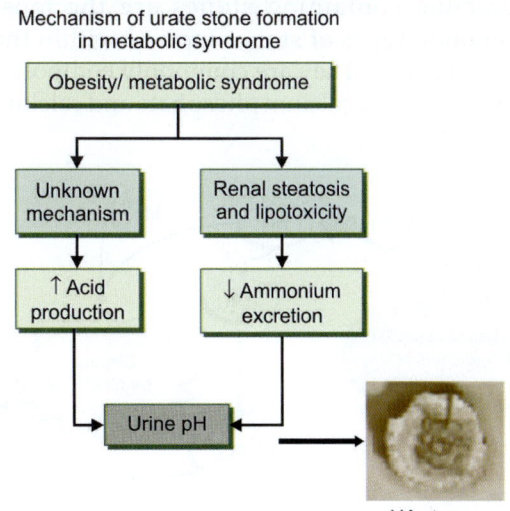

Mechanism of urate stone formation in metabolic syndrome

Obesity/ metabolic syndrome

Unknown mechanism — Renal steatosis and lipotoxicity

↑ Acid production — ↓ Ammonium excretion

Urine pH

UA stones

Fig. 49.1: Mechanisms involve increased uric acid production and acidic urine

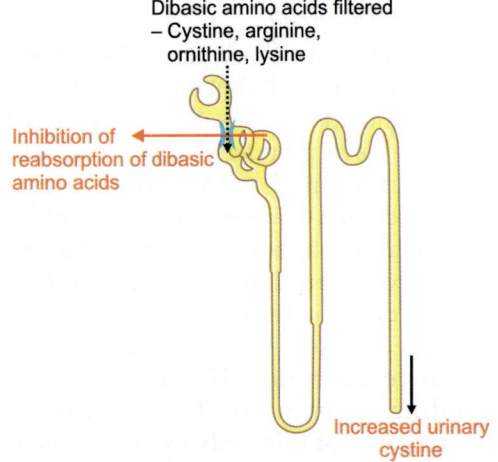

Fig. 49.2: Mechanism of increased urinary cystine excretion. The urinary excretion of dibasic amino acids like cysteine increase because of defective reabsorption in the proximal tubule

Types of Calculi

The human body can produce a variety of types of stones. The more common types of stones include calcium, uric acid, struvite and cystine.There are other stones that while unique, are rarely seen in clinical practice.

1. Calcium Stones

Calcium containing stones are the most common types of stones formed within the urinary tract. They are commonly composed of a mixture of calcium phosphate and calcium

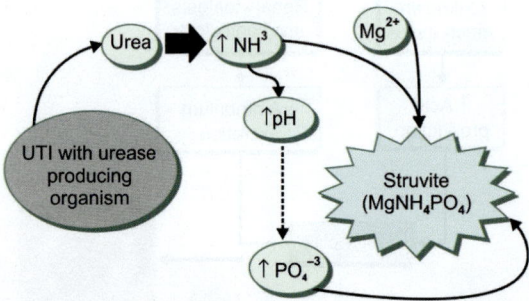

Fig. 49.3: Infection-related stone formation. Showing how Mg, NH_3 and PO_4 combine in presence of acidic urine

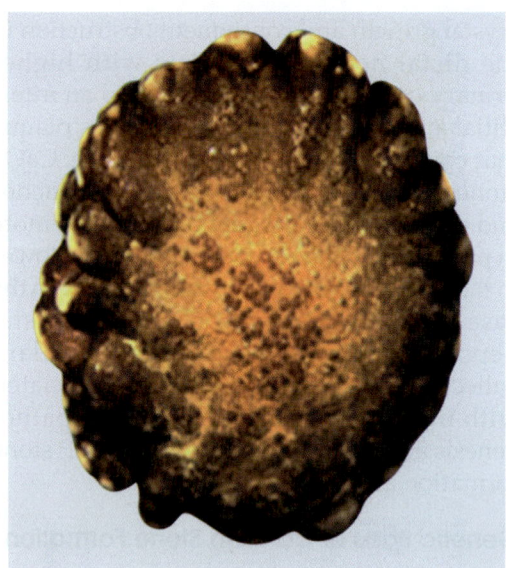

Fig. 49.4: Calcium oxalate monohydrate stone. Note the color and rough texture of calcium oxalate stone

oxalate. Among the different calcium stones are calcium oxalate monohydrate (Fig. 49.4), calcium oxalate dihydrate and calcium phosphate. They are rough, dirty brown in color and have sharp surface projections and edges.

2. Uric Acid Stones (Fig. 49.5)

Most common cause of these stones is low urine pH, associated with obesity, diabetes and metabolic syndrome. They are usually numerous rounded and vary in size. Since they are radiolucent, they are not visible in X-ray. Medical therapy by xanthine oxidase inhibitors prevent convertion of hypoxanthine to xanthine and to uric acid. The hypoxanthine is more soluble in alkaline urine and alkalinization of the urine helps to dissolve the pure uric acid stones over a long time.

3. Struvite Stones (Fig. 49.6)

These are also called infectious stones or magnesium ammonium phosphate stones. They are caused by urease splitting organisms.

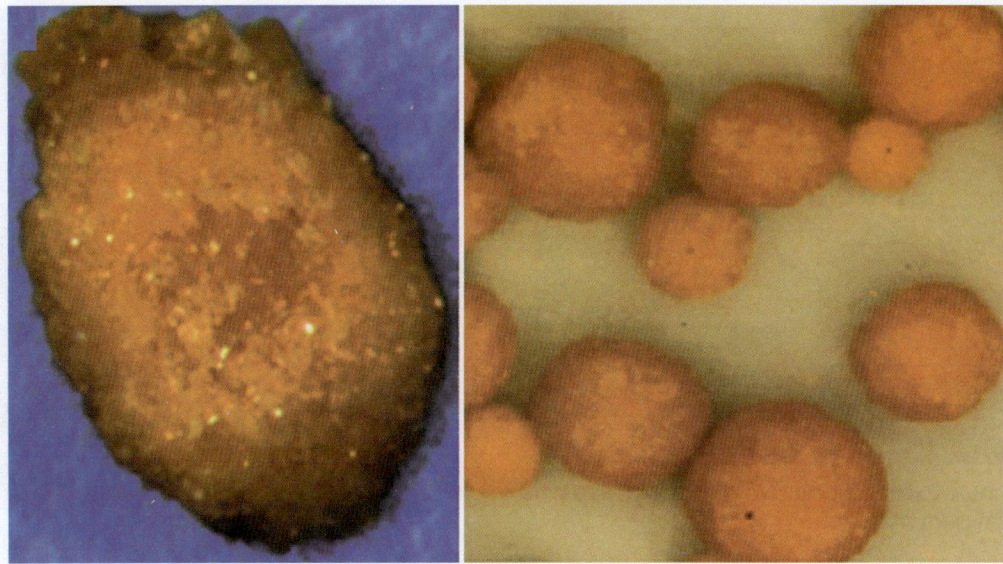

Fig. 49.5: Uric acid calculi. *Note:* Varying size and globular nature of multiple uric acid calculi

They are bulky with rounded edges and generally soft. Depending on the calcium content, they may be faintly radiopaque. Treatment is by complete stone removal and eradication of infection. Medical management

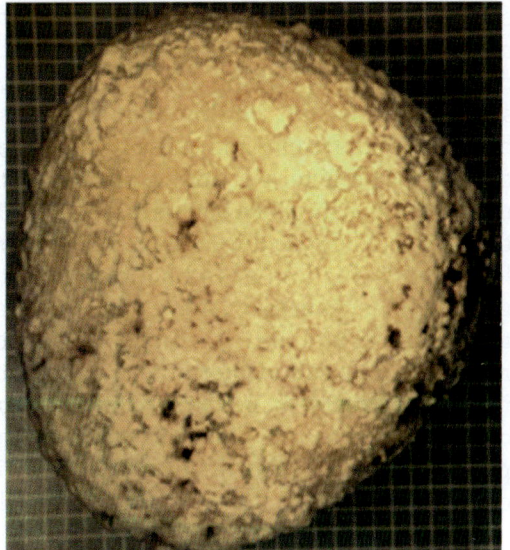

Fig. 49.6: Struvite stone. *Note:* Rounded stone with no sharp edges. Composed of magnesium ammonium phosphate

is recommended in patients who have incomplete removal of stones or poor surgical candidates.

4. Cystine Stones (Fig. 49.7)

Cystine in the urine or cystinuria, is a relatively rare autosomal recessive inborn error of metabolism characterized by impaired reabsorption of four dibasic amino acids: Cystine, ornithine, lysine and arginine (COLA), from the renal tubules as well as the gastrointestinal tract. Only the basic amino acid, cystine, is associated with stone formation due to its poor solubility in urine. Patients with cystinuria (>250 mg/24-hour) produce supersaturated urine and are at risk for crystallization and stone formation. Cystine stones are densely radiopaque (Fig. 49.8).

5. Xanthine Stones (Fig. 49.9)

Xanthine stones are very rare and may result from a genetic disorder in patients with hereditary xanthinuria. They may have an inborn defect of the enzyme xanthine oxidase and xanthine dehydrogenase. Since allopurinol used to treat uric acid stones prevents

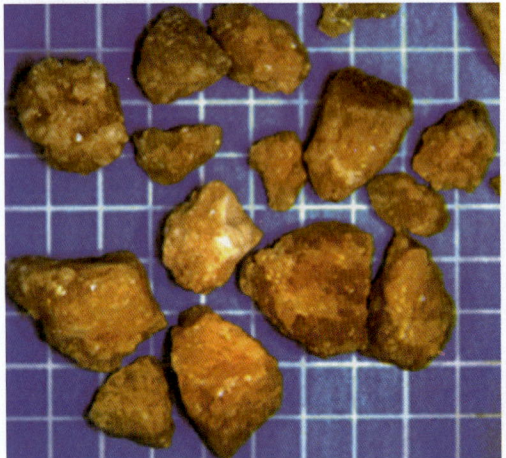

Fig. 49.7: Cystine stone. *Note:* Irregular size and shape of cystine stone

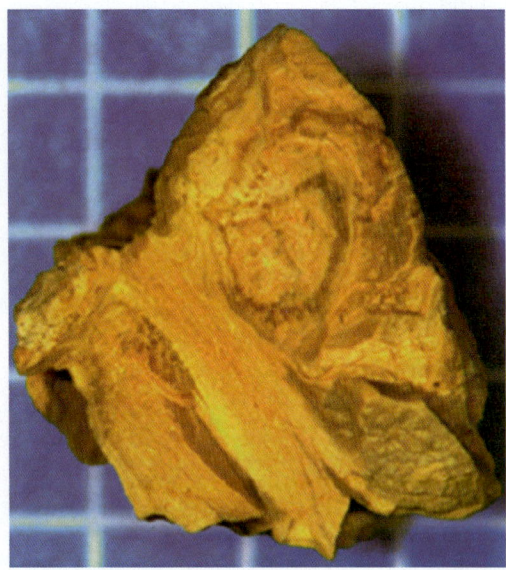

Fig. 49.9: Xanthine stone. Note the large stone roughly shaped like renal pelvis

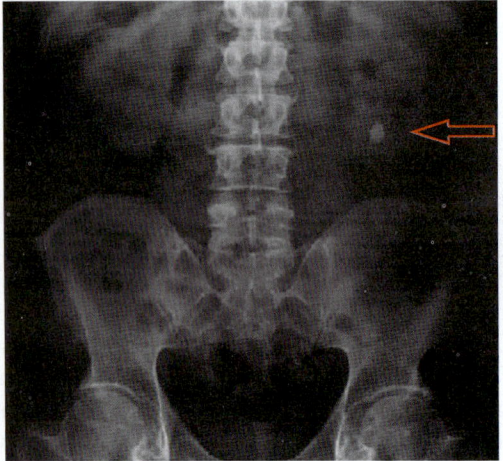

Fig. 49.8: Densely radiopaque single cystine calculus in left kidney

the conversion of xanthine to hypoxanthine and subsequently to uric acid, prolonged use of allopurinol may cause accumulation of xanthine and cause stones. These stones are large and radiolucent.

Symptoms

Stones in the urinary tract may remain asymptomatic and may be detected inciden-

tally during investigation for unrelated conditions or medical check up. The symptoms depend on the location, size and whether it is causing obstruction or irritation. The renal parenchyma has no pain fibers, the pain occurs due to irritation and spasm of ureter or obstruction of collecting system with distension and stretching of renal capsule. A stone of more than 5 millimeters can cause blockage of the ureter and cause typical renal colic. The characteristic and location of pain may change as the stone begins to move down the ureters. The pain due to renal colic may be localized to the loin or radiate from loin to groin. In men, pain may radiate to the groin or testicle and in women to the labia. The pain of renal colic intense and intermittent. The patent is not comfortable in any position and keeps changing the posture. This is in contrast to the pain in appendicitis where, the pain is constant and patient prefers not to move at all.

Other symptoms of kidney stones are:
a. Hematuria (red, pink, or brown urine)
b. Vomiting
c. Nausea

d. Discolored or foul-smelling urine (if infection is associated)

e. Chills

f. Fever

g. Frequency of micturition

h. Oliguria

i. Dysuria/strangury (if the stone is in bladder)

Diagnosis

Medical History

A detailed medical history to identify environmental and systemic factors should be undertaken. Systemic abnormalities include intestinal disease, disorders of calcium homeostasis such as primary hyperparathyroidism, conditions accompanied by extra-renal 1,25(OH)2D production such as granulomatous diseases, obesity, type II diabetes, recurrent urinary tract infection, bariatric surgery, medullary sponge kidney, and use of various drugs. Fluid intake and diet play a crucial role in the formation of kidney stones. Low fluid intake, high dietary salt and protein consumption are the most common dietary aberrations that increase the risk of nephrolithiasis.

Laboratory Diagnosis

Diagnosis of kidney stones requires a complete health history assessment and a physical exam. Other tests include: Urinalysis especially to check for crystals, bacteria, blood, and white cells. Blood tests for sugar, blood urea nitrogen (BUN), creatinine, uric acid, calcium, phosphorus and electrolytes are done to assess kidney function. The following imaging studies are done as indicated to identify the size, position and to rule out obstruction.

i. Ultrasound of the kidney

ii. Abdominal X-rays

iii. Intravenous urogram (IVU)

iv. Retrograde pyelogram

v. Abdominal CT scan

vi. MR urogram

Further laboratory investigations include urine metabolic evaluation, stone analysis, serial blood examination and imaging studies. Algorithmic approach to stone disease is shown in Flowchart 49.1. Analysis of renal stone provides valuable information for the diagnosis, type of stone and choosing correct treatment.

Treatment

When the patient presents acutely with severe pain or colic, prompt therapy with non-steroidal anti-inflammatory drug (NSAID) may be necessary. Opioids are avoided if the patient has recurrent bouts of colic since they may cause drug dependence. Concomitant use of an α-adrenoceptor blocker such as doxazosin, or a calcium antagonist, such as nifedipine is useful as they relax the ureter can improve the likelihood of spontaneous passage of distal ureteric stone. Metabolic screening is done following the resolution of the acute episode in those patients with a previous or family history, or who are thought to be at higher risk.

From a practical point of view, it is worthwhile classifying the newly diagnosed stone as follows:

i. 'Indeterminate' activity (newly diagnosed asymptomatic calculus which is not causing pain, hematuria, obstruction or infection).

General measures, observation and review at 6 months/earlier (if symptoms occur).

ii. 'Silent' (stone remaining asymptomatic, not showing increase in number/size, and not causing pain, hematuria, obstruction or infection after observation period of 6 months).

General measures, observation, medical measures if indicated and follow-up only.

iii. 'Metabolically' active (stone remaining asymptomatic but showing increase in number or size on review).

Needs medical measures if indicated and further investigations.

Flowchart 49.1: Algorithmic approach to renal stone disease

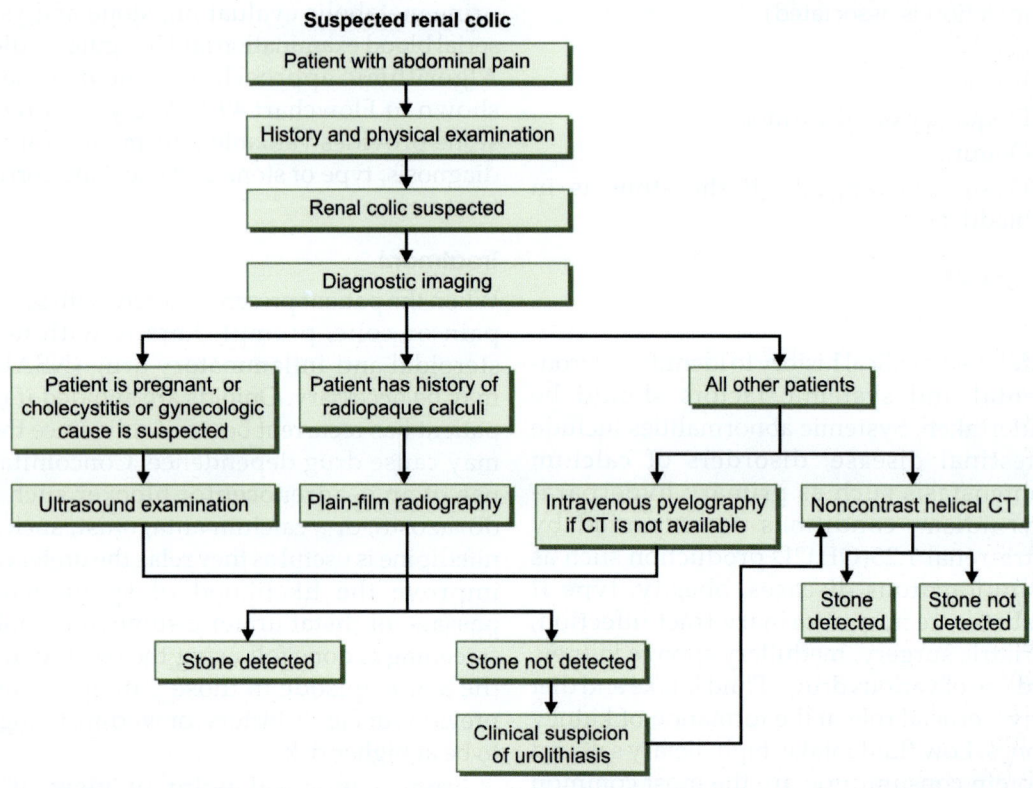

iv. 'Surgically' active (stone causing symptoms, recurrent pain, hematuria, infection or obstruction).

Such stones are to be removed by appropriate means.

General Measures

General management of recurrent kidney stones includes increased water intake, diet and lifestyle changes. Mediterranean diet, which comprises higher proportion of fruit, vegetables, low-fat dairy products and whole grains together with restricted intake of meat, sweets and sugar containing beverages is recommended.

Pharmacological Treatment

Pharmacological treatment is needed in most recurrent calcium kidney stone formers as well as in specific stone-forming populations such as UA, cystine, and infection-induced stones due to the lack of availability and/or consensus regarding the effectiveness of dietary restrictions.

Thiazide diuretics or their analogs are recommended in patients with recurrent or active disease. They help to lower urinary calcium excretion in recurrent calcium stone formers and reduce recurrence. Thiazides are effective in treating hypercalciuria and reducing stone recurrence regardless of the underlying pathophysiological mechanism. The optimal effect of thiazides is achieved when combined with low-salt diet with sufficient potassium supplementation. Potassium citrate/citric acid buffer solutions alkalinize the urine, lower urinary calcium excretion and reduce urinary CaOx, CaP, and UA deposition. In addition, alkali and thiazide use reduces the bone loss and fracture by increasing bone mineral density in the kidney stone patients.

Allopurinol treatment reduces urinary UA excretion as well as stone recurrence in hyperuricosuric calcium stone formers. Since multiple metabolic abnormalities may coexist in hyperuricosuric patients, combined thiazide and allopurinol treatment is more effective in reducing stone events compared with either treatment alone.

Acetohydroxamic acid is the only drug approved for the treatment of infection related kidney stones. This medication causes an irreversible inhibition of the enzyme urease, therefore attenuating the rise in both urinary pH and NH_4. This treatment should be used only if eradication of infection with antibiotics is ineffective even after surgical removal of the infection related stone.

Many options are available for the management of surgically active and symptomatic stones. Most stones can be managed by non-surgical methods using ultrasound or laser lithotripsy.

i. Extracorporeal shockwave lithotripsy (ESWL): It is a non-surgical treatment and the procedure involves administering shock waves focused on the stone from outside the body to break it into small fragments. This treatment can be recommended for stones less than 20 mm in size. The powdered stone fragments are passed through the natural passage. Contraindications are pregnancy or concurrent anticoagulation.

ii. Renal stones that do not respond to ESWL can be treated by flexible uretero-renoscopy (URS), if they are <20 mm and are accessible by ureteroscopy.

iii. Stones that are 20 mm or larger or situated in a calyceal diverticulum or a lower pole calyx, and inaccessible are better treated by percutaneous nephrolithotomy (PCNL).

iv. For bladder stones, cystolithotripsy can be performed through the cystoscope.

Open surgical methods are rarely practiced now. They are pyelolithotomy, nephrolithotomy, ureterolithotomy, cystolithotomy and urethrolithotomy.

Conclusion

The evaluation of kidney stone formers requires an extensive medical history to identify metabolic, environmental, dietary and/or genetic factors contributing to stone formation. Various imaging studies are available for follow-up of stone burden, but CT scan has become the gold standard modality for the initial assessment of patients with renal colic. Laboratory studies including urinalysis, stone composition analysis and serum and urinary chemistries are valuable for identifying environmental and metabolic processes contributing to stone disease, and in guiding initial and follow-up therapy.

(*Acknowledgments:* Pictures of renal stones. *Courtesy:* Louis Herring and Co, Orlando, Florida, USA.)

Asymptomatic Urinary Abnormalities

• MK Mohandas • R Kasi Visweswaran

Asymptomatic urinary abnormalities include asymptomatic hematuria, proteinuria, pyuria and bacteriuria either alone or in combination. Relevance of this topic is increasing in the current period as many urinary abnormalities are detected during routine health programs. Even though, asymptomatic abnormalities are benign most often, these may be the only pointer towards serious underlying conditions.

Isolated Microhematuria

Microhematuria is the presence of 3 or more RBCs/HPF. Significant microhematuria is the presence of >3 RBCs/HPF in 3 centrifuged urine samples. The most common causes of isolated microhematuria are glomerular diseases like IgA nephropathy, Alport's syndrome and thin basement membrane disease. Lower urinary tract bleeding usually produces gross hematuria with clots. The degree of hematuria often bears no correlation with the severity of the underlying condition. The initial assessment of microhematuria should be done in a freshly voided, clean catch midstream urine sample. If the urine specimen has been obtained by catheterization, urethral trauma itself can result in microhematuria. For the detection of microhematuria, the best sample is the first voided morning urine specimen.

From history, benign causes should be ruled out like contamination with menstrual blood, hematuria precipitated by strenuous exercise or sexual activity. History of trauma is also important. One should also ask for symptoms of urinary tract infection like fever, dysuria, or history of pharyngitis. Family history of renal disease, high myopia or deafness could point to hereditary nephritis as the probable cause of hematuria. Even if the history is not suggestive, urine culture and sensitivity should be done. The morphology of RBCs helps to differentiate glomerular from non-glomerular bleeding. In general more than 80% of RBCs will be dysmorphic in glomerular bleeding, whereas more than 80% of RBCs will be isomorphic in lower urinary tract bleeding. If a glomerular cause is suspected, a renal biopsy is the next step particularly if hypertension, proteinuria or abnormal serum creatinine value is present. Biopsy can be deferred and patient may be followed up if none of these are present. In any adult presents with persistent isolated hematuria, which is nonglomerular and/or associated with passage of clots, a detailed urological evaluation including IVU and cystourethroscopy should be done.

Isolated Proteinuria

Occurrence of proteinuria in the absence of hematuria, leukocyturia, abnormal urinary sediment, hypertension, impaired renal function, and urologic or other systemic abnormalities is called isolated proteinuria. The amount of proteinuria is usually less than 1 g/day but never more than 2 g. It is not a rare finding in the general population and is more common in children and adolescents. The prevalence is higher in girls than in boys. Isolated proteinuria can be classified into benign and pathological. Benign conditions can be subclassified as follows.

1. Functional Proteinuria

This usually occurs in association with fever, strenuous exercise, exposure to severe cold, emotional stress, congestive heart failure and seizures. This is benign, disappears with the correction of the precipitating event and is secondary to an alteration in the renal hemodynamics.

2. Idiopathic Transient Proteinuria

It is usually seen in children and young adults. On follow-up testing, it disappears spontaneously. Therefore follow-up urine testing of at least two or three urine samples is required to establish the diagnosis.

3. Orthostatic Proteinuria

This is the most common cause of isolated proteinuria in young adults. This is found in adolescents but is rare in persons above 30 years of age. Proteinuria occurs only in the upright position and disappears in the supine position. This condition has an excellent long-term prognosis. The degree of proteinuria does not exceed 1–1.5 g/day and in children the amount of proteinuria is usually less than 1 g/day. The diagnosis is established by the orthostatic or the postural test. The patient is asked to pass urine just before retiring to bed and the urine is discarded. After remaining supine all night, the entire urine sample is collected in the recumbent position the next morning. This is the supine or recumbent collection. After this, the urine samples are collected while the patient is ambulatory over the next 12–16 hours. The final sample is collected just before the patient retires to bed. This is the upright collection. In true postural proteinuria, the upright proteinuria will be >150 mg and the recumbent proteinuria will be <150 mg. Orthostatic proteinuria is usually transient in majority of cases, while it is fixed in others. Fortunately in most cases it disappears within 10–20 years of follow-up. For children with this condition annual follow-up is recommended. The long-term prognosis is found to be good even after 20–50 years.

4. Intermittent Proteinuria

Subjects with intermittent proteinuria have significant amount of protein in some of their urine samples without any renal or systemic illness.

Pathological causes of isolated proteinuria can be subclassified into:

a. *Persistent isolated proteinuria:* This accounts for about 10% of isolated proteinuria in young adults. The proteinuria persists for 3–6 months and has a worse prognosis compared to other forms of isolated proteinuria. This form of proteinuria should be investigated further with renal biopsy. On biopsy, 70% of individuals have normal histology or minor glomerular lesions like mild mesangial proliferation with or without focal sclerosis. Focal or diffuse proliferative glomerulonephritis is seen in 20% while 5% have interstitial nephritis. On long-term follow-up over 10–20 years, 50% develop hypertension and 20% ESRD. An increase in quantitative proteinuria and development of hypertension or microhematuria on follow-up are poor prognostic signs in this group of patients. So, such patients are followed-up at regular intervals for evidence of progressive renal insufficiency.

b. *Glomerular diseases with minimal inflammation:* Isolated proteinuria even without any glomerular inflammation occurs in pathological conditions like diabetes or amyloidosis.

Asymptomatic Bacteriuria

Asymptomatic bacteriuria is defined as isolation of a specified quantitative count of bacteria in an appropriately collected urine specimen from an individual without symptoms or signs of urinary tract infection. The quantitative counts are different for voided clean catch specimens and catheterized specimens.

- For asymptomatic women, bacteriuria is defined as two consecutive clean-catch voided urine specimens with isolation of the same bacterial strain in counts $\geq 10^5$ CFU/ml.
- For asymptomatic men, bacteriuria is defined as a single, clean-catch, voided urine specimen with one bacterial species isolated in a quantitative count of $\geq 10^5$ CFU/ml.
- For any asymptomatic patient, bacteriuria is defined as a single catheterized urine specimen with one bacterial species isolated in counts $\geq 10^5$ CFU/ml.

For an optimal clean-catch midstream urine, contact of the urinary stream with the skin and mucosa of external genitalia should be minimized and the urine collected directly into the sterile container. Females should be instructed to separate the labia and permit the urine flow directly from the urethra to the container. In uncircumcised males, the foreskin should be retraced and the glans cleaned and dried before collecting the sample. Initial stream of the voided specimen should be discarded so that the urethral contaminants are flushed out. The midstream urine is collected in a sterile container. The urine sample should be sent immediately to the microbiology laboratory since bacteria continue to proliferate in the warm urine, resulting in misleading increased bacterial

counts. If immediate transfer to the laboratory is not possible, the container should be transported in iced water or stored in a refrigerator at 4°C.

Screening for or treating asymptomatic bacteriuria is necessary only in pregnant ladies, those undergoing urological intervention and renal transplant recipients before and during the first 3 months following surgery. Asymptomatic bacteriuria in the above group of patients must be treated as UTI with appropriate antibiotics since the risk of developing pyelonephritis is high. Follow-up cultures are essential to confirm eradication of the organism from the urinary tract. Pregnant women have higher chances of developing pyelonephritis or pre-eclampsia if asymptomatic bacteriuria remains untreated. The chances of intrauterine growth retardation and prematurity are high for the fetus. Treatment before any urological intervention is necessary since any mucosal injury in presence of asymptomatic bacteriuria increases the risk of sepsis. Since transplant recipients are heavily immunosuppressed during the early postoperative period, asymptomatic bacteriuria should be treated. In other situations, aggressive treatment of asymptomatic bacteriuria is not warranted but should be on follow-up.

Isolated Pyuria

Pyuria is defined as presence of 10 or more WBCs per cubic mm in a centrifuged urine specimen or 3 or more WBCs in an uncentrifuged sample. It is important to ensure that a clean-catch midstream urine specimen is taken to redue the risk of contamination. Contamination of the urine sample often occurs from vaginal leukocytes or vaginal secretions in women. Urinary tract infection, the commonest cause of pyuria is associated with positive urine culture. When pyuria occurs in the absence of apparent bacterial infection, the condition is called 'isolated pyuria'. This is encountered commonly in the following situations (Table 50.1).

Table 50.1: List of conditions associated with isolated pyuria

1. Partially treated urinary tract infection/sepsis
2. Polycystic kidney disease/tubulointerstitial diseases
3. Pregnancy
4. Renal transplant rejection
5. Chronic interstitial nephritis
6. Nephrolithiasis/foreign body
7. Uroepithelial tumor/urinary fistulas
8. Painful bladder syndrome/interstitial cystitis/radiation cystitis
9. Prostatitis/pelvic infection/intra-abdominal infections
10. Infection with atypical organisms/tuberculosis/trichomonas/fungal
11. Sexually transmitted diseases (chlamydia/gonorrhea/syphilis)
12. Viral infections (genital herpes, adenovirus, HP virus, BK polyomavirus, HIV, CMV)
13. Autoimmune diseases (SLE/Kawasaki disease)
14. Drugs (NSAIDs, PPIs, aspirin, diuretics, antibiotics)

[HP: Human papilloma, HIV: Human immunodeficiency virus
CMV: Cytomegalovirus, SLE: Systemic lupus erythematosus
BK: The initials of the renal transplant recipient from whose urine, the polyomavirus was isolated in 1971

A urine culture and a genital swab culture can help rule out urinary and genital infections respectively. For the detection of genitourinary tuberculosis, 3 early morning urine samples should be tested for acid-fast staining and culture, Mantoux testing and plain X-ray abdomen for calcification will also give corroborative evidence. Allergic interstitial nephritis is usually associated with eosinophiluria, which can be detected with special stains like Wright's stain.

In addition to these isolated abnormalities, hematuria, proteinuria and pyuria can also occur in combination. Such combinations usually signify the presence of more severe underlying conditions than when they occur alone.

Miscellaneous

Diet in Renal Diseases

• MA Muthusethupathy • Suguna Rajendran • Aruna Sathyapriya

Dietetics play a key role in the management of various renal diseases. Despite the various types of food and fluids ingested, the volume and composition of body fluids is maintained constant. Since the kidneys are the main organs that excrete the metabolic waste , it is essential that diet must be modified when the kidneys are diseased (Fig. 51.1). The major components of our normal diet are carbohydrates, proteins, fats, water, vitamins, fibers and minerals. These components contribute to body weight as follows: Water 60%, proteins 17%, fats 14%, minerals 6% and carbohydrates 3%. The chief aim of food is to provide adequate energy for growth and everyday activities. Energy requirements are calculated according to body weight, gender, physiological status and nature of work for any individual. Normal requirement of energy is 30–40 kcal/kg body weight/day. The diet should contain the various components in the following proportion—carbohydrates 70%, fats 20%, and proteins 10%. The proportion of these components in normal diet and their energy yields for a 50 kg individual is given in Table 51.1.

The carbohydrates and fats are ultimately broken down to CO_2 and H_2O and liberate

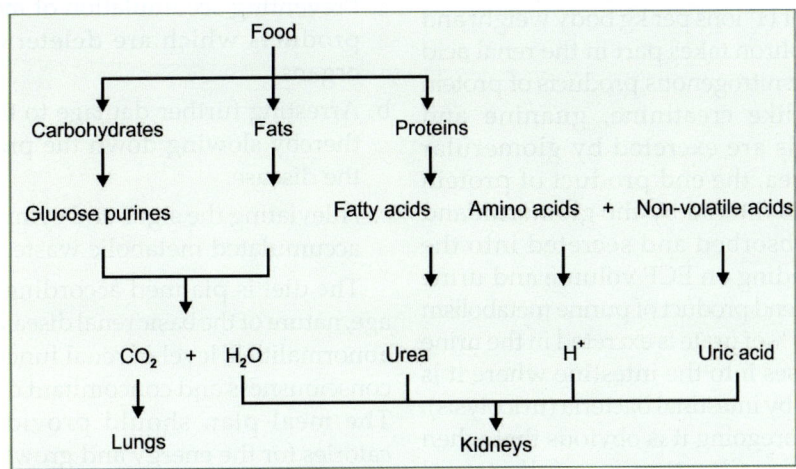

Fig. 51.1: Role of kidney in eliminating waste products derived from metabolism of food

Table 51.1: Proportion of carbohydrates, proteins and fats in normal diet and their energy yield for a 50 kg individual

Components (g)	Total amount required (kcal)	Energy in diet	Composition
Carbohydrates	350 (7 g/kg)	1400 (4 kcal/g)	70%
Proteins	50 (1 g/kg)	200 (4 kcal/g)	10%
Fats	45 (0.9 g/kg)	400 (9 kcal/kg)	20%

ATP for energy requirements. The proteins are broken down to urea and non-volatile acids like phosphoric and sulphuric acids. The nucleic acid breakdown results in the formation of uric acid. The CO_2 is excreted through the lungs. The water, urea, uric acid and H^+ ions depend on the kidneys for elimination.

The kidneys are very efficient in conserving water by concentrating the urine or excreting the excess water by diluting the urine. The major portion of the renal energy consumption is for reabsorbing filtered sodium. Since sodium is the chief in determining the body fluid volume, the kidney conserves or excretes sodium depending on the state of fluid balance. Since potassium is the chief intracellular cation and the ratio of intracellular to extracellular potassium determines the excitability of cells, potassium balance is very important for the organism. Kidneys conserve or excrete potassium depending on the composition of the body fluids. The acid load per day amounts to 1–2 mmol of H^+ ions per kg body weight and the entire nephron takes part in the renal acid excretion. The nitrogenous products of protein breakdown like creatinine, guanine and succinic acids are excreted by glomerular filtration. Urea, the end product of protein metabolism is filtered by the glomeruli and partially reabsorbed and secreted into the tubule depending on ECF volume and urine flow rate. The end product of purine metabolism is uric acid. 75% of urate is excreted in the urine and 25% passes into the intestine where it is broken down by intestinal bacteria (uricolysis).

From the foregoing it is obvious that when the glomerular filtration rate falls (renal failure), there is likely to be:

a. Accumulation of urea and other nitrogenous products leading to uremia.

b. Accumulation of hydrogen ions leading to metabolic acidosis.

c. Inability to excrete excess water leading to hyponatremia and fluid overload.

d. Inability to excrete excess of sodium leading to hypertension and pulmonary edema.

e. Inability to excrete uric acid leading to hyperuricemia and gout.

f. Inability to excrete phosphate leading to renal osteodystrophy.

g. In later stages, inability to excrete potassium leading to hyperkalemia.

Role of Dietetics in Renal Diseases

The aim of dietetics in renal disease is to adjust or change the diet in such a way that the perturbations of fluids and electrolytes caused by renal disease are minimised. This can be achieved by:

a. Preventing accumulation of metabolic end products which are deleterious to vital organs.

b. Arresting further damage to the nephrons thereby slowing down the progression of the disease.

c. Alleviating the signs and symptoms due to accumulated metabolic waste.

The diet is planned according to patient's age, nature of the basic renal disease, associated abnormalities, level of renal function, level of consciousness and concomitant drug therapy. The meal plan should provide adequate calories for the energy and growth needs and make the meal palatable.

The major five syndromes of renal disease which require modification in diet are:

1. Acute renal failure (AKI)
2. Chronic kidney disease stages 3–5 (earlier chronic renal failure)
3. Acute nephritic syndrome
4. Nephrotic syndrome
5. Renal stone disease

1. Diet in AKI (ARF)

During the oliguric phase of AKI, excretion of water, electrolytes and nitrogenous and products are diminished resulting in fluid overload, hyperkalemia, azotemia and acidosis. Hyperkalemia is more prominent if acidosis and hypoxia accompany the peripheral circulatory failure and in hypercatabolic states of AKI. During the diuretic phase the excretion of water, electrolytes and other solutes are increased. Contrary to the hyperkalemia of oliguric phase, dangerous levels of hypokalemia may occur during diuretic phase.

The diet should be planned according to the phases of AKI. In the oliguric phase, intake of salt, potassium, fluids and proteins are restricted and calories supplied mainly from carbohydrates and fats. Once, diuretic phase sets in, the intake of fluids should be 300–500 ml more than the total output during the previous 24 hours. Potassium/sodium supplementation may be necessary in hypokalemia/hyponatremia.

Calories

The daily calorie requirement is maintained at 30 kcal per kg body weight. Since proteins are to be restricted, adequate calories are provided by increasing carbohydrate combined with a normal or low fat diet. Intake of 100 g of sugar per day has a marked protein sparing effect. Up to 300 g of sugar can be advised if there is significant weight loss.

Proteins

Protein restriction is essential in renal failure to prevent accumulation of urea, uremic symptoms and to arrest further progression of the disease. Approximately 0.5/0.6 g/kg of proteins (50% of the normal requirement) is sufficient in AKI. Care is taken to provide essential amino acids within this allowance of proteins; therefore 60% of the proteins provided should be of high biological value. Eggs, milk, meat, fish and chicken are rich in high biological value protein. Parenteral administration of essential amino acids routinely to all cases of AKI is not advocated.

Fluids

Retention of excess water will lead to hyponatremia and other complications. If the patient is anuric, intake of fluids should equal insensible loss from the skin and respiratory tract minus the amount of water produced by metabolism. This generally would amount to 300–500 ml/day. In patients who are oliguric, fluid intake equivalent to volume of urine output + 500 ml is often adequate. If the patient with oliguria has symptoms of pulmonary edema, rigorous fluid restriction is essential (300 ml/day). In the diuretic phase, depending on the output, fluid intake can be liberalized. The best way to assess the adequacy of fluid therapy is monitoring daily weight. A daily weight loss of 0.2–0.3 kg is ideal in the oliguric phase. Any weight gain calls for further restriction of salt and water.

Sodium

Salt retention manifests as fluid overload and hypertension. In patients, who have signs of fluid overload, salt-free diet is advocated. In the diuretic phase, salt intake can be liberalized to prevent dehydration and hypovolemia.

Potassium

Since hyperkalemia is a life-threatening condition, food rich in potassium should be avoided totally. Fruits, except apple and pineapple, and vegetables, most of the greens are rich sources of potassium and should be avoided. Vegetables may be used after removal of potassium as follows. They are sliced and soaked in warm water for 45–60 minutes to remove potassium and the water is discarded.

A simple diet containing 100 g of butter, 100 g of glucose, 25 g of custard powder in 300 ml of water is advocated in some hospitals. Liquid diet schedule for a sick patient of AKI is given in Tables 51.2 and 51.3. A stable patient may be advised diet is given in Tables 51.4 and 51.5.

2. Diet in Chronic Kidney Disease (CKD)

In CKD stages 3, 4 and 5, there is irreversible renal damage and the nephron mass is reduced. Sclerosis occurs and the kidneys are smaller and sclerosed. Conservative management with diet forms the mainstay of therapy in the earlier phases of the disease. Such therapy helps in arresting or delaying the progression of the disease. Glomerular hyperperfusion and intraglomerular hypertension may be the two main factors, which favor progression of renal failure leading to sclerosis of the glomeruli. Proteins and lipids also contribute towards hyperperfusion and intraglomerular hypertension thereby accelerating the process of sclerosis. Dietetics can therefore play a key role in arresting the progression of the disease.

Calories

The normal caloric requirement is 30 kcal/kg body weight. In CKD, proteins and fats are restricted and maximum calories are obtained from carbohydrates. For chronic renal failure patients, 85% of calories are obtained from carbohydrates, 10% from fats and only 5% from proteins.

Proteins

Dietary proteins are restricted to 0.5–0.6 g/kg/day of high biological value protein from early renal failure when the creatinine is over 177 mmol/L or 2 mg/dl. Protein restriction not only limits urea production but also restricts the consumption of phosphates. Low protein diet reduces the metabolic breakdown of sulfur-containing amino acids and prevents the acidosis.

Fluids

In chronic renal failure, when urine output is good, it is maintained at 2.5–3.0 liters per day

Table 51.2: Liquid diet for a sick patient of ARF

Proteins	– 20 g (energy: 1597 kcal)		Fluids: 500 ml	Salt: Nil	
Food	Amount	Proteins (g)	Energy (kcal)	Sodium (mEq)	Potassium (mEq)
Milk	450 ml	14.4	302.0	3.1	16.2
Egg	1 no	6.4	83.0	2.7	1.8
Arrowroot flour	25 g	0.1	83.5	-	0.1
Unsalted butter	100 g	-	729.0	-	-
Glucose	100 g	-	400.0	-	-
Total		**20.9**	**1597.0**	**5.8**	**18.1**

Table 51.3: Meal plan (liquid diet) for ARF (Ryle's tube feeding)

6 am	Milk + egg + glucose	100 ml
9 am	Arrowroot porridge (prepared with milk, glucose and butter)	100 ml
1 pm	Arrowroot porridge	100 ml
5 pm	Milk + glucose + butter	100 ml
9 pm	Arrowroot porridge	100 ml

Table 51.4: Solid diet for a stable patient with ARF

Proteins—20.0 g   Sodium—7.5 mEq   Potassium—23.0 mEq
Fluids—500 ml   Salt—nil   Energy—1800 kcal

S.no.	Food	Amount	Protein (g)	Calories (kcal)	Sodium (mEq)	Potassium (mEq)
1.	Milk	200 ml	6.2	140	1.4	7.2
2.	Curds	50 ml	1.4	30	0.6	1.7
3.	Egg white	1 no.	3.2	16	2.8	1.3
4.	Cereal	100 g	6.3	350	0.4	3.0
5.	Vegetables	100 g	1.2	40	1.6	1.8
6.	Fruits	50 g	0.2	30	0.3	0.9
7.	Potato	50 g	0.7	44	03.	3.0
8.	Oil	50 g	-	450	-	-
9.	Sago	100 g	0.2	350	0.1	4.1
10.	Sugar	75 g	-	300	-	-
11.	Marie biscuits	2 nos	0.6	50	-	-
	Total		**20.0**	**1800**	**7.5**	**23.0**

Table 51.5: Meal plan (solid diet) for ARF

6 am	Milk 50 ml, with sugar
8 am	Sago uppuma or sago halwa
11 am	Fruit: Apple 1 small (or any other low potassium fruit taken from the exchange list, *see* Table 51.15)
1 pm	Rice: 1½ cups (50 g of uncooked rice)
	Curds 50 ml, vegetable fry 50 g (select from the list of low potassium vegetables, *see* Table 51.14)
	egg white, 1 no.
4 pm	Milk 100 ml, with sugar
	Marie biscuits—two
8 pm	Rice: 1½ cups
	Pepper water, 50 ml
	Potato puttu of 50 g of potato
10 pm	Sago or arrowroot porridge, 100 ml

Note: For vegetarians instead of one egg white, milk 100 ml can be given.

since maximum urea clearance occurs with this urine volume. In oliguric patients, fluids are restricted to urine output plus 300–500 ml/day.

Sodium

Salt restriction is advised only if the patient has symptoms of sodium retention such as hypertension or edema. In chronic interstitial nephritis, patients may have salt wasting tendency. In such cases, the salt intake should be liberal (6–10 g/day) so as to prevent hypovolemia and worsening of renal failure. Advice on salt intake is individualized in patients with chronic renal failure.

Potassium

Though hyperkalemia of rapid onset is not seen commonly in CKD due to compensatory factors, potassium restriction is advised in moderate and advanced cases.

Calcium and Phosphates

Hypocalcemia and hyperphosphatemia occur in CKD leading to renal osteodystrophy. High biological value proteins are also rich in phosphates. Dietary phosphate binders like calcium carbonate powder are necessary for the management of calcium and phosphate disorders of renal failure.

Table 51.6: Diet for CRF patient

Protein—30 g | Energy—2000 kcal | Fluids and salt, as per requirement

S. no.	Food	Amount	Protein (g)	Energy (kcal)	Sodium (mEq)	Potassium (mEq)
1.	Milk	300 ml	9.4	200	2.1	10.8
2.	Curds	100 ml	3.0	60	1.4	3.3
3.	Egg white	2 nos	6.4	30	5.7	2.7
4.	Cereals (rice)	150 g	9.6	530	0.8	4.5
5.	Vegetables (average)	100 g	1.2	50	1.6	1.8
6.	Fruits (average)	50 g	0.2	23	0.3	0.8
7.	Sago	100 g	0.2	350	0.1	0.1
8.	Sugar	75 g	-	300	-	-
9.	Oil	50 g	-	450	-	-
	Total		**30.0**	**2000**	**12.0**	**24.0**

Table 51.7: Meal plan for CRF patient

6 am	Milk, 100 ml, with sugar
8 am	Idlis two or Idiyappam (3–4 no), or appam two or rice upma 1½ cups, or aval upma with cereal 50 g Onion chutney or sugar 3 teaspoons and butter 1 teaspoon
11 am	Apple or guava 50 g or 1 small, or any other low potassium fruit 50 g, marie biscuits 2
1 pm	Rice 1½ cups of cooked rice (50 g of uncooked rice), curds 50 ml, egg white 1 no., vegetables 50 g (chosen from the list of low potassium group), sago papads 2 or 3 (homemade without salt)
4 pm	Sago halwa or sago upma, 1½ cups, milk 100 ml
8 pm	Same as lunch
10 pm	100 ml milk with sugar

Note: For vegetarians, instead of two eggs white, cheese 27 g or panneer or cottage cheese 35 g can be added. Two eggs white can be exchanged with a whole egg or with some other non-vegetarian item in the meat exchange

A 30 g protein model diet for chronic renal failure patients is given in Tables 51.6 and 51.7.

3. Diet in Acute Nephritic Syndrome

Monitoring urine output, daily weight, and blood pressure recording are essential for regulation of fluid balance. Caloric requirement is 30–40 kcal/kg body weight. In patients with renal failure, protein is restricted to 0.6 g/kg/day. In patients with fluid retention/overload, fluid intake restricted to 300–500 ml and is liberalized when urine output increases. Salt restriction is indicated for edema and hypertension. Potassium is restricted if the patient has renal failure or is oliguric.

4. Diet in Nephrotic Syndrome

In nephrotic syndrome, the dietary modifications should aim at improving hypoproteinemia

and correct hyperlipidemia. Normal intake of 30–40 kcal/kg is recommended. Contrary to the earlier practice of giving high protein diet of 1.5–2.0 g/kg/kg body weight, a normal protein diet (0.8–1 g/kg) is advised in nephrotic syndrome now. This diet helps in preventing further glomerular injury due to excess protein intake. Moreover high protein diet always poses a problem for restricting salt. Fluids can be liberal when there is no edema and increased urine output. Otherwise fluids are restricted to the volume of urine output plus 300 ml. Salt intake is restricted to 2 g per day till the edema subsides. Since these patients are on diuretics, hypokalemia may occur and potassium supplements may be necessary. If patients have renal failure also, protein restricted diet as in chronic renal failure is advised. A 60 g protein diet chart for nephrotic patient is given in Tables 51.8 and 51.9.

5. Diet in Renal Stone Disease

The dietary modifications depend on the type and composition of the stone. Generally a high intake of fluids (3–5 L/day) to make the urine dilute and enhance urinary flow is advised. The urine flow may wash out the particles of gravel from the urinary tract. Most renal stones are composed of calcium oxalate. Though it appears rational to restrict both calcium and oxalate in the diet, studies have shown that calcium-restricted diet leads to increased incidence of new urinary stones.

The probable reason for this pathological finding is that reduced dietary calcium leads to increased absorption of oxalate from the GI tract, thus resulting in increased oxalate in the urine and formation of oxalate stones. We therefore advise restriction of oxalate in the diet and allow moderate calcium intake. In urate stone disease, it is necessary to reduce purines in the diet.

For Oxalate Restriction

Avoid greens especially spinach, amaranth, drumstick leaves, curry leaves, beetroot, sweet potatoes, tapioca, drumstick, plantain flower, plantain green, nuts like almond,

Table 51.8: Diet for nephrotic syndrome

Proteins—60 g	Fluids—500 ml		Salt—nil		Energy—2000 kcal	
S.no. Food		Amount	Protein (g)	Energy (kcal)	Sodium (mEq)	Potassium (mEq)
1.	Milk	250 ml	8.0	168	1.7	9.0
2.	Curds	100 ml	3.0	60	1.4	3.3
3.	Egg white	4 nos	12.8	64	11.3	5.2
4.	Red gram dal	25 g	5.6	84	0.3	9.1
5.	Bengal gram	30 g	5.0	108	0.5	6.2
6.	Rice	200 g	12.8	692	0.9	6.1
7.	Idlis	3 nos	4.8	144	0.4	5.6
8.	Vegetables	200 g	2.8	74	3.2	3.6
9.	Khova (casein)	25 g	5.0	103	-	-
10.	Fruit	50 g	0.2	23	0.3	0.9
11.	Sugar	30 g	-	120	-	-
12.	Oil	40 g	-	360	-	-
	Total		**60.0**	**2000**	**20.0**	**49.0**

Table 51.9: Meal plan for nephrotic syndrome

Morning	Milk 100 ml with sugar
Breakfast	Idlis 3 nos, or chapatis—2 to 3 nos, or bread—3 slices or rava or vermicelli upma 1½ cups, egg white—1 no. with chutney or sambar or jam and butter
10 am	Milk khova 25 g
1 pm	Rice 3 cups, sambar 50 ml, curds 50 ml, egg whites 2 nos, vegetables 10 g, fry or curry, fruits 50 g of any variety
4 pm	Bengal gram sundal 50 g
	Coffee or tea—100 ml with 50 ml of milk
8 pm	Rice 3 cups, sambar 50 ml, curds 50 ml, egg white 1 no., vegetables 100 g
10 pm	Milk 100 ml

Notes: 1. For vegetarians instead of 3 eggs white, khova, cheese 48 g or paneer 53 g can be taken.

2. Since the diet already contains 500 ml of fluids, no more liquid in any form is allowed.

3. Four eggs white can be exchanged with other non-vegetarian item given in the meat exchange, *see* Table 51.12.

gingelly seeds and cashew-nuts, green chillies, fruits like amla, currants, figs, jackfruit, and mango (ripe), beef muscle, tea, beer, etc.

For Purine Restriction

Avoid beans, dry fish, meats, oat meals, peas dry, poultry, seafood, spinach which contain 50–150 mg purine/100 g, brain, kidney, liver, meat extracts, mushrooms, cardinos which contain 150 mg purines/100 g).

Food exchange lists: A food exchange list is utilized to offer variety to the diet (Tables 51.10 to 51.16).

Foods to be avoided: The following foods are rich in potassium and therefore be avoided in renal failure: Nuts, jaggery, instant coffee powder, coca, chocolate, coconut, tender coconut water, coriander powder, coffee, etc.

Table 51.10: Central exchange list

S.no.	Name of the foodstuff	Amount (g)	Protein (g)	Carbohydrates (g)	Fat (g)	Na (mEq)	K (mEq)	Energy (kcal)
1.	Rice parboiled	50	3.2	40	0.2	0.2	1.5	173
2.	Raw rice	47	3.2	36.8	0.2	0.2	0.9	162
3.	Jowar	30.8	3.2	22.4	0.6	0.1	1.0	107
4.	Oats	23.5	3.2	14.8	1.8	0.02	2.1	88
5.	Ragi	43.8	3.2	31.5	0.6	0.2	4.6	144
6.	Rice flakes	48.4	3.2	37.4	0.6	0.2	1.9	167
7.	Semolina	30.8	3.2	23.0	0.2	0.3	0.7	107
8.	Vermicelli	36.8	3.2	28.8	0.1	0.13	1.3	130
9.	Wheat flour	26.4	3.2	18.3	0.4	0.23	2.1	90
10.	Maida flour	29.0	3.2	21.4	0.3	0.12	1.0	101
11.	Bread (2 slices)	41.0	3.2	21.3	0.3	-	1.3	100
12.	Idlis (two)	90.0	3.2	19.0	0.1	0.3	3.7	96
13.	Cornflakes	38.0	3.2	32.9	0.2	10.8	1.5	144
14.	Sweet biscuits	50.0	3.2	36.0	7.6	-	-	225

Table 51.11: Milk exchange list

S.no.	Name of the foodstuff	Amount (g)	Protein (g)	Carbohydrates (g)	Fat (g)	Na (mEq)	K (mEq)	Energy (kcal)
1.	Milk (3% fat)	200 ml	6.4	8.8	8.2	1.39	7.2	134
2.	Curds	206 ml	6.4	6.2	8.3	2.9	6.9	124
3.	Cheese	27 g	6.4	1.7	6.7	7.7	0.7	94
4.	Cottage cheese	35 g	6.4	0.4	7.3	0.2	0.33	93
5.	Skimmed milk powder	17 g	6.48.7	-	4.4	5.84		61
6.	Whole milk powder	25 g	6.4	9.5	6.7	60.0	7.9	124
7.	Khova	32 g	6.4	8.0	8.3	-	-	132
8.	Cream	89 g	6.4	3.2	32.0	11.4	0.04	318

Table 51.12: Meat exchange list

S.no.	Name of the foodstuff	Amount (g)	Protein (g)	Carbohydrates (g)	Fat (g)	Na (mEq)	K (mEq)	Energy (kcal)
1.	Egg whole	48	6.4	-	6.4	2.7	1.8	83
2.	Egg white (2)	70.4	6.4	-	-	5.7	2.8	32
3.	Chicken	25	6.4	-	0.2	0.7	2.1	27
4.	Fish (average)	32	6.4	2	2.4	0.7	1.2	34
5.	Mutton	35	6.4	-	4.7	0.5	2.4	68
6.	Liver	32	6.4	-	1.0	1.0	1.3	34
7.	Prawns	34	6.4	0.3	0.3	1.0	2.3	30
8.	Crab	72	6.4	2.4	0.8	6.6	3.3	43
9.	Duck	30	6.4	-	1.4	2.6	2.5	39
10.	Beef	28	6.4	-	0.7	0.6	1.5	32
11.	Pork	34	6.4	-	1.5	0.8	2.3	39

Table 51.13: Dal exchange list

S.no.	Name of the foodstuff	Amount (g)	Protein (g)	Carbohydrates (g)	Fat (g)	Na (mEq)	K (mEq)	Energy (kcal)
1.	Red gram dal	27	6.0	15.6	0.5	0.3	7.64	91
2.	Bengal gram dal	29	6.0	17.3	1.6	0.9	5.4	108
3.	Black gram dal	25	6.0	14.9	0.4	0.43	5.1	87
4.	Green gram	25	6.0	14.2	0.3	0.3	5.4	83
5.	Green gram dal	25	6.0	15.0	0.3	0.3	7.4	87
6.	Bengal gram	35	6.0	21.3	1.8	0.6	7.3	126
	roasted	27	6.0	15.7	1.4	-	-	100
7.	Green peas	83	6.0	13.2	0.1	0.3	1.7	77
8.	Dry peas	31	6.0	18.0	0.3	5.8	5.8	98
9.	Roasted groundnuts	23	6.0	6.1	9.2	4.1	4.1	131
10.	Soya beans	14	6.0	2.9	2.7	-	-	61

Table 51.14: Vegetables exchange list (potassium content)

Group I	Group II	Group III
K content	K content	K content
<100 mg/100 g	101–200 mg/100 g	>200 mg/100 g
Fenugreek leaves	Bittergourd	Amaranth
Beetroot	Brinjal	Corriander leaves
Radish, pink	Cauliflower	Drumstick leaves
Snake gourd	Cabbage	Spinach
Bottle gourd	French beans	Colacasia
Beans	Ladies finger	Potato
Field beans	Onion stalks	Sweet potato
Cucumber	Plantain flower	Tapioca
	Green plantain	Yam
Green mango	Pumpkin	Cluster beans
Ridge gourd	Green tomato	Paruppu keerai
Peas chow-chow		

Table 51.15: Fruits exchange list (potassium content)

Group I	Group II	Group III
K content	K content	K content
<100 mg/100 g	101–200 mg/100 g	>200 mg/100 g
Apple	Jackfruit	Gooseberries
Guava	Pomegranate	Apricot
Papaya	Tomato	Banana
Pear		Lemon
Pineapple		Cherries
		Sweet lime
		Mango
		Plums
		Sapota
		Custard apple
		Peach

Table 51.16: Condiments and spices exchange list

S.no.	Condiment/spice	Quantity (g)	Potassium (mg)	Sodium (mg)
1.	Dry chillies	19	100	2.67
2.	Green chillies	47	100	3.00
3.	Coriander powder	10	100	3.20
4.	Cumin seeds	10	100	12.60
5.	Fenugreek seeds	19	100	3.61
6.	Turmeric powder	3	100	0.75

Tropical Nephropathy

• **Santhosh Varughese** • **Suceena Alexander**

INTRODUCTION

The countries between tropic of cancer in the north and tropic of capricorn in the south are the tropical countries. Several developing nations in this region are plagued with numerous environmental problems like poor sanitation, pollutants and infections, social issues like illiteracy and lower socioeconomic status and health related problems. Inadequate access to medical care, malnutrition, infections and higher maternal and fetal mortality rates are the main health related problems. Kidney diseases are also very common in the tropics. In addition to the kidney diseases encountered worldwide, certain unique kidney diseases in this region are discussed under the heading 'tropical nephropathies' in this chapter.

Kidney Diseases in the Tropics

Common tropical nephropathies may be grouped as follows.

I. *Tropical Nephropathies due to Infections*

Protozoal infections: Malaria, filariasis, schistosomiasis.

Viral infections: Hantavirus, dengue hemorrhagic fever, hepatitis B, hepatitis C, HIV associated nephropathies.

Bacterial infections: Tuberculosis, Hansen's disease, Salmonella infections, Shigella infections, Brucellosis.

Spirochetal infections: Leptospirosis

II. *Tropical Nephropathies due to Toxins*

Snake envenomation, insect stings, plant toxins (including indigenous medication), ethylene glycol, methanol, formic acid.

III. *Miscellaneous Tropical Nephropathies*

Post-infectious (or infection related) glomerulonephritis, other glomerular diseases, nephrolithiasis, Takayasu's aortoarteritis, some specific tropical nephropathies.

Renal Disease in Malaria

Malaria is caused by Plasmodium group of organisms and is an endemic disease of the tropical regions. Infections with *P. falciparum* and occasionally *P. vivax* cause acute kidney injury (AKI). Infections with *P. malariae* and to a lesser extent *P. falciparum* cause glomerulopathy.

Almost two-thirds of severe *P. falciparum* malaria may develop AKI by the end of the first week. AKI is commonly non-oliguric and lasts for about two weeks. The malarial parasite invades erythrocytes of all ages causing severe parasitemia. The rupture of parasitized erythrocytes release merozoites into circulation. These in turn invade other RBCs perpetuating infection. The stiff cell membrane of parasitized cell and the highly viscous cytoplasm adhere to the vascular endothelium by surface projections. These contain adhesion proteins, of which *P. falciparum* erythrocyte membrane protein 1 (PfEMP-1) is the most important adhesion protein. Severe hemolysis is common and may lead to "blackwater fever". The degree of sequestration of parasitized erythrocytes correlates with morbidity and mortality. Apart from these mechanical changes, there are immunologic changes that result in cytokine release, activation of complement and coagulation cascades and contribute to severity of illness. Electrolyte abnormalities of sodium, potassium, calcium and phosphorus and metabolic acidosis may also accompany AKI. Treatment of severe falciparum malaria is supportive combined with specific antimalarial therapy, usually intravenous artemisinins. Either peritoneal dialysis or hemodialysis may be employed to tide over the AKI. Despite all efforts, the mortality remains about 40%. Delay in treatment, degree of parasitemia, concomitant gram negative septicemia and multiorgan involvement are associated with increased mortality. *P. vivax* associated AKI is usually milder and results from intravascular fluid depletion and hemolysis. In communities where G6PD deficiency is common, drug-induced hemolysis in patients with glucose-6-phosphate dehydrogenase (G6PD) deficiency is a major contributor for development of AKI.

Malarial glomerulopathy (quartan malarial nephropathy) is an important cause of nephrotic syndrome in tropical Africa and develops weeks after the onset of fever. Proteinuria is accompanied by hypoalbuminemia, hypertension and renal dysfunction. Less than half of these patients have microscopic hematuria. The serum complements are normal. Renal histology is that of membrano-proliferative glomerulonephritis with IgG, IgM and C3 deposits. Antimalarial therapy is ineffective and the course is progressive, with progressive decline in renal function resulting in end stage renal disease (ESRD). The glomerulopathy resulting after *P. falciparum* infection is transient and resolves after infection settles.

Leptospiral AKI

Leptospira belong to the spirochetal group of organisms. *Leptospira interrogans* complex causes leptospirosis which is the most common zoonotic illness worldwide. It is particularly common in the tropics. There are 30 serogroups and 240 serotypes that are pathogenic. Of the myriad animal hosts described, rodents and specifically rats have been most commonly implicated. The hosts harbor large number of Leptospira in their kidneys which are shed via their urine for many years. Although they are very delicate organisms, a moist environment or stagnant water, not exposed to direct sunlight allows the Leptospira to survive outside a host. Humans get infected when they come into contact with infected urine containing the Leptospira. The organisms enter the body through abrasions in the skin or even intact mucosa. Farmers, fishermen, sewage workers and those exposed to contaminated water are at highest risk of infection. Others can also get infected with accidental exposure to urine of infected rodents or animals.

Young males are most commonly affected and the incidence of infection peaks during the monsoon season. Most infections are sub-clinical and self-limiting but the disease can sometimes be fatal. A week or two after infection, there is initially a syndrome of high fever with chills and rigor, headache and severe myalgia. This initial phase is called the leptospiremic phase. This is followed a few days later by recurrence of symptoms accompanied by cholestatic jaundice and renal involvement. This latter phase is called Weil's syndrome. Hypercatabolic AKI may occur in up to 85% of cases. AKI is usually non-oliguric and mild, especially in anicteric patients. However, severe disease is accompanied by oliguric AKI. The duration of AKI may last up to several weeks. Initial mild proteinuria with hyaline and granular casts precedes onset of azotemia. Hypokalemia, hypomagnesemia and hypophosphatemia occur due to tubular loss in about half the patients.

Leptospiral invasion of kidney tissue results in AKI. The organisms bind to 'toll-like receptors' and initiate an immune response characterized by activation of inflammatory pathways, release of cytokines and chemokines. The organisms also release endotoxins and enzymes. The leptospiral endotoxin has a glycoprotein component that inhibits Na^+-K^+ ATPase and $Na^+-K^+-Cl^-$ cotransporter. This is responsible for urinary potassium loss and hypokalemia. There is also a reduction in expression of Na^+H^+ exchanger isoform 3 and aquaporin 1 in the proximal tubule, which is responsible for acidosis and polyuria. Altered systemic hemodynamics similar to that occurring in sepsis is also seen. The resultant interstitial nephritis and tubular necrosis is the underlying pathology in leptospiral AKI. The plasma levels of TNF correlate with the degree of renal dysfunction. Serum level of procalcitonin is usually elevated.

Patients with severe hypotension are more likely to develop renal and pulmonary complications. Pulmonary hemorrhage and acute respiratory distress syndrome (ARDS) are associated with poor prognosis. The hypotension is due to profound systemic vasodilatation, fluid shift to muscles, relative intravascular volume deficit and renal vasoconstriction. They respond to careful intravenous fluid resuscitation, which must be done with central venous pressure monitoring so as not to precipitate acute pulmonary edema.

Diagnosis is established either by culturing blood or urine on Fletcher's or Stuart's semisolid media. Since the organisms are very delicate, special precautions are needed for culture. The diagnosis can be made by detection of anti-Leptospira antibodies of titre >1:400 or a fourfold rise in titre. Macroscopic agglutination test is used for rapid screening but its specificity is low. The gold standard in serology is the microscopic agglutination test. Other less commonly used serologic tests are different types of enzyme-linked immunosorbent assay (ELISA). At present, nucleic acid based testing is available only for research purposes.

Mild cases of leptospirosis recover spontaneously. Treatment includes supportive care with intravenous fluid administration and correction of electrolyte imbalance. Antimicrobial treatment of intravenous benzyl penicillin (1,500,000 units every 6 hours) or oral doxycycline (100 mg twice daily) for 7 days shortens the duration of febrile illness. Patients with severe AKI need dialysis, especially when hypercatabolic. In those with multiorgan dysfunction on inotropic support, intermittent hemodialysis may not be possible. Slow (or sustained) low efficiency daily dialysis (SLEDD) or continuous renal replacement therapy (CRRT) may be required. CRRT may enhance removal of cytokine and inflammatory mediators hastening recovery. Daily dialysis offers better chances of survival in comparison to an alternate day schedule. Apart from multiorgan dysfunction, other poor prognostic markers are older age, superadded infections, altered sensorium, pulmonary complications, hyperkalemia, hyperbilirubinemia and diarrhea.

Scrub Typhus Infection-associated AKI

Rickettsial infection due to *Orientia tsutsugamushi* occurs by subcutaneous inoculation of organisms by infected trombiculid mite larvae. The resultant scrub typhus infection has been growing in importance and is endemic in Asia. If untreated, the mortality may be as high as 30%. The predominant cause of disease is widespread vascular endothelial cell injury. Until recently, AKI due to scrub typhus was not known to be common. Urinary abnormalities may be seen in 70–80% of infected persons. AKI develops in about half of them due to acute tubular necrosis or tubulointerstitial nephritis. Twice daily doxycycline (100 mg) administered orally or intravenously is the drug of choice. Azithromycin may be used if the former is not tolerated.

Schistosomal Nephropathy

Seven pathogenic blood flukes, belonging to Schistosoma species affect humans. Of these, *S. mansoni* causes glomerulonephritis in about 20% of those affected while it occurs in less 2–5% of *S. haematobium* infected patients. It commonly affects young males, schistosomal nephropathy presents with pedal edema and ascites in additional to hepatosplenomegaly. Half the patients have hypertension. Other features are hypocomplementemia and bland urinary sediment. Demonstration of eggs in the stool or egg-containing granulomas in rectal or liver biopsies is diagnostic. Five different glomerular pathological patterns are known and result from varied immune response to parasitic antigens and localization of immune complexes in the glomerulus. This is due to portocaval shunting causing blood to bypass the liver. Treatment is largely ineffective. Accompanying Salmonella infections must be looked for and treated.

S. haematobium commonly infests the peri-vesical venous plexus of the lower urinary tract where the adult worm lives and lays eggs. Early infection usually manifests with "terminal" hematuria (hematuria occurring at the last part of void) and/or pyuria when the eggs are excreted in the urine. If severe, the hematuria may be seen throughout micturition. In chronic infection, the eggs get trapped and granulomatous inflammation and ulceration

of the bladder mucosa results. There may also be pseudopolyps formation in the walls of bladder and ureters. Cystoscopy and biopsy reveal presence of eggs. At this stage, prompt treatment will prevent fibrotic changes. Untreated, the disease progresses to fibrosis and calcification of the bladder wall. These patients present with increased frequency of micturition and dysuria. Radiological evaluation with ultrasonography and intravenous urography may reveal ureteric strictures, hydronephrosis and bladder wall irregularities. Long-standing obstructive disease leads to progressive renal dysfunction and ESRD. In places like Egypt, schistosomial affectation of the lower urinary tract contributes to 20% of ESRD.

Recurrent urinary tract infection may result from secondary bacterial infection. If there is exposure to tobacco and other carcinogens, bladder malignancy may result. S haematobium infection may also cause genital lesions in both sexes.

Filarial Nephropathy

Filarial worms live predominantly in the host's lymphatics. Glomerulopathies may be caused by *Wuchereria bancrofti, Loa loa, Onchocerca volvulus* and *Brugia malayi.* Infection is common in India and the rest of South Asia. *W. bancrofti* and *B. malayi* cause fever and presence of adult worm in the lymphatics cause lymphedema. Onchocerciasis, loiasis and brugiyan infections may be associated with proteinuria, microscopic hematuria and hypertension in up to a quarter of those affected. Varied glomerular pathology may be seen. Diffuse basement membrane thickening is a common finding. Glomerular disease results from deposition of circulating immune complexes. Non-nephrotic proteinuria and microscopic hematuria improves by treatment with diethylcarbamazine. Those with frank nephrotic syndrome usually have unrelenting decrease in renal function.

Chyluria

Chyluria is passage of milky white urine which may be accompanied by hematuria. It is due to leakage of lymph from rupture of dilated retroperitoneal lymphatics into the urinary tract. Chyluria is associated with *W. bancrofti* infestation and is often asymptomatic except for passing 'milky' urine. Occasionally, chyluria may lead to chronic protein loss and malnutrition and a propensity to develop infections. Diethylcarbamazine therapy and low fat diet help in more than three-fourths of cases. Resistant cases require sclerotherapy for the retroperitoneal lymphatics using povidone iodine or silver nitrate. Very rarely surgical treatment may be required.

Mycobacterial Renal Disease

Tuberculosis **(See Chapter 32)**

Tuberculosis (TB) is an important public health problem in the topical developing countries. Urogenital TB represents 27% of extra-pulmonary cases. Involvement of the kidneys may either be a localized genitourinary illness or part of disseminated (or miliary) tubercular infection. The topic is covered in a full chapter.

Hansen's Disease (Leprosy)

Hansen's disease caused by *Mycobacterium leprae*, has been on the wane. Renal involvement was common earlier and was responsible for the mortality. With effective control measures, the incidence of Hansen's disease and renal involvement are coming down. Histologically, renal involvement may occur in about 50% cases but clinically diagnosed glomerulo-nephritis is present in less than 2% patients. It is seen mostly in multibacillary disease and when there are episodes of erythema nodosum leprosum. Asymptomatic urinary sediment is most common. Nephrotic syndrome, acute nephritis and even rapidly progressive renal failure may sometimes occur. There is hypo-complementemia and circulating cryoglobulins may sometimes be demonstrated. The patho-genic antigen may be either a mycobacterial antigen or a non-mycobacterial antigen from a coinfection. Antibody response to dapsone used for therapy has also been implicated. While the glomerular disease does not respond to treatment, oral steroids are beneficial in improving renal function during erythema nodosum leprosum episodes. Both tuberculosis and leprosy may also cause secondary amyloidosis.

Hantavirus Infection

Hemorrhagic fever with renal syndrome caused by Hantaviruses is being increasingly recognized. The first Hantavirus isolate, 'Thottapalayam virus' was cultured in 1964 from Vellore, Tamil Nadu. Infected rodents are the natural hosts and harbor chronic infection. Accidental infection of humans occurs on inhaling contaminated aerosols of urine, faeces and saliva. In humans, the illness presents with a flu-like prodrome with symptoms of fever, headache, abdominal pain, vomiting and myalgia. There is cytokine response, complement activation and vascular endothelial cell injury. These result in hypovolemia, decreased perfusion of the kidney and acute tubular necrosis. In severe disease, there may be proteinuria with hematuria and leukocyturia. Treatment is supportive.

Dengue Virus Infection

Dengue virus is transmitted by the mosquito, *Aedes aegypti*, the yellow fever mosquito. The virus may cause no symptoms in about half of infected persons. After an incubation period of up to 2 weeks, viremia is followed by release of cytokines. The acute febrile illness (dengue fever) is characterized by intense myalgia, retro-orbital headache and leukopenia. Severe or reinfection results in both dengue hemorr-hagic fever (DHF) and dengue shock syndrome (DSS) which can lead to AKI.

AKI occurs in about 5% of severe dengue infection. It accompanies hypotension and rhabdomyolysis, or hemolysis and is a high risk for mortality. Three-fourths of patients with severe dengue infection may have proteinuria. Mesangial proliferation and immune complex deposition are seen on biopsy. Treatment is supportive and usually self-limiting.

Toxic Tropical Nephropathies

Of the toxic tropical nephropathies, the most important are snake envenomation, insect stings and plant toxins (including indigenous medication).

Nephropathy Associated with Snake Envenomation

As per the estimates of the World Health Organization, there are more than 2.5 million venomous snakebites occurring each year. Of these, renal involvement occurs secondary to bites from snakes of classes Viperidae (Russell's viper, saw-scaled viper, rattlesnakes) and Colubridae (boomslang, *Bothrops jararaca*) which are hemotoxic. The seasnakes (Hydrophidae) cause myotoxicity, rhabdomyolysis and renal failure. Bites by Russell's viper and saw-scaled viper (*Echis carinatus*) are common in India. AKI occurs in 13 to 32% of bites. *In vitro* experiments with venom fragments have shown an initial decrease in cardiac output due to the action of thromboxane A_2. This is followed by decrease in renal blood flow and glomerular filtration rate caused by nitric oxide and prostaglandin I_2. In addition, hemoglobinuria, systemic hemorrhage, activation of complement and release of reactive oxygen species lead to prolonged renal hypoperfusion resulting in tubular damage and AKI. Peptides in the snake venom directly affect various steps in the coagulation and fibrinolytic cascades causing disseminated intravascular coagulation. If AKI occurs without any of the above events, direct nephrotoxicity of snake venom is considered.

The possible mechanisms of direct injury are:

a. Metalloprotease causing proteolysis of extracellular matrix.
b. Apoptosis of vascular endothelial cells.
c. Phospholipase A_2 causing membrane injury and tubular necrosis.
d. Stimulation of hypothalamus—pituitary and immune axes.
e. Increased secretion of ACTH, corticosteroid and ADH.

The renal pathology is usually acute tubular necrosis and in severe cases, acute cortical necrosis. Several other glomerular and interstitial changes have been described.

The earliest symptoms occurring within a few minutes are pain and edema of the bitten part. This may progress to involve the whole limb. Hypotensive shock from hypovolemia is seen in 35%. Blood loss results from continuous bleeding from fang marks, hematemesis, melena, hemoptysis and bleeding into muscles, fascial compartments, serous cavities or subarachnoid space. The kidney is usually an "innocent bystander" and oliguric AKI usually sets in within a few hours of bite. Onset of AKI may be delayed by up to four days after the bite. In about 40% of Russell's viper envenomation cases, pain in renal angle precedes oliguria and may indicate propensity to develop AKI. This may be a clinical symptom to watch out for. AKI lasts for two to three weeks. The prognosis is poor in the elderly, those with delay in obtaining proper medical help, severe hemorrhagic complications and cortical necrosis. Immobilization, quickly transport to the nearest hospital and early anti-venom administration are key to effective recovery. The dose of antivenom depends on the persistence of envenomation as evidenced by prolongation of clotting time. In rare situations where antivenom is unavailable or patient develops severe allergic reaction to the antivenom, plasmapheresis may be offered. Other supportive therapies include blood transfusions, maintenance of electrolyte balance and maintenance of good urinary output with alkalinization of urine. In severe AKI, either peritoneal dialysis or hemodialysis may be used till renal recovery.

Bee, Wasp, and Hornet Stings induced Nephropathy

Honey bees, wasps and hornets are stinging insects common in the tropics. A large dose of venom is delivered when a person is stung by a swarm of bees. This results in an acute syndrome of varied symptoms including diaphoresis, vomiting, diarrhea, hypotension and alteration of sensorium. The components of the venom like melittin and phospholipase A_2 cause hemolysis, whereas histamine, serotonin, and acetylcholine cause rhabdomyolysis. Hemolysis, rhabdomyolysis as well as direct nephrotoxicity of the venom may cause acute tubular necrosis. Treatment is supportive.

Plant Toxin-induced Nephropathy

In recent times, more and more plant toxins are being recognized as having potential of inducing nephropathy. This is as an important cause of renal disease in the tropical region. Plant toxins causing nephropathy is a unique condition in which the exposure may be intentional as part of regional food habits (e.g. djenkol beans, mushrooms), or medicinal (e.g. impila, cat's claw) or there may be accidental ingestion. Many plant/plant products are consumed under the wrong notion that 'all plant products are 'natural' and therefore harmless'. A partial list of known plant nephrotoxins from India and their corresponding toxicity are listed in Table 52.1. Un-regulated, scientifically unproven indigenous medicines are popular and thriving on advertisements in lay press in the developing world. These medicines are prescribed by men practicing 'traditional' medicine, who feed on the ignorance of economically challenged people with inadequate access to healthcare and high cost of modern medicines. They are becoming increasingly popular even in the developed nations. Some of these medicines may have the potential to be nephrotoxic. This has been seen in the high incidence of toxic AKI and mortality in sub-Saharan Africa. Chinese herbal nephropathy is another such toxic nephropathy. Potentially poisonous plants may also be mistakenly identified as medicinal herbs by untrained workers. The toxicology of many of the indigenous medicines are yet unknown and hence, they are perhaps best avoided. AKI due to plant toxins is treated by immediate avoidance of the suspected offender and supportive care including dialysis. While AKI is usually suggested by temporal association, the impact of plant toxins on development of chronic interstitial nephropathy is still unknown.

Chemical nephrotoxins from accidental occupational exposure (e.g. chromic acid and accidental consumption or consumption with suicidal intention (e.g. copper sulfate, ethylene glycol, formic acid) are also important nephrotoxins in the tropical region. A high index of suspicion with immediate initiation of treatment

Table 52.1: Known plant nephrotoxins in India—a partial list (modified)			
Plant	*Active molecule*	*Renal manifestations*	*Other manifestations*
Averrhoa bilimbi (irumban puli)	Oxalic acid	Intratubular obstruction	AKI
Cleistanthus collinus (Oduvan)	Cleistanthin A & B, collinusin, dyphylline	Acute tubular necrosis	Hypotension, hypokalemia, arrhythmias
Dioscorea quartiniana (yam)	Dioscorine, dioscin	Acute tubular necrosis	Convulsions
Thevetia peruviana (yellow oleander)	Cardiac glycosides	Acute tubular necrosis, mesangiolysis	Liver failure, arrhythmias

is vital for survival. Delay in access to medical care is associated with development of multiorgan failure and very high mortality.

Conclusion

In the tropical regions of the earth, in addition to globally occurring conditions, we encounter certain unique kidney diseases. Infections like malaria, leptospirosis and tuberculosis, toxins from snake envenomation, insect stings and plant toxins, and several other conditions cause characteristic nephropathies that are encountered only in this region. Knowledge of these distinct "tropical nephropathies", clinical presentation, pathology, preventive measures and treatment, is crucial when dealing with these conditions in medical practice.

Ischemic Renal Disease

• Jacob George

INTRODUCTION

Kidneys are vital organs and their dysfunction leads to higher morbidity and mortality. They are highly vascular and receive nearly one-fifth of the cardiac output. Decreased blood flow to the kidneys can result in hypertension (renovascular hypertension) and may be a cause of progressive renal damage with a fall in glomerular filtration rate (GFR). When decrease in GFR is related to decreased blood flow to the kidney, the condition is termed ischemic renal disease (IRD) or ischemic nephropathy. Thus in IRD, there will be an accumulation of nitrogenous waste products like urea and creatinine in the blood, whereas in pure renovascular hypertension, though hypertension is present, blood urea and serum creatinine may not be elevated.

Etiology

The usual causes of IRD are shown in Table 53.1. The commonest cause in those above the age of fifty years is atherosclerosis of the renal arteries or abdominal aorta. It is often associated with evidence of generalized atherosclerosis with multiple organs being involved. In those below the age of fifty, aortoarteritis (Takayasu's arteritis) is more common. Fibromuscular dysplasia often

Table 53.1: Causes of ischemic renal disease

1. Atherosclerosis
2. Vasculitis (aortoarteritis)
3. Fibromuscular dysplasia
4. Coarctation of aorta
5. Atheroembolic renal disease
6. Congenital vascular anomalies

involves females less than 40 years. Though atheroembolic disease classically represents cholesterol embolization to the micro-circulation of the kidneys and other organs generally following an invasive arterial procedure in an atherosclerotic vessel, it can also rarely occur spontaneously or following anticoagulation.

When to Suspect IRD?

A high index of suspicion is necessary to diagnose IRD. In the early stages, there is reduced renal blood flow which can be associated with a progressive fall in GFR. As for most chronic renal diseases, symptoms can occur quite late, when the GFR falls <30 ml/min, with symptoms of fatigue, anorexia, nausea, vomiting, edema and breathlessness. While these symptoms are common to most causes of end-stage renal disease, one has to rely on other evidences for diagnosing IRD as the underlying etiology. When atherosclerotic renal disease is the etiology, there will be evidence of generalized atherosclerosis. History of claudication, previous coronary artery disease or cerebrovascular accidents may be present. Physical examination may reveal thickened arterial vessel wall, absent peripheral pulses (dorsalis pedis, posterior tibial, radial or ulnar. Presence of especially systolodiastolic renal bruit or femoral should raise the suspicion of an underlying IRD, especially if there is otherwise unexplained renal dysfunction. Diabetic patients are more prone for diffuse atherosclerosis (macro-angiopathy). Diabetic patients having renal failure, edema, proteinuria and retinopathy are more likely to have diabetic nephropathy. However, associated IRD may also be suspected especially in the presence of the above mentioned additional features. If a diabetic patient with renal failure does not have significant edema, proteinuria or retinopathy, the possibility of IRD as a cause of renal failure is high. The broad term 'diabetic kidney disease' is used for patients with diabetes mellitus and related renal diseases including diabetic nephropathy, IRD and other non-glomerular diabetic diseases.

Another clue to the presence of IRD could be a sudden deterioration of renal functions following use of drugs blocking renin-angiotensin-aldosterone system (RAAS blockers) like ACE inhibitors or angiotensin II receptor blockers. In diabetes, there is over-activity of RAAS system. The angiotensin II is a potent vasoconstrictor of the efferent glomerular arteriole. In IRD, the glomerular efferent arteriolar constriction is important in maintaining the intraglomerular capillary pressure and angiotensin II plays an important role here. As RAAS blockers can affect the action of angiotensin II, the intra-glomerular pressure can decrease resulting in a fall in GFR with renal failure and occasionally oligoanuria. This is particularly important in diffuse atherosclerotic narrowing

involving both renal arteries. If an elderly diabetic develops an unexplained deterioration in renal function, IRD should be ruled out.

Development of sudden onset of breathlessness in the absence of significant edema or heart disease is termed 'flash pulmonary edema'. Patients with bilateral renal artery narrowing are prone for decreased natriuresis. As they often have hypertension with left ventricular hypertrophy, the left ventricular compliance is decreased and hence any sudden rise in blood pressure could trigger pulmonary edema. Such patients also may warrant tests to confirm IRD.

Patients with IRD may have 'resistant hypertension'. Hence, IRD should be considered in patients with unexplained renal failure presenting with resistant hypertension. Table 53.2 shows the clinical situations where IRD should be suspected.

Table 53.2: Clinical clues to presence of ischemic renal disease

1. Diabetic patients with renal failure in absence of edema, proteinuria or retinopathy
2. Renal failure in patients with history of CAD, CVA, POVD
3. Sudden onset of renal failure following RAAS blockers
4. Renal failure with flash pulmonary edema
5. Age more than 50 with unexplained renal failure
6. Resistant hypertension in unexplained renal failure
7. Ultrasound showing size disparity of kidneys/duplex ultrasound (Doppler) showing evidence of compromised renal arterial flow

INVESTIGATIONS

When a clinical suspicion of IRD is made based on the above mentioned clues, investigations to rule out other possible causes of renal failure as well as to confirm the presence of IRD are warranted. Table 53.3 mentions some of the relevant investigations.

Urinalysis is usually unremarkable though mild proteinuria may occasionally occur if angiotensin II levels are high. Presence of

Table 53.3: Investigations in ischemic renal disease

1. Urine protein and deposits
2. Blood urea, serum creatinine, serum potassium
3. Ultrasound of kidneys
4. Doppler ultrasound of proximal and distal renal arteries
5. Conventional renal angiography
6. Magnetic resonance angiography of renal arteries
7. Isotope study and captopril renogram

significant proteinuria with microscopic hematuria should raise the possibility of an associated independent renal disease. As the GFR is reduced with significantly compromised blood flow, blood urea and serum creatinine may be raised. Hypokalemia may occur because of high aldosterone levels in those with no significant renal failure. Ultrasound may show normal or small sized kidneys with disparity in size of >1.5 cm between the two kidneys. Although this can occur with other causes of CKD, Doppler ultrasound scan will show evidence of compromised blood flow in the renal artery or major branches. The proximal Doppler criteria include a peak renal systolic velocity >200–300 cm/sec and a relative renal artery velocity >3.5 times that seen in the aorta. The distal Doppler criteria include pulsus parvus et tardus pattern due to dampening of blood flow, an increased acceleration time and changes in the resistivity index. Measurement of the resistivity index is important as they can predict response to interventional therapy. Resistivity index <0.7 may suggest benefit from intervention, whereas a resistivity index >0.8 suggests that significant renal parenchymal damage has occurred and interventions may be futile. Conventional angiography is the gold standard for demonstrating anatomical renal artery stenosis. It will be possible to measure the pressure gradient between the pre and post stenotic segments of the renal artery during the procedure. Presence of collaterals can also be seen in long-standing obstruction (Fig. 53.1). Conventional contrast

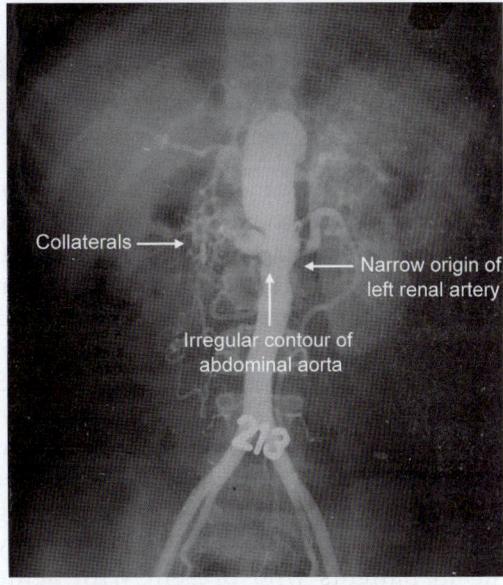

Fig. 53.1: Aortogram showing nonvisualized right kidney with plenty of collaterals suggesting long-standing right renal artery occlusion in a case of aortoarteritis with ischemic renal disease

Labels on figure: Collaterals; Narrow origin of left renal artery; Irregular contour of abdominal aorta

angiography may not be safe in advanced renal failure due to risk of contrast nephrotoxicity. Carbon dioxide angiography can be used in renal failure, but is technically difficult and resolution of anatomical features suboptimal. Plain magnetic resonance angiography or using contrast (gadolinium) can also be used but may give false positive reports. Gadolinium should be avoided if the GFR is <30 ml/min due to the risk of nephrogenic systemic fibrosis. Study of isotope renogram using technetium labeled DTPA after administration of ACEI, captopril (captopril renogram) will show a significant fall in GFR compared to pre-captopril level. Although this test may help to assess the functional significance of renal artery stenosis, is not useful in patients with renal failure due to poor renal uptake of the isotope. Presence of significant proteinuria, kidney size <8 cm, high resistivity index in Doppler scan, absence of significant gradient across the stenotic segment during angiography are suggestive of poor response to interventional therapy.

MANAGEMENT

Management of IRD includes medical, interventional and surgical options.

1. Medical Management

Most patients require medical management of blood pressure. The choice of antihypertensive drugs may have to be individualized. Management of diabetes, dyslipidemia, associated atherosclerosis, cardiovascular and peripheral vascular disease are undertaken using standard protocols. The role of RAAS blockers in IRD has been relooked recently. Formerly it was felt that RAAS blockers have to be avoided due to the risk of further compromised renal blood flow with resulting worsening of renal functions. This is especially true in patients who present with acute worsening of renal functions following RAAS blockade. Calcium channel blockers, β-blockers and diuretics are to be preferred here. However, in long-standing IRD with stable renal failure, RAAS blockers could be tried initially, especially in patients where the control blood pressure is difficult. However, these groups of drugs should be used cautiously under careful monitoring. Blood urea, serum creatinine and serum potassium should be monitored if possible twice weekly for the first 2 weeks. Thereafter, once a month for the next 3 months followed by every 3 months thereafter and continued if the patient is stable. It should be avoided in patients in whom compliance and follow-up cannot be ensured. If serum creatinine rises by more than 30% or potassium values exceed 5.5 mEq/L, RAAS blockers should be withdrawn because such patients are at high risk of cardiovascular, cerebrovascular and progressive renal damage. Often a combination with other antihypertensive drugs may be needed to achieve the target blood pressure of 140/90 mm.

Statins help to retard progression of atherosclerosis and in patients with diabetes. Though its protection against cardiovascular disease in advanced CKD has not been proved, statins are recommended in atherosclerotic IRD. Antiplatelet drugs (aspirin) may also be needed.

2. Interventional Management

Percutaneous renal angiography followed by interventional therapy in the form of renal angioplasty or stenting are the common interventional therapies available. The role of angioplasty has been questioned recently since the long-term benefits with regard to control of hypertension and retarding progressive renal damage has not been shown in several cases despite successful demonstration of improvement of renal blood flow. This is because permanent renal parenchymal damage may have occurred especially in long standing cases. Thus, patients with significant proteinuria, small kidneys, high resistivity indices are unlikely to benefit. This is especially true in atherosclerotic IRD and in diabetics. Angioplasty has been shown to be most promising in fibromuscular dysplasia, probably due to the relatively short duration. Recent worsening of renal functions following RAAS blockers, recurrent flash pulmonary edema, resistant hypertension, progressive renal dysfunction and recent onset of severe hypertension are other situations where intervention may have a role. Adverse effects include arterial perforation, thrombosis and atheroembolic renal disease.

3. Surgical Correction

This may be attempted in selected cases where angioplasty/stenting may not be feasible and in patients who may be likely to benefit from restoration of blood flow. Options include bypassing the obstruction by splenorenal or hepatorenal anastomosis or by using synthetic grafts. Renal autotransplantation of the ischemic kidney to another site using the iliac artery as done in conventional allograft renal transplantation can also be considered.

Aging and Kidneys

• Muthu Jayaraman

Aging is a programmed biological process associated with small transcriptional difference in many genes. It is also called 'senescence' which means 'irreversible growth arrest'. Cellular or replicative senescence is the key element of aging. Aging plays an active role in fibrogenesis and atrophy of renal tissue. With aging, kidneys become smaller, granular and irregular. The cortex becomes thinner. In addition changes like nephrosclerosis, reduction in GFR occur. The morphological and functional changes in different age groups of normal aging kidney are summarised in Table 54.1.

Radiologically, the kidney size is 10% less after 40 years and 30% less after 80 years. Cortical cysts start appearing by 40 years of age in more than 50% of the population. These cysts are benign, filled with yellow fluid and they may represent dilated tubules or tubular diverticulae. The kidney volume also shrinks with age with the loss of volume occurring mainly at the cortical region. The medulla maintains its volume and vascularity.

The number of glomeruli in each normal adult kidney varies from 3.3 lakhs to 1.1 million. The number of glomeruli in adults is predetermined at 36 weeks of gestation. 25% of population have less than 5 lakhs per kidney, another 25% have more than 7.4 lakhs per kidney. Females have 15% less than males. The number of functioning glomeruli starts decreasing at the rate of about 7000 per year, after age of 18 years.

Table 54.1: The change in morphological and functional characteristics in normal aging					
Parameter and change according to age	20 years	30 years	50 years	70 years	90 years
Renal mass	50 g at birth	400 g	-	300 g	-
Nephrosclerosis	<3%	< 3%	30%	50–70%	50–70%
Total kidney volume	100%	105%	100%	90 %	85%
Renal cortex	100%	100%	95%	85%	75%
Renal medulla	100%	110%	120%	115%	125%
GFR	100%	100%	85%	70%	60%
Serum creatinine	1 mg%	1 mg%	1 mg%	1 mg %	1 mg%
Renal plasma flow	-	650 ml/min	530 ml/min	430 ml/min	350 ml/min

With aging, glomeruli also start undergoing sclerosis: 10% are sclerosed by 40 years of age and the percentage increases as age advances. This process starts as basement membrane thickening, increase in mesangial volume and progressing to matrix sclerosis (Fig. 54.1). The approximate percentage of sclerotic glomeruli can be calculated as [(age/2) – 10]. Since the sclerosis mainly affects the superficial cortex, the cortex becomes thinner. In the glomeruli that have undergone global sclerosis, the tuft shrinks and disappears and the blood is shunted directly from the afferent to efferent arterioles. One-third to two-thirds of the remaining glomeruli may be normal or enlarged.

Tubules and interstitium also undergo senescent changes. The size and number of tubules decrease and the tubules are dilated with intratubular cast formation. Tubulo-interstitial infiltration with macrophages and lymphocytes and lead to fibrosis. Sclerosis of cortical, interlobular, and arcuate arteries also occurs. The density of peritubular capillary network also decreases. Thus, arteriolo-sclerosis and nephrosclerosis with ischemic atrophy of glomeruli, tubules and interstitium are the features of aging kidney (Fig. 54.2).

Together with the structural changes in the aging kidneys, the functions are also altered. Renal plasma flow (RPF) in young male is about 650 ml per minute. After 40 years of age, it decreases by 10% per decade and in elderly it is only around 350 ml per minute. Glomerular filtration rate (GFR): The GFR falls at a rate of 0.87 ml per minute per year after the age of 40 even in a normal person. Therefore, the GFR may fall from 120 ml/min at the age of 40 to about 60 ml/min by 100 years. Functional reserve is maintained at 15% since 36% of glomeruli maintain the adequate GFR in spite of age. Thus, normal decline in GFR per se is not of great significance since the elderly do not develop ESRD during their normal lifespan because of this. Even though the GFR comes down with age, the serum creatinine is maintained at normal level, since the muscle mass is reduced and less creatinine is produced. So, serum creatinine level may not truly indicate the fall in GFR in elderly. It is

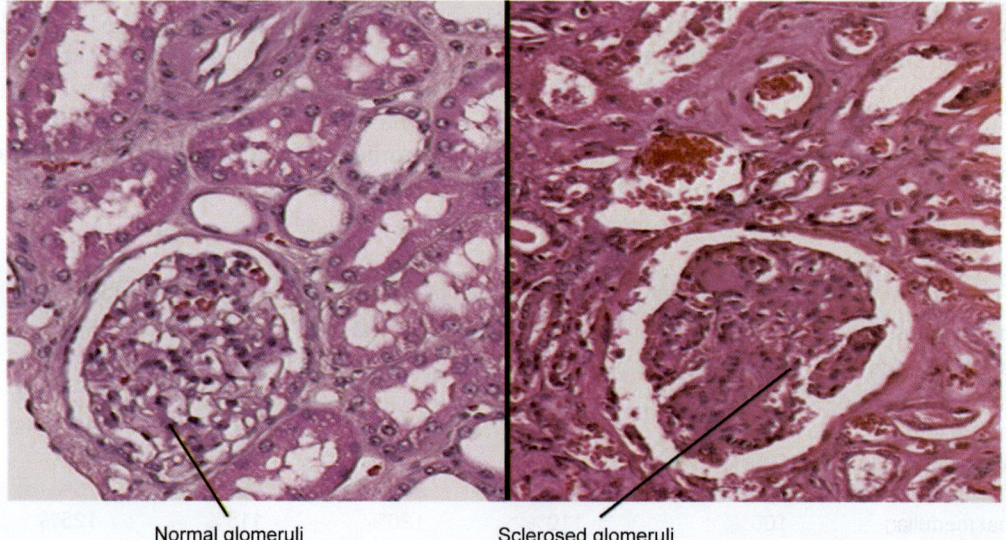

Normal glomeruli   Sclerosed glomeruli

Fig. 54.1: Normal and sclerosed glomerulus under high power. *Note:* Showing normal glomerulus (left). In the right hand side, glomerulus shows expanded mesangial matrix, reduced number of cells and the capillary lumens are occluded

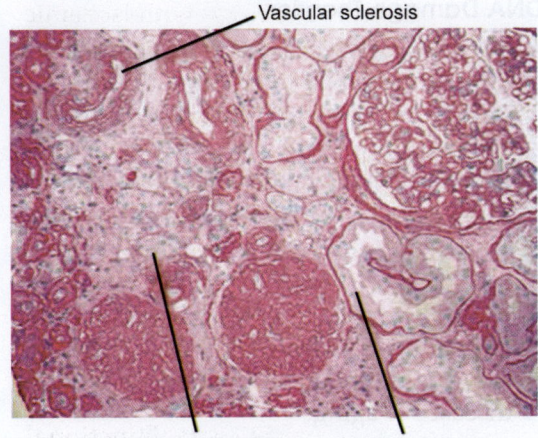

Fig. 54.2: The aging changes in the tubules, interstitium, and vasculature. *Note:* Tubular atrophy, tubulointerstitial infiltrates and vascular sclerosis in the renal histology

necessary to calculate the GFR based on any standard formula and not depend on the absolute value of creatinine as explained in the example. The estimated GFR (eGFR) calculated by Cockroft-Gault formula for different age groups assuming the same body weight and serum creatinine level in normal males and females in Table 54.2. Other formulas like MDRD formula and CKD (EPI) equations are also available for calculation of GFR from serum creatinine, age, sex, body weight, race, sex and other parameters. Accurate and actual measurements of GFR may be higher than the values obtained by calculation of e-GFR.

In the elderly, inability to concentrate and dilute urine is an important manifestation of tubular dysfunction and is due to a combination:

a. Interstitial damage
b. End organ resistance
c. Decreased production of hormones
d. Decreased insertion of aquaporin channels (apical AQP-2) involved in water reabsorption.

This results in nocturia, disorders of water metabolism and altered pharmacokinetics of drugs. Distal tubular sodium reabsorption is reduced leading to sodium wasting and dysnatremia. At the same time, potassium excretion in urine diminishes resulting in hyperkalemia. Acid excretion and bicarbonate handling are relatively normal.

The response of the vascular system to various hemodynamic changes in kidney is also altered in elderly people. The vasodilatory effect is blunted and the vasoconstrictor response is exaggerated and more sustained in the elderly. Therefore, the elderly cannot tolerate hemodynamic alterations as compared to younger individuals.

In the urinary tract, tone and motility of ureters are not greatly affected with age but micturition dysfunctions are common. The common problems are retention of urine or presence of excessive residual urine in bladder after micturition. The common causes are autonomic neuropathy, urethral obstruction due to prostatic enlargement or bladder contractile dysfunction in males. Abnormalities like prolapse uterus with incontinence,

Table 54.2: Normal estimated GFR in different age groups					
Serial no.	Age (years)	Serum creatinine (mg%)	Body weight (kg)	eGFR male (ml/min)	e-GFR female (ml/min)
1.	30	0.9	60	102	86.5
2.	40	0.9	60	92.5	78.7
3.	50	0.9	60	83.3	70.8
4.	60	0.9	60	74.0	62.9
5.	70	0.9	60	64.8	55.8
6.	80	0.9	60	55.5	47.2
7.	90	0.9	60	46.3	40.0

hormonally dependent changes in vaginal pH resulting in stricture urethra or other urinary tract abnormalities are common in women. Weak sphincter and inadequate pelvic support in women are other problems in women. Comorbidities like stroke, immobility, diabetes, prolonged catheter use and lower urinary tract infection may result in lower urinary symptoms and chronic infection.

Pathogenesis and Theories of Aging

Biological mechanisms leading to aging is not clearly known. The important factors implicated are:
a. Genetic factors
b. Molecular changes
c. Mitochondrial dysfunction
d. Oxidative stress
e. Shortening of the telomeres (ends of chromo-somes) signaling the onset of replicative senescence.
f. DNA damage and insufficient repair
g. Accumulation of glycation end products and cross-linking of proteins (such as collagen).

The Signaling Pathways in Aging

KLOTHO is an anti-aging gene which supresses aging through a variety of mechanisms. It has a favorable role in antioxidation, anti-senescence, anti-autophagy, and modulation of signaling pathways. KLOTHO levels decrease in aging and this leads to abnormal signaling, promotes profibrotic genes/proteins, stimulates fibrosis and mediates RAAS signaling reduced production of KLOTHO protein has been observed in aging and in patients with chronic renal failure which may be responsible for the degenerative processes like arteriosclerosis, osteoporosis and skin atrophy seen in these conditions. As KLOTHO level falls, fibroblast growth factor 23 (FGF23) increases resulting in fibrosis. Oxidative stress is caused by reduced anti-oxidant activity, increased ROS and decreased scavenging thereby leading to accumulation of advanced glycation end products (AGEs).

DNA Damage Theories

a. *DNA damage/repair theory:* Accumulated damage to DNA over time, inhibits the ability of cells to function. Defective expression of genes adds to the overall process of aging and leads to cell death.
b. *Free radical/oxidation theory:* Free radicals wreck havoc at a cellular level. They fuse the lipids and proteins, break off cell membrane proteins, disrupt nuclear membrane and destroy the cell identity. They cause damage to immune cells and predispose to other diseases of aging.
c. *Mitochondrial DNA theory:* Mitochondria are involved in cellular respiration. The inner membrane of mitochondria, being metabolically very active, is an important site of formation of highly reactive oxygen species. Injury to the mitochondrial genome paves the way for age related degenerative changes.
d. *Radiation theory:* Radiation increases rate of FR generation in cells from H_2O molecules. Ultraviolet and infrared radiation contribute significantly to photo-aging due to dermal connective tissue destruction, accelerate the aging of skin cells and possibly the whole body.

Built-in Breakdown Theory

Built-in breakdown theories are based on direct consequence of genetic programming built into the genome and cellular structure.
a. *Disposable soma theory:* The cells in the body are somatic or germline cells (cells of the sexual, reproductive system). By 'natural selection', Somatic cells to support and maintain gametes essential for reproduc-tion. Energy is spent to ensure minimum damage to molecular structures such as DNA and to ensure that the animal remains in sound condition through its natural reproductive age. Nature does not see the need to keep organism alive well past its time of procreation.

b. *Genetic theory:* The capacity of human cells to divide is limited. Cell senescence is genetically programmed and cells are actively metabolizing. This theory suggests that aging is predetermined in the genome. Surface membrane expresses a protein which inhibits DNA synthesis in older cells but not in young cells.

c. *Immunological theory:* The effectiveness of the immune system peaks at puberty and gradually declines. The quality, effectiveness and quantity of T cells, begins to decline after puberty. Since immunity based primarily on T cells, defective T cell function predisposes to susceptibility to infections and autoimmune phenomena in the elderly. Antibodies may lose their effectiveness and cause cellular stress and eventual death.

d. *Telomere theory:* Telomeres form caps at the ends of the chromosomes and function as caps preventing chromosomes from fusing together. Telomere length influences the stability of genetic information and successive cell division shortens the length of telomeres. The functional genes near the telomeres are lost. There is close correlation between telomere length and longevity.

Other Theories (Exogenous and Environmental)

a. *Nutritional factors and calorie restriction:* Reduction in calorie intake has established benefits relating to longevity. An inverse relationship has been established between metabolic rate, pulse rate and average lifespan of mammals.

b. *Advanced glycation end products (AGEs):* Glycation (earlier known as 'glycosylation') is the process by which glucose is irreversibly attached to the protein molecule and modifies its structure and function. It is implicated in genomic changes contributing to aging.

c. *Accumulation of metabolic waste products:* Accumulation of damaged macromolecules contribute to aging.

Even though the changes in the structure and function of the kidneys are not pathological, they may predispose to or precipitate many diseases. Decrease in GFR less than 60 ml/meter is a risk factor for CKD, coronary and cerebrovascular events. Inability to remove from the system of toxic substances and drugs, lead to drug toxicity and needs modification of drug dosing. Congestive cardiac failure is common as a result of the aging kidney's inability to regulate fluid volume and salt excretion. Immunosenescence can lead to infections and parenchymal injury. Bladder dysfunction with residual urine results in recurrent urinary tract infections, leading to acute and chronic infective interstitial nephritis. Due to vascular changes, renal perfusion is decreased which may result in acute ischemic injuries like ATN even with mild hypotension and dehydration.

Common Renal Disorders in the Elderly

CKD

Over 60% of elderly have a GFR less than 60 ml/min. However, the serum creatinine is not altered and is stable around 1 mg%. In differentiating aging *vs* CKD, the context is more important. They can be differentiated from CKD patients as follows. Regardless of age, if the GFR is less than 45 ml/min with albuminuria of 50–500 mg per day for more than 3 months, it can be labelled as CKD.

In CKD there is more rapid fall in GFR as compared to the elderly. Significant proteinuria is commonly seen in CKD. Aging *per se* does not lead to ESRD, but CKD patients, invariably progress to ESRD. In elderly with CKD, often diseases like diabetes, hypertension, vasculitis may be associated.

The prevalence of CKD in elderly is variable and is emerging as an important health care issue and economic concern.

The clinical implications of CKD in elderly are in the accurate assessment of GFR. Assessing the renal functional status by regular tests like serum creatinine, creatinine clearance may be fallacious. KDOQi guidelines recommend equation using creatinine and cystatin (CKD–EPI cr–cys) as an acceptable alternative to assess GFR.

Hypertension

The optimum BP in the elderly remains uncertain. Studies have shown that aggressive control of BP may lead to hypotension, syncope, acute kidney injury, hypokalemia and hyponatremia. The goal for systolic BP in elderly should be less than 140 mmHg and never less than 120 mm Hg.

Most of the elderly need more than two drugs. The first choice is a combination of calcium channel blocker (CCB) with thiazide. It must be remembered that thiazides may cause hyponatremia because of sodium loss in urine. If the BP is not well controlled, CCB combined with angiotensin converting enzyme inhibitors (ACEI) or angiotensin receptor blocker (ARB) and thiazide can be used. Combination of ACEI and ARB is not preferred. β-blockers are avoided as they increase central aortic pressure and reduce peripheral BP.

Acute Kidney Injury

Acute kidney injury is a common clinical problem in elderly as they are highly vulnerable. Numerous factors like age-related low GFR, associated comorbid conditions, risk of dehydration due to lack of thirst, inadequate handling of sodium and water by the aging kidneys, urinary tract obstruction, bladder dysfunction, retention of urine, and use of multiple drugs for other conditions ('polypharmacy') predispose to AKI. Alterations of renal and hepatic handling of many drugs occur in the elderly and result in raised drug levels resulting in AKI.

The incidence of both types of AKI, community acquired and hospital acquired are higher in the elderly. More than 50% of patients over the age of 65 years develop AKI during the ICU stay and the mortality ranges from 20 to 80%.

The etiology of AKI in ICU is variable between various countries. The common causes in the West are:

- Septic shock — 60%
- Heart disease — 44%
- Polytrauma — 19%
- Liver disease/HRS — 10%
- Heart surgery — 6%
- Unrecognized — 20%

The causes of spectrum of AKI in India are different:

- Sepsis — 36%
- Age related — 10.4%
- Hepatic causes — 6.1%
- Malaria, dengue, leptospirosis — 6.4%
- Drugs — 5.6%
- Snakebite — 2%
- RPGN — 1.8%
- H1N1 viral infection — 1.2%
- Poisoning — 1%
- Multiple myeloma — 1.6%

Acute kidney injury is classified as prerenal, intrarenal, and postrenal according to the causative factors. As in other age groups, prerenal causes include hypovolemia or hypotension due to any cause leading to renal hypoperfusion and prerenal failure. Hypovolemia could be due to loss of fluids from the body or redistribution of the intravascular fluid. Hypotension could be related to dehydration, cardiac failure, shock or pericardial effusion. If not corrected promptly, the condition may progress to established AKI often due to acute tubular necrosis (ATN). Nearly one-third of all cases of AKI in the elderly are due to ATN. Other intrarenal causes commonly seen in the elderly are:

- Rhabdomyolysis due to prolonged immobilization/stroke.
- Urosepsis caused by obstruction and catheter use (associated with high mortality of more than 80%).
- Vascular problems like atherosclerosis, thromboembolism caused by atrial fibrillation and myocardial infarction.

- ANCA associated vasculitis causing AKI is six times more common in those over the age of 75 years.
- Hyperosmolar states and associated electrolyte imbalances increase the chances of falls and subsequent AKI.

Postrenal causes account for about 9% of all cases. Common conditions are urethral obstruction following prostatic enlargement or stricture urethra. In women, pelvic malignancies and urethral strictures due to hormonal imbalances are the common cause of urethral obstruction.

AKI following surgery accounts for nearly 30% of all cases of AKI in the elderly. The contributing factors are associated cardiac problems, sepsis, use of nephrotoxic drugs and contrast agents. Many drugs are nephrotoxic in elderly individuals, more so in diabetic and hypertensive patients.

Making a diagnosis of AKI in elderly may be challenging. The routine use of serum creatinine as the marker of renal function is not reliable in elderly, as the production of creatinine is less due to lack of muscle mass. The level also fluctuates with hydration, vascular status, fever, muscle trauma, liver disorder and volume overload. Biomarkers like cystatin C, NGAL, KIM and IL-18 are useful in assessing renal functional status. Kidney biopsy is useful to make a histological diagnosis. It is indicated whenever cause of AKI is not obvious, there is delayed recovery from AKI, when parenchymal lesion is suspected or when a treatable cause is suspected. Kidney biopsy is safe in elderly, and should be performed by experiences personnel under ultrasound or CT guidance.

Some of the issues seen during RRT for AKI in elderly are hemodynamic instability, autonomic dysfunction, hypotension, cardiovascular events, and arrhythmias. The outcome in ICU patients requiring dialysis is poor and the mortality rate may be around 30 to 80%. Nearly 30% may not recover renal function and may remain dialysis dependent. Hemodialysis can be safely performed in stable elderly patients. However, the complication rates may be higher. Other options like sustained low efficiency dialysis (SLED) or continuous renal replacement therapy (CRRT) can be performed. Associated problems in elderly patients alter the overall outcome.

Nephrotic Syndrome (NS)

NS is not uncommon in the elderly. Secondary NS is more common (56%). The common secondary causes are hypertension, diabetes mellitus, malignancy related, systemic lupus erythematosus, infection related or primary NS. Among the primary, membranous nephropathy is more common.

Inappropriate Prescriptions

There is strong evidence today about the harm due to indiscriminate use of proton pump inhibitors (PPIs). It should be de-prescribed only for seven days. Patients should be counseled against self treatment with PPIs and many other drugs.

Renal Replacement Therapy (RRT) for Elderly

Age is not a limitation for dialysis and the number of patients getting dialysis beyond the age of 75 is increasing. Vascular access like AVF, vascular graft and central venous catheterization can be used in these patients. Although there are added risks like infection, maturity of AV fistula, early closure, hypotension and hypoglycemia during dialysis, the survival on dialysis has improved. Dialysis gives increase in survival advantage and better quality of life compared to untreated uremia.

Transplantation for Elderly

Number of candidates above the age of 65 years listed for transplant is very low. Although the survival of elderly after transplantation is favorable, availability of donor kidneys and priority given to an younger individual, and comorbidities in the elderly restrict their selection from the pool of potential recipients. The rejection is less common in the elderly. However, coronary artery disease and infection account for the higher mortality.

In this chapter, the morphologic and functional changes of normal aging process, biochemical and molecular changes and the common renal problems in elderly are explained. Special issues in the elderly which need special attention are briefly described.

Drugs and Kidney

• R Ram • N Sai Sameera

Drug-induced kidney damage is a common but often unrecognized problem. It accounts for up to 20% cases of AKI and may be involved in about 15% of cases of CKD. Because of certain unique characteristics, the kidneys are highly vulnerable to injury by drugs and toxins. The blood flow to the kidneys is up to 25% of the cardiac output and 90% of the blood flow is distributed to the cortex. Thus, each gram of renal cortex receives 3.5–4.0 ml blood every minute and is the highest blood flow in any organ system. The high endothelial surface area due to two sets of capillary systems predisposes the kidney to endothelial cell damage. Because of this rich blood supply, the tubules and interstitium are exposed to toxins to a much greater extent than the other tissues. In addition to this, toxic metabolites accumulate as a result of drug handling and metabolism in the kidney. Within the kidney, the medulla is especially vulnerable because of very high concentrations of the drug reached during the process of urinary concentration. Since many drugs and their metabolites are handled in the kidney by varying combination of glomerular filtration, tubular reabsorption, secretion or excretion all parts of the kidneys can be damaged by drugs, chemicals, toxins and

natural products. As many drugs are excreted by the kidneys, their high concentration in the tubular lumen may contribute to damage.

Drugs induce renal damage by different mechanisms. Causes like vascular occlusion (oral contraceptives), volume depletion (diuretics), loss of renal autoregulation (prostaglandin inhibitors and ACEI/ARBs) or increased catabolism (steroids) are the important prerenal factors. Immune mediated damage may occur leading to renal vasculitis (penicillamine), glomerular injury (NSAIDs, gold, penicillamine) or allergic interstitial nephritis (allopurinol, rifampicin). Number of drugs may cause direct toxicity to renal tubule resulting in tubular necrosis of acute papillary necrosis. Finally, drugs can also cause partial or complete obstruction to urinary tract leading to renal damage. Tubular blockage due to crystalluria occurs following treatment with sulphonamides and antiviral drugs, acyclovir and indinavir. NSAIDs may lead to papillary necrosis and drugs like methysergide, retroperitoneal fibrosis.

The body handles drugs by absorption, distribution, metabolism and excretion. The drug handling by the body is also significantly altered when the kidney function is deranged.

Absorption

In the case of orally administered drugs, gastrointestinal absorption is necessary for ensuring adequate drug action. Ammonia production occurs in the stomach in chronic renal failure, concomitant with urea accumulation and hydrolysis. Ammonia buffers hydrochloric acid, causing an increase in gastric pH leading to reduced absorption of drugs such as ferrous sulfate, folic acid, pindolol, and cloxacillin which depend on absorption at acidic pH. Diuretic resistance is reported to occur in the nephrotic syndrome and congestive cardiac failure as a consequence of poor intestinal absorption through edematous mucosa. Other more probable explanations are reduction in renal blood flow or binding to tubular protein.

Distribution

Protein binding of drugs is affected in renal impairment. This may lead to alterations in the plasma concentrations of a number of acidic compounds that compete for binding sites on albumin and other plasma proteins. The following are lists of influence of renal impairment on drugs binding to proteins.

a. *Reduced drug binding in renal impairment:* Barbiturates, clofibrate, diazepam, dicloxacillin, furosemide, methotrexate, phenytoin, salicylates, theophylline.

b. *Increased drug binding in renal impairment:* Imipramine.

c. *Unaltered drug binding in renal impairment:* Dapsone, D-tubocurarine, indomethacin, metoclopramide, quinidine, trimethoprim.

Metabolism

Uremia may affect drug metabolism and reduces the non-renal clearance of drugs such as acyclovir, aztreonam, moxolactam, cefotaxime, captopril, cimetidine, and metoclopramide (Table 55.1).

Renal Excretion

Polar (water-soluble) drugs generally remain in the tubular fluid and are excreted in the urine, while non-polar drugs are reabsorbed by passive diffusion down their concentration gradient into plasma. Organic acids (e.g. penicillins, cephalosporins, salicylates, frusemide, and thiazides) and organic bases (e.g. amiloride, procainamide, and quinidine) undergo active tubular secretion. Drugs like probenecid interact and inhibit tubular secretion of other drugs, e.g. penicillins, cephalosporins, and frusemide.

The renal excretion of some drugs also depends on the pH of urine. The pK is the pH at which 50% of the drug is ionized. If an organic acid has a pKA less than 7.5, increasing urine pH increases the amount of ionized drug and its excretion. Similarly, in the case of organic bases with a pKB greater than 7.5, decreasing the urinary pH increases the excretion. These principles underlie the

Table 55.1: Uremia and drug metabolism

Drug	Effect of metabolite	Metabolite
Acebutalol	Selectivity	N-acetyl analogue
Allopurinol	Rash	Oxypurinol
Codeine	Prolongation of analgesia, respiratory depression	Morphine
Clofibrate	Muscle damage, neuropathy	Chloro phenoxy isobutyric acid
Nitrofurantoin	Peripheral neuropathy	Nitrofurantoin metabolite
Morphine	Prolongation of analgesia	Morphine 6 glucuronide
Pethidine	Seizures	Norpethidine
Propoxyphene	Cardiotoxicity	Norpropoxyphene
Sulfonamides	Rash	Acetyl sulfonamide

rationale for alkaline diuresis in the treatment of salicylate poisoning. Most drugs that are eliminated by the kidney display first-order kinetics. First-order kinetics is a chemical reaction in which the rate of decrease in the number of molecules of a substrate is proportional to the concentration of substrate molecules remaining. In first-order reactions involving two substances, only one of the concentrations affects the rate. It is also called first-order reaction.

Renal Hemodynamics

A rapid reduction in drug clearance may result from acute renal failure associated with hypovolemia. Nonsteroidal anti-inflammatory agents alter GFR by inhibiting prostaglandin synthesis. Angiotensin-converting enzyme (ACE) inhibitors and angiotensin receptor antagonists (blockers) may diminish GFR significantly under circumstances such as dehydration or renovascular disease by lowering glomerular efferent arteriolar tone. The clearance of drugs by hemodialysis and hemofiltration follows first-order kinetics. In hemofiltration, drugs with a molecular weight less than that of inulin (5200 Da) will pass through, in hemodialysis most drugs with a molecular weight of less than 500 Da (which includes most antibiotics) will be cleared, but drugs such as vancomycin, amphotericin, and erythromycin behave differently with respect to hemofiltration/hemodialysis (Fig. 55.1).

Drug Dosing in Renal Failure

Dosage modification is required for those drugs with predominantly renal route of excretion in patients with renal dysfunction. The dose modification is made by calculating the creatinine clearance or eGFR rather than the serum creatinine values. It is not normally necessary to reduce the initial loading dose. The aim is to achieve the optimal therapeutic level of drug as in individuals with normal renal function. There are three ways of modifying the maintenance doses of drugs in patients with renal failure.

1. Dose reduction
2. Interval extension
3. By combining dose reduction with interval extension.

Since the clearance of the drug occurs by renal and non-renal routes, the total drug clearance is the sum of renal clearance + non-renal clearance. Drug clearance by the kidney is directly proportional to creatinine clearance.

In this calculation it is assumed that the non-renal clearance remains constant.

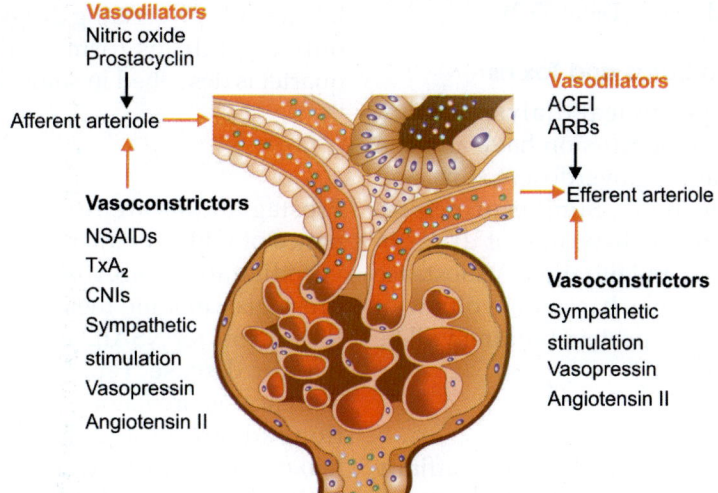

Fig. 55.1: Drugs acting on affrent and efferent arterial tone

The estimated drug clearance = Estimated renal clearance + Normal non-renal clearance

$$\text{Estimated renal clearance} = \frac{\text{Normal renal clearance for the drug} \times \text{Calculated creatinine clearance}}{100 \text{ ml/min}} \qquad \text{(Equation 1)}$$

In a patient with renal insufficiency,

$$\text{Maintenance drug dose} = \frac{\text{Regular maintenance dose} \times \text{Estimated drug clearance}}{\text{Normal drug clearance}} \qquad \text{(Equation 2)}$$

But this is not true in renal failure because gastrointestinal absorption and metabolism of drugs may also be altered. Therefore, when a drug with a narrow therapeutic window is used, the therapeutic drug monitoring by measuring plasma levels periodically should be used to guide drug dosing.

Calculating the Drug Dose in Patients on Dialysis

Dialysis affects the clearance of drugs depending on the volume of distribution of the drug, degree of protein binding and non-renal clearance. The clearance of the drug by dialysis will be high if the volume of distribution is <1 L/kg, if it is not highly protein bound and if the non-renal clearance is <400 ml/meter. In general, booster doses of such drugs should be are administered immediately following dialysis to maintain therapeutic blood levels (Table 55.2).

Poisoning due to Drugs and Toxins

Hemodialysis, peritoneal dialysis, hemofiltration, and hemoperfusion have all been used to eliminate drug overdose, toxins, and poisons from the body. Similar principles apply to those for the handling of drugs in therapeutic dialysis and filtration. A substance which is water-soluble, has a low volume of distribution and low protein binding will be cleared more efficiently.

Hemoperfusion

This technique imipenem relies on the affinity of the adsorbent for a toxin. Activated charcoal or polystyrne exchange resins are used in a column arranged like an artificial kidney. It is possible to combine hemoperfusion preceding filtration or dialysis in series. This is particularly useful for toxins with a low volume of distribution. Since heparin may also be adsorbed into the perfusion column additional doses of 2000 units per hour may be needed.

Drug-induced Renal Toxicity

Drug-induced renal toxicity is depicted in Table 55.3.

Four groups of drugs commonly used clinically causing nephrotoxicity are called the 'nephrotoxic quartet'. They are, NSAIDs, aminoglycosides, ACEIs/ARBs and radio-contrast agents. Many other drugs are also nephrotoxic and a combination of more than one nephrotoxic drugs invariably produces renal damage. Hence, great care should be taken while prescribing drugs. In this chapter, only the 4 drugs forming the nephrotoxic quartet is described in some detail.

1. *Nonsteroidal Anti-inflammatory Drugs (NSAIDs)*

Prostaglandins are responsible for maintenance of GFR by causing afferent arteriolar vasodilatation. NSAIDs cause inhibition of prostaglandins and thereby decrease the GFR. Risk factors for NSAID-induced injury include hepatic disease, renal disease, HTN, DM, diuretic use, circulatory compromise, dehydration, advanced age, myeloma. Increased leukotriene causes increased recruitment and activation of lymphocytes and thus cause alteration of permeability of glomerular

Table 55.2: Dosage modification of some of the commonly used drugs in renal failure

Name	User dose	>50	10–50	<10	Dialysis
Ampicillin/ sulbactam	1.5–3 g q6h	No change	Q8–12 h	q24h	HD: Dose after HD CAPD: q24h
Cefepime	1–2 g IV q8h	No change	q12–24 h	q24h	HD: 1–1.5 g after HD CAPD:1–2 g 48h
Cefotaxime	1–2 g IV q8h	q8–12 h	q12–24 h	q24h	HD: 1 g after HD CAPD: 0.5–1 g qd
Ceftazidime	1–2 g q8h	q8–12 h	q24–48 h	q48h	HD: 1 g after HD CAPD: 0.5 g qd
Ciprofloxacin PO	250–750 mg q12h	No change	(<30) q24h	q24h	HD, CAPD: 250–500 mg after dialysis
Ciprofloxacin IV	200–400 mg q12h	No change	(<30)q24h	q24h	HD, CAPD: 200–400 mg after dialysis
Levofloxacin PO, IV	250–500 mg qd	No change	250 mg q24–48 h	250 mg q48h	HD, CAPD: 250 q48h
TMP-SMX PO	1 tab bd	No change	(<30) 50%	Not recommended	HD: 50%
Imipenem	500 mg IVq6h	No change	250 mg q6–12 h	125–250 mg q12h	HD: Dose after HD CAPD:125–250 mg q12h
Meropenem	1 g IVq8h	No change	1 g q12h	0.5 g q12 h	HD: Dose after HD CAPD: 0.5 g q12h
Piperacillin/ tazobactam	3.375 gq6h	No change	2.25 g q6h	2.25 g q8h	HD:2.25 g q8h + 0.75 g after HD, CAPD:2.25g q8h
Tetracycline	250–500 mg q6h	q8–12 h	q12–24 h	q24h	Avoid
Amphotericin	0.4–1 mg/kg/dy	No change	No change	q24–48h	HD:No change CAPD: q24–48 h
Fluconazole	200–400 mg qd	No change	50%	50%	HD: Extra 200 mg After HD.CAPD:50%
Voriconazole IV	6 mg/kg q12 h × 2 then 4 mg/kg IV q12h	No change	Not recommended (toxic vehicle may accumulate, use PO route)	Not recommended (toxic vehicle may accumulate, use PO route)	Not recommended (toxic vehicle may accumulate, use PO route)
Acyclovir PO	200–800 mg q4–6 h	No change	(<25)q8h	q12h	HD: After HD
Acyclovir IV	5–12.4 mg/kg q8h	No change	q12–24 h	2.5 mg/kg q24h	HD: After HD CAPD:2.5 mg/kg q24h
Ganciclovir IV	5 mg/kg q24h	2.5–5 mg/kg q24h	0.6–1.25 mg/kg q24h	0.625 mg/kg 3 time a week	HD: 0.6 mg/kg after HD 0.625 mg/kg 3 time a week

membrane and causes nephrotic syndrome—minimal change disease and membranous nephropathy. The effects of NSAIDs are represented in Fig. 55.2.

Aminoglycosides

Aminoglycosides are highly charged, polycationic, hydrophilic drugs that cross biological membranes to a little extent. They are not

Table 55.3: Drug-induced renal toxicity

Mechanism	Drugs
Alteration of intrarenal hemodynamics and decrease in renal perfusion	NSAID, ACE inhibitors, ARBs, diuretics, tacrolimus, interleukins, cyclosporine, contrast media, norepinephrine, angiotensin receptor blockers, cocaine, mitomycin C, tacrolimus, estrogen, quinine
Acute interstitial nephritis with or without glomerulopathy	Antibiotics: Ciprofloxacin, cephalothin, methicillin, penicillin G, ampicillin, oxacillin, rifampicin NSAIDs, glafenin, ASA, fenoprofen, naproxen, phenylbutazone, piroxicam, tolemetin, zomepirac, contrast media, sulfonamides, thiazides, phenytoin, furosemide, allopurinol, cimetidine, omeprazole, phenindione
Heme pigment-induced toxicity	Cocaine, lovastatin, ethanol
Hypersensitivity angiitis	Ampicillin, penicillin, sulfonamides
Thrombotic microangiopathy—hemolytic uremic syndrome	Cyclosporine, mitomycin C, oral contraceptives, cocaine, quinine
Acute tubular necrosis	NSAIDs, glafenin, contrast media, acetaminophen, cyclosporine, aminoglycosides, cephalothin, amphotericin B, rifampicin, vancomycin, pentamidine, cisplatin, IV immunoglobulin, dextran, maltose, sucrose, mannitol, heavy metals
Tubular obstruction	Sulfonamides, methotrexate, methoxyflurane, triamterene, acyclovir, ethylene glycol, protease inhibitors

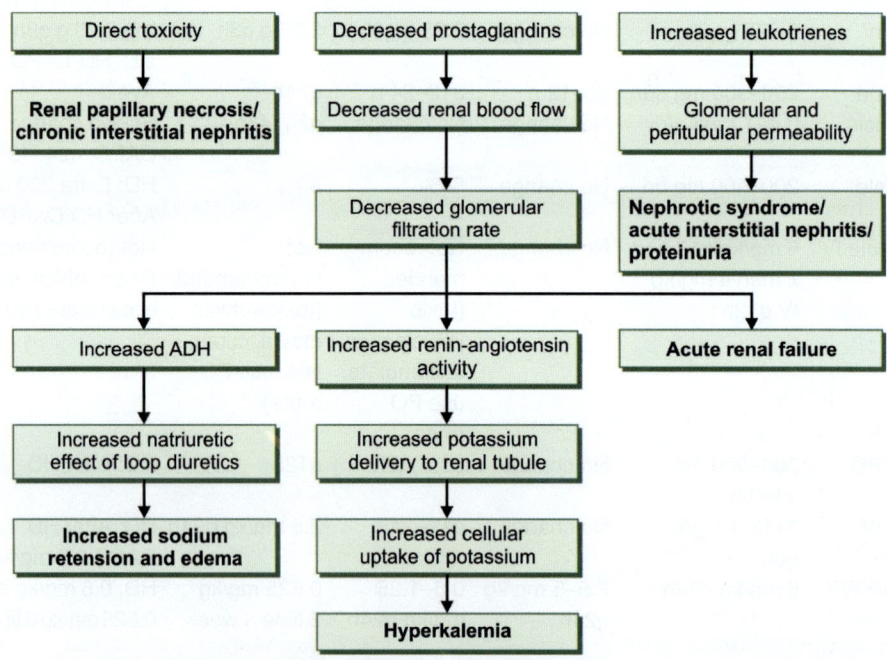

Fig. 55.2: Effects of NSAIDs

metabolized but are eliminated, unchanged, almost entirely by the kidneys. Aminoglycosides are filtered by the glomerulus at a rate equal to water. After entering the luminal fluid of proximal renal tubule, a small but toxicologically important portion of the filtered drug is reabsorbed and stored in the proximal tubule cells by negatively charged phospholipid-binding sites. After charge-mediated binding, the drug is taken up into the cell in small invaginations of the cell through megalin. Within 1 hour of injection, the drug is located at the apical endocytotic vesicles. These vesicles fuse with lysosomes, sequestering the unchanged aminoglycosides inside those organelles. A small part of the internalized aminoglycosides is shuttled to the Golgi complex. Once trapped in the lysosomes of proximal tubule cells, amino-glycosides electrostatically attached to anionic membrane phospholipids interfere with the normal action of some enzymes (i.e. phospho-lipases and sphingomyelinase). In parallel with enzyme inhibition, undigested phospho-lipids originating from the turnover of cell membranes accumulate in lysosomes, where they are normally digested and form myelin bodies.

The dosage calculation for amikacin is shown as an example. The loading dose remains the same (7.5 mg/kg body weight). A rough guide to drug maintenance dosage will be for a GFR of 21–50 ml/min, 5–6 mg/kg every 12 hours, for GFR of 10–20 ml/min, 3–4 mg/kg every 12 hours and for a GFR of <10 ml/min, 2 mg/kg every 24–48 hours.

ACE Inhibitors and ARBs

Acute renal dysfunction appears to be related to loss of postglomerular efferent arteriolar vascular tone and in general, is reversible after withdrawing the ACE inhibitor. In addition, ACE inhibition treatment has been associated exceptionally with membranous glomerulo-pathy and an acute interstitial nephritis with eosinophilia. When arterial pressure or body fluid volumes are sensed as sub-normal, the renin-angiotensin system is activated and plasma renin activity and angiotensin II levels increase as in renal artery stenosis, dietary sodium restriction or sodium depletion as during diuretic therapy, congestive heart failure, cirrhosis, and nephrotic syndrome. When activated, this renin-angiotensin system plays an important role in the maintenance of glomerular pressure and filtration through preferential angiotensin II-mediated constric-tion of the efferent arteriole. Thus, under such conditions the kidney becomes sensitive to the effects of blockade of the renin-angiotensin system by angiotensin I converting enzyme inhibitor or angiotensin II receptor antagonist.

Radiocontrast Agents

Contrast nephropathy, a major cause for AKI and often occurs about 24–72 hours of contrast exposure, peak around 3–5 days with decreasing

S.no.	Risk factor	Methods to reduce toxicity
	Table 55.4: Prevention of aminoglycoside nephrotoxicity	
1.	Advanced age	Dose modification based on eGFR and monitor RFT
2.	Comorbidities—diabetes mellitus, leukemia, chronic kidney disease, chronic liver disease, obstructive jaundice, hypoalbuminemia	Dose modification based on eGFR and monitor RFT
3.	Reduced effective circulatory volume—hypotension, sepsis, heart failure	Maintain adequate hydration. Dose modification based on eGFR and monitor RFT
4.	Concomitant medications—NSAIDs, ACEI, cisplatin, cyclosporine, clindamycin, vancomycin	To avoid these drugs concomitantly
5.	Elevated plasma drug concentrations	Once daily large dosing of drug, avoid long treatment course
6.	Type of aminoglycoside	Nephrotoxicity with gentamicin > tobramycin > amikacin > netilmycin. (Netilmycin is also nephro-toxic but the least of the lot)

creatinine in 7–10 days after exposure. The two major theories for contrast-induced nephrotoxicity are that ATN is caused by renal vasoconstriction resulting in medullary hypoxia, possibly mediated by effects of viscosity and by alterations in nitric oxide, endothelin, and/or adenosine, and that ATN is a direct result of the cytotoxic effects of the contrast agents on tubular cells. Prerenal factors or intratubular obstruction contribute to the pathogenesis as demonstrated by FeNa <1. Most patients are nonoliguric. The urinary sediment shows muddy brown granular and epithelial cell casts and free renal tubular epithelial cells. However, the absence of these urinary findings does not exclude the diagnosis.

Risk factors like chronic kidney disease, diabetes mellitus, multiple myeloma, intravascular volume depletion, recent exposure to radiocontrast agents, use of high osmolar and ionic compounds predispose to higher chances of nephrotoxicity. Low osmolal agents are useful in reducing the chances of contrast-induced nephrotoxicity. They include: iohexol, ioversol and iopamidol (nonionic) or Ionic agent—ioxaglate with osmolality 500 to 850 mOsm/kg. Iodixanol is iso-osmolal with plasma and is nonionic. If the volume of contrast is lower (<125 ml), the chances of damage are minimized though are not fully eradicated. But diabetic patients with a serum creatinine concentration >5 mg/dl may be at risk even with smaller volumes (20 to 30 ml) of contrast.

Prevention

High Risk Patients

a. Patients with eGFR <60 ml/min/1.73 m^2 with significant proteinuria
b. Patients with eGFR <60 ml/min/1.73 m^2 and comorbidities—diabetes, heart failure, liver failure, or multiple myeloma.
c. Patients with eGFR <45 ml/min/1.73/m^2 in absence of proteinuria or comorbidities.

d. Patients with eGFR <45 ml/min/1.73 m^2 and have proteinuria and diabetes or other comorbidities and all patients with eGFR <30 ml/min/1.73 m^2 should be considered at highest risk.

Preventive Measures

a. *Avoid NSAIDs and volume depletion:* To use low osmolar and isoosmolar, nonionic contrast at low dose and avoid multiple interventions at same time to space 24–48 hours between procedures.

b. *Hydration*
   i. Outpatients—3 ml/kg over one hour pre-procedure and 1 to 1.5 ml/kg/hour during and for four to six hours post-procedure, with administration of at least 6 ml/kg post-procedure.
   ii. Inpatients—1 ml/kg/hour for 6 to 12 hours pre-procedure, intra-procedure, and for 6 to 12 hours post-procedure.

Isotonic saline appears to be better than more hypotonic fluids (i.e. one-half isotonic saline). Bicarbonate provides no additional benefit to saline, needs to be compounded and is more expensive.

c. *N-acetylcysteine:* 1200 mg one hour before and one hour after angiography and then twice daily for four days has been used but not conclusively proved to be useful. Since it is relatively free of major side effects, it is used often.

Unsupervised drug usage and consumption of drugs/powders/other preparations in other systems of treatment could also be important causes of acute or chronic renal damage. Drug/toxin-induced renal damage is a common cause of iatrogenic AKI. Judicious use of drugs, appropriate dose modification depending of the level of renal function and avoiding nephrotoxic drugs or drug combinations in high risk patients reduces the incidence of drug-induced renal failure.

Obesity and Kidney

• Narayan Prasad

INTRODUCTION

Non-communicable diseases are emerging as major health problems over the last two decades with the decline in infectious diseases. Decrease in physical activity, increase in time spent on sedentary activities, prosperity, abundance of food and high calorie food intake lead to obesity. Obesity affects more than one in two adults and one in six children indicating spread of obesity epidemic at a fast pace. The definition of obesity is based on body mass index (BMI) which is defined as weight in kilograms divided by the square of the height in meters. The definition and different classes of obesity has been summarized in Table 56.1 and obesity associated kidney diseases in Table 56.2. Waist circumference (WC) and a waist-hip ratio (WHR) reflect visceral fat, it has been used as an important parameter to define obesity. WC of more than 102 cm and WHR of 0.9 for men and more than 88 cm and more than 0.8 respectively for women has been found superior to BMI to define obesity.

Chronic kidney disease (CKD) affects around 10% of the population worldwide. Obese individuals are more prone to kidney diseases than non-obese individuals. A very strong association between obesity and CKD has emerged. High BMI ranks as one of the strongest risk factors for new-onset CKD. Obesity is also a risk factor for diabetes, hypertension, dyslipidemia, hyperuricemia which are associated with CKD. Obesity and overweight also influence the progression of the kidney disease. Weight reduction, calorie restriction and increased physical activity may slow down the progression of the kidney disease.

Association of Obesity and CKD

Obesity is associated with:
a. New-onset CKD
b. Progression of CKD

Table 56.1: BMI-based definitions of obesity	
Normal weight	BMI 18.5–24.9 kg/m^2
Overweight	BMI 25–29.9 kg/m^2
Obesity	BMI ≥30 kg/m^2
Class 1 (or grade 1) obesity	BMI 30–34.9 kg/m^2
Class 2 (or grade 2) obesity	BMI 35–39.9 kg/m^2
Class 3 (or grade 3) or morbid obesity	BMI ≥40 kg/m^2

Table 56.2: Obesity-related kidney diseases
1. Chronic kidney diseases (CKD)
2. Obesity-related glomerulopathy (ORG)
3. Kidney stones
4. Kidney cancers

c. Occurrence and progression of proteinuria

d. Lower eGFR

e. Faster decline of GFR to end stage renal disease (ESRD).

Elevated BMI levels and class II obesity or more have been associated with more rapid progression in patients with pre-existing CKD. Compared to individuals with normal BMI, the relative risk for ESRD increases from 1.87 in overweight individuals to 7.07 in those with class 3 obesity and is an independent risk factor for ESRD. Higher WC and WHR are associated with albuminuria and poorer renal outcomes. Obesity may affect kidney function through mechanisms unrelated to cardio-vascular and metabolic effects of obesity.

Obesity-related Glomerulopathy (ORG)

With recognition of obesity as pandemic, incidence of ORG has also increased. ORG is a distinct entity featuring proteinuria, glomerulo-megaly, progressive glomerulosclerosis and renal functional decline in an obese patient. The incidence of ORG has increased by 10-fold from 0.2% in 1986–1990 to 2.0% in 1996–2000 and the trend is continuing. As per renal biopsy studies, it was noted that ORG occurs not only in morbid obesity but also in class 1, 2, 3 obesity. Glomerulomegaly and focal and segmental glomerulosclerosis (FSGS) are the two important events in the renal histology.

Pathology of ORG

Structural changes occur in morbid obesity much earlier than the onset of proteinuria. ORG is a pathological process characterized by glomerulomegaly which may or may not be associated with FSGS. It is a milder, more indolent form of FSGS. If present, FSGS is often the perihilar type (Fig. 56.1). The glomerulo-megaly due to hyperfiltration injury is not always directly proportional to the BMI and may occur in less obese individuals as well. Presence of lipid deposits in mesangial and tubular cells may be observed. The mean glomerular diameter in patients with ORG is

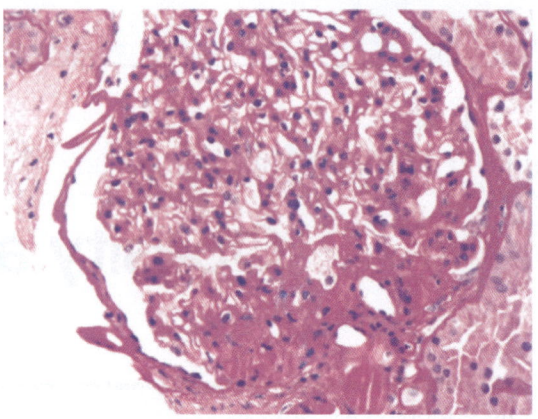

Fig. 56.1: Light microscopy showing glomerulo-megaly and focal segmental glomerulosclerosis. Single enlarged glomerulus with perihilar sclerosis involving about 30% of the glomerular capillary tuft (periodic acid–Schiff, original magnification × 400)

higher than that of non-obese age and sex-matched normal controls. In contrast to idiopathic FSGS, the segmental sclerosis in ORG typically affects the hypertrophied glomeruli and often perihilar in distribution. Only lesser number of glomeruli may be involved as compared to primary FSGS. The predilection of perihilar distribution indicates greater ultrafiltration pressure at the afferent than that at the efferent end of the glomerular capillary bed. Increased glomerular volume and decreased numerical density of podocyte has been observed. Decrease in podocyte number and increase in podocyte foot process length reflect initial adaptive hypertrophic responses which ultimately lead to podocyte depletion and development of segmental sclerosis. Half of the ORG patients have changes in glomeruli similar to diabetes like thickening of glomerular basement membrane, mesangial matrix expansion, and mesangial cell prolifera-tion without any evidence of glucose intolerance.

Immunofluorescence and Electron Microscopy Findings in ORG

Under immunofluorescence, nonspecific trapping of C3 and IgM may be seen in areas of sclerosis. There is also decrease in expression of insulin-like growth factor 1 (IGF-1) and increase in gene expression of cytokines like interleukin-6. Under electron microscopy, protein and lipid droplets in podocytes and endoplasmic reticulum of mesangial cells are seen. These changes suggest oxidative and cellular stress. Foot process effacement is relatively milder in ORG than primary FSGS.

ORG may occur superimposed on other glomerular diseases. Evaluation of obese patients with proteinuria revealed classical ORG in only 40% of patients and remaining 60% had unrelated pathology like diabetic nephropathy or other glomerular diseases. Rarely acute interstitial nephritis and acute tubular necrosis have been also detected. The interstitial fibrosis and tubular atrophy are less severe compared to primary FSGS.

Obesity and Nephrolithiasis

Higher body weight, high BMI, weight gain over time, higher baseline WC and diabetes are associated with the following risk factors for nephrolithiasis:

a. Lower urine pH → inversely related to body weight
b. Increased urinary oxalate → calcium oxalate stones
c. Increased urinary uric acid → uric acid/calcium stones
d. Increased urinary sodium
e. Increased urinary phosphate → calcium phosphate/mixed stone
f. Insulin resistance (calcium stones/renal ammonium production)
g. Hyperinsulinemia (increase urinary calcium excretion → calcium stones)
h. Metabolic derangements (calcium stones formation in kidney)
i. Defect in renal acid excretion → hypocitraturia → calcium nephrolithiasis.

Obesity and Kidney Cancer

There is a strong association between obesity and various types of malignancies, particularly renal cancers. For every 5 kg/m² higher BMI, the risk of renal cancers increase by 25% in both men and women across populations from different parts of the world.

Increased levels of growth factors such as insulin and insulin-like growth factor 1 (IGF-1), sex hormones such as estrogen, altered adipocytokine levels such as leptin and adiponectin may be responsible. Low-grade inflammation, oxidative stress, altered intestinal flora and microbiomes are also considered as other factors contributing to the higher incidence of cancers.

Pathophysiology

The mechanism by which obesity leads to CKD has been shown in Fig. 56.2. Obesity leads to CKD through both direct as well as indirect mechanisms. The direct pathophysiological effects are an alteration in renal hemodynamics, hyperfiltration, inflammatory state and adipokines. The GFR, renal plasma flow (RPF) and filtration fraction (FF) are initially higher in overweight than in the lean subjects. Afferent arteriolar vasodilation and increase in transcapillary hydraulic pressure difference increase GFR and hyperfiltration in these patients. Moreover, the proximal sodium reabsorption is increased which leads to decreased sodium delivery to macula densa, activation of tubuloglomerular feedback leading to preglomerular vasodilatation and more hyperfiltration.

Obesity and Hormonal and Neurohormonal Changes

Salt retention occurs due to high leptin and low adiponectin levels, hyperinsulinemia and alteration in baroreflexes activate renal sympathetic nervous system (SNS). Simultaneously there is activation of the renin-angiotensin system (RAAS) and increase in angiotensin II levels. Increased synthesis of RAAS components occurs in the fat cells in obese patients. Efferent arteriolar vasoconstriction by RAAS activation increases transcapillary hydraulic glomerular pressure.

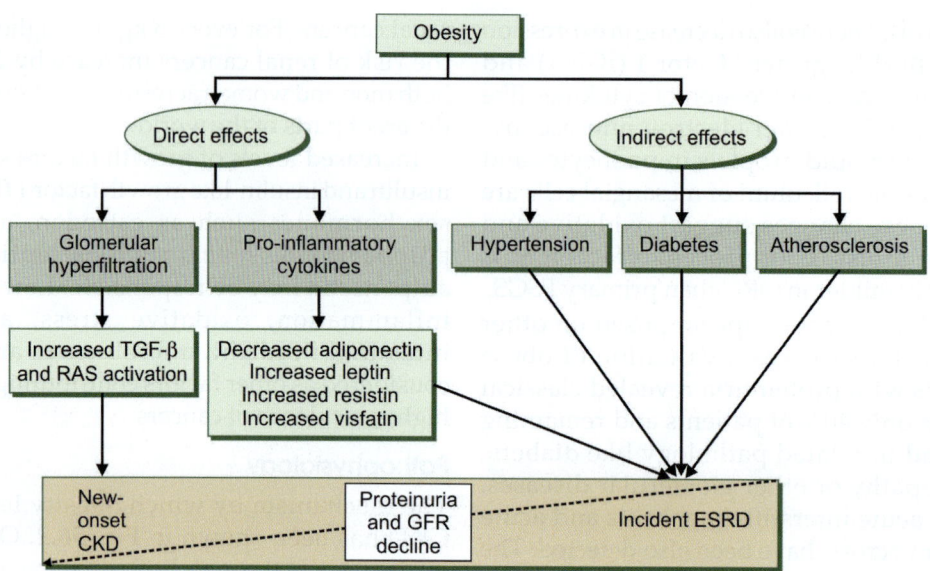

Fig. 56.2: Pathophysiology showing direct and indirect effects of adiposity on incident and new-onset CKD

Adipose Tissue and Endocrine Changes

Adipose tissue acts like an endocrine organ and is a pleiotropic source of hormones and chemokines, collectively called adipokines. The paracrine effects of adipokines have effects on the kidneys. Adipokines such as leptin, adiponectin, and resistin affect cellular hypertrophy, extracellular matrix and renal fibrosis. Visceral adipose tissue contributes to the highest level of inflammation, hyperinsulinemia and insulin resistance. Adipocytes synthesize proinflammatory and proatherogenic cytokines like TNF-α, angiotensin II, and IL-6. High leptin and low adiponectin levels lead to a proinflammatory state, fibrosis, proximal tubular sodium absorption, effacement of podocytes and albuminuria. High aldosterone levels in obesity lead to glomerular hyperfiltration and podocyte injury through free radicals.

All adaptive changes in obesity lead to glomerulomegaly and hyperfiltration. Since the numbers of nephrons are fixed at birth and are independent of body size, increase in GFR leads to increase in single nephron GFR and individuals with less number of nephrons carry maximum risk of glomerular hypertrophy. This maladaptive state of afferent arteriolar dilatation leading to increase in intracapillary pressure, hyperfiltration maladaptation of podocytes leads to glomerular hypertrophy and glomerulosclerosis. Glomerulosclerosis occurs when foot process of podocyte enlarges and detaches from the basement membrane resulting in proteinuria followed by sclerosis of glomeruli. Indirectly obesity increases the risk of diabetes, hypertension, and atherosclerosis and thus increases the risk of CKD. The understanding of the genetic contributors for CKD in obesity may enable effective therapeutic intervention in the future.

Clinical Presentation

In early stages of obesity, there may not be any clinical manifestation relating to CKD. Patients usually present with isolated subnephrotic proteinuria with normal urine sediment with or without renal dysfunction.

Even in those cases with nephrotic range proteinuria (>3.5 g/day), typical clinical features of NS edema, hypoalbuminemia and hyperlipidemia are absent. The main differential diagnosis in such cases is primary FSGS. The salient features which differentiate between the two are enumerated in Table 56.3.

Persistent proteinuria in obese patients is surrogate marker of ORG, however, other causes of proteinuria should be excluded. Hypertension and dyslipidemia are the other common associations. The podocyte injury in ORG is maladaptive and differs from idiopathic FSGS. The handling of the proteins by the tubule may also be different from the classical nephrotic syndrome patient. The age of the patient, level of proteinuria, serum creatinine at presentation determine the progress of the disease and up to 10 to 33% of patients reach ESRD by 10 years. The prognosis of FSGS related to obesity is better than primary FSGS. A strong association of nephrolithiasis and renal cancer has emphasized the need to screen for these diseases.

Treatment

The best treatment is primordial prevention by a nationwide campaign among children and adolescents to prevent risk factors for obesity.

Weight reduction: Weight loss leads to the reduction in glomerular hypertrophy, proteinuria, blood pressure, lipid levels, inflammation and improves insulin resistance. Nonsurgical strategy of weight loss is low calorie diet. Renal benefits in terms of reduction in proteinuria and obesity-related glomerular hyperfiltration. Weight loss by low calorie diet leads to increase in feutin A and adiponectin levels. High fiber diet promotes the growth of short-chain fatty acid producing bacteria in the intestine which help to reduce inflammation and thereby the progression of the disease. Physical activity and exercises will also enable weight reduction. Metformin along with physical exercise shows a better metabolic control.

The usage of anti-obesity agents like orlistat and sibutramine may help in weight reduction but multiple side effects, especially in cardiovascular patients limit its use.

RAAS blockade helps to decrease in proteinuria. Ramipril exerts greater anti-proteinuric effect in obese and overweight patients than in those with normal BMI. The drugs that block renin-angiotensin system has

Table 56.3: Differences between ORG and idiopathic FSGS		
Characteristic	*ORG*	*Primary FSGS*
Onset	middle-aged adults	Children and young adults
Clinical manifestations	Slowly progressive	Sudden onset
Proteinuria and serum albumin	Subnephrotic proteinuria with normal serum albumin levels. Full NS uncommon	Nephrotic range proteinuria in most patients Hypoalbuminemia and full NS common
Clinical course	Slower progression than primary FSGS	Faster progression
Focal sclerosis like FSGS	Fewer than in primary FSGS	More frequent
FSGS variants	Perihilar variant	Not otherwise specified, tip and collapsing variants more common
Glomerulomegaly	Present in all cases	Variable
Foot process effacement	Usually <50% glomerular surface area	Usually >50% glomerular surface area
Renal survival	Better. 50% survival at 10 years	Worse than ORG. Only 25% survival at 10 years

renoprotective effect by reducing glomerular hyperfiltration and antifibrogenic effects and are used in obesity and ORG. Mineralo-corticoid receptor activation has a key role in obesity and the metabolic syndrome.

Bariatric Surgery

Weight loss can be achieved effectively with bariatric surgery. Resolution of nephrotic syndrome in patients with biopsy proven FSGS and normalization of proteinuria after bariatric surgery has been reported. Long-term stabilization of renal function, improve-ments in blood pressure, better glycemic control, favorable changes in metabolic and inflammatory markers and improvement in quality of life have been observed after bariatric surgery and weight reduction in patients with obesity-related glomerulopathy. However, bariatric surgery may be followed by severe renal complications, such as nephrolithiasis, oxalate nephropathy and acute kidney injury.

Conclusion

The prevalence of obesity and ORG has increased with changes in sedentary lifestyles and food habits in recent past.ORG patients do not show clinical pictures of nephrotic syndrome despite having nephrotic range proteinuria mainly because of maladaptive changes happening with podocyte at glo-merular bed and slow indolent course of the disease. Obesity may be associated with development and progression of CKD, nephrolithiasis and kidney cancers as well. The weight loss with hypocaloric diet, weight reducing agents with careful monitoring of side effects, ACE inhibitor and ARB, and bariatric surgery may slow and show regression of the ORG.

More research is needed in the future about markers of kidney injury to predict CKD in obesity. The pathophysiology of disease progression without any significant proteinuria needs to be explored and the effect of calorie restriction or bariatric surgery on ORG reversal needs to be systematically studied. There is a need for large prospective controlled trials on therapeutic intervention in obesity. Further studies are needed on the influence of obesity on other renal disorders like diabetic kidney disease and glomerulonephritis. Better survival of obese patients on maintenance hemodialysis has been observed and faster decline of renal function in obese renal transplant recipient has also been reported.

Renal Biopsy

• R Kasi Visweswaran

INTRODUCTION

Renal biopsy is an important investigation and it helps us to visualize the pathologic changes in kidney. This is useful for classifying renal diseases systematically into various types, understanding the pathogenesis and deciding the treatment. A carefully performed renal biopsy, studied by appropriate stains under light and immunofluorescent microscopy is sufficient in most clinical situations. In the first half of the 20th century, an open wedge biopsy was the only option. During the later half of the last century the liver biopsy technique using Vim Silverman's needle, the Franklin's modification of Vim Silverman needle and spring-loaded biopsy needles were used. The kidney was localized with the help of plain X-ray and the biopsy site was marked on the X-ray. The corresponding site was marked on the back of the patient. A fine needle was used to assess the depth of the kidney from the skin. The movement of the needle with respiration helps to confirm entry into the renal capsule. Biopsy was then taken from the same site. With the advent of ultrasonography the depth and position of the kidney can be marked and the procedure done with relative case. Compact biopsy guns are used commonly in Fig. 57.1. With real time ultrasound, the biopsy needle can be passed

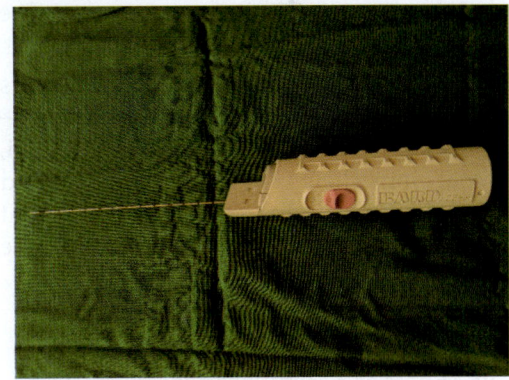

Fig. 57.1: Biopsy gun. Spring-loaded device which can perform the biopsy after the needle tip is properly positioned and the gun 'fired'

through the biopsy port of the ultrasound probe. By this the success rate is nearly hundred percent and complications negligible. Now, transjugular endovascular biopsy procedures are available.

Renal biopsy is done for the diagnosis of mainly five groups of disorders.

A. *Nephrotic syndrome:* Generally, all adults with nephrotic syndrome are advised to undergo renal biopsy initially itself. In the case of children, a biopsy is considered after the initial course of steroids only for those in whom use of more powerful immunosuppressive drugs are contemplated. If facilities are not locally available, a primary physician is justified in trying a 6–8-week course of steroids in even adults before considering renal biopsy. Indications for renal biopsy in nephrotics are:

i. Onset below 1 year or above 16 years.

ii. Nephritic onset of nephrotic syndrome.

iii. Non-nephrotic proteinuria with or without hematuria.

iv. Steroid dependent, frequently relapsing or cases with steroid side effects (where more powerful immunosuppressive drugs are considered).

B. *Steroid-resistant nephrotic syndromes* (irrespective of age): These should be subjected to renal biopsy before considering more powerful immunosuppressive drugs.

C. *Dialysis dependent AKI:* In patients remaining dialysis dependent even 6–8 weeks after apparent presentation as AKI, renal biopsy helps to identify the cause and reversibility. It helps to identify the patient and decide the treatment plan in the following groups:

i. Ischemic of tubular injury

ii. Toxic type of renal damage

iii. Whether patchy cortical necrosis has occurred

iv. Whether total renal cortical necrosis has occurred

v. Presence of intratubular deposits or crystals delaying recovery

vi. Unsuspected pre-existing disease.

D. *Diagnosis of "obscure" renal failure/rapid worsening of renal function:* Many patients may present with no apparent or obvious reason for renal failure. Many of the cases may be related to use of nephrotoxic drugs/toxins/"natural" products, undetected early systemic illness (lupus nephritis, vasculitis, paraproteinemias or renal failure in diabetes). Although renal biopsy is not routinely advised in a diabetic with overt proteinuria and gradual loss of renal function over the years, if the urine sedi-

ments show RBCs or sudden worsening of proteinuria or renal dysfunction occurs, renal biopsy is indicated. Renal biopsy helps to confirm if the diabetic person has a non-diabetes related renal disease in addition to diabetic nephropathy. When a patient has rapid worsening of renal function in whom obstructive uropathy and bilateral renal artery stenosis and use of drugs acting on renin angiotensin system is excluded, renal biopsy becomes mandatory for diagnosis.

E. *Evaluation of renal dysfunction in transplanted kidney:* Biopsy is useful tool to assess the cause of postrenal transplant renal dysfunction. It helps to diagnose various causes of postrenal transplant renal dysfunction.

i. Acute rejection

ii. Chronic rejection

iii. Cyclosporine nephrotoxicity

iv. Acute tubular necrosis

v. *De novo* or recurrence of the disease in the transplant.

Procedure

For biopsy of 'native' kidney, appropriate pre-biopsy work up and preparation are essential to optimize the safety. Preliminary investigations including urinalysis, complete blood count, blood sugar and renal functions are performed. This is followed by ultrasonography to confirm that the patient has two kidneys of near-normal size, shape and position. The test of coagulation including bleeding time, clotting time, plalelet count, activated partial thromboplastin time and prothrombin time should be normal. Blood pressure should be controlled on drugs in hypertensive patients (DBP <95 mm Hg). Urine should be sterile.

The contraindications for renal biopsy include solitary kidney (except under special situations), infected kidney, renal neoplasms, uncontrolled blood pressure, systemic bleeding tendency, advanced uremia, obesity and non-cooperative patient.

The procedure and steps are explained to the patient before taking an informed consent. Instructions are given to hold the breath for a short while when asked for during the procedure. The patient is positioned prone with a comfortable sand bag or pillow under the upper abdomen. The site and depth from skin to the lower pole of the left kidney with the breath held inspiration is marked with the help of ultrasound. The skin is prepared, draped and local anesthetic infiltrated from the skin puncture site up to the renal capsule (renal capsule is a pain sensitive structure). The various structure traversed by the needle can be assessed because of its varying resistance. The biopsy gun is prepared and cocked. Small stab incision is made on the skin using a no. 11 blade to enable the biopsy needle to penetrate the skin easily. If real time ultrasound guidance is used, the needle of the biopsy gun is advanced with the patient holding breath in deep inspiration for the desired length and the gun is fired. In a fraction of a second, the biopsy gun is withdrawn and the patient asked to breath normally. By exposing the cutting needle of the biopsy gun, the specimen of renal tissue is carefully recovered. Inspection under the operating microscope or hand lens helps to confirm presence of glomeruli which appear as red dots. A small portion (3–4 mm) with a few glomeruli is separated and preserved in transport medium or sent to the lab immediately in ice cold saline for immunofluorescence. Another small cortical core is preserved in glutaraldehyde solution for electron microscopy (if needed) and the remaining part of the sample sent for light microscopy in formaline-saline or Bouin's fluid. If there is any doubt about the adequacy of the number of glomeruli, the procedure is repeated and a second core obtained. EM study is necessary only for diagnosis of certain specific diseases. Special stains including PLA2R antigen can be performed with the specimen for light microscopy.

Firm external pressure with the palm is applied over the biopsy site for 15–20 minutes to minimize chances of perirenal hematoma. The patient is advised bed rest for 8–12 hours. Pulse and blood pressure are monitored. An abdominal binder may be used for the first few hours or till the urine sample is clear. Patient is instructed to collect urine sample in separate bottles observe for development of hematuria. Patient is instructed to be up and about after the first 12 hours. Some centers perform the procedure as a 'Day procedure' and the patient is discharged after a few hours.

Transient microscopic hematuria is universal after renal biopsy. Macroscopic hematuria. Pain, perinephric hematoma. Arteriovenous fistula, large intrarenal or perinephric hematoma and infections are rare. Onset of severe hypertension shortly after the biopsy may suggest subcapsular hematoma compressing the renal parenchyma ("Page kidney"). Embolization of the AV fistula may be needed for persistent hematuria with loss of large volumes of blood, requiring repeated transfusions.

Processing of Tissue

An adequate biopsy should contain at least 8 glomeruli and 1 blood vessel. In diffuse disease, as in membranous glomerulo-nephritis, even a single glomerulus may be adequate for making a diagnosis. In focal lesions, the greater the member of glomeruli sampled, the greater is the probability of a definite diagnosis. Renal tissue is studied by light microscopy with special stains (hematoxylin and eosin, modified silver stain (periodic acid/methenamine or Jone's stain / PAS or PLA2R). Tissue for light microscopy is embedded in paraffin and sectioned using a fine microtome into 2–3 micron thin sections. Hematoxylin and eosin (H&E) stains are useful for overall assessment of interstitium, infiltrating cells especially eosinophils and fibrin. PAS accentuates the basement membrane, matrix material, defines the brush border of proximal tubular cells, areas of hyalinosis and protein precipitates including cryoglobulin. The basement membrane is best visualized by a silver stain, usually the Jone's stain. Areas of fibrosis and collagen deposition are well delineated by Masson's trichrome stain.

In immunofluorescence study, the fresh renal biopsy specimen is sectioned with freezing microtome, treated with antibody to immunoglobulins or complement components or proteins. Since immunoglobulins are themselves antibodies, the reagents used for immunofluorescence are antibodies to the antibodies. They get attached to the corresponding immunoglobulins in the biopsy specimen. Fluorescein conjugated antibodies directed against IgG, IgA, IgM and complement components are commonly used. Since the antibodies are tagged with fluorescein, their position and intensity can be assessed by viewing through fluorescent microscope.

Tissue for electron microscopy is fixed in 1% osmium tetroxide. The tissue is then dehydrated, embedded and sectioned to 60–90 Å thin sections, stained with uranyl acetate or lead citrate to enhance contrast. Electron microscopy helps to study the changes in the kidney at cellular and sub-cellular levels.

Interpretation of Renal Biopsy

While interpreting hematoxylin and eosin-stained renal biopsy slide under low power, it will be possible to scan the slide overall and count the glomeruli. A minimum of 8 glomeruli should be present to consider the specimen as adequate. The tubules, interstitium and blood vessels can also be identified under low power. Under higher magnification, the glomeruli are studied in detail. The 3 resident cells in the glomerulus are mesangial, endothelial and epithelial cells. Glomeruli are studied with reference to cellularity, capillary lumen, capillary wall, crescents, adhesion of the glomerular capillary tuft to the parietal epithelial cell, mesangium and intraglomerular blood vessels. The appearance of normal renal biopsy and minimal change glomerulonephritis will be identical under light microscopy (Fig. 57.2). It will be possible to identify conditions like glomerulosclerosis (Fig. 57.3), thickening of basement membrane (membranous nephropathy) (Fig. 57.4), proliferative glomerulonephritis, crescentic glomerulonephritis (Fig. 57.5), necrotizing glomerulonephritis (Fig. 57.6), vasculitis (Fig. 57.7), wireloop lesions of lupus nephritis, amyloidosis (Fig. 57.8) or nodular inter-capillary glomerulosclerosis (Kimmelstiel-Wilson lesion) of diabetic nephropathy (Fig. 57.9) by light microscopy. The capillary wall consists of an endothelial cell layer, basement membrane and visceral epithelial cell layer. The term 'endocapillary' is used to denote the endothelial, mesangial and visceral epithelial cells. The term 'extracapillary' represents the surrounding parietal epithelial cell forming the Bowman's capsule.

The terms "diffuse", "focal", "global" and "segmental" signify the distribution of specific changes. The term "diffuse" is used

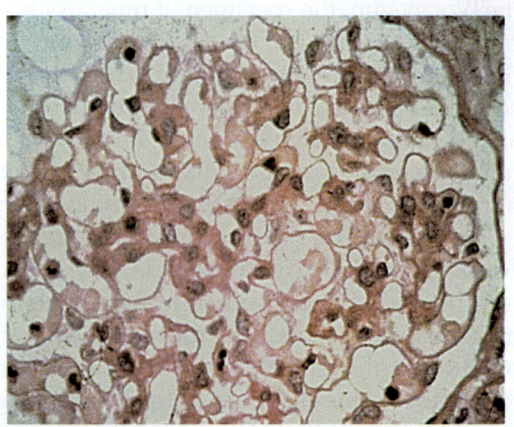

Fig. 57.2: Normal glomerulus (high power). *Note:* Single glomerulus cellularity is normal, capillary walls appear thin and capillary lumens patent throughout. In minimal change also, the light microscopy will be normal

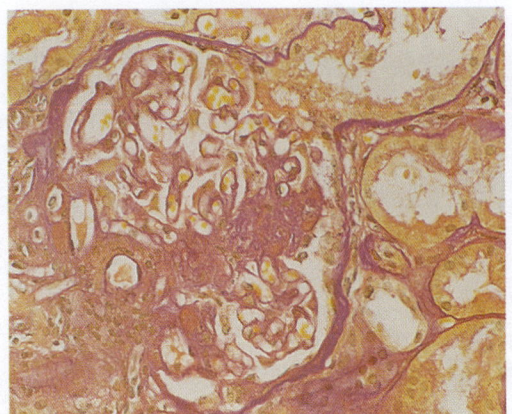

Fig. 57.3: Segmental (focal) glomerulosclerosis. *Note:* Single glomerulus showing sclerosis involving less than 50% of the glomerular area. The rest of the glomerulus is relatively normal. In the area of sclerosis, the morphology of the glomerulus is lost. If the involvement is affecting less than 50% of the glomeruli in the whole biopsy, the label of 'focal' can be applied

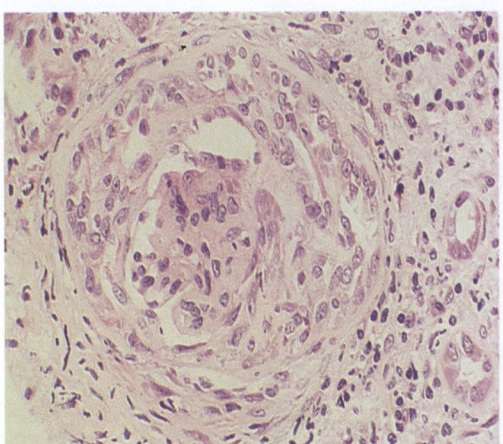

Fig. 57.5: Glomerulus with crescent. *Note:* Single glomerulus showing parietal cell proliferation forming a circumferential crescent which is about 10 cell layers thick and composed of proliferated cells—cellular crescent. The Bowman's space and capillaries are compressed

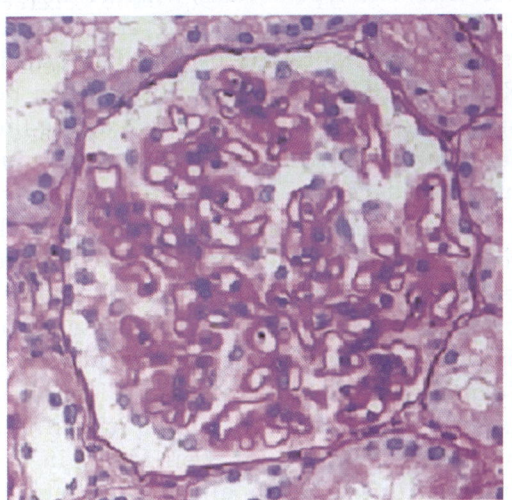

Fig. 57.4: Membranous nephropathy (H & E stain). *Note:* There is no increase in cellularity and the glomerular basement membrane is uniformly thickened

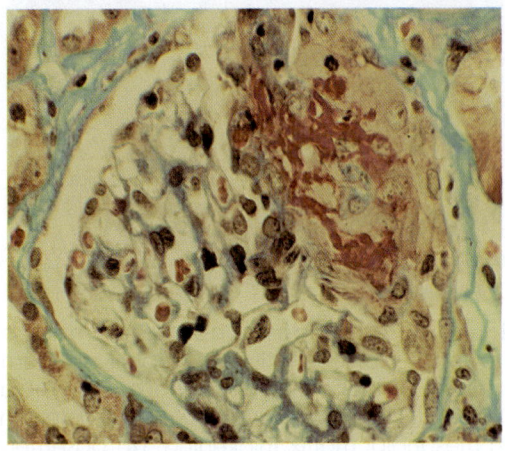

Fig. 57.6: Necrotising glomerulonephritis. *Note:* About one-third of the glomerulus is completely damaged with bleeding in the glomerular capillary tuft. The rest of the glomerulus is relatively normal

when more than 50% of the glomeruli in the biopsy are involved. If the involvement is less than 50% of the glomeruli, it is called "focal". If more than 50% of the glomerular tuft area is involved, it is termed global, and if it is less than 50% of the area of the glomerulus, it is called "segmental". Therefore, the term "focal and segmental glomerulosclerosis" means less than 50% of the glomeruli in the biopsy specimen and less than 50% of the area of the

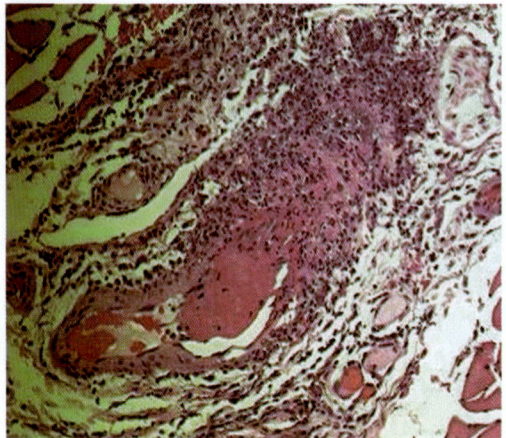

Fig. 57.7: Blood vessel in vasculitis. *Note:* Blood vessel in the kidney showing necrotising vasculitis and perivascular cuffing by inflammatory cells

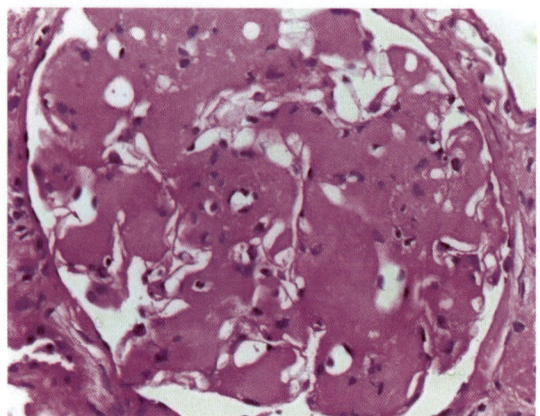

Fig. 57.9: Nodular intercapillary glomerulosclerosis (KW lesion). *Note:* Mesangial increase and nodular sclerosis caused by intraglomerular hypertension, renal vasodilatation or from ischemic injury due to hyaline narrowing of intrarenal blood vessels

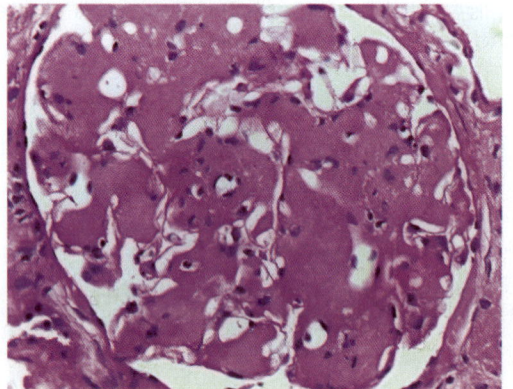

Fig. 57.8: Amyloidosis (confluent mass of amyloid). *Note:* Faintly eosinophilic uniform extracellular deposition throughout. Glomerular changes: (1) Capillary narrowing, (2) tuft distortion, (3) mesangial matrix thickening, (4) basement membrane widening, (5) tubules and interstitium also show uniform extracellular deposition

glomerular tuft show evidence of sclerosis. 'Sclerosis' means collapse and scarring of capillary loop. 'Crescent' is formed by the proliferation of parietal epithelial cells. A crescent may be circumferential, segmental, sclerosed of fibrotic.

After studying the glomerulus, attention is paid on the tubules, interstitium, and the blood vessels. The integrity of the tubular cells, status of tubular basement membrane, presence, and type of casts, whether tubular cells are necrosed, regenerating, or entrapped in area of interstitial fibrosis can be studied. Rejection of transplanted kidney can be suspected if there is "tubulitis" where the tubules are infiltrated with lymphomononuclear cells.

Normally, the tubules are arranged back to back with no space between them. The potential space between the tubules represents the interstitium. The presence of space between tubules represents interstitial edema. Infiltrating cells can also be identified in the interstitium in acute interstitial nephritis. Presence of eosinophils in the interstitium suggests allergic interstitial nephritis. Areas of fibrosis and infiltration by lymphomononuclear cells can also be seen in the interstitium in chronic interstitial nephritis and cyclosporine nephrotoxicity. If blood vessels are included in the biopsy, lesions like intimal fibrosis, proliferation, thickness of muscle layer, perivascular cuffing and reduplication of internal elastic lamina can be identified.

The distribution of immune deposition can be studied by direct immunofluorescence. The distribution may be mesangial or in the capillary wall and the pattern may be either 'granular' (Fig. 57.10), linear (Fig. 57.11) or Pauci-immune (no significant deposits). Combinations of IgG, IgM, C3, C1q may be seen in lupus nephritis. This is call 'full house' immune deposition. In IgA nephropathy, only IgA and rarely C3 are seen in immunofluorescence. C3 glomerulopathy is associated with mainly C3 deposits in the glomerular capillaries. It is also possible to identify the immune complexes by immunohistochemistry from the paraffin block sent for light microscopy (Fig. 57.12).

Renal biopsy is a very useful investigation if performed for the right indication by experienced person. In 50–60% of instances, the renal biopsy may lead to a change in the working diagnosis and treatment. Biopsy of native kidney helps to identify the precise renal disease and unsuspected systemic diseases like multiple myeloma, SLE, amylodosis or even diabetes mellitus are diagnosed by renal biopsy. Presently, it is the

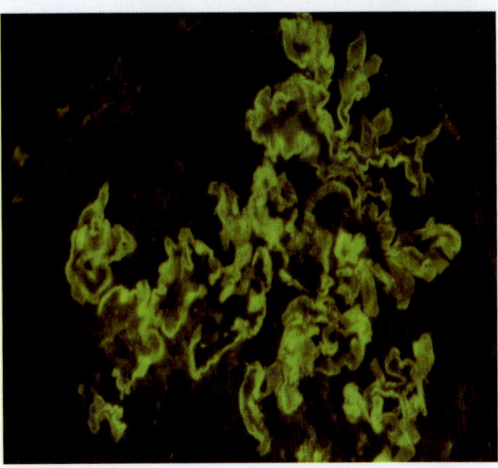

Fig. 57.11: Linear immune deposits (direct immuno-fluorescence). Direct immunofluorescence showing staining for immunoglobulin in a linear (ribbon-like) pattern along the capillary loops

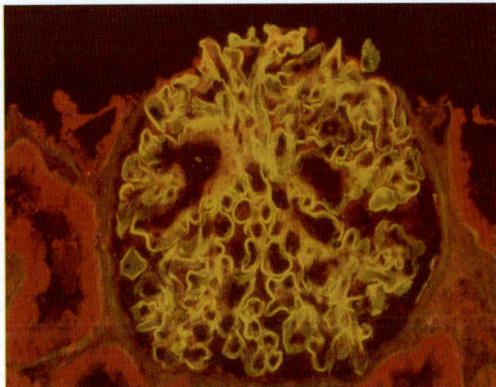

Fig. 57.12: Immunohistochemistry-linear staining. Immunohistochemistry staining of light microscopy sample showing linear staining along glomerular capillary wall

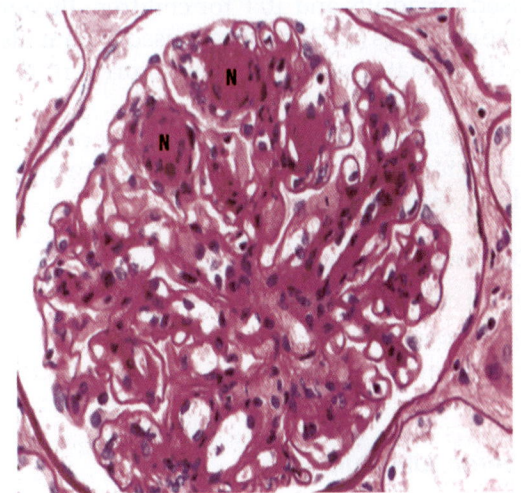

Fig. 57.10: Granular immune deposits (direct immunofluorescence). Direct immunofluorescence showing staining for immunoglobulin in a granular pattern along the capillary loops

best way to confirm rejection and determine the diagnosis and management in renal transplant dysfunction. With the advent of ultrasonography and the use of biopsy gun, renal biopsy has become a safe procedure in experienced hands. The complications are often minor in the form of small peri-renal hematoma or self-limiting microscopic hematuria.

Common Urological Instrumentations

• Suresh Bhat

URETHRAL INSTRUMENTATION—GENERAL

Aseptic technique: For all instrumentation procedures, the attending clinician should wear sterile gloves. The penis, scrotum and the perineum are cleaned with an antiseptic solution and the area is draped with sterile towel. In females, vulva is cleansed and labia held apart to reduce contamination. Catheters or instruments are lubricated before use. The male urethra is lubricated by instilling at least 10 ml of a water-soluble lubricant or anesthetic jelly through the external meatus using the blunt tipped nozzle. The approximate volume of the male urethra is 10 ml and 2% Xylocaine jelly is commonly used. Lubricant must be introduced into the urethra gently and slowly to avoid an undesirable spasm of the external urethral sphincter. Adequate anesthetic effect is achieved in 2–5 minutes. In women, the catheter dipped in sterile lubricant/local anesthetic is sufficient. Slow intravenous injection of a tranquilizing drug such as diazepam or barbiturate administered 30–45 minutes before instrumentation allays apprehension. Diazepam also relieves spasm of external sphincter. General anesthesia should be used in children, apprehensive patients and when painful procedures are necessary. Short-acting barbiturate (thiopental) is ideal for short procedures. Instrumentation is always uncomfortable and may be painful especially when the instrument passes through the prostatic urethra. The procedure should be performed gently to avoid trauma.

Instruments are commonly calibrated according to the French (F) scale. Each number on the scale equals 0.33 mm. For example, the number 24 in a 24 F catheter indicates the outer diameter of 8 mm. The number 24 represents the outer circumference of the catheter. Size 14 to 18 F Foley's catheters are commonly used for adults and 10 F for children. Bigger size catheters (22 F or 24 F) are used in patients with hematuria, with a view to prevent the catheter block by clots.

Urethral catheterization and care of the catheter: Catheters are used for diagnostic as well as therapeutic purposes.

Diagnostic Purposes

a. To calibrate the urethra
b. To assess the amount of residual urine
c. To introduce contrast medium in the bladder for cystography.

Therapeutic Purposes

a. To relieve urinary retention
b. To evacuate blood and clots from the bladder.
c. Postoperative drainage following bladder and urethral surgery.

Types of Catheters

a. Ordinary rubber catheter (Jaque's catheter) of varying size from 3F to 12 F maybe used only for 'in and out' catheterization.

b. Foley's catheter is available in sizes varying from 8 to 24 F. The maximum capacity of the bulb is noted in the catheter. However, it is not necessary to inflate the bulb fully since it may cause discomfort to the patient. The two-way Foley's catheter is used for routine drainage and three-way catheter for continuous bladder irrigation especially in patients with hematuria to prevent clot formation in the bladder. Three-way catheters are used after prostatectomy for continuous bladder irrigation.

c. Malecot's catheter is used for suprapubic drainage of the bladder in patients with difficult urethral catheterization and for postoperative drainage of the bladder following bladder and prostatic surgery. It is also used as a nephrostomy tube, for drainage of obstructed kidneys.

Technique of Catheterization

With aseptic precautions, the urethra is lubricated and anesthetized by using local anesthetic jelly. Penile clamp is applied to retain the jelly in the urethra for five minutes. The patient is directed to relax and breathe in and out gently during the procedure. The catheter is often held in the right hand and the penis is held up vertically with the left hand. This is to straighten the urethra which is otherwise is S-shaped. Catheter is introduced into the urethra and advanced gently. There may be a resistance at the level of external sphincter after which it will slide easily through the prostatic urethra into the bladder. Mid catheter urine sample is collected for culture and sensitivity. The bulb of the Foley's catheter is inflated with 10 to 15 ml of sterile water. An overdistended balloon within the bladder, causes pressure over the trigone resulting in an urge to pass urine. It also induces spasm and suprapubic pain due to

trigonal and rectal as well as reduction in the outflow channel. Since the volume marked in the Foley's catheter is the maximum capacity of the bulb, it is not necessary to over inflate the bulb for routine indwelling catheterization. Forceful insertion should be avoided as it may cause urethral trauma.

If the catheterization is unsuccessful, trocar cystostomy under local anesthesia is to be done. The area just above the pubic symphysis is anesthetized, a small incision is made in the skin and the trocar is pushed down into the distended bladder. A 16 F Foley's catheter is introduced into the bladder through the trocar and is connected to the urobag for a closed drainage. This procedure is preferably done under ultrasound guidance to avoid injury to the bowel. It is advisable to fix the catheter to the lower abdomen or to the upper thigh with an adhesive plaster. Catheterization is done under antibiotic cover to prevent bacteremia. Secretions from the urethra may get inspissated at the level of external urethral meatus and impede the free drainage leading to urethritis or abscess. The meatus is cleaned with antiseptic solution to clear the space between meatus and catheter for the unimpeded drainage of the secretions every day (urethral toilet). If the catheter is blocked by blood clots or debris, the block is removed by flushing the catheter using sterile normal saline or mild antiseptic solution like dilute povidone iodine. Urinary tract infection is promptly treated with appropriate antibiotics. When a Foley's catheter made of latex and coated with silicone is used for long-term/permanent drainage, it is to be changed every month or two. Otherwise, suprapubic cystotomy is done to reduce the urethral complications. Silastic Foley's catheter can be retained for up to 3 months.

Catheterization is easier in females. After the area is prepared, the labia are held apart and the lubricated catheter is passed into the external meatus and advanced gently. Catheterization may be difficult in obese women, those with adductor spasm in lower extremities and in those with hypospadias or intravaginal urethral meatus. Lithotomy position may help easy identification of the meatus and catheter insertion. In some children, short general anesthesia may be required. Often, 10 F Foley's catheter is used for continuous drainage in children.

Urinary tract infection, urethral injury and bleeding are the usual complications. Injury to the prostate gland may occur in patients with enlarged prostate. Urethral abscess and fistula formation may occur in paraplegic patients on long-term catheter drainage. A defective Foley's catheter bulb may get deflated automatically or fail to deflate leading to self-retained Foley's catheter. Ultrasound-guided puncture of the bulb may be tried to deflate the balloon.

Condom Drainage

Condom drainage is a useful form of urinary drainage in unconscious patients with urinary incontenence or in patients with paraplegia and reflex neurogenic bladder. It helps to prevent soiling of linen and bed with urine. Condom catheters are often used. The catheter can be improvised easily by connecting a urobag to the tip of a condom that is punctured appropriately. The condom is applied and it is fixed over the shaft of penis.

Urethral Dilatation

The instruments used for calibrating and dilating the urethra are urethral sounds, bougie and dilators. They are also measured in the French scale. Urethral sounds are metallic instruments shaped to the curve of urethra. They differ from the dilator in having a flattened tip, and were originally used in the diagnosis of bladder stones. Urethral bougies are soft, pliable dilators used to dilate narrow strictures. Urethral dilators are metal instruments similar to the urethral sound but with blunt and rounded tip. These instruments should be used only by experienced persons.

Cystoscopy and Urethroscopy

Cystoscopy and urethroscopy are important procedures for the evaluation and treatment of urological diseases. Cystourethroscopy and related procedures allow the urologist to observe and diagnose diseases of the urinary tract. Some of the important cystoscopic techniques include visualization of the bladder, endoscopic procedures in the bladder, passage of a catheter or stent into the ureter for retrograde pyelography or for drainage of obstructed kidneys, passage of a stone basket for ureteral stone retrieval and biopsy. Endoscopic procedures are contraindicated in the presence of acute urethritis, prostatitis or cystitis. Nowadays, flexible cystoscopy is available. This is less painful and can be performed as an office procedure. This is useful in the follow-up of bladder cancer.

Litholapaxy and Lithotripsy

Litholapaxy is an endoscopic procedure in which bladder stones are crushed using a lithotrite, and the stone fragments are evacuated from the bladder. In lithotripsy, the bladder stones are disrupted by electro-hydraulic shock waves or ultrasound waves. These waves are generated outside the body and transmitted to the stone by a special probe introduced through the cystoscope. Holmium laser is currently the preferred energy source for breaking stones. The fragments are then evacuated from the bladder. In children and in adults with larger bladder stones, percutaneous cystolithotripsy is preferred. This is to prevent urethral injury.

Ureterorenoscopy

Ureterorenoscopy is the procedure in which the interior of ureter and renal pelvis are inspected using the ureterorenoscope. It is a long delicate instrument passed through the bladder into the ureter and renal pelvis. General or epidural anesthesia is required for this procedure. With refinements in technology, slender ureteroscopes are available that can be used even in children. Ureterorenoscopy is useful in the management of ureteric stones, stones in renal pelvis or major calyces, superficial tumors in these areas and ureteric stricture. Ureteroscopy may be associated with complications like ureteric injury or perforation. Flexible ureterorenoscopy with lithotripsy using Holmium YAG laser is currently the best treatment modality for caliceal stones less than 1–2 cm. This procedure is called retrograde intrarenal surgery (RIRS). This is equally good for renal pelvic stones <2 cm. In patients on antiplatelets or anti-coagulants, this is the preferred modality as these drugs need not be stopped.

Percutaneous Renal Procedures

Percutaneous renal procedures are done by establishing a track through the skin in the loin to the kidney. Through this track, the nephroscope is passed into the kidney. Manipulations are done through the nephroscope and its accessories. Indications for this procedure are: (1) Drainage of an obstructed and infected kidney as in hydronephrosis and pyo-nephrosis, (2) removal of renal calculus, (3) fulguration of small tumors in the renal calyx and pelvis. Stones larger than 2 cm are better removed using percutaneous nephro-lithotomy (PCNL). Superficial tumors in the kidney may be managed via percutaneous approach. However, the morbidity associated with this procedure is higher and includes bleeding, collecting system injury, urinary leak, hydrothorax, adjacent organ injury like liver, spleen intestine, etc. To reduce the morbidity, refinements in the technology and techniques have lead to the development of miniPERC, microPERC which utilize smaller sized instruments.

Extracorporeal Shock Wave Lithotripsy (ESWL)

This is a noninvasive method of treating stones within the kidney and ureter by using external lithotriptors. The stone is accurately localized and shock waves are propagated through the soft tissues toward the stone. Repeated shock waves progressively fragment the stone into smaller particles. The fragmented particles are passed out along with urine and can be facilitated by diuretic therapy, α-blockers like tamsulosin, calcium channel blockers. Patients with stones smaller than 2 cm are the ideal candidates for this procedure. Pregnancy is an absolute contraindication. Urine should be sterile. Failure of this may need PCNL or flexible ureteroscopy to remove the stone.

Index